Coding and Reimbursement for Hospital Outpatient Services

Second Edition

Susan Von Kirchoff, MEd, RHIA, CCS, CCS-P

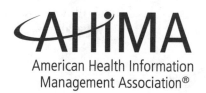

AHIMA

American Health Information
Management Association®

ISBN 1-58426-191-9
AHIMA Product No. AC206308

Melanie A. Endicott, MBA/HCM, RHIA, CCS, CCS-P, Technical Reviewer
Katie Greenock, Assistant Editor
Carol M. Spencer, RHIA, Technical Reviewer
Melissa Ulbricht, Editorial/Production Coordinator
Pamela Woolf, Project Editor
Ken Zielske, Director of Publications

AHIMA strives to recognize the value of people from every racial and ethnic background as well as all genders, age groups, and sexual orientations by building its membership and leadership resources to reflect the rich diversity of the American population. AHIMA encourages the celebration and promotion of human diversity through education, mentoring, recognition, leadership, and other programs.

American Health Information Management Association
233 North Michigan Avenue, 21st Floor
Chicago, Illinois 60601-5800
www.ahima.org

Contents

About the Author

Susan Von Kirchoff, MEd, RHIA, CCS, CCS-P. Susan has seen most aspects of the healthcare environment. She has 12 years of health information experience in the areas of ICD-9-CM and CPT-4 coding for inpatient and outpatient coding and reimbursement. She has authored the first Certified Coding Specialist manual sold throughout the United States and has also spoken nationally for many AHIMA constituent state association and Healthcare Financial Management Association meetings.

As a member of the BKD Health Care Group located in Little Rock, Arkansas, Susan provides reimbursement consulting services for hospitals and physician practices including ambulatory payment classification (APC) reimbursement, Medicare-severity DRGs (MS-DRGs), and evaluation and management (E&M) analyses. She also provides case management medical necessity training and assists home health facilities in their documentation, admission criteria, and compliance efforts.

With a Masters in Education and a BS degree in Health Information Management from Arkansas Tech University, Russellville, Susan is a Registered Health Information Administrator (RHIA), Certified Coding Specialist (CCS), Certified Coding Specialist-Physician-based (CCS-P), and an active member of the Arkansas Health Information Management Association, where she serves as President. Susan is also a member of the Healthcare Financial Management Association.

Preface

Coding and Reimbursement for Hospital Outpatient Services has been written for coding practitioners who have Current Procedural Terminology (CPT) coding knowledge and experience.

The reimbursement material is specific to the hospital outpatient setting; that is, to hospitals paid under the Medicare outpatient prospective payment system (OPPS). However, most of the coding guidelines are applicable to both the hospital outpatient and physician practice settings because the guidelines were compiled from official coding and clinical resources that apply to both facilities and practitioners.

The case studies at the end of each chapter in the second part of this book are followed by thought-provoking questions for further review for some of the more common outpatient services. The answers to the case studies are based on the codes and modifiers that would be assigned on behalf of a facility.

The coding process involves a combination of skills, and readers are expected to have basic knowledge of medical terminology, body systems, disease processes, and outpatient procedures. The author has established the following objectives to assist readers as they use this book:

- To provide a basic introduction to outpatient coding requirements

- To introduce typical difficulties with interpreting and coding outpatient procedures

- To illustrate how to apply coding guidelines to ensure accurate code assignment

- To identify the documentation necessary for code assignment

This book is divided into three parts. Part I, Understanding the Outpatient Prospective Payment System (OPPS), contains the first two chapters. Chapter 1, Overview of Coding and Reimbursement under OPPS, provides information on outpatient versus inpatient care, legislative background, the evolution of the hospital OPPS, and ambulatory surgical center (ASC) payment groups versus ambulatory payment classification (APC) payment groups. Chapter 2, Outpatient Claims Preparation and Processing, contains information on the steps for claims preparation, billing requirements related to APCs, and steps for claims processing.

Part II, Coding under OPPS, contains chapters 3–12. Chapters 3–11 each provide definitions, coding guidelines, and documentation requirements for a specific body system: integumentary; musculoskeletal; respiratory; cardiovascular, hemic, and lymphatic; digestive; urinary and male genital systems, reproductive system, and intersex surgery; female genital; nervous; and eye and auditory. Chapter 12, Ancillary Services and Departments, contains medical visit coding guidelines and documentation requirements for ancillary services and departments.

Each chapter in part II contains actual operative reports from real-life cases. (All identifiers have been removed or changed for confidentiality and privacy.) The questions following each case study were developed to challenge and test the knowledge gleaned from the material.

Part III, Ensuring Coding and Billing Integrity under OPPS, contains three chapters. Chapter 13, APCs and Data Quality, addresses chargemaster data quality, coding specialist data quality, and using information technology for APC data quality. Chapter 14, Coding and Incomplete Clinical Data, addresses the issues involved with substandard documentation, physician queries, and coding issues not officially addressed. The chapter appendix contains readings on ethics in coding and the physician query process. And Chapter 15, APC Compliance Strategies, presents a detailed discussion of compliance relative to patient access, medical staff, patient financial services, the chargemaster team, ancillary departments, the laboratory department, and the HIM department.

This book also includes two appendices. Appendix A presents glossary terms and acronyms; and Appendix B contains an answer key for the case study exercises presented in chapters 3–11. The answers to the case studies are based on the codes and modifiers that would be assigned on behalf of a facility.

Coding and Reimbursement for Hospital Outpatient Services must be used with the current edition of *Current Procedural Terminology (CPT 2008)* (code changes effective January 1, 2008), published by the American Medical Association or HCPCS Level II codes, current as of December 31, 2007. A file containing the most current versions of the HCPCS Level II codes can be found under the Utilities/Miscellaneous heading at the following CMS Web site: www.cms.hhs.gov/HCPCSReleaseCodeSets.

The Web sites listed in this book were current and valid as of the date of publication. However, Web page addresses and the information on them may change or disappear at any time and for any number of reasons. Users are encouraged to perform their own general Web searches to locate any site addresses listed here that are no longer valid.

Acknowledgments

We are grateful to the following individuals for serving as technical reviewers of the first edition of *Coding and Reimbursement for Hospital Outpatient Services*:

Eleanor Ann Joseph, MPA, RHIA, CPHQ, CHP, CCS, CCS-P, CPC
Karen D. Lockyer, RHIT, CPC
Leona M. Thomas, MHS, RHIA
Kathy C. Trawick, EdD, RHIA

And would like to also thank the following individuals for serving as reviewers of this edition:

Melanie A. Endicott, MBA/HCM, RHIA, CCS, CCS-P.
Carol M. Spencer, RHIA
Martha Hurtado, RHIA
Barbara Abbadini Garner, RHIT
Leah A. Grebner, MS, RHIA, CCS
Mary Dudash-White, MA, RHIA, CCS

We would also like to thank the first edition author Lolita M. Jones, RHIA, CCS.

Part I

Understanding the Outpatient Prospective Payment System (OPPS)

Chapter 1

Overview of Coding and Reimbursement under OPPS

On August 1, 2000, the outpatient prospective payment system (OPPS) replaced fee-for-service Medicare reimbursement with a fixed, prospectively-determined payment system for products and services provided by outpatient treatment facilities. On January 1, 2008, a major revision to OPPS was introduced. The revisions to the ambulatory payment classification (APC) Medicare reimbursement methodology was in response to the recent growth explosion of Medicare expenditures paid for hospital outpatient services over the past few years without regard to quality or the impact on the health of the Medicare beneficiary. With the calendar year (CY) 2008 OPPS update, two recurring themes are prevalent: Medicare beneficiaries must receive services that are medically necessary; and services must be rendered by hospitals in the most efficient manner. The overriding theme is quality of care, which will result positively on the health of the Medicare beneficiary. These initiatives may be summed up by the term *value-based purchasing*. The OPPS rule in CY 2008 introduced the Hospital Outpatient Quality Data Reporting Program (HOP QDRP), which will impact reimbursement in CY 2009; however, measure reporting is required in CY 2008. The Centers for Medicare & Medicaid Services (CMS) (formerly known as the Health Care Financing Administration, or HCFA) believes it is important to initiate specific payment approaches to explicitly encourage efficiency in the hospital outpatient setting, which they believe will control future growth in the volume of OPPS services.

The impact of these recent OPPS changes in this complex APC reimbursement methodology has re-established the importance of accurate coding and reporting for reimbursement. Furthermore, the line between charging and coding has become blurred as the coders' role intersects with the billers' role in healthcare organizations. Aligning billing and coding expertise, defining and providing clear expectations, and requiring ongoing education help to ensure accurate, compliant billing. Facilities often struggle with how to clearly delineate which codes are reported by the charge description master (CDM) and which codes are reported by the Health Information Management (HIM) coding staff. Accurate, complete, and compliant coding continues to be a top priority.

Based on the APC system, the reimbursement methodology for the OPPS requires coders to have advanced clinical knowledge for accurately reporting diagnosis codes, as well as a proficient and comprehensive knowledge of complex procedures crossing many medical specialties. Furthermore, the coder requires an advanced understanding of the International Classification of Diseases, 9th Revision, Clinical Modification (ICD-9-CM), as related in particular to medical necessity coding. Finally, the coder of today requires in-depth understanding of numerous procedure coding and classification systems including the American Medical Association (AMA)'s Current Procedural Terminology (CPT) and CMS' Healthcare Procedural Coding System (HCPCS—pronounced "hick picks") coding systems. These comprise level I and level II procedure codes and are required for reporting on all Medicare claims. The APC is derived from this code as well as many other factors incorporated to the APC assignment. The coder of today, coding under OPPS, not only needs to understand correct coding, but also must have a clear understanding of the Correct Coding Initiative (CCI) edits, status indicators, and other complexities of the APC reimbursement system. These complexities will be further described throughout this book; and when appropriate, the coder's role related to these will be highlighted.

Legislative Background

The Medicare program was established in 1965 by an act of Congress. As the Medicare statute was originally enacted, Medicare payment for both inpatient and outpatient hospital services was based on hospital-specific, reasonable costs attributable to serving Medicare beneficiaries. Later, the law was amended to limit payment to the lesser of a hospital's reasonable costs or to its customary charges. With increases in the demand for healthcare services, the introduction of new technologies, the structure of the health insurance industry, and inflationary economic factors, healthcare costs soared under the cost-based payment methodology. The government responded by exploring measures to contain healthcare costs, the principle of which was the introduction of prospective payment. Further refinement of this system is in place with the most significant changes introduced in CY 2008.

1983 Social Security Amendments

The Social Security Amendments of 1983 (Public Law 98-21) completely revised the cost-based payment system for most hospital inpatient services by enacting section 1886(d) of the Social Security Act (SSA). This section provided for a prospective payment system (PPS) for acute inpatient hospital stays, effective with hospital cost-reporting periods beginning on or after October 1, 1983.

Although payment for most inpatient services became subject to a PPS, hospitals continued to receive payment for outpatient services based on hospital-specific costs, which provided little incentive for efficiency of services. At the same time, advances in medical technology and changes in practice patterns were bringing about a shift in the site of medical care from the inpatient to the outpatient setting.

During the 1980s, Congress took steps to control the escalating costs of providing outpatient care by legislating a number of different payment methods for specific types of hospital outpatient services. These methods included:

- Fee schedules for clinical diagnostic laboratory tests, orthotics, prosthetics, and durable medical equipment (DME)

- Composite rate payment for dialysis for persons with end-stage renal disease (ESRD)

- Payments based on blends of hospital costs and the rates paid in other ambulatory settings such as separately certified ambulatory surgical centers (ASCs) or physician offices for certain surgery, radiology, and other diagnostic procedures

Nevertheless, Medicare payment for services performed in the hospital outpatient setting remained largely cost based.

The Omnibus Budget Reconciliation Acts of 1986 and 1990

In the Omnibus Budget Reconciliation Act of 1986 (OBRA 1986) (Public Law 99-509) and the Omnibus Budget Reconciliation Act of 1990 (OBRA 1990) (Public Law 101-508), Congress required the secretary of Health and Human Services (HHS) to develop a proposal to replace the then-current hospital outpatient payment system with a PPS and to submit a report to Congress on the proposed system.

In OBRA 1986, Congress also paved the way for development of a PPS, under section 9343(g), by requiring fiscal intermediaries (FIs) to require hospitals (effective July 1, 1987) to report claims for services under the HCPCS coding system. FIs are insurance companies or third-party payers that have a contract with CMS to process hospital outpatient claims for services that the hospitals provide to Medicare beneficiaries.

HCPCS coding enabled CMS to determine what specific procedures, services, and supplies are being billed. For those procedures that are not covered under HCPCS (level II codes), CMS contracted with the AMA and established rights to use the CPT coding system (level I codes). Both of these levels comprise the HCPCS codes reported, which are the basis for payment under the APC system.

- Level I codes are those in the AMA's CPT coding system comprising medical and surgical diagnostic and therapeutic procedures, as well as evaluation and management (E/M) codes for all medical and surgical physician specialties. These are also referred to as category I codes. In addition, category III codes are used for reporting to Medicare and these are new temporary codes for emerging technologies, services, and procedures. (Note: Category II codes used for performance measurement are not used by CMS in the OPPS at this time).

- Level II codes (or National Codes) are alphanumeric codes in the A0000–V9999 code range, which CMS created to classify services or supplies not found in CPT. Before 1983, there was no uniform way for healthcare providers to code materials and supplies for reimbursement. A sampling of categories include medical and surgical supplies, codes specific to hospital OPPS, DME, drugs, orthotics and other implantable devices, other temporary codes, dental, and ambulance.

Today, HCPCS Level I and II codes are required for reporting various services, supplies, and materials provided to Medicare and Medicaid beneficiaries. HCPCS Level I codes are published by the AMA, are updated annually, and become effective each January. In addition, new HCPCS Level II codes are developed throughout the year, and CMS notifies healthcare providers by printing the new codes (and their effective dates) in the Medicare carrier and FI bulletins, usually quarterly. Please note that not all payers accept HCPCS Level II codes.

The Balanced Budget Act of 1997

The Balanced Budget Act of 1997 (BBA) (Public Law 105-33), enacted on August 5, 1997, contains a number of provisions that affect Medicare payment for hospital outpatient services. The BBA provided for implementation of a PPS for most hospitals for outpatient services furnished on or after January 1, 1999, and for cancer hospitals that are excluded from inpatient PPS for services furnished on or after January 1, 2000. Implementation of the hospital outpatient PPS was delayed until August 1, 2000, due to Year 2000 (Y2K) system concerns.

The BBA required that the outpatient PPS include inpatient services covered under Part B for beneficiaries who are entitled to Part A benefits, but who have exhausted their Part A benefits or otherwise are not in a covered Part A stay.

However, section 1833(t)(1)(B) specifically excludes PPS coverage of the following services, which must be paid under separate fee schedules:

- Ambulance services
- Physical therapy
- Occupational therapy
- Speech-language services
- Pathology services
- Diagnostic and screening mammography
- Lab services paid under the Clinical Diagnostic Laboratory Fee Schedule (CLFS)
- Services for beneficiaries with end-stage-renal disease (ESRD) paid under the ESRD composite rate
- Services and procedures that require an inpatient stay, which are paid under the hospital inpatient prospective payment system (IPPS).
- Maryland hospitals (only for services paid under cost containment waiver)
- Critical access hospitals
- Hospitals located outside of the 50 states, District of Columbia, and Puerto Rico
- Indian Health Service hospitals

In addition, the secretary of HHS was required to develop a classification system for covered outpatient services, which should consist of groups arranged so that the services within each group are comparable clinically and with respect to the use of resources.

In addition, section 1833(t)(1)(B) authorized:

- Specific data requirements for establishing relative payment weights, which were to be based on median hospital costs determined by data from the most recent available cost reports
- A portion of the Medicare payment and the beneficiary copayment attributable to labor and labor-related costs be adjusted for geographic wage differences
- The establishment of other adjustments, such as outlier adjustments or adjustments for certain classes of hospitals, which are necessary to ensure equitable payments

All adjustments are required to be made in a budget-neutral manner. This section concludes with the requirement that a control on unnecessary increases in the volume of covered services be established.

The Balanced Budget Refinement Act of 1999

The Balanced Budget Refinement Act of 1999 (BBRA 1999) made major changes that affected the then-impending hospital outpatient PPS, including the following:

- Providing that the secretary of HHS make payment adjustments for covered services whose costs exceed a given threshold (that is, an outlier payment)
- Requiring that the secretary of HHS establish transitional pass-through payments for certain medical devices, drugs, and biologicals
- Providing that OPPS include as covered outpatient services implantable prosthetics and DME, and diagnostic x-ray, laboratory, and other tests associated with those implantable items

- Limiting the variation of costs of services within each payment classification group by providing that the highest median (or mean cost, if elected by the secretary of HHS) for an item or service within the group cannot be more than two times greater than the lowest median (or mean) cost for an item or service within the group. The provision allows the secretary of HHS to make exceptions in unusual cases, such as for low-volume items and services.

- Requiring that at least annual review of groups, relative payment weights, and wage and other adjustments be made by the secretary of HHS to take into account changes in medical practice, the addition of new services, new cost data, and other relevant information and factors. (The SSA further requires the HHS to consult with an expert outside advisory panel composed of an appropriate selection of provider representatives who will review the clinical integrity of the groups and weights and advise the secretary accordingly. The panel may use data other than those collected or developed by the HHS for the review and advisory purposes.)

- Limiting the coinsurance amount for a procedure performed in a year to no more than the hospital inpatient deductible for that year

Transitional Adjustment to Limit Decline in Payments

In certain situations, CMS has provided for transitional adjustments to limit needed payment reductions under the hospital OPPS. For example, the median per diem cost for community mental health centers (CMHCs) historically has greatly exceeded the median per diem cost for hospital-based partial hospitalization programs (PHPs). Furthermore, the costs for CMHCs have fluctuated significantly from year to year, while the costs for hospital-based PHPs have remained relatively constant. In CY 2003, CMS identified that CMHCs may have been increasing and decreasing their charges in response to Medicare payment policies, hence allowing for reimbursement of inappropriate outlier payments. In CY 2006, CMS reviewed various alternatives to balancing the cost-to-charge ratio (CCR) and median per diem cost for CMHCs. A 15 percent reduction in payments was adopted as the best alternative to strike an appropriate balance between the median PHP and CMHC data and to reduce the risk of any adverse impact on access to mental health services that might result from a large single-year rate reduction.

For CY 2007, CMS calculated the PHP per diem payment rate using the same updated methodology that was adopted in CY 2006 and made an additional 15 percent reduction to the combined hospital-based and CMHC median per diem cost used to establish the CY 2006 per diem PHP payment. Through the outpatient code editor (OCE), when the payment for specified mental health services provided by one hospital to a single beneficiary on one date of service, based on the payment rates associated with the APCs for the individual services, would exceed the per diem PHP payment (listed as APC 0033—Partial Hospitalization), those specified mental health services are assigned to APC 0034, which has the same payment rate as APC 0033, and the hospital is paid one unit of APC 0034.

Hold Harmless Provisions

Covered hospital outpatient services furnished in a calendar year from January 1, 2006 through December 31, 2008, for which the PPS amount is less than the pre-BBA amount, are increased by 95 percent of the difference for services furnished during 2006, 90 percent of the difference for services furnished during 2007, and 85 percent of the difference for services furnished during 2008, if the hospital falls under one of the following categories.

- Located in a rural area
- Less than 100 beds

- Not a sole community hospital
- Not an essential access community hospital

The hold-harmless provision applies permanently to cancer centers and children's hospitals to the proportion of their pre-BBA payment relative to their costs.

Hospital Outpatient Prospective Payment System

In response to OBRA 1986 and OBRA 1990 requirements to develop a hospital outpatient PPS, CMS examined systems that were in place or under development and entered into a cooperative agreement with 3M-Health Information Systems, a healthcare information systems (IS) vendor, to develop a reimbursement system for outpatient services.

Development of an APC Reimbursement System

The present APC system, which is the heart of the OPPS, evolved from an earlier 3M system known as ambulatory patient groups (APGs). The initial APG system was followed by an updated version known as Version 2.0. After the release of Version 2.0, CMS revised the APGs based on more recent Medicare data. These revisions constitute what is now called the ambulatory payment classification system based on APC groups, which Medicare implemented on August 1, 2000.

Services within the APC system are identified by HCPCS codes and descriptions. The composition of the APC groups rests on two premises:

- The procedures within each group must be similar clinically.
- The procedures must be similar in terms of resource costs.

Example 1: APC group 0003, Bone Marrow Biopsy/Aspiration, contains CPT codes 38220 and 38221, both of which describe bone marrow procedures.

APC 0003	**Bone Marrow Biopsy/Aspiration**
(HCPCS Code)	*(HCPCS Code Description)*
38220	Bone marrow aspiration
38221	Bone marrow biopsy

Example 2: APC group 0158, Colorectal Cancer Screening: Colonoscopy, contains HCPCS Level II codes G0105 and G0121, both of which describe colon cancer (CA) screening.

APC 0158	**Colorectal Cancer Screening: Colonoscopy**
(HCPCS Code)	*(HCPCS Code Description)*
G0105	Colon CA screen; high-risk individual
G0121	Colon CA screen; not high-risk individual

Example 3: APC group 0170, Dialysis, contains CPT codes 90935 and 90945 and HCPCS Level II code G0257, all of which describe dialysis.

APC 0170	**Dialysis**
(HCPCS Code)	*(HCPCS Code Description)*
90935	Hemodialysis, one evaluation
90945	Dialysis, one evaluation
G0257	Unscheduled or emergency dialysis in a hospital

How the APC Groups Were Constructed

3M-Health Information Systems created APGs by combining procedure codes and diagnosis codes into groups that were clinically related, such as all codes for repair of fractured legs, and analyzing claims data to determine if the codes that were clinically similar also used resources in similar ways (for example, surgical repair would likely be more resource-intensive than closed manipulation and casting). The resources examined were based on a sample of Medicare claims for outpatient services.

The costs that were calculated using billed charges and department CCRs included direct costs as well as the overhead for performing the services. The APGs were clustered into significant surgical and nonsurgical procedures, medical visits in both clinics and emergency departments, and ancillary services. Other groups captured incidental services that would not be paid separately and procedures for which no payment is made, such as services specifically excluded from Medicare payment by statute.

This process of revising 3M-Health Information System's APGs resulted in the development of hundreds of mutually exclusive and exhaustive service categories called ambulatory payment classification groups, or APCs.

The items and services within an APC group cannot be considered comparable with respect to the use of resources if the highest-cost item or service within a group is more than two times greater than the lowest-cost item or service within the same group.

In general, the five criteria for compilation of APC groups are as follows:

- **Resource homogeneity**: The amount and type of facility resources (for example, operating room time, medical surgical supplies, and equipment) that are used to furnish or perform the individual procedures or services within each APC should be homogeneous. That is, the resources used are relatively constant across all procedures or services, even though resource use may vary somewhat among individual patients.

- **Clinical homogeneity**: The definition of each APC group should be clinically meaningful. That is, the procedures or services included within the APC group relate generally to a common organ system or etiology, have the same degree of extensiveness, and utilize the same method of treatment (surgical, endoscopic, and so forth). For APCs, the definition of clinical meaningfulness relates to the medical rationale for differences in resource use.

- **Provider concentration**: If a particular service is offered in only a limited number of hospitals, the impact of payment for the service is concentrated in a subset of hospitals. Therefore, it is particularly important to have an accurate payment level for services with a high degree of provider concentration. Conversely, the accuracy of payment levels for services that are offered routinely by most hospitals does not bias the payment system against any subset of hospitals. Thus, differences in the resource requirements for individual services within an APC are of less significance when all the services within the APC are offered routinely by most hospitals because the impact of the difference should average out at the hospital level.

- **Frequency of service**: Unless CMS found a high degree of provider concentration, it avoided creating separate APC groups for services that are performed infrequently. It is difficult to establish reliable payment rates for low-volume APC groups. Therefore, CMS assigned the codes to the APC that was the most similar in terms of resource use and clinical coherence.

- **Minimal opportunities for upcoding and code fragmentation**: The APC system is intended to discourage using a code in a higher-paying group to define a case. That is, putting two related codes, such as the codes for excising a lesion of 1.1 cm and one of 1.0 cm, in different APC groups may create an incentive to exaggerate the size of the lesions to justify the incrementally higher payment. APC groups based on subtle distinctions would be susceptible to this kind of upcoding. Therefore, CMS kept the APC groups as broad and inclusive as possible without sacrificing resource or clinical homogeneity.

In general, HCPCS codes that are nonspecific (such as 20999, Unlisted procedure, musculo-skeletal system, general) were assigned to the lowest-paying APC that was consistent with the clinical characteristics of the service.

Composite APCs Under OPPS

Composite APCs reflect an evolution in CMS's approach to payment under the OPPS. Where the claims data showed that combinations of services were commonly furnished together, composite APCs were established under which CMS would pay a single rate for the service reported with a combination of HCPCS codes on the same date of service (or different dates of service) rather than continuing to pay for these individual services under service-specific APCs.

Encounter-based composite APCs for CY 2008 could move the OPPS toward possible payment based on an encounter or episode-of-care basis. This could perhaps enable CMS to use more valid and complete claims data, create hospital incentives for efficiency, and provide hospitals with significant flexibility to manage their resources that do not exist when payment for services is on a per-service basis. As such, these proposed composite APCs may serve as a prototype for future creation of more composite APCs, through which OPPS payment could be provided for other types of services in the future. Composite APCs are further discussed later in this book.

When evaluating new services for payment under the OPPS, CMS uses all information available regarding the clinical characteristics of procedures and the expected hospital resource costs. CMS reserves new technology APC assignments for those services where there is not an appropriate clinical APC for the new service. In many cases, new HCPCS codes describe services that are similar to existing services that are paid under the OPPS and for which cost data is available from hospital claims. CMS follows the claims data closely and carefully reviews the new technology and clinical APC assignments of relatively new OPPS services for each update year when new claims data become available.

Reporting Hospital Quality Data under OPPS

In the CY 2007 OPPS/ASC final rule, CMS indicated an intent to establish, in CY 2009, an OPPS Reporting Hospital Quality Data for Annual Payment Update (RHQDAPU) program modeled after the current IPPS RHQDAPU program. CMS states that the quality of hospital outpatient services would be most appropriately and fairly rewarded through the reporting of quality measures developed specifically for application in the hospital outpatient setting. As required by statute, consensus was reached by affected parties, as the measures were identified as appropriate for reporting on hospital outpatient care in collaboration with professionals and providers with experience in hospital outpatient settings as well as with the Hospital Quality Alliance (HQA), a hospital-industry led, public-private collaboration established to promote public reporting on hospital quality of care.

CMS finalized the specifications for these 10 measures and released them publicly on August 28, 2007. In addition, these 10 measures have gone through the National Quality Forum (NQF) steering committee process. Therefore, for hospitals to receive the full OPPS payment update for services furnished in CY 2009, in the CY 2008 OPPS/ASC proposed rule (72 FR 42800), CMS proposed to require that hospital outpatient settings submit data on 10 measures, effective with hospital outpatient services furnished on or after January 1, 2008. These measures are discussed later in this chapter on page 17.

Payment Status Indicators

To implement the OPPS, Medicare assigns a payment status indicator (SI) for every code in the HCPCS and CPT coding systems to identify how the service or procedure described by the code would be paid under the hospital OPPS.

The status indicators (SIs) that CMS assigns to HCPCS codes and APCs under the OPPS indicate whether a service represented by a HCPCS code is payable under the OPPS or another payment system, whether adjustments to payment are required, or if other particular OPPS policies apply to the code.

CMS assigns one and only one SI to each APC and each HCPCS code. Each HCPCS code that is assigned to an APC has the same SI as the APC to which it is assigned.

The software that controls Medicare payment looks to the SIs attached to the HCPCS codes and APC groups for direction in claims processing. Therefore, SI assignment has significance for the payment of services. (See Table 1.1 for the 2008 OPPS SIs and their explanations and Table 1.2 for a list of the 2008 OPPS SIs for *some* of the CPT and HCPCS Level II codes.)

Table 1.1.   **2008 payment status indicators for the hospital OPPS**

Indicator	Item/Code/Service	Explanation
A	Services furnished to a hospital outpatient that are paid under a fee schedule/payment system other than OPPS; for example: • Ambulance services • Clinical diagnostic laboratory services • Nonimplantable prosthetic and orthotic devices • Epoetin (EPO) for ESRD patients • Physical, occupational, and speech therapy • Routine dialysis services for ESRD patients provided in a certified dialysis unit of a hospital • Diagnostic mammography • Screening mammography	Not paid under OPPS. Paid by fiscal intermediaries/MAC under a fee schedule/payment system other than OPPS. Not subject to deductible or coinsurance.
B	Codes that are not recognized by OPPS when submitted on an outpatient hospital Part B bill type (12x and 13x)	Not paid under OPPS. • May be paid by intermediaries/MACs when submitted on a different bill type (for example, 75x [CORF]), but not paid under OPPS. • An alternate code that is recognized by OPPS when submitted on an outpatient hospital Part B bill type (12x and 13x) may be available.
C	Inpatient procedures	Not paid under OPPS. Admit patient; bill as inpatient.
D	Discontinued codes	Not paid under OPPS. Not paid under Medicare.
E	Items, codes, and services: • That are not covered by Medicare based on statutory exclusion • That are not covered by Medicare for reasons other than statutory exclusion • That are not recognized by Medicare but for which an alternate code for the same item or service may be available • For which separate payment is not provided by Medicare	Not paid under OPPS or any other Medicare payment system.
F	Corneal tissue acquisition; Certain certified registered nurse anesthetist (CRNA) services and Hepatitis B vaccines	Not paid under OPPS. Paid at reasonable cost.

(Continued on next page)

Table 1.1.   **(Continued)**

Indicator	Item/Code/Service	Explanation
G	Pass-through drugs and biologicals	Paid under OPPS; separate APC payment includes pass-through amount.
H	Pass-through device categories	Separate cost-based pass-through payment; not subject to copayment.
K	(1) Nonpass-through drugs and biologicals (2) Therapeutic radiopharmaceutical (3) Brachytherapy sources (4) Blood and blood products	(1), (2), (3), (4) Paid under OPPS; separate APC payment.
L	Influenza vaccine; pneumococcal pneumonia vaccine	Not paid under OPPS. Paid at reasonable cost; not subject to deductible or coinsurance.
M	Items and services not billable to the fiscal intermediary	Not paid under OPPS.
N	Items and services packaged into APC rates	Paid under OPPS. However, payment is packaged into payment for other services, including outliers. Therefore, there is no separate APC payment.
P	Partial hospitalization	Paid under OPPS; per diem APC payment.
Q	Packaged services subject to separate payment under OPPS payment criteria	Paid under OPPS; Addendum B displays APC assignments when services are separately payable. (1) Separate payment based on OPPS payment criteria. (2) If criteria are not met, payment is packaged into payment for other services, including outliers. Therefore, there is no separate APC payment.
S	Significant procedure, not discounted when multiple	Paid under OPPS; separate APC payment.
T	Significant procedure, multiple procedure reduction applies	Paid under OPPS; separate APC payment.
V	Clinic or emergency department visit	Paid under OPPS; separate APC payment.
X	Ancillary service	Paid under OPPS; separate APC payment.
Y	Nonimplantable durable medical equipment	Not paid under OPPS. All institutional providers other than home health agencies bill to durable medical equipment regional carrier (DMERC).

Source: November 27, 2007, *Federal Register*.

Table 1.2.   **2008 OPPS status indicators for selected CPT and HCPCS codes**

Code	SI	Abbreviated Code Description
11603	T	Excision, malignant lesion, trunk, arms, or legs + marg 2.1–3 cm
19290	N	Place needle wire, breast
23472	C	Reconstruct shoulder joint
27096	B	Inject sacroiliac joint
65771	E	Radial keratotomy
70336	S	Magnetic image, jaw joint
73130	X	X-ray exam of hand
77057	A	Mammogram, screening
90581	N	Anthrax vaccine, subcutaneous
90658	L	Flu vaccine, 3 yrs, intramuscular
99281	V	Emergency department visit
C2616	K	Brachytherapy source, Yttrium-90
J1743	G	Injection, idursulfase

(Continued on next page)

Table 1.2.   (Continued)

Code	SI	Abbreviated Code Description
E2326	Y	Breath tube kit
G0129	P	Partial hospital program service
V2785	F	Corneal tissue processing

For FY 2008, comment indicators are to reference which codes are new and active for specific HCPCS. Comment indicator "New code, interim APC assignment; comments" will be accepted on the interim APC assignment for the new code. In addition to "CH," active HCPCS code in current year and next calendar year, status indicator or APC assignment has changed; or active HCPCS code will be discontinued at the end of the current calendar year.

Description of the APC Groups

Each APC group consists of a cluster of services provided during a particular outpatient procedure. Each service or procedure within the APC group is identified by a HCPCS code. Inclusion in an APC group means that services are similar both clinically and in use of resources.

APC Grouping Logic

CMS defines each outpatient service under the PPS by a HCPCS code and classifies it into either an APC group for which an OPPS payment rate is established or a nonpayment category of services that are excluded from the outpatient PPS. A weight is associated with each APC group.

Procedures and services assigned a nonpayment classification include:

- Services that can be provided only on an inpatient basis
- Codes or services that are not covered by Medicare
- Procedures and services paid under fee schedules or another payment method

The APC system consists of hundreds of groups of services that are covered under the hospital outpatient PPS. In CY 2008, the APCs, represented by a four digit number, range from 0001 to 9508 for a total of 795, ranging from the lowest payment of $.21 to the highest payment of $ 25,040.37. There are five composite APCs. It is anticipated that these will increase in future years. To calculate the APC payment, the calculation includes the following:

- Relative weight
- Payment weight
- Status indicator (covered earlier)
- National unadjusted copayment
- Minimum unadjusted copayment

Relative weight is a number that reflects the expected resource consumption for cases associated with each APC—relative to the average of all APCs—that is used in determining payment. Where a payment weight has been established to maintain consistency in using a median for calculating unscaled weights representing the median cost of some of the most frequently provided services, such as the median cost of the mid-level clinic APC, use proposed APC 0606 to calculate unscaled weights. Following the standard methodology for calculating APCs and utilizing the CY 2008 median for APC 0606, CMS assigned APC 0606 a relative payment weight of 1.00 and divided the median cost of each

APC by the median cost for APC 0606 to derive the unscaled relative payment weight for each APC. Note: The choice of the APC on which to base the relative weights for all other APCs does not affect the payments made under the OPPS because the weights are scaled for budget neutrality.

Example: The following is an excerpt from the 2008 APC data ("SI" is the status indicator, "Rel. Wt." is the relative weight, "Pay. Rate" is the payment rate, "Natl. Coin." is the national unadjusted coinsurance, and "Min. Coin." is the minimum unadjusted coinsurance):

APC	HCPCS	APC Description	HCPCS Description	SI	Rel. Wt.	Pay. Rate	Natl. Coin.	Min. Coin.
0100		Cardiac Stress Tests		X	2.5547	162.72	41.44	32.54

0179T	64 lead ecg w tracing
93017	Cardiovascular stress test
93024	Cardiac drug stress test
93025	Microvolt t-wave assess
Q0035	Cardiokymography

For the above excerpt, the ancillary service (status indicator "X") APC group 0100 contains CPT codes 0179T, 93017, 93024, and 93025, and HCPCS Level II code Q0035, all of which are cardiac stress test–related services.

Relative Weights

Section 1886 of the SSA requires the HHS to develop relative payment weights for covered groups of hospital outpatient services. Calculating OPPS payment rates consists of calculating relative resource cost and calculating budget neutrality adjustments, which are applied to estimates of resource cost and the conversion factor to create a budget-neutral PPS. The medians were converted to payment weights by dividing the median for each APC (a group of HCPCS codes) by the median cost for APC 606, the mid-level outpatient visit APC in CY 2008. By assigning APC 606 a relative payment weight of 1.3226, hospitals can easily compare the relative relationship of one APC to another. Next, CMS divided the median cost for each APC by the median cost for APC 606 to derive the relative payment weight for each APC.

Example: The 2008 relative weight for APC 0100, Cardiac Stress Tests, is 2.5547. Thus, APC 0100 is considered to be a more resource-intensive APC group than APC 606, which has a relative weight of 1.3226.

APC	Group Title	SI	Relative Weight	Payment Rate	National Unadjusted Copayment	Minimum Unadjusted Copayment
	Cardiac Stress Tests	X	2.5547	162.72	41.44	32.54

Conversion Factor

The SSA requires CMS to establish a conversion factor each calendar year to determine the Medicare amounts for each covered group of services. The prospective payment rate set for each APC is calculated by multiplying the APC's relative weight by a conversion factor.

Example: The 2008 relative weight for APC 0100, Cardiac Stress Tests, is 2.5547, and the CY 2008 conversion factor is $63.69. Thus, the CY 2008 payment rate for APC 0100 is $162.72 ($63.69 x 2.5547).

Calculation of Medicare Payment Amount and Copayment Amount

A Medicare payment amount is calculated for every APC group. The Medicare payment amount takes into account wage index and other applicable adjustments and applicable beneficiary deductible amounts. The Medicare payment amount calculated for an APC group applies to all the services classified within that group.

Example: For APC group 0100, Cardiac Stress Tests, the CY 2008 payment rate is $162.72.

APC	Group Title	SI	Relative Weight	Payment Rate	National Unadjusted Copayment	Minimum Unadjusted Copayment
0100	Cardiac Stress Tests	X	2.5547	162.72	41.44	32.54

A copayment amount is calculated annually for each APC group. The copayment amount calculated for an APC group applies to all the services classified within that group.

Example: For APC group 0100, Cardiac Stress Tests, the CY 2008 national unadjusted copayment amount was $41.44.

APC	Group Title	SI	Relative Weight	Payment Rate	National Unadjusted Copayment	Minimum Unadjusted Copayment
0100	Cardiac Stress Tests	X	2.5547	162.72	41.44	32.54

The transition of all APC groups to the standard Medicare copayment rate (20 percent of the wage-adjusted APC payment rate) will be gradual. For those APC groups for which copayment is currently a relatively high proportion of the total payment, the process will be correspondingly lengthy. Thus, the SSA offers hospitals the option of electing to reduce copayment amounts and to advertise these reduced rates.

The SSA requires the HHS to establish a procedure under which a hospital, before the beginning of a year, can reduce the copayment amount otherwise established for some or all hospital outpatient department services to an amount not less than 20 percent of the hospital OPPS amount.

Example: For APC group 0100, Cardiac Stress Tests, the CY 2008 minimum unadjusted copayment amount was $32.54. Thus, if a hospital elected to reduce the copayment amount for the services that group to APC 0100, the reduced copayment amount could not be less than $32.54.

APC	Group Title	SI	Relative Weight	Payment Rate	National Unadjusted Copayment	Minimum Unadjusted Copayment
0100	Cardiac Stress Tests	X	2.5547	162.72	41.44	32.54

The statute further provides that the election of a reduced copayment amount applies without change for the entire year.

The SSA provides that deductibles cannot be waived and no reduction in copayment elected by the hospital may be treated as a bad debt.

A hospital may make the election to reduce copayments on a calendar year basis. It must notify its FI of its election to reduce copayments no later than ninety days prior to the start of the calendar year. This 90-day notification requirement is necessary to give the intermediaries sufficient time to make the systems changes required to implement the hospital's election. The hospital's notification must be in writing and specifically identify the APC groups to which the hospital's election applies and the copayment level (within the limits identified below) the hospital has selected for each group.

A hospital may elect to reduce the copayment amount for any or all APC groups. However, it may not elect to reduce the copayment amount for some, but not all, services within the same APC group.

Example: A hospital cannot elect only to reduce the copayment amount for a cardiac drug stress test (code 93024) without electing to reduce the copayment amount for all the other services (codes 0179T, 93017, 93025, and Q0035) assigned to APC 0100.

APC	HCPCS	APC Description	HCPCS Description	SI	Rel. Wt.	Pay. Rate	Natl. Coin.	Min. Coin.
0100		Cardiac Stress Tests		X	2.5547	162.72	41.44	32.54

    0179T   64 lead ecg w tracing
    93017   Cardiovascular stress test
    93024   Cardiac drug stress test
    93025   Microvolt t-wave assess
    Q0035   Cardiokymography

A hospital may not elect for an APC group a copayment amount that is less than 20 percent of the adjusted APC payment rate for that hospital. In determining whether to make such an election, hospitals should note that the national copayment amount under this system, based on 20 percent of national median charges for each APC, may yield copayment amounts that are significantly higher or lower than the copayment the hospital has previously collected. This is because the median of the national charges for an APC group, from which the copayment amount is ultimately derived, may be higher or lower than the hospital's historic charges. CMS advises that hospitals, in determining whether to exercise the option of electing lower copayment and the level at which to make the election, carefully study the annual copayment amounts for each APC group in relation to the copayment amount the hospital has previously collected.

Composite APCs

The changes in CY 2008 represent the beginning of a shift in CMS's overall approach to payment under the OPPS. CMS is moving away from service-specific payments by expanding the packaging of individual services into APC groups and creating encounter-based APCs that will pay a single rate for a combination of specific services.

Elimination of Certain APCs through Expanded Packaging of Ancillary Services

Currently, there are a number of services that are not paid separately but are packaged into the APC rate for their related procedure or services. For CY 2008, CMS is looking to create more incentives for the efficient delivery of services and, hence, is expanding the number of services that will be packaged into larger APC groups. CMS is packaging payment for HCPCS codes associated with the following ancillary services:

- Guidance Services
- Image Processing Services
- Intraoperative Services
- Imaging Supervision and Interpretation Services
- Diagnostic Radiopharmaceuticals
- Contrast Agents
- Certain Observation Services (excluding instances where observation care is a major component of the encounter). Observation service composite APC is titled Level I and Level II Extended Assessment and Management composite APC.

This policy will be implemented in a budget-neutral manner by redistributing outpatient dollars to all other services. While this does not result in immediate savings for the Medicare program, CMS believes elimination of separate payments for these procedures will reduce growth in the volume of services provided in the outpatient setting over the longer term.

Combining Certain APCs into New, Encounter-Based APCs

As mentioned earlier in this chapter, CMS is creating a new type of APC called a composite APC. These new APCs would differ significantly from the current APCs in that composite APCs are encounter-based and a single payment would be made when a certain combination of HCPCS codes are reported on the same date of service, rather than paying for individual services under service-specific APCs.

For CY 2008, CMS is establishing a total of five composite APCs:

- APC 8000: Cardiac Electrophysiologic Evaluation and Ablation Composite
- APC 8001: LDR Prostate Brachytherapy Composite
- APC 8002: Level I Extended Assessment & Management Composite
- APC 8003: Level II Extended Assessment & Management Composite
- APC 0034: Mental Health Services Composite

Quality Reporting

As required by law, CMS has established a quality measure reporting program called the Hospital Outpatient Quality Data Reporting Program (HOP QDRP) that will measure a hospital's outpatient quality of care. Providers will be required to submit data on seven (reduced from the proposed ten) outpatient measures, effective for hospital outpatient services furnished on or after April 1, 2008, in order to be eligible to receive the full OPPS payment update in CY 2009. Noncompliant providers in CY 2008 will receive the OPPS update reduced by 2.0 percentage points in CY 2009.

The seven measures CMS is requiring for the initial implementation of the HOP QDRP have been endorsed by the National Quality Forum (NQF) and include:

- Emergency Department (ED) Transfer Acute Myocardial Infarction (AMI)-1—Aspirin at Arrival
- ED-AMI-2: Median Time to Fibrinolysis
- ED-AMI-3: Fibrinolytic Therapy Received Within 30 Minutes of Arrival

- ED-AMI-4: Median Time to Electrocardiogram (ECG)
- ED-AMI-5: Median Time to Transfer for Primary Percutaneous Coronary Intervention (PCI)
- PQRI #20: Perioperative Care: Timing of Antibiotic Prophylaxis
- PQRI #21: Perioperative Care: Selection of Prophylactic Antibiotic

Marketbasket CY 2008

The final rule provides a full market basket update of 3.3 percent. Including adjustments for budget neutrality, the conversion factor will increase by approximately 3.6 percent from $61.468 in CY 2007 to $63.694 in CY 2008.

Outlier Payments

The final rule will decrease the outlier fixed-dollar threshold from $1,825 in CY 2007 to $1,575 in CY 2008. Therefore, under the final rule, outlier payments will be provided when the cost of furnishing a service exceeds 1.75 times the APC payment amount and exceeds the APC payment rate plus a $1,575 fixed-dollar threshold.

Adjustment for Area Wage Differences

As part of the methodology for determining prospective payments to hospitals for outpatient services, the SSA requires the HHS to determine a wage adjustment factor to adjust the portion of payment and copayment attributable to labor-related costs for relative differences in labor and labor-related costs across geographic regions in a budget-neutral manner.

CMS decided that using the hospital IPPS wage index as the source of an adjustment factor for geographic wage differences for the hospital outpatient department PPS was both reasonable and logical, given the inseparable, subordinate status of the outpatient department within the hospital overall.

The hospital IPPS wage index reflects the following:

- Total salaries and hours from short-term, acute care hospitals
- Home office costs and hours
- Fringe benefits associated with hospital and home office salaries
- Direct patient care contract labor costs and hours
- The exclusion of salaries and hours for nonhospital-type services such as skilled nursing facility (SNF) services, home health services, or other subprovider components that are not subject to the PPS

CMS updates the wage index values used to calculate hospital outpatient department PPS Medicare payment and beneficiary copayment amounts on a calendar year basis. In other words, the hospital IPPS wage index values that are updated annually on October 1st will be implemented for the hospital outpatient department PPS on the January 1st immediately following. CMS uses this schedule so that wage index changes are implemented concurrently with any other revisions, such as changes in the APC groups resulting from new or deleted CPT codes that are implemented on a calendar year basis.

Example: Here is the 2008 wage index value for the urban area of Ann Arbor, Michigan, which includes its constituent counties of Lenawee, Livingston, and Washtenaw.

Urban Area (Constituent Counties)	Wage Index

Ann Arbor, Michigan
    Lenawee, Michigan
    Livingston, Michigan
    Washtenaw, Michigan
	1.0678

Example: Here is the 2008 wage index value for the nonurban area in Iowa, which would include any counties that are not located in an urban area of Iowa.

Nonurban Area	Wage Index
Iowa	0.8615

Labor-Related Portion of Hospital Outpatient Department PPS Payment Rates

In calculating payments to hospitals under the hospital IPPS, the labor-related portion of expenses within the standardized amounts used to establish the prospective payment rates is multiplied by the hospital wage index value to offset regional wage differences.

To adjust the APC payment rates and beneficiary copayment rates for outpatient services for geographic wage variations, CMS proposed to use the same labor-related percentage (60 percent) it used initially to standardize costs for geographic wage differences. When intermediaries calculate actual payment amounts, they multiply the prospectively determined APC payment rate and copayment amount by that labor-related percentage to determine the labor-related portion of the base payment and copayment rates that are to be adjusted using the appropriate wage index factor. Then the labor-related portion is multiplied by the hospital's IPPS wage index factor, and the resulting wage-adjusted labor-related portion is added to the nonlabor-related portion, resulting in wage-adjusted payment and copayment rates. Next, the wage-adjusted copayment amount is subtracted from the wage-adjusted APC payment rate and the result is the Medicare payment amount for the service or procedure. Even when a hospital elects to discount the copayment, the full copayment amount is assumed for purposes of determining Medicare program payments.

Example: This example shows how an FI would calculate the wage-adjusted payment for a cardiovascular stress test (CPT code 93017) with an APC 0100 payment rate of $162.72 that is performed in the outpatient department of a hospital located in Ann Arbor, Michigan. The copayment amount for the procedure is $41.44.

CPT/ HCPCS Code	SI	Code Description	APC	Relative Weight	Payment Rate	National Unadjusted Copayment	Minimum Unadjusted Copayment
93017	X	Cardiovascular stress test	0100	2.557	162.72	41.44	32.54

Urban Area (Constituent Counties)	Wage Index

Ann Arbor, Michigan
    Lenawee, Michigan
    Livingston, Michigan
    Washtenaw, Michigan
	1.0678

The steps for calculating a wage-adjusted payment are as follows:

1.	APC payment rate	$162.72
2.	Labor percentage	.60 (60%)
3.	Labor-related portion	$97.63
4.	Nonlabor-related portion (Step 1 - step 3)	$65.09
5.	Wage-adjusted labor portion (step 3 x wage index value 1.0678)	$104.25
6.	Adjusted APC payment (step 4 + step 5)	$169.34

Thus, under the OPPS, Ann Arbor hospitals will receive $169.34 for cardiovascular stress tests coded and billed as code 93017.

Outlier Adjustment

The BBRA of 1999, requires that the HHS make an additional payment (that is, an outlier adjustment) for outpatient services for which a hospital's charges, adjusted to cost, exceed a fixed multiple of the outpatient PPS payment as adjusted by pass-through payments. The HHS determines this fixed multiple and the percent of costs above the threshold that is to be paid under this outlier provision. The statute sets a limit on projected aggregate outlier payments.

Under the statute, projected outlier payments may not exceed an "applicable percentage" of projected total payments. Outlier payment costs are simulated using several different fixed-dollar thresholds holding the 1.75 multiple constant until the total outlier payments equal 1.0 percent of the aggregated total OPPS payments.

Example: Following is the computation of an outlier payment adjustment for a sample hospital. To compute the adjustment, the following data are required:

Total charges for all covered services	$3,000.00
Outpatient cost to charge ratio	0.987564
Total OPPS payments on claim	$992.90

The steps for calculating the outlier payment for a sample claim are:

1.	Total charges for all covered OPPS services on bill	$3,000.00
2.	Outpatient cost to charge ratio	0.987564
3.	Computed costs for OPPS services	$2,962.69
4.	Total OPPS payments on claim	$992.90
5.	OPPS outlier threshold (line 4 x 2.5)	$2,482.25
6.	Amount of costs over threshold (line 3 - line 5)	$480.44
7.	Outlier payment (line 6 x .75)	$360.33

APC System Updates

In accordance with the amendments enacted by the BBRA of 1999, for implementation effective January 1 of each year, CMS annually reviews and updates the APC groups, the relative payment weights, and the wage and other adjustments that are components of the outpatient PPS to take into account changes in medical practice, changes in technology, the addition of new services, new cost data, and other relevant information and factors.

CMS updates the wage index values used to calculate program payment and copayment amounts on a calendar year basis, adopting, effective for services furnished each January 1, the wage index value established for a hospital under the IPPS the previous October 1

The SSA also requires the HHS to update annually the conversion factor used to determine APC payment rates. The 2006 conversion factor for the OPPS was $59.511; the 2007 conversion factor for the OPPS was $61.551; and the 2008 conversion factor for the OPPS is $63.694.

CPT and HCPCS Code Changes

The composition of all the APC groups is expected to remain essentially intact from one year to the next, with the exception of the few changes that may be necessary as a consequence of annual revisions to HCPCS and CPT codes. CMS does not routinely reclassify services and procedures from one APC to another but, instead, makes the changes based on evidence that a reassignment would improve the group(s) either clinically or with respect to resource consumption.

All changes in APC groups must be budget neutral, and changes in APC groups will only be made through notice and comment in the *Federal Register* when the annual outpatient PPS update is implemented.

CMS follows certain conventions when, as a result of annual HCPCS and CPT revisions, it must add new services to the hospital outpatient PPS. As part of the notice and comment process accompanying the annual update of the outpatient PPS, CMS assigns a newly-created code to the existing APC that, in the judgment of its medical advisors, is the most similar clinically and in terms of resource requirements to the new service. Because a new service will not have any charge history or cost data associated with it, classification of a new service to an existing APC group will not alter the APC payment rate, relative weight, and program payment and copayment amounts that have been established for that APC group. The new service will assume the same payment rate, relative weight, and program and copayment amounts that have been established for the APC group to which it is classified.

If the annual revision of HCPCS or CPT results in the deletion of a code or service that is classified in an APC group under the outpatient PPS, CMS removes that service from the APC group and discontinues paying for it under the outpatient PPS.

If the code is revised so that it no longer belongs in the APC to which it was originally assigned, the revised code is placed in an APC that better matches the new description. As in the case of an entirely new code, no cost data would be available for the revised code, so it will be assigned the weight, program payment rate, and copayment rate of the codes in the new APC.

CMS will not create an APC for an entirely new code but will assign the new code for at least two years to an existing group, while accumulating data on its costs relative to the other codes in the APC.

Services Excluded from the Hospital OPPS

Section 1833(t)(1)(B)(i) of the Act authorizes the Secretary to designate the hospital outpatient services that are paid under the OPPS. While most hospital outpatient services are payable under the OPPS, section 1833(t)(1)(B)(iv) of the Act excludes payment for ambulance, physical and occupational therapy, and speech-language pathology services, for which payment is made under a fee schedule.

Section 614 of Public Law 108-173 amended section 1833(t)(1)(B)(iv) of the Act to exclude payment for screening and diagnostic mammography services from the OPPS. The Secretary exercised the authority granted under the statute to also exclude from the OPPS those services that are paid under fee schedules or other payment systems. Such excluded services include, for example, the professional services of physicians and nonphysician practitioners paid under the Medicare Physician Fee Schedule (MPFS); laboratory services paid under the clinical diagnostic laboratory fee schedule (CLFS); services for beneficiaries with end stage renal disease (ESRD) that are paid under the ESRD composite rate; and services and procedures that require an inpatient stay that are paid under the hospital IPPS. Services that are excluded from payment under the OPPS are set forth in Sec. 419.22 of the regulations.

Under Sec. 419.20(b) of the regulations, the types of hospitals and entities that are excluded from payment under the OPPS are specified. These excluded entities include Maryland hospitals, but only for services that are paid under a cost containment waiver in accordance with section 1814(b)(3) of the Act; critical access hospitals (CAHs); hospitals located outside of the 50 States, the District of Columbia, and Puerto Rico; and Indian Health Service (IHS) hospitals.

Maryland Hospital Cost Containment Services

Certain hospitals in Maryland qualify for payment under the state's payment system. The OPPS-excluded services are limited to those paid under the state's payment system. Any other outpatient services furnished by Maryland hospitals are paid under the OPPS.

Indian Health Service Hospital Outpatient Services

The outpatient services provided by IHS hospitals will continue to be paid under separately established rates that are published annually in the *Federal Register*.

Critical Access Hospital Outpatient Services

CAHs are excluded from the OPPS because they are paid under a reasonable cost-based system. A CAH is located in a rural area, provides 24-hour emergency care services, and has an average length of stay of 96 hours or less. In addition, it is located more than 35 miles from another hospital or CAH; or in areas with mountainous terrains or only secondary roads, or it is more than 15 miles from another medical facility. Alternatively, it has been certified by the state as being a necessary provider of healthcare services to residents in the area.

Ambulance Services and Physical/Occupational/Speech Therapy

Ambulance services, physical and occupational therapy, and speech–language pathology services are paid for under fee schedules in all settings.

Services Already Paid for under Fee Schedules or Other Payment Systems

Certain services are already paid for under fee schedules or other payment systems including, but not limited to, screening mammographies, services for patients with end-stage renal disease (ESRD) that are paid for under the ESRD composite rate, laboratory services paid for under the clinical diagnostic laboratory fee schedule, and DME, prosthetics, orthotics, and supplies (DME-POS), including prosthetic devices and implants paid for under the DMEPOS fee schedule when the hospital is acting as a supplier of these items. For example, an item such as a walker that is given to the patient to take home but also may be used while the patient is at the hospital is billed to the DME regional carrier rather than paid for under the hospital outpatient PPS. To receive payment for DME under Medicare, a hospital must obtain a supplier number and meet the other requirements set by applicable Medicare rules and regulations.

Example: The SI "A" appears for the following laboratory and equipment/supply codes because these codes are not paid for under the OPPS. Rather, these codes are paid by the FIs under a fee schedule or payment system other than OPPS.

Code	SI	Abbreviated Code Description
81005	A	Urinalysis
90901	A	Biofeedback training, any method
E0445	A	Oximeter, noninvasive

Inpatients of a Skilled Nursing Facility

Hospital outpatient services furnished to SNF inpatients as part of their resident assessment or comprehensive care plan, and thus included under the SNF PPS, that are furnished by the hospital under arrangement are billable only by the SNF, regardless of whether the patient is in a Medicare Part A SNF stay.

Inpatient Procedures

Inpatient procedures are not classified in an outpatient APC group, and no payment is provided for them under the hospital outpatient PPS. CMS will deny payment for claims that are submitted for these procedures furnished as outpatient services because such procedures, when performed on an outpatient basis, are not considered safe or appropriate and, thus, do not qualify as reasonable and necessary under Medicare rules.

Some procedures by their nature require inpatient care. Open abdominal surgery requires a postoperative recovery period, for example, to ensure that bowel function resumes. Certain major surgeries require monitoring in an intensive care unit until the patient's neurological or other function returns. Other surgeries involve large or delicate surgical wounds that require monitoring, skilled dressing changes, and fluid replacement. These procedures obviously require inpatient care and performing them on an outpatient basis would clearly jeopardize patient health and safety. Other procedures are not as clearly defined as inpatient, but CMS has classified them as such because they are performed on an inpatient basis virtually all the time for the Medicare population because of either their invasive nature, the need for postoperative care, or the underlying physical condition of the patient.

The inpatient list specifies those services that are only paid for when provided in an inpatient setting. These are services that require inpatient care because of the nature of the procedure, the need for at least twenty-four hours of postoperative recovery time or monitoring before the patient can be safely discharged, or the underlying physical condition of the patient.

Example: The SI "C" appears for the following CPT codes because they are on the Medicare inpatient-only list:

CPT/HCPCS	Status Indicator	Description
69535	C	Remove part of temporal bone
69554	C	Remove ear lesion
69950	C	Incise inner ear nerve

CMS Web site to the home page is www.cms.hhs.gov/home/medicare.asp.

CMS uses the following criteria when reviewing procedures to determine whether they should be moved from the inpatient list and assigned to an APC group for payment under the OPPS:

- Most outpatient departments are equipped to provide the services to the Medicare population.

- The simplest procedure described by the code may be performed in most outpatient departments.

- The procedure is related to codes that CMS has already removed from the inpatient list.

In the November 27, 2007, *Federal Register*, CMS specified additional criteria.

The following is a summary of the major changes included in the CY 2008 OPPS/ASC proposed rule:

- The methodology used to recalibrate the proposed APC relative payment weights

- The proposed payment for partial hospitalization services, including the proposed separate threshold for outlier payments for CMHCs

- The proposed update to the conversion factor used to determine payment rates under the OPPS

- The proposed retention of our current policy to use the IPPS wage indices to adjust for geographic wage differences, the portion of the OPPS payment rate, and the copayment standardized amount attributable to labor-related cost

- The proposed update of statewide average default CCRs

- The proposed application of hold harmless transitional outpatient payments (TOPs) for certain small rural hospitals

- The proposed payment adjustment for rural sole community hospitals

- The proposed calculation of the hospital outpatient outlier payment

- The calculation of the proposed national unadjusted Medicare OPPS payment

- The proposed beneficiary copayments for OPPS services

CMS publishes a Medicare inpatient-only list every year when the annual OPPS updates are published in the *Federal Register*. For example, for the CY 2008 OPPS update, the Medicare inpatient-only list was published in the November 27, 2007, *Federal Register*. (See www.cms.hhs.gov/hospitaloutpatientPPS/HORD/list.asp for more information.)

The fact that a procedure is included in an APC group under the hospital OPPS does not necessarily mean that it may only be performed in an outpatient setting. In every case, CMS expects the surgeon and the hospital to assess the risk to the individual patient and to act in the patient's best interests.

CMS notes that its designation of a service as inpatient-only does not necessarily preclude it from being furnished in a hospital outpatient setting; rather, it means only that Medicare will not make payment for the service when it is furnished to a Medicare beneficiary in that setting. This leaves the beneficiary liable for payment when the procedure is, in fact, performed in the outpatient setting. CMS hopes that hospitals will advise beneficiaries of the consequences when procedures on the inpatient list are provided as outpatient services (that is, denial of Medicare payment with concomitant beneficiary liability).

The Medicare inpatient-only list is used to govern payment for Medicare-covered outpatient services furnished by hospitals to Medicare beneficiaries. The list represents national Medicare policy and is binding on FIs and quality improvement organizations, as well as on hospitals and Medicare-participating ASCs.

Medicare payment policy and rules are not binding on employer-provided retiree coverage that may supplement Medicare coverage. However, Medigap insurers must follow Medicare's coverage determinations. CMS notes that services included in the outpatient PPS and assigned to an APC may be performed on an inpatient basis when the patient's condition warrants inpatient admission.

Outpatient Care Prior to an Inpatient Admission

Preadmission diagnostic services and other preadmission services prior to an inpatient admission, although outpatient services, are not paid under OPPS.

Preadmission Diagnostic Services

Effective for services furnished on or after January 1, 1991, diagnostic services (including clinical diagnostic laboratory tests) provided to a Medicare beneficiary by the admitting hospital or an entity wholly owned or operated by the hospital (or by another entity under arrangements with the hospital) within three days prior to the date of the beneficiary's admission are deemed to be inpatient services and included in the inpatient payment unless there is no Part A coverage. An entity is wholly owned or operated by the hospital if the hospital is the sole owner or operator. The three-day window provision does not apply to ambulance services.

> **Example:** If a patient is admitted on a Wednesday, services provided by the hospital on Sunday, Monday, or Tuesday are included in the inpatient Part A payment.

For services provided on or after October 31, 1994, for hospitals and units excluded from the IPPS (such as psychiatric hospitals), this provision applies only to services furnished within one day prior to the date of the beneficiary's admission.

Revenue codes are used to group HCPCS codes to services or items in FL 42 of the UB-04.

For this provision, diagnostic services are defined by the presence on the bill of the following revenue and/or HCPCS codes:

Revenue	Description
254	Drugs incident to other diagnostic services
255	Drugs incident to radiology
30X	Laboratory
31X	Laboratory pathological
32X	Radiology diagnostic
341	Nuclear medicine, diagnostic
35X	CT scan
40X	Other imaging services
46X	Pulmonary function
48X	Cardiology, with HCPCS codes 93015, 93307, 93308, 93320, 93501, 93503, 93505, 93510, 93526, 93541, 93542, 93543, 93544, 93561, or 93562
53X	Osteopathic services
61X	MRT
62X	Medical/surgical supplies, incident to radiology or other diagnostic services
73X	EKG/ECG
74X	EEG
92X	Other diagnostic services

The Internet address for the CMS revenue code crosswalk is www.cms.hhs.gov/HospitalOutpatientPPS/03_crosswalk.asp#TopOfPage.

Other Preadmission Services

Effective for services furnished on or after October 1, 1991, nondiagnostic outpatient services that are related to a patient's hospital admission and provided by the hospital or an entity wholly owned or operated by the hospital (or by another entity under arrangements with the hospital) to the patient during the three days immediately preceding the date of the patient's admission are deemed to be inpatient services and included in the inpatient payment. This provision applies only when the patient has Part A coverage; it does not apply to ambulance services.

For services provided on or after October 31, 1994, for hospitals and units excluded from the IPPS, this provision applies only to services furnished within one day prior to the date of the beneficiary's admission.

Preadmission services are related to the admission when furnished in connection with the principal diagnosis that necessitates the patient's admission as an inpatient (that is, when the outpatient principal diagnosis is the same as the inpatient principal diagnosis). Thus, whenever Part A covers an admission, hospitals may bill nondiagnostic preadmission services to Part B as outpatient services only if they are not related to the admission.

Services Included in the Hospital OPPS

Services that are included within the OPPS system are all hospital outpatient services that have not been identified for exclusion as described above. Among the types of services that CMS has classified into APC groups for payment under the hospital OPPS are:

- Supplies
- Implantable items
- Drugs, pharmaceuticals, and biologicals
- Surgical procedures
- Radiology, including radiation therapy
- Clinic visits
- Scheduled interdisciplinary team conferences
- Emergency department visits
- Critical care
- Limited follow-up services
- Diagnostic services and other diagnostic tests
- Surgical pathology
- Cancer chemotherapy
- Cancer hospitals
- Cancer hospitals that are excluded from IPPS
- Services for patients who have exhausted their Part A benefits
- Distinct parts of hospitals that are excluded under IPPS
- Services furnished to SNF patients that are not packaged into SNF consolidated billing
- Certain preventive services furnished to healthy persons
- Antigens, vaccines, splints, and casts
- Partial hospitalization for the mentally ill

- Inpatient procedures for patients who expire
- Observation services

Supplies

Supplies such as surgical dressings that can be used during surgery or other treatments in the hospital outpatient setting are also on the DMEPOS fee schedule. When they are used in the hospital outpatient setting, payment for such supplies is packaged into the APC payment rate for the procedure or service with which the items are associated.

> **Example:** Under the OPPS, when a hospital bills Medicare for an endoscopic procedure, such as a diagnostic colonoscopy, and a supply item, such as a disposable endoscope sheath, payment for the sheath is packaged (SI "N") into the surgical service APC (SI "T") payment the hospital receives for the colonoscopy. For code A4270, then, the SI "N" means that the disposable endoscope sheath will not be paid for separately under OPPS. The sheath is considered a supply and payment for supplies furnished by an ASC in connection with a surgical procedure is bundled into the payment for the surgical procedure for which the supplies are required. Reporting for all services and procedure is required even though payment is not made.

Code	SI	Abbreviated Code Description
A4270	N	Disposable endoscope sheath, each
45378	T	Diagnostic colonoscopy

Source documents and contents: The following documents may contain information about the supplies used: operative report/procedure note, visit note.

Coding from source documents: There are times when use of a particular supply drives the payment of the case into a higher-paying APC, so when coding outpatient cases it is important to review the medical record for the supplies used. Supplies are typically captured by the charge description master (CDM) codes; however, it is a prudent practice for coders to be aware of those supplies which impact APC payment.

> **Example:** Under the OPPS, when a hospital uses supplies such as lasers or heater probes to control bleeding via a sigmoidoscope, the APC payment rate is higher.

CPT/ HCPCS Code	SI	Code Description	APC	Relative Weight	Payment Rate	National Unadjusted Copayment	Minimum Unadjusted Copayment
45330	T	Sigmoidoscopy flexible; diagnostic, with or without collection of specimen(s) by brushing or washing (separate procedure)	0146	5.0972	324.66	-----	64.93

CPT/ HCPCS Code	SI	Code Description	APC	Relative Weight	Payment Rate	National Unadjusted Copayment	Minimum Unadjusted Copayment
45334	T	Sigmoidoscopy, flexible; with control of bleeding (for example, injection, bipolar cautery, unipolar cautery, laser, heater probe, stapler, plasma coagulator)	0147	8.7031		-----	110.87

Implantable Items

Implantable items range from corneal tissue to various prosthetic devices, shunts, pumps, and other devices. Some of these items are packaged into APC groups; others are reimbursed separately.

Packaged Implantables

Costs for the following items are included in hospital outpatient PPS payment rates (that is, the item is classified to the APC group that includes the service to which the item relates):

- Prosthetic implants (other than dental) that replace all or part of an internal body organ (including colostomy bags and supplies directly related to colostomy care)

- Replacement of these implants/devices

Implantable DME

Implantable items are used in performing diagnostic x-rays, diagnostic laboratory tests, and other diagnostic tests.

> **Example:** Under the OPPS, when a hospital bills Medicare for an aqueous shunt placement procedure, such as insertion of a Molteno shunt, and also bills for the Molteno aqueous shunt, payment for the shunt is packaged (SI "N") into the surgical service APC (SI "T") payment that the hospital receives for insertion of the aqueous shunt.

Note: According to CMS, as published in the November 27, 2007, *Federal Register*, hospitals may use CPT codes to report any packaged services ("N" status indicator codes) that were performed, consistent with CPT coding guidelines.

Code	SI	Abbreviated Code Description
L8612	N	Aqueous shunt prosthesis
66180	T	Aqueous shunt to extraocular reservoir

Separately Reimbursable Implantables

CMS does not package payment for corneal tissue acquisition costs into the payment rate for corneal transplant surgical procedures. Rather, it makes a separate payment for these acquisition costs based on the hospital's reasonable costs incurred to acquire corneal tissue.

Example: Under the OPPS, when a hospital bills Medicare for the processing of corneal tissue, the hospital is paid a reasonable cost rate (SI "F"). However, the hospital also receives a separate payment for the corneal transplant procedure itself under a surgical service APC (SI "T") payment group.

Code	SI	Abbreviated Code Description
V2785	F	Corneal tissue processing
65755	T	Corneal transplant

Some items may be candidates for the transitional pass-through payment, which would entitle the hospital to a separate payment for the item in addition to a payment for the service to which the item relates. The BBRA of 1999 required that for the OPPS, the HHS must establish transitional pass-through payments for certain high-cost medical devices, drugs, and biologicals. The purpose of this provision was to ensure that hospitals did not experience tremendous losses under the OPPS during the initial implementation phase.

Example: Under the OPPS, a device category transitional pass-through payment (SI "H") will be made to the hospital for the implantable device The hospital also will receive the surgical service APC (SI "T") payment for the spinous process distraction device surgery itself.

Code	SI	Abbreviated Code Description
C1821	H	Interspinous process distraction device (implantable)
0171T	T	Insertion of posterior spinous process, lumbar, single level

Source documents and contents: The following documents may contain information about the implantable items used: manufacturer's label, operative report/procedure note, visit note.

Coding from source documents: There are times when insertion of a particular implant drives the payment of the case into a higher-paying APC, so it is important to review the medical record for the implant(s) inserted or replaced during the surgical procedure. Following are some implantable items that can trigger higher APC payments: infusion pumps, venous access ports, penile implants, neurostimulators, electrodes, generators, and stents.

Drugs, Pharmaceuticals, and Biologicals

In many instances, CMS packaged the cost of drugs, pharmaceuticals, and biologicals into the APC payment rate for the primary procedure or treatment with which they are used.

Example: Under the OPPS, use of the drug Kenalog (reported under its generic name with code J3301) is packaged (SI "N") into the payment for the injection procedure. In the case below, when Kenalog is injected into a joint, the surgical service APC (SI "T") payment includes both the injection procedure and the drug.

Code	SI	Abbreviated Code Description
J3301	N	Triamcinolone acetonide injection
20610	T	Drain/inject, joint/bursa

Additional payment for some drugs, pharmaceuticals, and biologicals may be allowed under a separate APC payment rate. For example, thrombolytic agents and chemotherapeutic agents would yield separate payments.

Example: Under the OPPS, the upper gastrointestinal (GI) endoscopic submucosal injection of Botox for esophageal spasms would yield a separate APC payment (SI "K") for the Botox in addition to the surgical service APC (SI "T") payment for the endoscopic injection.

Code	SI	Abbreviated Code Description
J0585	K	Botulinum toxin a per unit
43236	T	Upper GI scope w/submucosal injection

Some drugs and biologicals may be candidates for the transitional pass-through payment, which would entitle the hospital to a separate payment for the item in addition to a payment for the service to which the item relates.

Example: The SI "G" appears for the following CPT codes because they are on the transitional pass-through list:

Code	SI	Abbreviated Code Description
C9239	G	Inj. Temsirolimus
C9352	G	Neuragen nerve guide, per cm
C9353	G	Neurawrap nerve protector, cm
C9354	G	Veritas collagen matrix, cm
C9355	G	Neuromatrix nerve cuff, cm

Source documents and contents: The following documents may contain information about the drugs, pharmaceuticals, and biologicals used: physicians' orders, medication sheets, clinical notes, operative reports, procedure notes, visit notes.

Coding from source documents: The medical record should be reviewed carefully because use of a particular drug, pharmaceutical, or biological sometimes generates a separate APC or transitional pass-through payment.

Surgical Procedures

The OPPS contains APC payment groups for numerous surgical procedures including, but not limited to

Ablations	Endoscopies	Ligations
Amputations	Excisions	Ostomies
Biopsies	Explantations	Reconstructions
Catheterizations	Fusions	Reductions
Debridements	Graft applications	Repairs
Destructions	Implantations	Revisions
Device applications	Incisions	Shavings
Dilations	Injections	Stabilizations
Drainages	Intubations	Transections

Here are some of the most commonly performed outpatient procedures, all of which are assigned to the surgical service OPPS SI "T."

Code	SI	Abbreviated Code Description
11400	T	Removal of skin lesion
12031	T	Layer closure of wound(s)
19120	T	Removal of breast lesion
25605	T	Treat fracture radius/ulna
28296	T	Correction of bunion
29881	T	Knee arthroscopy/surgery
31625	T	Bronchoscopy w/biopsy(s)
43239	T	Upper GI endoscopy, biopsy
45385	T	Lesion removal, colonoscopy
52000	T	Cystoscopy
58120	T	Dilation and curettage
62311	T	Inject spine lumbar/sacral (caudal)
66984	T	Cataract surgery w/lens, 1 stage
69436	T	Create eardrum opening

Source documents and contents: The following documents may contain information about the surgical procedures performed: operative reports, procedure notes, visit notes, clinical notes.

Coding from source documents: The medical record should be reviewed carefully because the surgical approach, the operative technique, and/or the complexity of the surgical procedure sometimes generate a higher-paying APC or multiple APC payments.

Example: Under the OPPS, the APC payment is higher when a clavicle is removed through an arthroscopic approach than when removed through an open approach.

CPT/HCPCS Code	SI	Code Description	APC	Relative Weight	Payment Rate
23120	T	Open partial claviculectomy	0050	29.1900	1859.23
29824	T	Arthroscopic distal claviculectomy	0041	28.7803	1833.13

Example: Under the OPPS, multiple payments are generated for APC 206 when a patient has multilevel transforaminal injections. An additional payment(s) for APC 206 is generated for every code 64484 reported on the claim.

CPT/HCPCS Code	SI	Code Description	APC	Relative Weight	Payment Rate
64484	T	Injection transforaminal lumbar/sacral add-on	0206	4.0964	260.92

Example: Under the OPPS, the APC payment is higher when an inguinal hernia is repaired laparoscopically versus through an open surgical approach.

CPT/HCPCS Code	SI	Code Description	APC	Relative Weight	Payment Rate
49500	T	Open repair inguinal, hernia initial, reduce	0154	30.6788	1.954.06
49650	T	Laparoscopic hernia repair, initial	0131	45.5317	2900.10

Radiology, Including Radiation Therapy

The OPPS contains APC payment groups for numerous radiology and radiation therapy services including, but not limited to:

Clinical brachytherapy
Clinical treatment management
Clinical treatment planning
Diagnostic imaging
Diagnostic nuclear medicine
Diagnostic ultrasound
Radiation oncology
Therapeutic nuclear medicine

Example: Below are examples of radiology and radiation therapy services. Some of these services are paid for as ancillary service APCs (SI "X"); others are paid for as significant procedure APCs (SI "S").

Code	SI	Abbreviated Code Description
71010	X	Chest x-ray
76001	N	Fluoroscope examination, extensive
76705	S	Echo exam of abdomen
78306	S	Bone imaging, whole body
79999	S	Nuclear medicine therapy

Source documents and contents: The following documents may contain information about the radiology and radiation therapy services performed: radiology reports, operative reports, procedure notes, visit notes, clinical notes.

Coding from source documents: Sometimes multiple codes are required for accurate APC payments of radiology or radiation therapy services. Thus, it is important to thoroughly review all the radiology and radiation therapy documentation.

Example: Under the OPPS, use of contrast dye triggers a higher APC payment for diagnostic imaging services.

CPT/HCPCS Code	SI	Code Description	APC	Relative Weight	Payment Rate
70450	S	CT scan head/brain w/o dye	0332	3.0109	191.78
70460	S	CT scan head/brain w/o dye	0283	4.3564	277.48

Example: Under the OPPS, ancillary service (SI "X") APC 263 is made for the radiological guidance used to place a needle wire radiologic marker into the breast for a breast biopsy. Payment for placement of the needle wire and guidance for needle wire is packaged (SI "N") into payment for the breast biopsy under surgical service (SI "T") APC 028.

CPT/HCPCS Code	SI	Code Description	APC	Relative Weight	Payment Rate
19125	T	Excision, breast lesion identified by radiologic marker	0028	20.6417	1314.75
19290	N	Place needle wire, breast	—	—	—
77032	N	Guidance for needle, breast	—	—	—

Example: Under the OPPS, a surgical service (SI "Q") payment is made for insertion of catheters and needles into the prostate to facilitate radiation therapy. Packaged services are subject to separate payment under OPPS payment criteria. If criteria is not met, payment is packaged into payment for other services, including outliers.

CPT/HCPCS Code	SI	Code Description	APC	Relative Weight	Payment Rate
55875	Q	Percutaneous/needle insertion, prostate	0163	36.0774	2297.91
77777	S	Apply interstitial radiation intermediate	312	8.5140	542.29

Example: Under the OPPS, a surgical service (SI "T") APC payment is generated for an epidural lysis on a single day, and no additional payment is made for the epidurography based on status indicator "N".

CPT/HCPCS Code	SI	Code Description	APC	Relative Weight	Payment Rate
62264	T	Epidural Lysis	0203	14.4879	922.79
72275	N	Epidurography			

Clinic and Emergency Department Visits

According to the *Medicare Hospital Manual*, section 442.7, "A visit is defined as direct personal contact between a registered hospital outpatient and a physician (or other person who is authorized by State licensure law and where applicable, by hospital staff bylaws to order or provide services for the patient) for purposes of diagnosis or treatment of the patient . . . . (Visits with more than one health professional, and multiple visits with the same health professional, that take place during the same session and at a single location with the hospital, constitute a single visit.)."

In 2007, CMS distinguished between two types of emergency departments: Type A emergency departments and Type B emergency departments. New codes were developed to identify hospital outpatient clinic and emergency department visits that meet the definition of Type B facilities. The codes will allow for tracking of resource costs of Type B emergency departments and determine how the costs for services provided in Type B emergency departments differ from the costs of clinic and Type A emergency department visits.

CMS recognizes that emergency departments continue to provide care to patients requiring less resource-intensive treatment, such as clinic-type patients who come to the emergency room for care. Therefore the creation of Type B differentiates a clinic-level visit performed in the ED from a Type A visit, which is considered emergent. The new codes for emergency visits provided in Type B emergency departments are as follows:

HCPCS Code	HCPCS Description
G0380	Lev 1 hosp type B ED visit
G0381	Lev 2 hosp type B ED visit
G0382	Lev 3 hosp type B ED visit
G0383	Lev 4 hosp type B ED visit
G0384	Lev 5 hosp type B ED visit

Type A emergency departments should continue to bill CPT codes 99281–99285 as they have been billed in the past.

A Type B emergency department is an emergency department that meets the definition of a "dedicated emergency department" in the *Federal Register*, 42 CFR 489.23 under the EMTALA regulations. It must meet one of the following requirements:

1. It is licensed by the State in which it is located under applicable State law as an emergency room or emergency department.
2. It is held out to the public (by name, posted signs, advertising, or other means) as a place that provides care for emergency medical conditions on an urgent basis without requiring a previously scheduled appointment.
3. During the calendar year immediately preceding the calendar year in which a determination under this section is being made, based on a representative sample of patient visits that occurred during that calendar year, it provides at least one-third of all of its outpatient visits for the treatment of emergency medical conditions on an urgent basis without requiring a previously scheduled appointment.

For CY 2007, CMS will reimburse at five payment levels for clinic and Type A emergency department visits, instead of the previous three payment levels. Type A emergency department visits will continue to be paid at the emergency department rates. Type B emergency department visits will be paid at clinic visit rates until additional data is collected to determine resources of cost utilized. There is no distinction between new and established patients.

Following are the codes for critical care in the emergency department:

HCPCS Code	HCPCS Description
99291	Critical care, evaluation and management of the critically ill or critically injured patient; first 30–74 minutes.
99292	Each additional 30 minutes.
G0390	Trauma response associated with hospital critical care services.

No changes to emergency room visit coding were applied in CY 2008; therefore, the G codes still apply.

National guidelines for E/M visit coding have not been implemented for CY 2008. Creating national guidelines has proven more difficult than initially anticipated, and some hospitals have expressed significant concerns about virtually all of the models CMS has discussed. CMS would not expect individual hospitals to necessarily experience a normal distribution of visit levels across their claims, although they would expect a normal distribution across all hospitals as currently observed and as would be expected if national guidelines were implemented. Until national guidelines are established, hospitals should continue using their own internal guidelines to determine the appropriate reporting of different levels of clinic and emergency department visits.

In the absence of national guidelines, CMS will continue to regularly reevaluate patterns of hospital outpatient visit reporting at varying levels of disaggregation below the national level to ensure that hospitals continue to bill appropriately and differentially for these services. CMS expects hospitals' internal guidelines to comport with these principles (the last five are new for CY 2008):

1. The coding guidelines should follow the intent of the CPT code descriptor in that the guidelines should be designed to reasonably relate the intensity of hospital resources to the different levels of effort represented by the code.
2. The coding guidelines should be based on hospital facility resources. The guidelines should not be based on physician resources.

3. The coding guidelines should be clear to facilitate accurate payments and be usable for compliance purposes and audits.

4. The coding guidelines should meet the HIPAA requirements.

5. The coding guidelines should only require documentation that is clinically necessary for patient care.

6. The coding guidelines should not facilitate upcoding or gaming.

7. The coding guidelines should be written or recorded, well-documented, and provide the basis for selection of a specific code.

8. The coding guidelines should be applied consistently across patients in the clinic or emergency department to which they apply.

9. The coding guidelines should not change with great frequency.

10. The coding guidelines should be readily available for FI (or, if applicable, Medicare Administrative Contractor) review.

11. The coding guidelines should result in coding decisions that could be verified by other hospital staff, as well as outside sources.

CMS provided clarification of some of the principles. The first principle states that coding guidelines should follow the intent of the CPT code descriptor to relate the intensity of resources to different levels of effort represented by the code, not that the hospital's guidelines need to specifically consider the three factors included in the CPT E/M codes for consideration regarding physician visit reporting. Regarding principle 2, hospitals are responsible for reporting the CPT E/M visit code that appropriately represents the resources utilized by the hospital, rather than the resources utilized by the physician. This does not preclude a hospital from using or adapting the physician guidelines if the hospital believes that such guidelines adequately describe hospital resources. Regarding principle 8, a hospital with multiple clinics (for example, primary care, oncology, wound care, and so forth.) may have different coding guidelines for each clinic, but the guidelines must be applied uniformly within each separate clinic. The hospital's assorted sets of internal guidelines must measure resource use in a relative manner, in relation to each other. For example, the hospital resources required for a Level 3 established patient visit under one set of guidelines should be comparable to the resources required for a Level 3 established patient visit under all other sets of clinic visit guidelines used by the hospital. Regarding principle 9, CMS would generally expect hospitals to adjust their guidelines less frequently than every few months and they believe it would be reasonable for hospitals to adjust their guidelines annually, if necessary. Regarding principle 10, hospitals should use their judgment to ensure that coding guidelines are readily available, in an appropriate and reasonable format. CMS would encourage fiscal intermediaries and Medicare Administrative Contractors to review a hospital's internal guidelines when an audit occurs. Regarding principle 11, hospitals should use their judgment to ensure that their coding guidelines can produce results that are reproducible by others.

The final APC payment groups for medical visits are constructed using CPT visit codes only; however, CMS still requires hospitals to provide accurate ICD-9-CM diagnosis coding on claims for payment under the OPPS, even though the ICD-9-CM diagnosis codes are not used in the APC grouping logic.

In developing medical visit APCs based on CPT visit codes only, CMS continues to group APCs based on the OPPS rate-per-service basis. Each APC represents the hospital median cost of the service. APC 0606 represents a mid-level clinic hospital visit (where Level III hospital clinic visits represent the most frequently furnished services) and CMS chose to scale all the hospital clinic relative weights. These collapsed CPT codes define hospital/clinic visits into five groups (0604, 0605, 0606, 0607, 0608). The final APC groups (and codes) for clinic visits are as follows:

APC	HCPCS	APC Description	HCPCS Description	SI	Rel. Wt.	Pay. Rate	Natl. Coin.	Min. Coin.
0604		Level 1 Hospital Clinic Visits		V	0.8388	53.43	—	10.69
	92012		Eye exam, established patient					
	99201		Office/outpatient visit, new					
	99211		Office/outpatient visit, est					
	G0101		CA screen; pelvic/breast examination					
	G0245		Initial foot exam PTLOPS					
	G0379		Direct admit hospital observation					
	G0380		Level 1 hosp type B ED visit					

APC	HCPCS	APC Description	HCPCS Description	SI	Rel. Wt.	Pay. Rate	Natl. Coin.	Min. Coin.
0605		Level 2 Hospital Clinic Visits		V	0.9964	63.46	—	12.69
	92002		Eye exam, new patient					
	92014		Eye exam and treatment					
	99202		Office/outpatient visit, new					
	99212		Office/outpatient visit, est					
	99213		Office/outpatient visit, est					
	99431		Initial care, normal new-born					
	G0246		Follow-up eval of foot PTLOPS					
	G0344		Initial preventive exam					
	G0381		Lev 2 hosp type B ED visit					

APC	HCPCS	APC DDescription	HCPCS Description	SI	Rel. Wt.	Pay. Rate	Natl. Coin.	Min. Coin.
0606		Level 3 Hospital Clinic Visits		V	1.3226	84.24	—	16.85
	92004		Eye exam, new patient					
	99203		Office/outpatient visit, new					
	99214		Office/outpatient visit, est					
	G0382		Lev 3 hosp type B ED visit					

APC	HCPCS	APC Description	HCPCS Description	SI	Rel. Wt.	Pay. Rate	Natl. Coin.	Min. Coin.
0608		Level 5 Hospital Clinic Visits		V	2.1740	138.47	—	27.69
	99205		Office/outpatient visit, new	Q				
	G0175		OPPS Service, sched team conf					
	G0384		Lev 5 hosp type B ED visit					

CMS realizes that although the E/M (992XX) codes assigned to these APCs appropriately represent different levels of physician effort, they do not adequately describe nonphysician resources. In the same way that each CPT code represents a different degree of physician effort, however, the same concept can be applied to each code in terms of differences in resource utilization.

Therefore, under the OPPS, CMS directed each facility to develop a system for mapping the provided services or combination of services furnished to the different levels of effort represented by the codes.

CMS holds each facility accountable for following its own system for assigning the different levels of CPT codes. As long as the services furnished are documented and medically necessary and the facility is following its own system, which reasonably relates the intensity of hospital resources to the different levels of HCPCS codes, CMS assumes that the facility is in compliance with these reporting requirements as they relate to the clinic/emergency department visit code reported on the bill. Thus, CMS would not expect to see a high degree of correlation between the code reported by the physician and that reported by the facility. The code reported by the facility needs to reflect the facility resources.

Exhibit 1.1 (at the end of this chapter) contains the recommendation for standardized hospital E/M coding of clinic services developed by the American Hospital Association (AHA) and the American Health Information Management Association (AHIMA). These recommendations are examples only and are not adopted by CMS.

> **Example:** Using Exhibit 1.1, the following hospital clinic visit would be coded and billed as a low-level hospital clinic visit, which would group to APC 604. The blood pressure measurement for this clinic patient is a form of "bedside diagnostic testing," and the range-of-motion shoulder testing is a form of a "single specialized clinical measurement or assessment."

Source documents and contents: The following documents may contain information about the clinic visit: visit note, clinical notes, progress notes. (See Figure 1.1 for a sample clinic visit note.)

Figure 1.1. Sample clinic visit note

Rheumatology Clinic
NOTE

May 28, 200X

Today, I had the pleasure of seeing Ms. Gill back in the Rheumatology Clinic. I had last seen her last summer when she was visiting the state. At that time, I injected her right shoulder for rotator cuff tendinitis. She said she had good relief until about March. She also had the left shoulder injected about November, and this also was good until about March. In March, she was treated with a short course of oral prednisone which did give some temporary improvement lasting 2–3 weeks, but her shoulder has been bothering her more since. It particularly is bothersome when dressing and sleeping. She is doing range-of-motion exercises but is unable to do strengthening exercises because of their effect on her muscle pain.

Current Medications:
Ascorbic acid
Calcium
Magnesium
Multivitamin
Naproxen
Propranolol
Serevent
Alpha lipoic acid
Flax seed oil

Physical Examination: Blood pressure 110/72, pulse 74

Ms. Gill was a pleasant woman who was in no acute distress. She did have pain with range of motion of the shoulders, particularly on the left; however, the range of motion was full. There was pain with resisted abduction and external rotation.

Impression: Rotator cuff tendinitis

Coding from source documents: Both the visit code mapping logic/criteria used by the hospital and the documented services provided during the clinic visit determine the hospital's receipt of a low-, mid-, or high-level hospital clinic visit APC payment. The hospital clinic visit code must be assigned based on the criteria and the medical records documentation provided.

Scheduled Interdisciplinary Team Conferences

For the OPPS, CMS developed a code for reporting those visits in which numerous physicians see a patient concurrently (for example, a surgeon, a medical oncologist, and a radiation oncologist for a cancer patient) to discuss treatment options and to ensure that the patient is fully informed. In this instance, each physician addresses the patient's care from a unique perspective.

When several physicians see a patient concurrently in the same clinic for the same reason, the hospital reports one clinic visit using an appropriate visit code even though each physician bills individually for his or her professional services.

CMS has established HCPCS Level II code G0175 for hospitals to use in reporting a scheduled medical conference with the patient involving a combination of at least three healthcare professionals, at least one of whom is a physician.

G0175   Scheduled interdisciplinary team conference (minimum of three, exclusive of patient care nursing staff) with patient present.

Under the OPPS, code G0175 is paid under high-level clinic visit APC 608.

Source documents and contents: The following documents may contain information about the clinic visit: visit note, clinical notes, team conference form/note. (See Figure 1.2. for a sample team conference note.)

Figure 1.2.   Sample team conference note

Geriatric Assessment Clinic
Interdisciplinary Team Conference

Patient: _____

Date: _____

Start time: _____
End time: _____
Total time spent in conference: _____ minutes

PATIENT SIGNATURE:

_____

TEAM MEMBERS' SIGNATURES:

_____

_____

_____

_____

_____

_____

TEAM RECOMMENDATION:

_____

_____

_____

_____

_____

_____

_____

_____

Coding from source documents: When reviewing the medical record, the following should be verified before assigning code G0175:

- The conference was a scheduled encounter
- The conference involved at least three healthcare providers, exclusive of patient care nursing staff
- The patient was in fact present during the conference.

APC Payment Groups under Emergency Department Visits

The final APC payment groups for medical visits are constructed using CPT visit codes only; however, CMS still requires hospitals to provide accurate ICD-9-CM diagnosis coding on claims for payment under the OPPS, even though the ICD-9-CM diagnosis codes are not used in the APC grouping logic.

In developing medical visit APCs based on CPT visit codes only, CMS expanded emergency visits into five groups with an additional two groups for critical care. The final APC groups (and codes) for emergency visits are as follows:

APC	HCPCS	APC Description	HCPCS Description	SI	Rel. Wt.	Pay. Rate	Natl. Coin.	Min. Coin.
0609		Level 1 Emergency Visits		V	0.7970	50.76	12.70	10.15
	99281		Emergency dept visit					

APC	HCPCS	APC Description	HCPCS Description	SI	Rel. Wt.	Pay. Rate	Natl. Coin.	Min. Coin.
0613		Level 2 Emergency Visits		V	1.3137	83.67	21.06	16.73
	99282		Emergency dept visit					

APC	HCPCS	APC Description	HCPCS Description	SI	Rel. Wt.	Pay. Rate	Natl. Coin.	Min. Coin.
0614		Level 3 Emergency Visits		V	2.0750	132.17	34.50	26.43
	99283		Emergency dept visit					

APC	HCPCS	APC Description	HCPCS Description	SI	Rel. Wt.	Pay. Rate	Natl. Coin.	Min. Coin.
0615		Level 4 Emergency Visits		Q	3.3377	212.59	48.49	42.52
	99284		Emergency dept visit					

APC	HCPCS	APC Description	HCPCS Description	SI	Rel. Wt.	Pay. Rate	Natl. Coin.	Min. Coin.
0616		Level 5 Emergency Visits		Q	4.9535	315.51	72.86	63.10
	99285		Emergency dept visit					

CMS realizes that although the E/M codes assigned to these APCs appropriately represent different levels of physician effort, they do not adequately describe nonphysician resources. However, in the same way that each CPT code represents a different degree of physician effort, the same concept can be applied to each code in terms of the differences in resource utilization.

Therefore, for the OPPS, CMS directed each facility to develop a system for mapping the provided services or combination of services furnished to the different levels of effort represented by the codes.

CMS holds each facility accountable for following its own system for assigning the different levels of CPT codes. As long as the services furnished are documented and medically necessary and the facility is following its own system, which reasonably relates the intensity of hospital resources to the different levels of HCPCS codes, CMS assumes that the facility is in compliance with these reporting requirements as they relate to the clinic/emergency department visit code reported on the bill. Therefore, CMS would not expect to see a high degree of correlation between the code reported by the physician and that reported by the facility. This is because the physicians must report the E/M codes using the official E/M guidelines that have been approved by the AMA and CMS.

Exhibit 1.2 contains the recommendation for standardized hospital E/M coding of emergency department services developed by the AHA and the AHIMA.

Example: Using Exhibit 1.2, the following hospital emergency department visit example would be coded and billed as a Level 3 Type A Emergency visit, which would group to APC 614. The cardiac monitoring that was performed is a Level 2 (Mid-Level) Intervention.

EMERGENCY ROOM RECORD EXAMPLE

CHIEF COMPLAINT: Heart palpations

PAST MEDICAL HISTORY: Ms. Hart is an 86-year-old female who states she had a very restless night feeling frequent irregularities of her heart. She states she has seen her personal physician, Dr. Polk, with this problem in the past, and he has prescribed metoprolol which she is currently taking at a dose of 25 mg b.i.d. This has not suppressed the activity, and she continues to be quite worried about it. She has no chest pain, no dyspnea, no dizziness, nausea, or diaphoresis.

PHYSICAL ASSESSMENT: Alert and appears in no distress. Skin is warm and dry. Lungs: Clear to auscultation bilaterally. Heart: Mostly regular rate and rhythm, but cardiac monitor shows initially fairly frequent premature atrial contraction. Later in the evaluation after the patient had taken additional dose of metoprolol 25 mg p.o., she was having no sensation of the ectopy, and there was no evidence of ectopy on the cardiac monitor. We note her initial blood pressure was quite elevated, and this also came down to a normotensive range. She has no prior history of hypertension.

TREATMENT PROVIDED: Cardiac monitoring was done. The patient was given metoprolol 25 mg p.o. I advised the patient that I believe she would benefit from increasing the metoprolol to 50 mg p.o. b.i.d., but she should watch for any side effects of significant bradycardia. She should follow up with her personal physician in one to two weeks to reassess this dosage.

I also advised the patient that this rhythm appears to be a low risk rhythm and tried to provide significant reassurance and advised her that the very concern over the rhythm may accentuate the rhythm. She is advised to avoid stimulating drugs, some of which she apparently had been taking in cold remedies, and she is advised to avoid caffeine.

DIAGNOSIS AT DISCHARGE: Cardiac arrhythmia

CONDITION ON DISCHARGE: Satisfactory

Source documents and contents: The following documents may contain information about the emergency department visit: emergency department record/sheet, visit note, clinical notes, triage form.

Coding from source documents: Both the visit code mapping logic/criteria used by the hospital and the documented services provided during the emergency department visit determine the hospital's receipt of a low-, mid-, or high-level emergency department visit APC payment. The emergency department visit code must be assigned based on the criteria and the medical record documentation provided.

Critical Care

CMS uses the CPT codebook definition of critical care, which is the direct delivery by a physician(s) of medical care for a critically ill or critically injured patient. A critical illness or injury acutely impairs one or more vital organ systems such that there is high probability of imminent or life-threatening deterioration in the patient's condition. Critical care involves high-complexity decision making to assess, manipulate, and support vital system function(s) to treat single or multiple vital organ system failure and/or to prevent further life-threatening deterioration of the patient's condition.

Hospitals must use CPT code 99291 to bill for outpatient encounters in which critical care services are furnished. For up to the first 30 minutes of critical care, the highest E/M level is billed 99285. If 30–74 minutes, then 99291, status indicator Q. Each additional 30 minutes is coded with 99292, status indicator "N"; however all codes are reported regardless of payment. Under the OPPS, CMS allows the hospital to use CPT 99291 in place of, but not in addition to, a code for a medical visit or an emergency department service. So it would be inappropriate for the hospital to code both an emergency department visit code, such as 99285, and critical care code 99291 for a single outpatient encounter.

> **99291**   Critical care, evaluation and management of the critically ill or critically injured patient; first 30–74 minutes

Code 99291 groups to significant procedure APC 617 (SI "S").

APC	HCPCS	APC Description	HCPCS Description	SI	Rel. Wt.	Pay. Rate	Natl. Coin.	Min. Coin.
0617		Critical Care		Q	7.3166	466.02	111.59	93.20
	99291		Critical care, first hour					
	99292		Each additional 30 minutes	N				

APC	HCPCS	APC Description	HCPCS Description	SI	Rel. Wt.	Pay. Rate	Natl. Coin.	Min. Coin.
0618		Trauma Response with Critical Care		S	5.1854	330.28	132.11	66.06
	G0390		Trauma response w/hosp critical					

If other services, such as surgery, x-rays or cardiopulmonary resuscitation, are furnished on the same day as the critical care services, CMS allows the hospital to bill for them separately. (See Exhibit 1.3. for CMS recommendations for critical care services.)

Source documents and contents: The following documents may contain information about critical care services: emergency department record/sheet, visit note, clinical notes, triage form.

Coding from source documents: The medical records documentation should be reviewed carefully to verify that the physician(s) documented the time he or she spent providing critical care services. Critical care code 99291 should be assigned only when the physician documents that he or she spent at least thirty minutes providing critical care services.

Limited Follow-Up Services

Examples of limited follow-up services include cast removal, cast replacement, dressing change, wound check, and suture removal.

Packaged services are those that are recognized as contributing to the cost of the services in an APC, but that CMS does not pay for separately. CMS did not include limited follow-up services in the packaged groups under the hospital outpatient PPS because of the difficulty in matching the costs of these services with their associated primary encounter in the CMS database.

CMS did not propose, nor did it include in the April 7, 2000, *Federal Register*, a provision for a global period for hospital outpatient services analogous to the global period affecting payments for professional services made under the Medicare physician fee schedule. As a result, hospitals can bill Medicare for follow-up care services rendered during a patient's postoperative period. For example, hospitals should bill for a patient who is seen in the hospital outpatient setting for suture removal ten days after a wound repair was performed.

For now under the OPPS, hospitals are to bill follow-up care using the appropriate CPT/HCPCS code based on the care rendered.

Source documents and contents: The following documents may contain information about the follow-up visit: emergency department record/sheet, visit note, clinical notes, triage form, operative report/procedure note.

Coding from source documents: The appropriate CPT or HCPCS Level II code should be assigned for the follow-up service documented. When a visit code must be used for the follow-up service, both the visit code mapping logic/criteria used by the hospital and the documented services provided during the visit determine the hospital's receipt of a low-, mid-, or high-level visit APC payment. When applicable, the visit code must be assigned based on the criteria and the medical records documentation provided.

Example: A Medicare outpatient is seen in the emergency department for removal of sutures (status post simple closure of 2-cm neck laceration). The sutures were removed, and the hospital coded the visit as a low-level emergency department visit (99281).

Diagnostic Services and Other Diagnostic Tests

The OPPS contains APC payment groups for numerous diagnostic services and other diagnostic tests including, but not limited to:

Allergen immunotherapy	Dialysis	Interviews
Audiological function tests	Echocardiography	Psychotherapy
Biofeedback	Electrophysiological studies	Pulmonary testing
Blood typing	Fertility procedures	Sleep testing
Cardiac catheterization	Gastric analysis	Vascular studies
Cardiography	Immunization administration for vaccines/toxoids	Neurostimulator analysis programming
Central nervous system assessment/tests	Injections	Psychiatric diagnostic assessment/tests

Example: Below are some of the most commonly performed diagnostic services, some of which are assigned to ancillary service APCs (SI "X"), significant procedure APCs (SI "S"), and surgical service APCs (SI "T").

Code	SI	Abbreviated Code Description
92960	S	Cardioversion electrical, external
93005	S	Electrocardiogram, tracing
93312	S	ECHO transesophageal
93526	T	RT & LT heart catheters
93797	S	Cardiac rehab
93975	S	Vascular study
94010	X	Breathing capacity test
94060	X	Evaluation of wheezing

Source documents and contents: The following documents may contain information about the diagnostic services and other diagnostic tests: emergency department record/sheet, visit note, clinical notes, triage form, operative report/procedure note, respiratory therapy note/sheet, cardiac catheterization report.

Coding from source documents: The medical record should be reviewed carefully because the complexity of the diagnostic test or service sometimes generates a higher-paying APC or multiple APC payments.

Example: The following diagnostic case would be coded as 94010 (Spirometry, including graphic record, total and timed vital capacity, expiratory flow rate measurement[s], with or without maximal voluntary ventilation) and assigned to an ancillary services (SI "X") APC group: A 65-year-old man is evaluated for increasing shortness of breath with exertion. He has a history of coronary heart disease and has been a cigarette smoker for 50 years. A spirogram is obtained to determine whether he has significant pulmonary dysfunction and to further separate this into predominantly restrictive or obstructive disease.

Example: The reports in Figure 1.3 describe an initial and a repeat chest x-ray performed on the same outpatient on the same date of service. These reports would be coded as 71010 and 71010–76, which are assigned to an ancillary service APC 0260 (SI "X").

Figure 1.3.   Radiology reports

RADIOLOGY—RETRIEVE X-RAY EXAM REPORT
Exam: PORT CHEST—AP/PA
Completed: 7/13/200X

FINAL REPORT

Exam #38613 chest 7/13/200X   8:00 AM

History: Rule out infiltrates

Findings: Portable supine chest from July 13, 200X, without comparisons

Impression: NG tube is coiled within the stomach. Normal cardiomediastinal silhouette. Mild left lower lobe atelectasis. Diffuse haziness of the right lung is due to rotation versus layering effusion. Left upper lobe is clear. Pulmonary vasculature is normal. No soft tissue abnormalities seen.

Exam: PORT CHEST—AP/PA 07/13/20XX

FINAL REPORT

7/13/200X   3:00 PM
History: Evaluate lung volumes and pleural effusion

Findings: Portable supine AP chest compared to film from earlier the same day. The patient is markedly rotated. There is a persistent left pleural effusion. The lungs are clear except for several areas of minimal subsegmental atelectasis. Lines and tubes project in stable position. Lung volumes are stable.

Impression: No interval change.

Surgical Pathology

The OPPS contains APC payment groups for surgical pathology services, including but not limited to, surgical pathology gross examination, surgical pathology microscopic examination, decalcification, special stains, determinative histochemistry, determinative cytochemistry, pathology consultations, immunocytochemistry, electron microscopy, and protein analysis of tissue.

Example: Here are some of the most commonly performed surgical pathology services:

Code	SI	Abbreviated Code Description
85097	X	Bone marrow interpretation
88300	X	Surgical path, gross
88302	X	Tissue exam by pathologist
88312	X	Special stains
88329	X	Path consult intraoperative
88358	X	Analysis, tumor

Example: The report in Figure1.4 describes fine needle aspiration of the pancreas. This report would be coded as 88173, which is assigned to an ancillary service APC 0343 (SI "X").

Code	SI	Abbreviated Code Description
88173	X	Cytopathology evaluation, FNA, report

Source documents and contents: The following documents may contain information about the surgical pathology services rendered: pathology report, cytology report, fine needle aspiration (FNA) reports, operative report/procedure note. (See Figure 1.4 for an FNA report.)

Figure 1.4.   Sample FNA report

Fine Needle Aspiration Report

SPECIMEN(S): 1 fine needle aspiration, pancreas

SPECIMEN ADEQUACY: Satisfactory for evaluation, but limited by low cellularity

CYTOLOGIC EXAMINATION: Negative for malignancy

CELL BLOCK FINDINGS: The cell block material is noncontributory.

COMMENTS: Recommend further evaluation. A few mucinous appearing cells are present. Further studies are advised if clinically warranted.

ADEQUACY ASSESSMENT: This aspirate was performed by the radiologist/clinician. Pass 1 inadequate for assessment.

CLINICAL HISTORY: Pancreatic mass

Coding from source documents: The medical record should be reviewed carefully because the complexity of the surgical pathology services sometimes generates a higher-paying APC or multiple APC payments.

Cancer Chemotherapy

Under the OPPS, there are two components to the APC payment for chemotherapy: one for the route of administration of the drug, and another for each chemotherapy drug.

The OPPS contains significant procedure APC (SI "S") payment groups for chemotherapy administration.

Code	SI	Abbreviated Code Description
96409	S	Chemotherapy, push technique
96413	S	Chemotherapy, infusion method

The chemotherapy drugs are paid under different APC groups based on the specific drug code that is reported and billed. Examples of chemotherapy drugs paid under the OPPS include:

Code	SI	Abbreviated Code Description
J9045	K	Carboplatin injection
J0150	K	Adenosine 6 MG injection
J1190	K	Dexrazoxane HCl injection
J9213	K	Interferon alfa-2a injection
J9265	K	Paclitaxel injection
J9280	K	Mitomycin 5 MG injection
J9340	K	Thiotepa injection

Source documents and contents: The following documents may contain information about the chemotherapy services rendered: operative report/procedure note, oncology note/record, physician's orders, medication sheet/record.

Coding from source documents: The medical record should be reviewed carefully because:

- The use of an infusion technique and another technique to administer the chemotherapy drug(s) sometimes generates the higher-paying APC.
- The administration of multiple drugs and/or specific drug dosage amounts sometimes generates multiple APC payments.

Cancer Hospitals That Are Excluded from IPPS

Although cancer hospitals that provide inpatient care to Medicare beneficiaries are not reimbursed under the IPPS, these same hospitals are reimbursed under the OPPS. Under the OPPS, services typically provided by cancer hospitals to Medicare beneficiaries include, but are not limited to, chemotherapy administration, infusion therapy, radiation therapy, clinical brachytherapy, vascular access device insertion/repair/replacement/removal, arteriovenous fistula-shunt creation/revision/repair, chemosurgery, malignant lesion excision/destruction/ablation, and lymph node biopsies/staging/excisions.

Services for Patients Who Have Exhausted Their Part A Benefits

Medicare payment under the hospital outpatient PPS is provided for certain services furnished to inpatients who have exhausted Part A benefits or otherwise are not in a covered Part A stay. Examples of services covered under this provision include diagnostic x-rays and certain other diagnostic services and radiation therapy covered under the SSA.

Distinct Parts of Hospitals That Are Excluded under IPPS

Distinct parts of hospitals that are excluded under the IPPS are included in the OPPS to the extent that outpatient services are furnished by the hospital. Examples of distinct parts of hospitals that are included under the OPPS are inpatient psychiatric units and inpatient rehabilitation units. For example, a hospital with an excluded inpatient psychiatric unit will have payment made under the OPPS for outpatient psychiatric services, including services provided to inpatients who are not in a covered Medicare Part A stay.

Services Furnished to SNF Inpatients That Are Not Packaged into SNF Consolidated Billing

The OPPS includes specific hospital outpatient services furnished to a beneficiary admitted to a Medicare-participating SNF who is not considered an SNF resident (for purposes of SNF consolidated billing with respect to those services that are beyond the scope of SNF comprehensive care plans).

The specific hospital outpatient services that are excluded from SNF consolidated billing are cardiac catheterization, computerized tomography (CT) scans, magnetic resonance imaging (MRI) scans, ambulatory surgery involving use of an operating room, emergency room services, radiation therapy, angiography, and lymphatic and venous procedures. In general, these are services that are commonly furnished by hospital outpatient departments and that SNFs would be unable to provide.

Certain Preventive Services Furnished to Healthy Persons

The OPPS includes certain preventive services that are furnished to healthy patients. The status indicators for the screening services vary from medical visits ("V"), significant procedures ("S"), and surgical services ("T").

Code	SI	Abbreviated Code Description
G0101	V	CA screen; pelvic/breast exam
G0104	S	CA screen; flexi sigmoidscope
G0105	T	Colorectal scrn; hi risk ind
G0106	S	Colon CA screen; barium enema
G0117	S	Glaucoma scrn hgh risk direc
G0118	S	Glaucoma scrn hgh risk direc
G0120	S	Colon ca scrn; barium enema
G0121	T	Colon ca scrn not hi rsk ind

Source documents and contents: The following documents may contain information about the preventive services rendered: operative report/procedure note, physician's orders, referral form, progress notes.

Coding from source documents: The medical record should be reviewed carefully because CMS has specific documentation requirements to justify the medical necessity of the screening services.

Example: Screening colonoscopies are covered for people at high risk for colorectal cancer once every 24 months. High-risk individuals are those people who have a close relative who has had colorectal cancer or an adenomatous polyp; a family history of adenomatous polyposis or hereditary nonpolyposis colorectal cancer; a personal history of adenomatous polyps or colorectal cancer; inflammatory bowel disease, including Crohn's disease; and/or ulcerative colitis.

The following operative report excerpts are excellent examples of documentation that supports the coding and billing of code G0105, colorectal cancer screening; colonoscopy on individual at high risk:

Case 1: "She is a high-risk patient with a family history of colon cancer, and breast cancer in herself."

Case 2: "Preoperative Diagnosis: Personal history of polyps; family history of colon cancer."

Case 3: "Preoperative Diagnosis: Family history of colon cancer in a first-degree relative, screening examination."

Antigens, Vaccines, Splints, and Casts

The Balanced Budget Act of 1997 (BBA) authorized CMS to implement a Medicare PPS for the following services, and, effective August 1, 2000, CMS implemented the OPPS for these services:

- Vaccines, splints, casts, and antigens provided by home health agencies (HHAs) that provide medical and other health services
- Vaccines provided by comprehensive outpatient rehabilitation facilities (CORFs)
- Splints, casts, and antigens provided to hospice patients for treatment of a nonterminal illness

HHAs, CORFs, and hospices are required to report the following codes (when applicable) to ensure that they are paid under the OPPS:

- Antigens: 95144–95149, 95165, 95170, 95180 and 95199

- Hepatitis B Vaccines: G0010, 90740, 90743, 90744, 90746, 90747

- Splints: 29105–29131, 29505, 29515

- Casts: 29000–29086, 29305, 29325–29445, 29450, 29700–29750, 29799

Partial Hospitalization for the Mentally Ill

A partial hospitalization program (PHP) is a distinct and organized intensive psychiatric outpatient day-treatment program designed to provide patients with profound and disabling mental health conditions with an individualized, coordinated, comprehensive, and multidisciplinary treatment program.

Patients eligible for the Medicare partial hospitalization benefit comprise two groups:

- Patients who have been discharged from a psychiatric hospital for whom partial hospitalization services are provided in lieu of continued inpatient treatment

- Patients who exhibit disabling psychiatric/psychological symptoms as a result of an acute exacerbation of a severe and persistent mental illness for whom the partial hospitalization services are provided in lieu of admission to an inpatient psychiatric hospital

The OPPS includes partial hospitalization services provided by a hospital to its outpatients or by a Medicare-certified community mental health center (CMHC). Partial hospitalization APC group 033 contains two HCPCS Level II codes that are assigned to status indicator "P."

APC	HCPCS	APC Description	HCPCS Description	SI	Rel. Wt.	Pay. Rate	Natl. Coin.	Min. Coin.
0033		Partial Hospitalization		P	—	—	—	—
	G0129		Partial hosp prog service					
	G0176		OPPS/PHP activity therapy					

The APC group 0033 payment for partial hospitalization services represents the facility's costs for overhead, support staff, and the services of clinical social workers (CSWs) and occupational therapists (OTs), whose professional services are considered to be partial hospitalization services for which payment is made to the facility.

Source documents and contents: The following documents may contain information about the PHP services rendered: intake assessment form, treatment plan, psychiatric progress note, certification statement, recertification statement.

As required by the SSA, admission to a partial hospitalization program is limited to patients whose physicians certify that:

- The individual would require inpatient psychiatric care in the absence of partial hospitalization services.

- An individualized, written plan of care has been established by a physician and is reviewed periodically by a physician.

- The patient is or was under the care of a physician.

This certification would be made when the physician believes that the course of the patient's current episode of illness would result in psychiatric hospitalization if the partial hospitalization services were not substituted.

The PHP must receive, upon admission, the initial physician certification that establishes the need for partial hospitalization. The first recertification is required as of the eighteenth day of services, and subsequent recertifications are required no less frequently than every 30 days.

Each recertification must address:

- The patient's response to the intensive therapy

- Therapeutic interventions provided by the active treatment program that make up partial hospitalization services

- Changes in functioning and status of the serious psychiatric symptoms that place the patient at risk of hospitalization

- Treatment plan and goals for coordination of services, such as community supports and less-intensive treatment options to facilitate discharge from the PHP

Coding from source documents: The medical record should be reviewed carefully because CMS has specific coding and billing requirements to justify the medical necessity of the PHP services.

Under the OPPS, the PHP claim must include a mental health ICD-9-CM diagnosis code and at least three partial hospitalization HCPCS codes for each day of service, one of which must be a psychotherapy HCPCS code. Below are CMS-approved partial hospitalization codes:

Description	HCPCS Code
Occupational therapy (partial hospitalization)	G0129
Activity therapy (partial hospitalization)	G0176
Education training (partial hospitalization)	G0177
Psychiatric general services	90801, 90802, 90875, 90876, 90899*
Individual psychotherapy	90816*, 90817*, 90818, 90819, 90821, 90822, 90823*, 90824*, 90826, 90827, 90828, 90829
Group psychotherapy	90849, 90853, 90857
Family psychotherapy	90846, 90847, 90849
Psychiatric testing	96101, 96116, 96118

* Brief psychotherapy codes that group to APC 0322

Inpatient Procedures for Patients Who Expire

The Medicare inpatient-only list specifies those services that are only paid when provided in an inpatient setting. On rare occasions, a procedure on this list must be performed to resuscitate or stabilize a patient with an emergent, life-threatening condition whose status is that of an outpatient and who dies before being admitted as an inpatient. For those rare and unusual cases, the surgical service APC payment group 0375 (Ancillary outpatient services when patient expires) is used to reimburse the hospital. (Note: If the patient has the inpatient procedure performed and is admitted as an inpatient, the hospital is paid under the IPPS.)

To be paid under APC 0375, hospitals must submit an outpatient claim for all services furnished, including the inpatient procedure code with modifier –CA appended.

CA	Procedure payable only in the inpatient setting when performed emergently on an outpatient who dies before admission

CMS believes that such patients would typically receive services such as those provided during a high-level emergency visit, appropriate diagnostic testing (x-ray, CT scan, EKG, and so on), and administration of intravenous fluids and medication prior to the surgical procedure. Because these combined services constitute an episode of care, separate payment is not allowed for other services furnished on the same date. This approach allows hospitals to submit an outpatient claim and receive payment; however, the payment is solely under APC 0375.

> **Example:** A patient seen in the emergency department has an intra-aortic assist device inserted percutaneously. After the procedure is performed, and before the patient can be admitted to an inpatient unit, the patient expires. The CPT code for the procedure, 33967, is assigned to an inpatient procedure status indicator "C." When the hospital submits the claim, modifier –CA must be appended to code 33967 for the hospital to receive the OPPS payment under APC 0375.

Code	SI	Abbreviated Code Description
33967	C	Insert intra-aortic percutaneous device

Source documents and contents: The following documents may contain information about the inpatient procedures performed on patients who expire: emergency department note/form, operative report, procedure note.

CMS requires that the patient's medical record contain all of the following information:

- Documentation that the reported HCPCS code for the surgical procedure with OPPS payment status indicator "C" (such as CPT code 33967) was actually performed

- Documentation that the reported surgical procedure with status indicator "C" was medically necessary

> **Examples:** A procedure assigned to inpatient procedure status indicator "C" under the OPPS is performed to resuscitate or stabilize a beneficiary who appears with or suddenly develops a life-threatening condition that is thoroughly documented in the medical record. The patient dies during surgery or postoperatively before being admitted.
>
> An elective or emergent surgical procedure payable under the OPPS is being performed. Because of sudden, unexpected intra-operative complications (which are thoroughly documented), the physician must alter the surgical procedure and perform a procedure with OPPS status indicator "C." The patient dies during the operation before he or she is admitted as an inpatient.

Coding from source documents: The medical record should be reviewed carefully because CMS has very specific coding and billing guidelines for inpatient procedures performed on patients who expire. These guidelines include the following:

- Procedure codes with status indicator "C" to which modifier –CA is not appended and that are submitted on an outpatient bill receive a line item denial, and no other services furnished on the same date are payable.

- When an outpatient undergoes a procedure that is on the inpatient list, and the patient subsequently is admitted to an observation bed, the procedure with status indicator "C submitted on an outpatient bill receives a line item denial. In such cases, no other services furnished on the same date are payable.

- If a pass-through drug or device is given a patient during the same encounter when a procedure billed with modifier –CA is performed, CMS wants the hospital to include these services on the claim that is submitted for the encounter. Although CMS would not pay separately for the pass-through items, it would use the data for future updates of the OPPS.

Observation Services

Observation services refers to the practice of placing a patient in a hospital area or room to be monitored while determining whether he or she needs to be admitted, have further outpatient treatment, or be discharged.

After 1983, many hospitals began to rely heavily on the use of observation services when quality improvement organizations (QIOs) (formerly called peer review organizations, or PROs) questioned admissions under the hospital IPPS. In some cases, however, patients were kept in "outpatient" observation for days or even weeks at a time. This resulted in excess payments from both the Medicare program and beneficiaries who generally paid a higher coinsurance. In recent years, the distinction between inpatient and outpatient care has been blurred by the retention of outpatients in the hospital overnight, sometimes for many days in a row. Medicare paid for observation services while the hospital determined whether an outpatient needed admission for further treatment. Frequently, patients did not understand that they were not inpatients until they were billed for 20 percent of outpatient charges as copayment.

In response to this practice, in November 1996, CMS issued instructions limiting covered observation services to no more than 48 hours except in the most extreme circumstances. CMS made it clear at that time that observation was not a means to make it possible to perform inpatient surgery on an outpatient basis; nor was it appropriate to retain chemotherapy patients in long-term observation.

Because observation is not provided as the sole service a patient receives, CMS packaged costs associated with observation into the median costs for the services (for example, surgery or chemotherapy) with which they were furnished under the OPPS.

Routinely billing an observation stay for patients recovering from outpatient surgery is not allowed under the hospital outpatient PPS, and there needs to be clear understanding of the definition of routine recovery and when a patient requires observation care. A diagnosis or condition should be documented to denote the change in the patient's status.

Observation services have been packaged and payment will be provided through a composite APC methodology when certain criteria apply. These composite APCs are for extended assessment and management, of which observation care is a component. The Outpatient Code Editor (OCE) will determine the payment for observation as packaged into a composite APC payment or packaged into payment for other separately payable services provided in the encounter. HCPCS code G0378, Hospital observation services, per hour, has been assigned a status indicator "N," meaning that its payment will always be packaged, either into one of the two composite APCs or, when the composite criteria are not met, into the payment for the major services on the claim. A qualifying diagnosis is no longer required, but, for the purpose of composite APC payment, all other criteria required in CY 2007 for separate observation care payment has been retained, including: a minimum number of 8 hours; a qualifying visit, direct admission to observation care, or critical care; and no "T" status procedure reported on the day before or day of observation services. The general reporting requirements for observation services have also been retained. These are the requirements related to the physician order and evaluation, documentation, and observation beginning and ending times.

Direct Admission to Observation

Payment for direct admission to observation will be made either under composite APC 8002 (Level I Prolonged Assessment and Management Composite) or under APC 0604 (Level 1 Hospital Clinic Visits). The composite APC will apply, regardless of the patient's particular clinical condition, if the hours of observation services (HCPCS code G0378) are greater than or equal to eight and billed on the same day as HCPCS code G0378, and there is not a "T" status procedure on the same date or day before the date of HCPCS code G0378. If the composite APC is not applicable, payment for HCPCS code G0379, Direct admission of patient for hospital observation care, may be made under APC 0604. In general, this would occur when the units of observation reported under HCPCS code G0378 are less than eight and no services with a status indicator "T" or "V" or Critical Care (APC 0617) were provided on the same day of service as HCPCS code G0379. The criteria for payment of HCPCS code G0379 under APC 0604 will be the same as in CY 2007. In cases where the criteria for payment under either APC are not met, HCPCS code G0379 is assigned status indicator "N."

Source documents and contents: The following documents may contain information about the observation services rendered: emergency department record, physician's orders, progress notes, nursing notes, diagnostic and therapeutic test results.

To bill for observation services, CMS requires meeting the following documentation criteria:

- Observation time begins at the clock time documented in the patient's medical record, which coincides with the time the patient is placed in a bed for the purpose of initiating observation care in accordance with a physician's order.

- The ending time for observation occurs either when the patient is discharged from the hospital or is admitted as an inpatient. The time when a patient is "discharged" from observation status is the clock time when all clinical or medical interventions have been completed, including any necessary follow-up care furnished by hospital staff and physicians that may take place after a physician has ordered that the patient be released or admitted as an inpatient. However, observation care does not include time spent by the patient in the hospital subsequent to the conclusion of therapeutic, clinical, or medical interventions, such as time spent waiting for transportation to go home.

- The beneficiary is under the care of a physician during the period of observation as documented in the medical record by admission, discharge, and other appropriate progress notes that are timed, written, and signed by the physician.

- The medical record includes documentation that the physician used risk stratification criteria to determine that the beneficiary would benefit from observation care. (These criteria may be published generally accepted medical standards or established hospital-specific standards.) Note: The manner in which documentation of risk stratification is made is at the discretion of the physician.

- Observation care is billed hourly for a minimum of eight hours up to a maximum of 48 hours. CMS would not pay separately for any hours a beneficiary spends in observation over 24 hours, but all costs beyond 24 hours would be packaged into the APC payment for observation services. Note: Observation services should be charged by the hour. If the number of hours is less than eight, payment is packaged into the associated clinic or emergency visit. If more than 24 hours of observation are billed, payment for any time over 24 hours is packaged into the payment for 8 to 24 hours of observation.

Table 1.3.   **Diagnosis codes required for observation services (APC 0339)**

For Chest Pain

411.1	Intermediate coronary syndrome
411.81	Coronary occlusion without myocardial infarction
411.0	Postmyocardial infarction syndrome
411.89	Other acute ischemic heart disease
413.0	Angina decubitus
413.1	Prinzmetal angina
413.9	Other and unspecified angina pectoris
786.05	Shortness of breath
786.50	Chest pain, unspecified
786.51	Precordial pain
786.52	Painful respiration
786.59	Other chest pain

For Asthma

493.01	Extrinsic asthma with status asthmaticus
493.02	Extrinsic asthma with acute exacerbation
493.11	Intrinsic asthma with status asthmaticus
493.12	Intrinsic asthma with acute exacerbation
493.21	Chronic obstructive asthma with status asthmaticus
493.22	Chronic obstructive asthma with acute exacerbation
493.91	Asthma, unspecified with status asthmaticus
493.92	Asthma, unspecified with acute exacerbation

For Heart Failure

391.8	Other acute rheumatic heart disease
398.91	Rheumatic heart failure (congestive)
402.01	Malignant hypertensive heart disease with heart failure
402.11	Benign hypertensive heart disease with heart failure
402.91	Unspecified hypertensive heart disease with heart failure
404.01	Malignant hypertensive heart and renal disease with heart failure
404.03	Malignant hypertensive heart and renal disease with heart and renal failure
404.11	Benign hypertensive heart and renal disease with heart failure
404.13	Benign hypertensive heart and renal disease with heart and renal failure
404.91	Unspecified hypertensive heart and renal disease with heart failure
404.93	Unspecified hypertensive heart and renal disease with heart and renal failure
428.0	Congestive heart failure, unspecified
428.1	Left heart failure
428.20	Unspecified systolic heart failure
428.21	Acute systolic heart failure
428.22	Chronic systolic heart failure
428.23	Acute on chronic systolic heart failure
428.30	Unspecified diastolic heart failure
428.31	Acute diastolic heart failure
428.32	Chronic diastolic heart failure
428.33	Acute on chronic diastolic heart failure
428.40	Unspecified combined systolic and diastolic heart failure
428.41	Acute combined systolic and diastolic heart failure
428.42	Chronic combined systolic and diastolic heart failure
428.43	Acute on chronic combined systolic and diastolic heart failure
428.9	Heart failure, unspecified

Composite APC Assignment Logic

The composite APCs are assigned according to precise rules as presented here and in Exhibit 1.4. Different criteria are used for Level I and Level II Extended Assessment and Management composite APCs. APC G0379 (Separate Direct Admit) has its own processing logic.

Extended Assessment and Management Composite APC Rules:

a) If the criteria for the composite APC are met, the composite APC and its associated SI are assigned to the prime code (visit or critical care).

b) Only one extended assessment and management APC is assigned per claim.

c) If the criteria are met for a level I and a level II extended assessment and management APC, assignment of the level II composite takes precedence.

d) If multiple qualifying prime codes (visit or CC) appear on the day of or day before G0378, assign the composite APC to the prime code with the highest separately paid payment rate; assign the standard APC to any/all other visit codes present.

e) Visits not paid under an extended assessment and management composite are paid separately.

> **Exception:** Code G0379 is always packaged if there is an extended assessment and management APC on the claim.

f) The SI for G0378 is always N.

g) Level I and II extended assessment and management composite APCs have SI = V if paid.

h) The logic for extended assessment and management is performed only for bill type 13x, with or without condition code 41.

i) Hours/units of service for observation (G0378) must be at least 8 or the composite APC is not assigned.

j) If a "T" procedure occurs on the day of or day before observation, the composite APC is not assigned.

k) Assign units of service = 1 to the line with the composite APC.

l) Assign the composite payment adjustment flag to the visit line with the composite APC and to the G0378.

m) If the composite APC assignment criteria are not met, apply regular APC logic for separately paid items, special logic for G0379, and the SI for G0378 = N.

Level II Extended Assessment and Management Criteria:

a) If there is at least one of a specified list of critical care or emergency room visit codes on the day of or day before observation (G0378), assign the composite APC and related SI to the critical care or emergency visit code.

b) Additional emergency or critical care visit codes (whether or not on the prime list) are assigned to their standard APCs for separately paid items.

Prime/List A Codes	Nonprime/List B Code	Composite APC
99284, 99285, 99291	G0378	8003

Level I Extended Assessment and Management Criteria:

a) If there is at least one of a specified list of prime clinic visit codes on the day of or day before observation (G0378), or code G0379 is present on the same day as G0378, assign the composite APC and related status indicator to the clinic visit or direct admission code.

b) Additional clinic visit codes (whether or not on the prime list) are assigned to their standard APCs for separately paid items.

c) Additional G0379, on the same claim, are assigned SI = N.

Prime/List A Codes	Nonprime/List B code	Composite APC
99205, 99215	G0379, G0378	8002

Separate Direct Admit (G0379) Processing Logic:

a) Code G0378 must be present on the same day

b) No SI = T, E/M, or C/C visit on the same day

c) Code G0379 may be paid under the composite 8002, paid under APC 604, or packaged with SI = N.

ASC Payment Groups versus APC Payment Groups

An ambulatory surgery center (ASC) is a provider whose sole purpose is to furnish services in connection with surgical procedures that do not require inpatient hospitalization. An ASC is either independent, or freestanding (not a part of a provider of services or any other facility), or operated by a hospital (under the common ownership, licensure, or control of a hospital).

Generally, there are two primary elements in the total cost of performing a surgical procedure:

- The cost of the physician's professional services for performing the procedure
- The cost of services furnished by the facility where the procedure is performed (for example, surgical supplies and equipment, and nursing services)

However, the ASC's reimbursement—by Medicare—for the costs of services furnished by the facility (that is, facility costs) is limited to surgical procedures designated by the HHS as appropriately performed on an inpatient basis in a hospital, but which also can be performed safely on an ambulatory basis in an ASC. The law ties coverage of ASC services under Part B to specified surgical procedures that are contained in a list developed and periodically revised by the HHS, that is, the ASC list. Medicare will not reimburse ASCs for facility costs associated with procedures not included on the ASC list.

Medicare still uses the ASC payment groups to reimburse ASCs for their facility costs, but it no longer uses them to reimburse hospitals.

Payment Methodology CY 2008

The Medicare Prescription Drug, Improvement, and Modernization Act of 2003 (MMA) required CMS to revise the ASC payment system no later than January 1, 2008.

The revised ASC payment system is based on the hospital OPPS. The standard ASC payment for most ASC-covered surgical procedures is calculated by multiplying the ASC conversion factor ($41.401 for CY 2008) by the ASC relative payment weight (based on the OPPS relative payment weight) for each separately payable procedure. Per the MMA, contractors will pay ASCs based on the lesser of the actual charge or the standard ASC payment rate. Payment rates for surgical procedures that are commonly performed in physicians' offices and for the technical component of covered ancillary radiology procedures cannot exceed the Medicare physician fee schedule (MPFS) nonfacility practice expense (PE) amount. Payment policies for drugs and biologicals and other covered ancillary services mirror the OPPS as well.

The complete lists of ASC-covered surgical procedures and ASC-covered ancillary services, the applicable payment indicators, payment rates for each covered surgical procedure and ancillary service before adjustment for regional wage variations, the wage- adjusted payment rates, and wage indices are available on the CMS Web site (www.cms.hhs.gov/ascpayment). See also instructions in the Medicare Claims Processing Manual, Chapter 14, Sections 30 and 40.

ASCs experience greater efficiencies in furnishing surgical services than hospital outpatient departments, resulting in surgical procedures being less costly when performed in that setting of care. In the CY 2008 OPPS/ASC final rule, CMS estimates that ASCs should be paid about 65 percent of the OPPS payment rates for the same surgical procedures.

When the ASC performs multiple surgical procedures in the same operative session that are subject to the multiple procedure discount, contractors pay 100 percent of the highest paying surgical procedures on the claim, plus 50 percent of the applicable wage-adjusted payment rate(s) for the other ASC-covered surgical procedures, subject to the multiple procedure discount furnished in the same session. In determining the ranking of procedures for application of the multiple procedure reduction, contractors shall use the lower of the billed charge or the ASC payment amount. The multiple procedure reduction is the last pricing routine applied to applicable ASC procedure codes.

ASC surgical procedures billed with modifier –73 or –52 shall not be subjected to further pricing reductions (that is, the multiple-procedure price reduction rules will not apply). The OPPS/ASC final rule for the relevant payment year specifies whether or not a surgical procedure is subject to multiple-procedure discounting for that year.

Addendum AA of the CY 2008 OPPS/ASC final rule, available at www.cms.hhs.gov/ASCPayment/04f_CMS-1392-FC(ASC).asp, indicates whether or not a surgical procedure is subject to multiple-procedure discounting for CY 2008. For more information, see the Medicare Claims Processing Manual, Chapter 14, Section 40.5.

Due to the significant changes in payment under the revised ASC payment system, CMS is providing a four-year transition to the fully implemented revised ASC rates. Accordingly, CY 2008 payment for surgical procedures on the CY 2007 list of covered surgical procedures will be made based on a blend of 75 percent of the CY 2007 rate and 25 percent of the revised ASC rate. For CY 2009, the blend will be 50/50, and for CY 2010, the blend will be made up of 25 percent of the CY 2007 rate and 75 percent of the revised ASC rate. The revised ASC rates will be fully implemented in CY 2011. Payment for covered surgical procedures added for ASC payment in CY 2008 or later and payment for covered ancillary services that are not paid separately under the existing ASC payment system will not be subject to a transition.

Exhibit 1.1. Recommendation for standardized hospital E/M coding of clinic services

Note: This is a sample model developed from prior fiscal years before E/M was expanded to 5 levels. The Hospital Evaluation and Management Coding Panel has sent recommendations to the Centers for Medicare & Medicaid Services for a standard Evaluation and Management coding model. The model would be designed to give objective and consistent industry-wide criteria for coding of emergency department, critical care, and clinic services.

Clinic visit: A patient who presents to the hospital clinic for services is registered and receives one or more of the clinical interventions listed here.

Level 1 (Low-Level) Interventions

At least one item below qualifies for low-level. Additional explanations, examples, and classifications appear in italics. The items listed here are performed by hospital staff, rather than by a physician.

Bedside diagnostic testing, unless tests are separately billed	*Examples: Dipstick urine testing, capillary blood sugar (Accu-Check, Dextrostick), Hemoccult, occult blood tests (Strep test is not included because it is separately billable.)*
Blood pressure recheck	
Clinical staff assessment (excluding physician)	*Example: Vitals, or chief complaint, or clinical assessment of symptom*
Flushing of Heplock	
Patient registration, room setup, patient use of room, room cleaning—covered by a separately billable procedure	
Routine simple discharge instructions	
Single specialized clinical measurement or assessment	*Example: Fetal heart tones, positional blood pressure readings, Snellan exam, and cardiac monitor rhythm strip performed by nurse*
Specimen collection(s), where nurse provides patient with instructions and patient self-collects, other than venipuncture (for example, midstream urine samples)	*Example: Nursing instruction of patient on proper specimen collection (for example, midstream urine, sputum); includes collection of specimen (not the performance of the lab test)*
Suture or staple removal	
Tuberculosis test check	
Wound care management (when not separately billable), not repaired—up to 25 sq cm	*Includes cleansing, assessment, measurement, photographing, ankle brachial index, and/or dressing of wound; includes Steri-Strips and other adhesives, eye patch, butterflies. (For multiple wounds, add the total size of all wounds.)*

Exhibit 1.1. (Continued)

Level 2 (Mid-Level) Interventions	
At least one item below qualifies for mid-level. Additional explanations, examples, and clarifications appear in italics. The items listed here are performed by hospital staff, rather than physician.	
Administration of oral, topical, rectal, PR, NG, or SL medication(s)	
Administration of single disposable enema	
Application of preformed splint(s)/elastic bandages/ sling(s), or immobilizer for nonfracture of nondisloca- tion injuries, when not separately billable as a procedure	*Preformed are off-the-shelf. If creating a splint from plas- ter or fiberglass or other material (custom-made splint), would have separate code. Splints are not billed sepa- rately. Splints, casting, and so on for fractures are sepa- rately billable and paid under the fracture management.*
Assist physician with examination	*Pelvic exam included here. Includes eye exam/slit lamp exam of eye. Nursing documentation must support assis- tance unless there is a hospital protocol regarding assis- tance with exam.*
Blood draw(s) through specialized vascular access device	
Care of device(s) or catheter(s) (both indwelling and in and out) (vascular and nonvascular) and/or ostomy device(s)—other than insertion or reinsertion	*Examples: Irrigation, assessment, flushing, adjustment, positioning, changing of bags, checking; examples of cath- eters/devices: Foley, ileal conduit, gastrostomy, ileostomy, colostomy, nephrostomy, tracheostomy, PEG tube, central lines, arterial lines, PICC lines*
First-aid procedures	*Examples: Control bleeding, ice, monitor vital signs, cool body, remove stinger from insect bite, cleanse and remove secretions*
Foreign body(ies) removal of skin, subcutaneous or soft tissue without anesthesia or incision, when not a sepa- rately billable procedure	
Frequent monitoring/assessment as evidenced by two sets of vital signs or assessments (including initial set), integral to current interventions and/or patient's condition	*Examples: Additional vital sign; assessment of cardiovas- cular, pulmonary, or neurological status; assessment of pain scale, pulse oxymetry, or peak flow measurement*
Oxygen administration—initiation and/or adjustment from baseline oxygen regimen	*Includes conversion to hospital-supplied oxygen with rate adjustments, as well as initiation of oxygen administration*
Specimen collection(s) other than venipuncture, per- formed by nursing staff (for example, cultures)	*Collection of specimen (not the performance of the lab test) (for example, throat culture collection)*
Wound care management when not separately billable, 26–50 sq cm	*Includes cleansing, assessment, measurement, photo- graphing, ankle brachial index, and/or dressing of wound; includes Steri-Strips and other adhesives, eye patch, butterflies (For multiple wounds, add the total size of all wounds.)*

(Continued on next page)

Exhibit 1.1. (Continued)

Contributory Factors for Clinic E/M Mode from Low-Level to Mid-Level or from Mid-Level to High-Level *Contributory factors* are services or other factors that, when present, may increase the E/M level from mid- to high-level. Only one factor is required. These factors apply only to the low-level and the mid-level. A high-level E/M may not be increased to critical care by a contributory factor. Additional explanations, examples, and clarifications appear in italics.	
Airway insertion (nasal, oral)	
Altered mental status	
Arrangements and/or social service intervention (includes required reporting)	*Examples: Arrangements and/or social intervention for child abuse, battery, elder abuse, and so on*
Scheduling/coordination of ancillary services	
Arrival/transfer via paramedic/ambulance	
Assessments or care related to multiple catheters or devices	*Examples of catheters/devices: Foley, gastrostomy, ileostomy, colostomy, tracheostomy, PEG tube, central lines, arterial lines, PICC lines*
Face-to-face patient education requiring 30–59 minutes	*Documentation will support the content of the education, time involved, and any factors that affected the time required. Examples include crutch training, diabetic teaching, counseling regarding diet, exercise, and other lifestyle changes.*
Isolation	
Patient acuity warrants simultaneous care by hospital staff (more than one-on-one)	
Patient discharge status other than home or discharge to facility other than originating facility (includes also admission to hospital inpatient or observation)	
Reporting to law enforcement or protective services (for example, gunshots)	
Special needs requiring additional specialized facility resources (for example, language/cognitive, communication impairment)—age appropriate	*Example: Patient requires use of an interpreter. However, if patient does not understand English, but nurse speaks the same language and is able to translate, no additional specialized resources are required and this would not qualify as a contributory factor.*

Exhibit 1.1.   (Continued)

Level 3 (High-Level) Interventions	
At least one item below qualifies for high-level. Additional explanations, examples, and clarifications appear in italics. The items listed here are performed by hospital staff, rather than physician.	
Assessment, crisis intervention, and supervision of imminent behavioral crisis threatening self or others	
Assistance with or performance of fecal disimpaction (manual disimpaction or multiple enemas)	
Continuous irrigation of eye using therapeutic lens (for example, Morgan lens)	
Face-to-face patient education requiring more than 60 minutes	*Documentation will support the content of the education, time involved, and any factors that affected the time required. Examples include crutch training, diabetic teaching, counseling regarding diet, exercise, and other lifestyle changes.*
Frequent monitoring/multiple assessments as evidenced by more than two sets of vital signs or assessments (including initial set) integral to current interventions and/or patient's condition	*Examples: Additional vital signs; assessment of cardiovascular, pulmonary, or neurological status; assessment of pain scale, pulse oxymetry, or peak flow measurement*
Nasotracheal (NT) or orotracheal (OT) suctioning	
Wound care management (when not separately billable), not repaired—51 sq cm or greater	*Includes cleansing, assessment, measurement, photographing, ankle brachial index, and/or dressing of wound. Includes Steri-Strips and other adhesives, eye patch, butterflies. (For multiple wounds, add the total size of all wounds.)*

Exhibit 1.2.   Recommendation for standardized hospital E/M coding of Emergency Department services

Note: This is a sample model developed from prior fiscal years before E/M was expanded to 5 levels. The Hospital Evaluation and Management Coding Panel has sent recommendations to the Centers for Medicare & Medicaid Services for a standard Evaluation and Management coding model. The model would be designed to give objective and consistent industry-wide criteria for coding of emergency department, critical care, and clinic services.

Emergency department visit: A patient who presents to the emergency department for services, is registered, and receives one or more of the clinical interventions listed here.

Level 1 (Low-Level) Interventions

At least one item below qualifies for low level. Additional explanations, examples, and clarifications appear in italics. The items listed here are performed by hospital staff, rather than a physician. Three or more of the interventions identified by an asterisk (*) qualify for mid-level (level 2). Each line item may only be used once toward this increase.

*Administration of oral, topical, rectal, PR, NG, or SL medication(s)	
*Administration of single disposable enema	
*Application of preformed splint(s)/elastic bandage(s)/sling(s), or immobilizer(s) for nonfracture or nondislocation injuries	*Preformed are off-the-shelf. Creation of a splint from plaster or fiberglass or other material would have separate code. Splints are not billed separately. Splints, casting, and so on for fractures are separately billable and paid under the fracture management.*
*Assisting physician with examination(s)	*Pelvic exam is included here. Includes eye exam/slit lamp exam of eye. Nursing documentation must support assistance, unless there is a hospital protocol regarding assistance with exam.*
*Bedside diagnostic testing, unless tests are billed separately	*Examples: Dipstick urine testing, capillary blood sugar *Accu-Check, Dextrostick, Hemoccult, occult blood tests (Strep test is not included because it is separately billable.)*
*Cleaning and dressing of a wound, single body area, not repaired (but includes butterflies)	*Examples: Steri-Strips and other adhesives, eye patch*
*First-aid procedures	*Examples: Control bleeding, ice, monitor vital signs, cool body, remove stinger from insect bite, cleanse and remove secretions*
*Flushing of Heplock	
Follow-up visit	*Definition: Patient instructed to return for wound check or suture removal or rabies injection series*
*Foreign body(ies) removal of skin, subcutaneous or soft tissue, without anesthesia or incision	
Initial clinical assessment	*Examples: Vitals, chief complaint, and clinical assessment of symptom. All elements must be present.*
Measurement/assessment of fetal heart tones	
Nursing visual acuity assessment (for example, Snellan exam)	

Exhibit 1.2. (Continued)

Specimen(s) collection other than venipuncture (for example, midstream urine samples, cultures)	*Example: Nursing instruction of patient on proper specimen collection (for example, midstream urine, sputum). Includes collection of specimen (not the performance of the lab test) (for example, throat culture collection)*

Level 2 (Mid-Level) Interventions

At least one item below qualifies for mid-level. Additional explanations, examples, and clarifications appear in italics. The items listed here are performed by hospital staff, rather than a physician. Three or more of the interventions identified by an asterisk (*) qualify for high-level (level 3). Each line item may only be used once toward this increase.

*Assistance with or performance of fecal disimpaction (manual disimpaction or multiple enemas)	
*Cardiac monitoring	*Includes one or more of the following: Physical assessment by the nurse after initiation of cardiac monitoring, and/or pulses, and/or heart sounds, and/or nursing interpretation of strips*
*Care of device(s) or catheter(s) (both indwelling and in and out) (vascular and nonvascular) and/or ostomy device(s)—other than insertion or reinsertion	*Examples: Irrigation, inspection, assessment, flushing, adjustment, positioning, changing of bags, checking; examples of catheters/devices: Foley, ileal conduit, gastrostomy, ileostomy, colostomy, nephrostomy, tracheostomy, PEG tube, central lines, arterial lines, PICC lines*
Frequent monitoring/assessment as evidenced by three sets of vital signs or assessments (including initial set) integral to current interventions and/or patient's condition	*Examples: Additional vital signs; assessment of cardiovascular, pulmonary, or neurological status; assessment of pain scale, pulse oximetry, or peak flow measurement*
*Insertion of nasogastric (NG) tube or oral gastric (OG) tube	
*Nasotracheal (NT) or orotracheal (OT) suctioning	
*Oxygen administration—initiation and/or adjustment from baseline oxygen regimen	*Includes conversion to hospital-supplied oxygen with rate adjustments, as well as initiation of oxygen administration*
*Traction setup	*Application of traction device for comfort (includes hair traction, Sager traction) prior to definitive treatment*

Contributory Factors for Emergency Department E/M Model from Low-Level to Mid-Level or from Mid-Level to High-Level

Contributory factors are services or other factors that, when present, may increase the E/M assignment by one level. Only one factor is required. These factors apply only to the low level and the mid-level. A high-level E/M may not be increased to critical care by a contributory factor. Additional explanations, examples, and clarifications appear in italics.

Airway insertion (nasal, oral)	
Altered mental status	
Arrangements and/or social service intervention (includes required reporting)	*Examples: Arrangements and/or social intervention for child abuse, battery, elder abuse, and so on*
Scheduling/coordination of ancillary services	

(Continued on next page)

Exhibit 1.2. (Continued)

Arrival/transfer via paramedic/ambulance	
Assessments or care related to multiple catheters or devices	*Examples of catheters/devices: Foley, gastrostomy, ileostomy, colostomy, tracheostomy, PEG tube, central lines, arterial lines, PICC lines*
Isolation	
Multiple nursing interventions—three or more different types of interventions. Only interventions identified by an asterisk apply.	*Example: Three bedside diagnostic tests would only be counted as one item because they are both included in one category. This example would not qualify as a contributory factor.*
Patient acuity warrants simultaneous care by hospital staff (more than one-on-one)	
Patient discharge status other than home or discharge to facility other than originating facility (includes also admission to hospital inpatient or observation)	
Reporting to law enforcement or protective services (for example, gunshots)	
Special needs requiring additional specialized facility resources (for example, language/cognitive, communication impairment)—age appropriate	*Example: Patient requires use of an interpreter. However, if patient does not understand English, but nurse speaks the same language and is able to translate, no additional specialized resources are required and this would not qualify as a contributory factor.*

Level 3 (High-Level) Interventions

At least one item below qualifies for high-level. Additional explanations, examples, and clarifications appear in italics. The items listed here are performed by hospital staff, rather than a physician.

Administration of multiple concurrent intravenous (IV) infusions (2 or more) through different lines or through one or more multiple lumen lines	*(Separately billable only for one line per encounter)*
Assessment, crisis intervention, and supervision of imminent behavioral crisis threatening self or others	
Assistance with or performance of sexual assault exam by hospital nursing staff	
Continuous irrigation of eye using therapeutic lens (for example, Morgan lens)	
Core temperature interventions (for example, heated or cooled IV fluids, heated or cooled gastric lavage, heated or cooled peritoneal lavage)	
Decontamination of hazardous material threatening life, limb, or function by irrigation of organs of special sense, or administration of antidotes or showering	
Monitoring and related attendance of moderate sedation	*Example: Monitoring and related attendance of "conscious sedation"*
Precipitous delivery of baby	

Exhibit 1.2. (Continued)

Continuous ongoing nursing assessments as evidenced by more than three sets (including initial set) of vital signs or assessments integral to current interventions and/or patient's condition	*Examples: Additional vital signs; assessment of cardiovascular, pulmonary, or neurological status; assessment of pain scale, pulse oximetry, or peak flow measurement*

Exhibit 1.3. Recommendation for standardized hospital evaluation and management coding of critical care services

Note: This is a sample model developed from prior fiscal years before E/M was expanded to 5 levels. The Hospital Evaluation and Management Coding Panel has sent recommendations to the Centers for Medicare & Medicaid Services for a standard Evaluation and Management coding model. The model would be designed to give objective and consistent industry-wide criteria for coding of emergency department, critical care, and clinic services. The following interventions qualify as critical care. Additional explanations, examples, and clarifications appear in italics. The items listed here are performed by hospital staff, rather than a physician.	
Interventions/care for critically ill or critically injured patients, for example: central nervous system failure; circulatory failure; shock, renal, hepatic, metabolic, and/or respiratory failure. This may include, but is not limited to, the following interventions:	*Examples of critically ill or critically injured patients include: cardiopulmonary arrest or near arrest related to primary cardiac or respiratory causes, drug overdose, hyper/hypothermia, trauma (including severe burns), and other shock events such as anaphylaxis, diabetic shock, internal bleeding, sepsis, etc.*
Assist in induction/monitoring of pharmaceutical-induced coma	*Examples: Barbiturate coma for status epilepticus*
Assist with rapid sequence intubation (that with provision/administration of sedative and/or paralytic agents) and/or airway management	*Examples: AMBU, frequent ETT suctioning, set up for tube thoracostomy and assist physician with procedure, assist physician in performance of emergent cricothyrotomy, tracheostomy, endotracheal intubation, chest tube insertion, or any other emergency airway*
Code team/crash team/trauma team intervention	*Multidisciplinary team approach to life- or limb-threatening situation. Some of the interventions will be separately billable, but this intervention requires additional facility resources with the activation and initiation of code interventions. Examples: Performance of cardiopulmonary resuscitation, application and use of external, percutaneous, or intracardiac pacemaker, setup for peritoneal lavage, resuscitation for hypothermia, CPR, defibrillation/emergent cardioversion, thoracotomy, pericardiocentesis*
Control of major hemorrhage such as for threatened exsanguination leading to hemodynamic instability	*Control of hemorrhage, for example, for major trauma, postsurgical, including monitoring, IV fluids, emergent administration of multiple concurrent blood products, and so on*
Irrigation, monitoring, and titration of thrombolytic agents and vasopressors	*Monitoring and potential intervention for clinical instability with regard to vasoactive drips or push, antiarrhythmics for life-threatening arrhythmias (for example, Nitroglycerin, Nitroprusside, dopamine, dobutamine, Levophed, Isuprel, amiodarone, Lidocaine, procainamide) and thrombolytic agents for acute myocardial infarction, strokes, pulmonary embolism (Streptokinase, TPA)*
Continuous and ongoing reassessment until stabilized, requiring immediate aggressive interventions in an unstable patient with potential for rapid deterioration and demonstrated instability	

Exhibit 1.4. Composite APC Rules

Extended Assessment and Management Composite APC Rules:

a) If the criteria for the composite APC are met, the composite APC and its associated SI are assigned to the prime code (visit or critical care).

b) Only one extended assessment and management APC is assigned per claim.

c) If the criteria are met for a level I and a level II extended assessment and management APC, assignment of the level II composite takes precedence.

d) If multiple qualifying prime codes (visit or CC) appear on the day of or day before G0378, assign the composite APC to the prime code with the highest separately paid payment rate; assign the standard APC to any/all other visit codes present.

e) Visits not paid under an extended assessment and management composite are paid separately.

Exception: Code G0379 is always packaged if there is an extended assessment and management APC on the claim.

f) The SI for G0378 is always N.

g) Level I and II extended assessment and management composite APCs have SI = V if paid.

h) The logic for extended assessment and management is performed only for bill type 13x, with or without condition code 41.

i) Hours/units of service for observation (G0378) must be at least 8 or the composite APC is not assigned.

j) If a "T" procedure occurs on the day of or day before observation, the composite APC is not assigned.

k) Assign units of service = 1 to the line with the composite APC.

l) Assign the composite payment adjustment flag to the visit line with the composite APC and to the G0378.

m) If the composite APC assignment criteria are not met, apply regular APC logic for separately paid items, special logic for G0379 and the SI for G0378 = N.

Level II Extended Assessment and Management Criteria:

a) If there is at least one of a specified list of critical care or emergency room visit codes on the day of or day before observation (G0378), assign the composite APC and related SI to the critical care or emergency visit code.

b) Additional emergency or critical care visit codes (whether or not on the prime list) are assigned to their standard APCs for separately paid items.

Prime/List A Codes	Nonprime/List B Code	Composite APC
99284, 99285, 99291	G0378	8003

Exhibit 1.4. (Continued)

Level I Extended Assessment and Management Criteria:

a) If there is at least one of a specified list of prime clinic visit codes on the day of or day before observation (G0378), or code G0379 is present on the same day as G0378, assign the composite APC and related status indicator to the clinic visit or direct admission code.

b) Additional clinic visit codes (whether or not on the prime list) are assigned to their standard APCs for separately paid items.

c) Additional G0379, on the same claim, are assigned SI = N.

Prime/List A Codes	Nonprime/List B code	Composite APC
99205, 99215	G0379, G0378	8002

Separate Direct Admit (G0379) Processing Logic:

a) Code G0378 must be present on the same day

b) No SI = T, E/M, or C/C visit on the same day

c) Code G0379 may be paid under the composite 8002, paid under APC 604, or packaged with SI = N.

Chapter 2

Outpatient Claims Preparation and Processing

Understanding how claims are prepared for payment depends on understanding how payment decisions and coverage determinations are made under OPPS. In addition, a detailed knowledge of ICD-9-CM diagnostic and HCPCS/CPT procedural coding is required. Use of modifiers, reporting of units of service, packaging under APCs, Correct Coding Initiative (CCI) edits, national coverage decisions (NCDs), and familiarity with the inclusions and exclusions are essential to understanding how OPPS reimbursement is accomplished.

Electronic Healthcare Transactions and Data Sets

The Administrative Simplification provisions of the Health Insurance Portability and Accountability Act of 1996 (HIPAA) Title II, required the Department of Health and Human Services (HHS) to establish national standards for electronic healthcare transactions and national identifiers for providers, health plans, and employers. It also addressed the security and privacy of health data. As the industry adopts these standards for the efficiency and effectiveness of the nation's healthcare system, that system will improve through the use of electronic data interchange.

On August 17, 2000, the final rule on Standards for Electronic Transactions and Code Sets was published in the *Federal Register* (65 FR 50312). In this rule, (the Transactions Rule), the Secretary of HHS adopted standards for eight electronic transactions and six code sets.

The transactions are

- Healthcare Claims or Equivalent Encounter Information
- Eligibility for a Health Plan
- Referral Certification and Authorization
- Healthcare Claim Status
- Enrollment and Disenrollment in a Health Plan
- Healthcare Payment and Remittance Advice
- Health Plan Premium Payments
- Coordination of Benefits

The code sets are:

- *International Classification of Diseases*, 9th Edition, Clinical Modification, Volumes 1 and 2
- *International Classification of Diseases*, 9th Edition, Clinical Modification, Volume 3 Procedures
- *National Drug Codes*; CMS-0003/5-F, page 8
- *Code on Dental Procedures and Nomenclature*
- *Health Care Financing Administration Common Procedure Coding System*
- *Current Procedural Terminology*, 4th Edition

Electronic Data Interchange

Electronic data interchange (EDI) refers to the electronic transfer of information in a standard format between trading partners. When compared with paper submissions, EDI can substantially lessen the time and costs associated with receiving, processing, and storing documents. The use of EDI can also eliminate inefficiencies and streamline processing tasks, which can in turn result in less administrative burden, lower operating costs, and improved overall data quality.

The healthcare industry recognizes the benefits of EDI, and many entities in the industry have developed proprietary EDI formats. However, with the increasing use of healthcare EDI standards, the lack of common, industry-wide standards has emerged as a major obstacle to realizing potential efficiency and savings (CMS n.d.). Available online at www.cms.hhs.gov/ HIPAAGenInfo/01_Overview.asp.

Claims Preparation

Background UB-04

The National Uniform Billing Committee (NUBC) approved the UB-04 as the replacement for the UB-92 in February, 2005. The NUBC was responsible for the design and printing of the UB-04 form. The UB-04 contains a number of improvements that resulted from nearly four years of research. The HIPAA Accredited Standards Committee (HIPAA ASC) 837 institutional electronic claim format is the version of the form currently in use by providers who submit claims electronically.

The UB-04 (Figure 2.1) is the basic hardcopy form, also known as form CMS-1450. The paper claim form required by CMS is only accepted from institutional providers such as hospitals, skilled nursing facilities, and home health agencies to list a few. Available online at www.cms.hhs.gov/ MLNProducts/downloads/ub04_fact_sheet_050207.pdf.

Figure 2.1. UB-04 form

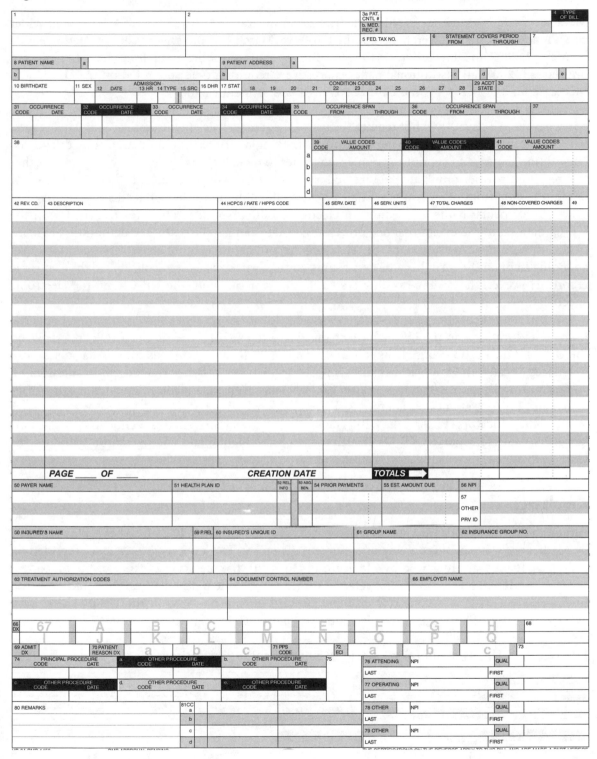

Transitional Period

Medicare fiscal intermediaries (FIs), Medicare Administrative Contractors (MACs), and provider clearinghouses were required to accept the UB-04 by March 1, 2007. The transitional period ended on May 22, 2007, to allow providers time to adjust operations for the new billing changes. However, on May 23, 2007, all institutional paper claims were required to be submitted on the UB-04 and Medicare no longer accepts the UB-92, even as an adjustment claim.

The UB-04 is a uniform institutional provider claim form suitable for billing multiple third-party payers. All payers will not require the use of the same data elements; rather, individual payers will determine the data requirements. A provider filing a UB-04 should retain a copy designated "Institution Copy" and submit the remaining copies to their FI/MAC, managed care plan, or other insurer. If a provider omits any required data, the FI/MAC will either ask for the missing data or obtain the data from other sources. The FI/MAC will maintain the data on its history record.

Data elements in the CMS uniform electronic billing specifications are consistent with the UB-04 data set to the extent that one processing system can handle both. The definitions are identical, although in some situations, the electronic record contains more characters than the corresponding item on the form because constraints on the form size are not applicable to the electronic record. However, the revenue coding system is the same for both the UB-04 and the electronic specifications.

The UB-04 incorporates the National Provider Identifier (NPI) as well as additional updates. Many data locations on the UB-92 have changed to a four-digit "type-of-bill" (TOB) reference on the UB-04. One of the major changes is the expansion of ICD-9-CM fields from 9 diagnoses to 18 diagnoses, located in FL 67 (Principal Diagnosis) to FL 67A-Q (Other Diagnosis). In addition, FL 76 (Admitting Diagnosis/Patient's Reason for Visit) has been expanded to FL 69 (Admitting diagnosis) and FL 70 (Patient's reason for visit).

The form locators (FLs) on the UB-04 claim form are referenced in this section to illustrate how key APC data are reported. UB-04 instructions for completion and coding can be found on the CMS Web site: www.cms.hhs.gov/Transmittals/downloads/R1104CP.pdf.

Coding

Although diagnosis codes are not used in the APC grouping process, ICD-9-CM codes are required by Medicare for hospital reporting of outpatient diagnoses. However, diagnosis codes reported on claims frequently are reviewed by Medicare FIs to verify the medical necessity of the outpatient services rendered. For example, if a cataract surgery CPT code were billed, an FI would expect to find a cataract diagnosis code (for example, 366.10) on the claim, as in the UB-04 claim form excerpt for diagnosis coding reporting shown in Figure 2.2.

Figure 2.2.   UB-04 claim form excerpt: Diagnosis coding reporting

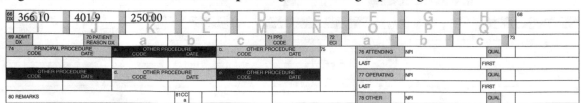

Coding conventions in the outpatient setting differ slightly from those in use in inpatient settings. The diagnosis identified in FL 67 on the claim need not be the principal diagnosis code based on the principal diagnosis definition under the inpatient diagnosis-related groups (MS-DRGs). Instead, for outpatient claims, the diagnosis code listed in FL 67 is the reason for the visit as identified at the time of the visit (for example, in billing for clinic and emergency department visits). A patient who attends several different clinics in one day should have separate claims submitted for each clinic visit because, currently, only one "reason for visit" diagnosis can be associated with each claim.

Under the OPPS, CPT and/or HCPCS Level II codes are required for reporting outpatient services and procedures. Numerous CPT and HCPCS codes are very specific and thus should be reported appropriately because each code could trigger an APC payment. (See Figure 2.3 for an excerpt from a UB-04 claim form.)

Figure 2.3.   UB-04 claim form excerpt: CPT/HCPCS code reporting

42 REV. CD.	43 DESCRIPTION	44 HCPCS / RATE / HIPPS CODE
320	DX X-RAY	71010
320	DX X-RAY	72040
320	CT SCAN	70459

Note: According to CMS, as published in the November 27, 2007, *Federal Register,* hospitals may use CPT codes to report any packaged services ("N" status indicator codes) that were performed, consistent with CPT coding guidelines. All services provided should be reported whether or not reimbursement is expected. The data collected by Medicare can impact future revisions to pricing, bundling, unbundling, and whether a service will continue to be packaged.

CMS is responsible for administering the Medicare, Medicaid, and State Children's Health Insurance Programs, as well as a number of health oversight programs. CMS gathers and formats data to support the agency's operations. Information about Medicare beneficiaries, Medicare claims, Medicare providers, clinical data, and Medicaid eligibility and claims is included. This data is made available to the public, subject to privacy release approvals and the availability of computing resources. The Medicare Provider Analysis and Review (MEDPAR) file contains records for 100 percent of Medicare beneficiaries who use hospital outpatient services. The records are stripped of most data elements that will permit identification of beneficiaries. The national file consists of approximately 12 million records. The data is extracted from the UB-04 fields.

The FL 42 (Revenue Code/REV. CD) allows a three- or four-digit code to be reported that identifies a specific accommodation, ancillary service, or billing calculation related to the services included on the bill. The FL 43 (Revenue Code description/DESCRIPTION) contains a narrative description or standard abbreviation for each revenue code category reported on the UB-04. A single UB-04 claim form has 450 lines for listing revenue codes and charges. More information about the UB-04 can be found online at www.cms.hhs.gov/ElectronicBillingEDITrans/15_1450.asp#TopOfPage.

Modifiers

After a CPT or HCPCS Level II code is assigned, a CPT or HCPCS Level II modifier may be needed to indicate that a service or procedure that has been performed has been altered by some specific circumstances but has not changed in its definition or code. The proper use of modifiers reduces the need for separate procedure listings to describe the modifying circumstance. When needed, the two-digit modifier is placed after the procedure code; for example, bilateral procedure modifier –50 is attached to inguinal hernia repair code 49505 to report a bilateral inguinal hernia repair.

Modifiers are required to meet at least one of the following criteria:

- Payment implications
- Future need for payment data for constructing an outpatient PPS
- Coding consistency and editing

On the claim form, a hyphen does not appear between the CPT/HCPCS code and the two-digit modifier. The hyphen is only used in instructional literature regarding modifiers. A maximum of two two-digit modifiers can be reported next to a single CPT/HCPCS code. The modifiers listed below include –50 (Bilateral Procedure), –LT (Left Side), and –59 (Distinct Procedural Service). The UB-04 claim form (Figure 2.4) illustrates modifier reporting. (See Exhibit 2.1 at the end of this chapter for the 2008 listing of modifiers required for Medicare hospital outpatient services.)

Figure 2.4.   UB-04 claim form excerpt: Modifier reporting

42 REV. CD.	43 DESCRIPTION	44 HCPCS / RATE / HIPPS CODE
360	OPERATING RM	49505**50**
360	OPERATING RM	28080**LT**
360	OPERATING RM	28080**LT59**

Units of Service

For each CPT or HCPCS Level II code assigned and reported on the UB-04 claim, a unit of service must be assigned. Service units are defined as the number of times the service or procedure being reported was performed. Hospitals are required to make a numerical entry in UB-04 FL 46.

Under the OPPS, each unit of service recorded in UB-04 FL 46 triggers a payment. Thus, CMS has created a second set of edits limiting the number of units allowed for each HCPCS code. For example, only "1" will be accepted in the unit's field for cataract surgery. However, for most services, the edit allows for the procedure to be performed a number of times in a day, with an upper limit to reduce obvious errors. Of course, hospitals should report only the actual number of times a procedure was performed, keeping in mind that CPT and HCPCS definitions sometimes specify the units.

For example, CPT code 11720, Debridement of nail(s) by any method; one to five, should be reported only once (unit of service "1") for any number of nails debrided between one and five, inclusive. If more than five nails are debrided, the appropriate code is 11721, Debridement of nail(s) by any method; six or more, which is billed only once (unit of service "1") in place of 11720. (See Figure 2.5.)

Figure 2.5.   UB-04 claim form excerpt: Service units section

42 REV. CD.	43 DESCRIPTION	44 HCPCS / RATE / HIPPS CODE	45 SERV. DATE	46 SERV. UNITS
510	CLINIC	11720	03262008	1

The Medicare outpatient code editor (OCE) is used by each Medicare FI to process all Medicare hospital outpatient claims. The OCE contains a series of units of service edits that are specific to the type of service billed. The premises used to arrive at a maximum number of units of service are based on knowledge of the human anatomy and an understanding of the standards of medical/surgical practice utilized in the development of the National Correct Coding Initiative (NCCI or CCI) edits, which are discussed later in this chapter.

Billing Requirements Related to APCs

CMS encourages hospitals to report all charges for all services on claims for Medicare payment so that the data on which the APC relative weights are set will fully reflect the relative costs of all services. As a matter of policy, however, CMS does not generally mandate the reporting of services under specific revenue centers but, rather, leaves that decision up to the hospitals.

CMS does not regulate what hospitals charge for hospital services and will not advise hospitals on how to determine the charge for an item or service.

Packaged Implantables

Although packaged implantable items generate no separate OPPS payment, these items must be coded. In 2005, CMS required hospitals to include device category "C" codes on claims when such devices were used in conjunction with procedures billed and paid for under the OPPS. The goal of CMS was to improve the quality of the claims data in support of their transition to the use of all single claims to establish payment rates for those APCs. Failing to bill and charge appropriately, either using "C" codes or revenue center codes, could lead to reduced payments to hospitals for Medicare outpatient services.

For example, if CPT code 36558 is reported, device category HCPCS Level II code C1751 is required.

36558:	Insertion of tunneled centrally inserted central venous catheter, without subcutaneous port or pump; age 5 years or older
C1751:	Catheter, infusion, inserted peripherally, centrally or midline (other than hemodialysis)

In 2008, in an initial step toward creating larger payment groups for hospital care, CMS has packaged payment for items and services in certain categories of HCPCS codes. Finalized packaged services include guidance, image processing, intraoperative services, imaging supervision, interpretation, diagnostic radiopharmaceuticals and contrast agents, and observation services. CMS will package payment either unconditionally (SI N) or conditionally, allowing separate payment if certain criteria are met (SI Q). Table 10, in the final rule (page 66659), contains a complete list of all codes in the final seven categories (available online at www.cms.hhs.gov/HospitalOutpatientPPS/HORD/list.asp#TopOfPage).

The OCE will determine SI Q with two edits levels. For level 1, if SI Q is reported on the same day as SI S, T, V, or X, payment for Q will be packaged. For level 2, payment for Q will be packaged if SI Q is reported on the same date as SI T.

Hospitals should continue to report all appropriate codes and charges for all services furnished, packaged or not. CMS emphasizes that there are no new billing requirements associated with this change in policy payment.

A hospital must report the C codes in FL 44 of the UB-04 claim form or the electronic equivalent. If one device is shown for one APC, that device would have to be billed on the claim for a service in that APC or the claim would be returned to the provider for correction. If more than one device is shown for one APC, the provider would be required to bill one of the device codes shown on the same claim with the service in that APC for the claim to be accepted. (See www.cms.hhs. gov/HospitalOutpatientPPS.)

Drugs, Pharmaceuticals, and Biologicals

In CY 2008, Medicare will reimburse drugs using average sales price plus 5 percent, which has integrated payments for both acquisition and overhead costs aggregate. The threshold for packaged drugs is less than $60. Anti-emetics remain exempt from the packaging requirement, along with intravenous immunoglobulin pre-administration reported with HCPCS code G0332.

CMS is also going to allow hospitals to report any HCPCS code for a Part B drug that is covered under OPPS, regardless of the unit determination in the HCPCS descriptor. Table 34 in the final rule lists previously unrecognized codes by moving the SI from B to K. CMS will continue to pay for transitional pass through drugs (SI G), separately payable drugs without pass through payments (SI K), vaccines (SI L, F), and orphan drugs (G).

Pharmacy systems typically have "sub-basements" that must be mapped to the charge description master in order for the HCPCS code to transfer to the UB-04 claim form.

CMS does not require hospitals to report a HCPCS code for every drug that is administered to a patient; however, to receive payment for a drug for which a separate payment is provided, hospitals have to bill for the drug using revenue code 636, Drugs requiring detailed coding, and report the appropriate HCPCS code for the drug. Status indicator (SI) "K" designates drugs for which separate payment is allowed.

Although CMS does not require hospitals to report HCPCS codes for packaged drugs, hospitals must continue to bill charges for packaged drugs by including the charge for packaged drugs in the charge for the procedure or service with which the drug is used or as a separate drug charge (whether it is separately payable). Reporting charges for packaged drugs is critical because packaged drug costs are used in calculating outlier payments. In addition, these charges are identified in the course of the annual OPPS updates when CMS calculates hospital costs for the procedures and services with which the drugs are used.

Hospitals should bill for packaged drugs that are assigned SI "N" using any of the following drug revenue codes, which are packaged revenue codes under the OPPS: 250, 251, 252, 254, 255, 257, 258, 259, 631, 632, or 633. Hospitals are not required to use HCPCS codes when billing for packaged drugs unless revenue code 636 is used.

Hospitals should use the UB-04 FL 46 to report multiples of the dosage identified in the HCPCS Level II drug code narrative descriptor. Fractions of the dose specified in the code descriptor may be reported as one unit or one additional unit, as appropriate. That is, if the amount of the drug administered to a patient is less than the amount described by the HCPCS Level II code, a hospital may bill for one unit.

> **Examples:** Adenosine 3 mg IV (J0150) is drawn from a 6-mg ampule and administered to convert a supraventricular arrhythmia. Report HCPCS code J0150 (Injection, Adenosine, 6 mg) with "1" unit of service, even though the entire 6 mg ampule dose was not administered.
>
> 500 mg of dexrazozane HCI (J1190) is administered. Report HCPCS code J1190, Injection, dexrazoxane HCI injection, 250 mg, with the number "2" as the unit of service to indicate that 500 mg of the drug was used.

Emergency Department Visits

If a surgical procedure is performed in the emergency department, the charge for the procedure must be billed with the emergency department revenue code. When an emergency department visit occurs on the same day the procedure is performed, a charge should be billed for the visit and a separate charge for the procedure. The physician may need to indicate that on the day a procedure or service identified by a CPT code was performed, the patient's condition required a significant, separately identifiable E/M service above and beyond the other service provided or beyond the usual preoperative and postoperative care associated with the procedure that was performed. Modifier –25 should be appended to the visit code if the procedure performed is a separately identifiable service.

Surgical Procedures

The elective cancellation of procedures is not reported. If multiple procedures were planned, only the procedure actually initiated is billed. A pattern of canceled procedures prompts medical review of the reasons for cancellation and may trigger review of the appropriateness of patient selection for outpatient surgery.

Injection/Infusion Therapy and Cancer Chemotherapy

For CY 2007, OPPS drug administration APCs have been restructured resulting in a six-level hierarchy where active HCPCS codes have been assigned according to their clinical coherence and resource use. In comparison to the CY 2006 payment structure that bundled payment for several instances of a type of service (nonchemotherapy, chemotherapy by infusion, noninfusion chemotherapy) into a per-encounter APC payment, the CY 2007 structure provided a separate APC payment for each reported unit of a separately payable HCPCS code.

In CY 2006, hospitals were instructed to bill for the first hour (and any additional hours) by each type of infusion service (nonchemotherapy, chemotherapy by infusion, noninfusion chemotherapy). In CY 2007, the first hour no longer existed. CPT codes allow for only one initial service per encounter, for each vascular access site, no matter how many types of infusion services are provided; however, hospitals will receive an APC payment for the initial service and separate APC payment(s) for additional hours of infusion or other drug administration services provided that are separately payable.

In CY 2006, hospitals providing infusion services of different types (nonchemotherapy, chemotherapy by infusion, noninfusion chemotherapy) received payment for the associated per-encounter infusion APC even if these infusions occurred during the same time period. In CY 2007, CPT instructions allowed reporting of only one initial drug administration service, including infusion services, per encounter for each distinct vascular access site, with other services through the same vascular access site being reported via the sequential, concurrent, or additional hour codes.

For CY 2008, Table 2.1 represents the final changes to the drug administration APC structure.

Table 2.1. CY 2008, Six-Level Drug Administration APC structure

CY 2008 APC Level	APC Status Indicator	CY 2008 APC Median	CPT/HCPCS Code	Description
0436 Level I	S	$16.21	90472	Immunization admin, each add
			90473	Immune admin oral/nasal
			90474	Immune admin oral/nasal addl
			90779	Ther/prop/diag/inj/inf proc
			95115	Immunotherapy, one injection
			96549	Chemotherapy, unspecified
0437 Level II	S	$25.13	90471	Immunization admin
			90761	Hydrate iv infusion, add-on
			90766	Ther/proph/dg IV inf, add-on
			90767	Tx/proph/dg addl seq IV inf
			90770	Sc ther infusion, addl hr
			90772	Ther/proph/diag inj, sc/im
			95117	Immunotherapy injections
			95144	Antigen therapy services
			95145	Antigen therapy services
			95146	Antigen therapy services
			95147	Antigen therapy services
			95148	Antigen therapy services
			95149	Antigen therapy services
			95165	Antigen therapy services
			95170	Antigen therapy services
			G0377	Administra Part D vaccine
0438 Level III	S	$51.22	90771	Sc ther infusion, reset pump
			90773	Ther/proph/diag inj, ia
			90774	Ther/proph/diag inj, iv push
			90775	Tx/pro/dx inj new drug addon
			96401	Chemo, anti-neopl, sq/im
			96402	Chemo hormon antineopl sq/im
			96405	Chemo intralesional, up to 7
			96406	Chemo intralesional over 7
			96415	Chemo, IV infusion, addl hr
			96417	Chemo IV infus each addl seq
			96423	Chemo ia infuse each addl hr
			96542	Chemotherapy injection
0439 Level IV	S	$105.38	96409	Chemo, IV push, sngl drug
			96411	Chemo, IV push, addl drug
			96420	Chemo, ia, push tecnique
0440 Level V	S	$114.64	90760	Hydration iv infusion, init
			90765	Ther/proph/diag IV inf, init
			90769	Sc ther infusion, up to 1 hr
			96521	Refill/maint, portable pump
			96522	Refill/maint pump/resvr syst

0441 Level VI	S	$149.34	96413	Chemo, IV infusion, 1 hr
			96416	Chemo prolong infuse w/pump
			96422	Chemo ia infusion up to 1 hr
			96425	Chemotherapy,infusion method
			96440	Chemotherapy, intracavitary
			96445	Chemotherapy, intracavitary
			96450	Chemotherapy, into CNS

As shown above, the placement of HCPCS codes into the six levels follows logical, clinically coherent principles and is consistent with both expected and observed differences in hospital resource costs, both across levels and within each level. For example, the first hour of chemotherapy infusion is assigned to Level VI, while additional hours of chemotherapy infusion are assigned to Level III. This structure is mirrored by the nonchemotherapy codes that show the first hour of nonchemotherapy infusion assigned to Level V, while additional hours of nonchemotherapy infusion are assigned to Level II.

Infusions Started Outside the Hospital

Hospitals may receive Medicare beneficiaries for outpatient services who are in the process of receiving an infusion at their time of arrival at the hospital, such as a patient who arrives via ambulance with an ongoing intravenous infusion initiated by paramedics during transport. Hospitals are reminded to bill for all services provided using the HCPCS code(s) that most accurately describe the service (s) they provided. This includes hospitals reporting an initial hour of infusion, even if the hospital did not initiate the infusion, and additional HCPCS codes for additional or sequential infusion services if needed.

Claims Processing

When a claim has been prepared, it is subject to verification and validation under the OCE and NCCI edits. Codes must be packaged into the correct APC groups and appropriate discounts applied to ensure accurate and timely reimbursement. Only when all of the editing and payment processing issues have been completed and there are no unresolved edits will the Medicare FI pay the claim.

Medicare Outpatient Code Editor

All hospital OPPS claims submitted to the Medicare FI are processed against the Medicare OCE edits.

The OCE is a computer software program used by FIs to detect incorrect coding and billing data and to determine whether the APC payment methodology applies to hospital outpatient UB-04 claims data. The occurrence of an OCE edit can result in one of six different dispositions, which help to ensure that FIs in various parts of the country are following similar claims-processing procedures. The dispositions are

- Claim rejection
- Claim denial
- Claim return to provider
- Claim suspension

- Line item rejection
- Line item denial

The two main functions of the OCE are to

- Edit claims data to identify errors and identify claim and line dispositions
- Assign an APC group number for each service covered under OPPS and return information to be used as input to the OPPS pricer (used to calculate the OPPS rate)

In general, the OCE performs all functions that require specific reference to CPT/HCPCS codes, CPT/HCPCS modifiers, and ICD-9-CM diagnosis codes. (See Exhibit 2.2. for a list of January 2008 OCE edits.)

National Correct Coding Initiative Edits

Under the OPPS, it is possible for a hospital to receive multiple APC payments for a single outpatient encounter. To ensure that overcoding does not inappropriately trigger multiple APC group payments, CMS has implemented the NCCI edits to prohibit fragmenting/unbundling of services through the inappropriate reporting of multiple CPT/HCPCS codes. CCI edits are applicable to claims submitted on behalf of the same beneficiary, provided by the same provider and on the same date of service. The hospital OPPS CCI edits are actually the Medicare OCE edits 19, 20, 39, and 40. There are two main types of CCI edits:

- The comprehensive/component edits that are applied to code combinations where one of the codes is a component of a more comprehensive code. In this instance, only the comprehensive code is paid. For example, 36415 (routine venipuncture) is a component part of code 36430, Transfusion, blood or blood components, and should not be billed separately. Similarly, code 94760 (pulse oximetry) should not be billed with surgical procedures for which it is a common monitoring technique.
- The mutually exclusive edits are applied to code combinations where it is considered to be either impossible or improbable for one of the codes to be performed with the other code. For example, code 93797, Physician services for outpatient cardiac rehabilitation; without continuous ECG monitoring, should not be billed simultaneously with code 93798, Physician services for outpatient cardiac rehabilitation with continuous ECG monitoring.

Other unacceptable code combinations also are included. One such combination consists of one code that represents a service "with" something and the other "without" that same thing. The edit is set to pay the lesser-priced service.

Although CCI edits are applied to the outpatient claim when it is submitted to the Medicare FI, most hospitals process their codes against the CCI edits before the claim is finalized and submitted for payment. Four of the OCE edits discussed above contain the CCI edits that CMS uses to ensure that hospitals are not unbundling/overcoding.

Since January 2008, the HOPPS CCI utilized by Medicare carriers has been available online at www.cms.hhs.gov/NationalCorrectCodInitEd/02_hoppscciedits.asp. (See Figure 2.6.)

Figure 2.6. Internet home page for hospital OPPS CCI edits
(http://www.cms.hhs.gov/NationalCorrectCodInitEd/02_hoppscciedits.asp)

National Correct Coding Initiative Edits for Hospital Outpatient PPS— Version 13.3 (Effective January 1, 2008)

Note: All CCI edits will be incorporated in the Outpatient Code Editor (OCE) with the exception of anesthesiology, E/M, mental health, and derma bond. In addition, CCI edits for computer aided detection (CAD) devices were removed from the 9.2 version of the OCE. They will be re-incorporated in a subsequent release.

Column 1/Column 2 Correct Coding Edits
(formerly Comprehensive/Component Edits)
- Surgery: Integumentary System -
  CPT CODES 10000-19999 (excel file zipped 171Kb)
- Surgery: Musculoskeletal System -
  CPT CODES 20000-29999 (excel file zipped 727Kb)
- Surgery: Respiratory, Cardiovascular, Hemic and Lymphatic Systems -
  CPT CODES 30000-39999 (excel file zipped 317Kb)
- Surgery: Digestive System -
  CPT CODES 40000-49999 (excel file zipped 353Kb)
- Surgery: Urinary, Male Genital, Female Genital, Maternity Care and Delivery Systems -
  CPT CODES 50000-59999 (excel file zipped 320Kb)
- Surgery: Endocrine, Nervous, Eye and Ocular Adnexa, Auditory Systems -
  CPT CODES 60000-69999 (excel file zipped 265Kb)
- Radiology Services -
  CPT CODES 70000-79999 (excel file zipped 92Kb)
- Pathology and Laboratory Services -
  CPT CODES 80000-89999 (excel file zipped 54Kb)
- Medicine Evaluation and Management Services -
  CPT CODES 90000-99999 (excel file zipped 97Kb)
- Category III Codes -
  CPT CODES 0001T-0099T (excel file zipped 4Kb)
- Supplemental Services -
  HCPCS LEVEL II Codes A0000-V9999 (excel file zipped 29Kb)

Mutually Exclusive Correct Coding Edits
- Surgery: Integumentary System -
  CPT CODES 10000-19999 (excel file zipped 68Kb)
- Surgery: Musculoskeletal System -
  CPT CODES 20000-29999 (excel file zipped 25Kb)
- Surgery: Respiratory, Cardiovascular, Hemic and Lymphatic Systems -
  CPT CODES 30000-39999 (excel file zipped 28Kb)
- Surgery: Digestive System -
  CPT CODES 40000-49999 (excel file zipped 13Kb)
- Surgery: Urinary, Male Genital, Female Genital, Maternity Care and Delivery Systems -
  CPT CODES 50000-59999 (excel file zipped 11Kb)
- Surgery: Endocrine, Nervous, Eye and Ocular Adnexa, Auditory Systems -
  CPT CODES 60000-69999 (excel file zipped 15Kb)
- Radiology Services -
  CPT CODES 70000-79999 (excel file zipped 40Kb)
- Pathology and Laboratory Services -
  CPT CODES 80000-89999 (excel file zipped 15Kb)
- Medicine Evaluation and Management Services -
  CPT CODES 90000-99999 (excel file zipped 14Kb)
- Category III Codes -
  CPT CODES 0001T-0099T (excel file zipped 2Kb)

Column1/Column 2 Edits (excerpt)

Column1/Column 2 Edits (excerpt)					
Column 1	Column 2	* = In existence prior to 1996	Effective Date	Deletion Date *=no data	Modifier 0=not allowed 1=allowed 9=not applicable
60000	36000		20021001	*	1
60000	36410		20021001	*	1
60000	37202		20021001	*	1
60000	60001		19970101	*	1
60000	62318		20021001	*	1
60000	62319		20021001	*	1
60000	64415		20021001	*	1
60000	64416		20030101	*	1
60000	64417		20021001	*	1
60000	64450		20021001	*	1
60000	64470		20021001	*	1
60000	64475		20021001	*	1
60000	69990		20000605	*	0

Packaging under the APC Groups

After the Medicare FI processes the OPPS claim through the OCE edits, the CPT/HCPCS codes that are assigned the SI "N" (packaged/incidental) are identified. FIs do not calculate a reimbursement amount for these incidental codes.

Packaged services are those that are recognized as contributing to the cost of the services in an APC, but that CMS does not pay for separately. CMS packaged into the APC payment rate for a given procedure or service any costs incurred to furnish the following items and services:

- Use of an operating suite
- Procedure room or treatment room
- Use of the recovery room or area
- Use of an observation bed (unless authorized for separate payment)
- Anesthesia
- Medical and surgical supplies and equipment
- Surgical dressings
- Supplies and equipment for administering and monitoring anesthesia or sedation
- Intraocular lenses
- Capital-related costs
- Costs incurred to procure donor tissue other than corneal tissue
- Various incidental services such as venipuncture

CMS also packaged the cost of many pharmaceuticals and biologicals within APC groups. It did this because many drugs are usually provided in connection with some other treatment or procedure. For example:

CPT/HCPCS Code	SI	Code Description
52281	T	Cystoscopy and treatment
51605	N	Preparation for bladder x-ray

If a hospital bills a cystoscopy (code 52281) and the preparation for bladder x-ray (code 51605), only code 52281 generates a payment because code 51605 has an "N" status under the OPPS. (See packaged service example in Figure 2.7.)

Figure 2.7. UB-04 claim form excerpt: Packaged service example

42 REV. CD.	43 DESCRIPTION	44 HCPCS/RATES	45 SERV. DATE	46 SERV. UNITS
360	OPERATING RM	52281	03262008	1
360	OPERATING RM	51605	03262008	1

Discounting of Payments under the OPPS

Separate payments are made for codes that are not designated as packaged. However, some codes have their OPPS payments discounted as discussed here.

Multiple Procedures

When more than one surgical procedure with payment SI "T" is performed during a single operative session, the full Medicare payment is made and the beneficiary pays the coinsurance for the procedure having the highest payment rate.

Fifty percent of the usual Medicare APC payment amount and beneficiary coinsurance amount would be paid for all other procedures performed during the same operative session to reflect the savings associated with having to prepare the patient only once and the incremental costs associated with anesthesia, operating and recovery room use, and other services required for the second and subsequent procedures. The reduced payment for multiple procedures would apply to both the beneficiary coinsurance and the Medicare payment.

> **Example:** When a hospital bills both bunion correction code 28292–LT and hammertoe repair code 28285–T3, as shown here, code 28292–LT is paid at 100 percent of the APC payment rate, but code 28285–T3 is paid at 50 percent of the APC payment rate. (See Figure 2.8. for a multiple surgery example.)

CPT/HCPCS Code	SI	Code Description	APC	Relative Weight	Payment Rate
28292	T	Correction of bunion	0057	20.8284	$1,326.64
28285	T	Repair of hammertoe	0055	20.8284	$1,326.64

Figure 2.8. UB-04 claim form excerpt: Multiple surgery example

42 REV. CD.	43 DESCRIPTION	44 HCPCS/RATES	45 SERV. DATE	46 SERV. UNITS
360	OPERATING RM	28292	03262008	1
360	OPERATING RM	28285	03262008	1

Discontinued Surgery

Modifier –73, Discontinued Outpatient Hospital/Ambulatory Surgery Center [ASC] Procedure Prior to the Administration of Anesthesia, identifies a procedure that is terminated after the patient has been prepared for surgery, including sedation when provided, and taken to the room where the procedure is to be performed, but *before* anesthesia is induced (whether local, regional block(s), or general anesthesia). To recognize the costs incurred by the hospital to prepare the patient for surgery, the hospital receives 50 percent of the payment, as indicated by modifier –73.

Example: A Medicare outpatient is scheduled to have arthroscopic left knee lateral meniscectomy (CPT code 29881) performed under general anesthesia. After the patient is taken to the operating room, but before the anesthesia is administered, the patient develops a cardiac arrhythmia. The procedure is cancelled, and the patient is taken to the recovery room. On the bill, the case is reported as 29881–73 and the hospital receives 50 percent of the APC payment for code 29881. (See Figure 2.9.)

CPT/HCPCS Code	SI	Code Description	APC	Relative Weight	Payment Rate
29881	T	Knee arthroscopy/surgery	0041	28.7803	$1,833.13

Figure 2.9. **UB-04 claim form excerpt: Preanesthesia discontinued surgery example**

42 REV. CD.	43 DESCRIPTION	44 HCPCS/RATES	45 SERV. DATE	46 SERV. UNITS
360	OPERATING RM	2988173	03262008	1
				1

Modifier –74 is used to indicate that a surgical procedure was started, but discontinued *after* the induction of anesthesia (whether local, regional block, or general anesthesia), or *after* the procedure was started (incision made, intubation begun, scope inserted) due to extenuating circumstances or circumstances that threatened the patient's well-being. To recognize the costs incurred by the hospital to prepare the patient for surgery and the resources expended in the operating room and recovery room, the hospital receives 100 percent payment, as indicated by modifier –74.

Example: A Medicare outpatient is scheduled to have a left excisional breast biopsy performed under local anesthesia. After the patient is taken to the operating room, and after the anesthesia is administered, she develops high blood pressure. The procedure is cancelled, and the patient is taken to the recovery room. On the bill, the case is reported as 19120–74 and the hospital receives 100 percent of the APC payment for code 19120. (See Figure 2.10.)

CPT/HCPCS Code	SI	Code Description	APC	Relative Weight	Payment Rate
19120	T	Removal of breast lesion	0028	20.6417	$1,314.75

Figure 2.10. **UB-04 claim form excerpt: Postanesthesia discontinued surgery example**

42 REV. CD.	43 DESCRIPTION	44 HCPCS/RATES	45 SERV. DATE	46 SERV. UNITS
360	OPERATING RM	1912074	03262008	1
				1

Modifier –52, Reduced Services, is used to indicate a procedure that did not require anesthesia but was terminated after the patient has been prepared for the procedure (including sedation when provided) and taken to the room where the procedure is to be performed. To recognize the costs incurred by the hospital to prepare the patient for surgery, the hospital receives 50 percent of the payment for the procedure, as indicated by modifier –52.

Example: A Medicare outpatient was scheduled to have a colonoscopy through a colostomy site without the use of anesthesia. After the patient was taken to the endoscopy suite, several attempts to intubate the colon were unsuccessful. The procedure was cancelled and the patient taken to the recovery room. On the bill, the case is reported as 44388–52 and the hospital receives 50 percent of the APC payment for code 44388. (See Figure 2.11.)

CPT/HCPCS Code	SI	Code Description	APC	Relative Weight	Payment Rate
44388	T	Colonoscopy thru stomach	0143	8.8486	$563.60

Figure 2.11. UB-04 claim form excerpt: No-anesthesia discontinued surgery example

42 REV. CD.	43 DESCRIPTION	44 HCPCS/RATES	45 SERV. DATE	46 SERV. UNITS
750	GI SERVICES	4438852	03262008	1
				1

Calculation of Final APC Payments

When all the editing and payment-processing issues have been completed, and if there are no unresolved edits, the Medicare FI pays the claim. The payment information is communicated to the hospital in either a hard-copy Medicare remittance advice statement or an 835 electronic transaction standard.

Hospitals should have a process in place to reconcile outpatient codes and APCs billed *against* outpatient codes and APCs paid (on the remittance statement) for Medicare. This will facilitate the hospital's identification of claims that have been under- or overpaid by the FI.

Example: Figure 2.12 reflects an actual UB-04 (with all identifiers changed) for a Medicare outpatient seen in the hospital ED for the following services:
82553	Creatinine kinase, MB fraction only
82550	Creatinine kinase
71010	Chest x-ray
72040	Cervical spine x-ray
70450	CT scan brain
99285–25	Level V ED visit
93005	EKG

Figure 2.12.   UB-04 claim form excerpt: Medicare Outpatient example

42 REV. CD.	43 DESCRIPTION	44 HCPCS/RATES	45 SERV. DATE	46 SERV. UNITS
270	MED–SURG SUPPLY			
270	MED–SURG SUPPLY		03262008	1
300	LABORATORY	82553	03262008	
301	LAB/CHEMISTRY	82550	03262008	
320	DX X-RAY	71010	03262008	
320	DX X-RAY	72040	03262008	
350	CT SCAN	70450	03262008	
450	EMERG ROOM	9928525	03262008	
730	EKG/ECG	93005	03262008	

Figure 2.12 reflects the actual Medicare explanation of benefits/remittance advice notice that details how each code was paid by Medicare. Lab codes 82550 and 82553 were paid under the Medicare clinical diagnostic lab fee schedule, so no APC groups are listed next to these codes:

HCPCS Code	Revenue Code	APC Modifier
82550	270	
82553	301	
71010	301	00260
72040	320	00260
70450	350	00332
99285	450	00616–25
93005	730	0099

Figure 2.13. Sample Medicare remittance notice for UB-04

Medicare Part-A
Explanation of Benefits (EOB)

Payee: USA Medical Center   Payor: TriSpan Health Services
                                                           3545 Lakeland Drive
                                                           Jackson, MS   342253046

SMITH, BO   Prv No: 1234556
Service From 01/2/2008 Thru 01/22/2008   RA Date: 02/19/2008

Pat#:	08776109	DRG Amt:	.00	Submit Chgs:	2,040.10
HIC:	687102140A	Outlier Amt:	.00	Covered Chgs:	2,040.10
ICN:	2038288184	Deduct Amt:	.00	Non-Covered Chgs:	.00
MRN:	897891938	Blood Deduct:	.00	Denied Chgs:	.00
		Co-I ns Amt:	173.38	Capital Amt:	.00
Cost Rpt Days:		Interest:	.00	Capital FSP Amt:	.00
Cov Days:		G-R Reduct:	.00	Capital HSP Amt:	.00
Non-Cov Days:		HCPCS Allow:	1,752.23	Capital DSH Amt:	.00
Outlier Days:		Pat Payment:	.00	Old Capital Amt:	.00
Co-Ins Days:		MSP Liab Met:	.00	Capital Outlier:	.00
		Primary Pay:	.00	Capital IME:	.00
DRG:	_____	SP Pass Thru:	.00	Capital Except:	.00
DRG Weight:	_____	Share:	.00	Indirect Teach:	.00
Per Diem:	_____	Prof Comp:	.00	Oper Hospital DRG:	.00
Reimb Rate:				Contractual Adj:	1,561.73
				Payment:	304.99

Type of Bill: Hospital / Outpatient (Part A)
Frequency: Admit Through Discharge Claim
Claim Status: _____ as Primary
Patient Status: _____ (or did not recover – Christian Science Patient)

Date	HCPCS	Rev_ APCs	Modifier Unit	Submit	Co-Ins	C/A	Payment
01/22/08				194.60	.00	194.60	.00
01/21/08	82550	270		48.50	.00	39.40	9.10
01/21/08	82553	301		70.00	.00	53.87	16.13
01/22/08	71010	301	00260	87.00	19.70	51.17	16.13
01/22/08	72040	320	00260	195.00	19.70	159.17	16.13
01/21/08	70450	350	00332	819.00	81.93	657.97	79.10
01/21/08	99285	450	00612 25	605.00	48.60	401.78	154.62
01/21/08	93005	730	0099	21.00	3.45	3.77	13.78

STATEMENT OF CERTIFICATION

This will certify that the above beneficiary-specific Explanation of Benefits (EOB) is a true print out of the Medicare standard format of the American National Standards Institute Accredited Standards Committee (ANSI ASC X12) 835 electronic remittance advice (835). The above EOB contains selected beneficiary-specific data elements from transmission which have not been edited, altered or manipulated in any way in order to support submission of Medicare payment supplemental insurance companies. The 835 remittance is to this provider electronically during the course of ordinary business by the fiscal intermediary.

Exhibit 2.1. 2008 listing of modifiers required for Medicare hospital outpatient services

Modifier(s)/
Official Reporting Guideline

–25   Significant, Separately Identifiable Evaluation and Management Service by the Same Physician on the Same Day of the Procedure or Other Service

Modifier –25 applies only to E/M service codes and then only when an E/M service was provided on the same date as a diagnostic medical/surgical and/or therapeutic medical/surgical procedure(s).

–50   Bilateral Procedure

This modifier is used to report bilateral procedures performed at the same operative session as a single line item. The appropriate five-digit code describing the first procedure should be reported. The performance of a second (bilateral) procedure is indicated by adding modifier –50 to the procedure code. Two line items must not be submitted to report a bilateral procedure.

–52   Reduced Services

Modifier –52 is used in those situations where discontinued procedure modifier –73 or modifier –74 would have been appropriate, but because the use of local, regional, or general anesthesia was not an inherent part of performing the procedure, modifier –52 is used to show that the procedure was discontinued. Modifier –52 is not used when a code is used to classify the extent of the procedure performed. If no code exists for what has been done, the intended code should be reported with modifier –52.

–58   Staged or Related Procedure or Service by the Same Physician During the Postoperative Period

Modifier –58 is reported to indicate the performance of a procedure or service during the same calendar day postoperative period. Modifier –58 should be reported for a procedure or service that is "planned prospectively at the time of the original procedure (staged); more extensive than the original procedure; or for therapy following a diagnostic surgical procedure."

–59   Distinct Procedural Service

Modifier –59 is used to identify procedures/services that are not normally reported together but may be performed under certain circumstances. This may represent a different session or patient encounter, different procedure or surgery, different site or organ system, separate incision, or separate injury (or area of injury in extensive injuries) not ordinarily encountered or performed on the same day by the same physician. This modifier is used to indicate that a procedure or service was distinct or independent from other services performed on the same day.

–73   Discontinued Outpatient Hospital Surgical Procedure (ASC) or Diagnostic Procedure/Service Prior to the Administration of Anesthesia

Modifier –73 is used for surgical procedures for which anesthesia (general, regional, or local) is planned and the procedure is discontinued *after* the patient has been prepared for the procedure and/or *before* the induction of anesthesia.

–74   Discontinued Outpatient Hospital/Ambulatory Surgery Center Procedure After Administration of Anesthesia

Modifier –74 is used for surgical procedures for which anesthesia (general, regional, or local) is planned and the procedure is discontinued *after* the administration of anesthesia.

–76   Repeat Procedure by Same Physician

This modifier is used to indicate that a procedure or service was repeated in a separate operative session on the same day. The procedure should be reported once and then again with modifier –76 added. This modifier may be reported for services ordered by physicians, but performed by technicians.

–77   Repeat Procedure by Another Physician

Modifier –77 is used to indicate that a basic procedure performed by another physician had to be repeated in a separate operative session on the same day. The procedure should be reported once and then again with modifier –77 added. This modifier may be reported for services ordered by physicians, but performed by technicians.

Exhibit 2.1.   (Continued)

–78	Return to the Operating Room for a Related Procedure During the Postoperative Period

Modifier –78 is used to indicate that another procedure was performed during the postoperative period of the initial procedure that was performed earlier in the same day. This modifier should be reported when the subsequent procedure relates to the first procedure and the subsequent procedure requires use of an operating room.

–79   Unrelated Procedure or Service by the Same Physician During the Postoperative Period

Modifier –79 is used to indicate that the performance of a procedure or service by the same physician during the postoperative period was unrelated to the original procedure performed earlier in the day.

–91   Repeat Clinical Diagnostic Laboratory Test

Modifier –91 is intended to identify a laboratory test that is performed more than once on the same day for the same patient when it is necessary to obtain subsequent (multiple) results in the course of the treatment.

–AE   Registered Dietitian

No specific guidelines are available from CMS at the time of publication.

–AF   Specialty Physician

No specific guidelines are available from CMS at the time of publication.

–AG   Primary Physician

No specific guidelines are available from CMS at the time of publication.

–AK   Non-Participating Physician

No specific guidelines are available from CMS at the time of publication.

–AR   Physician Provider Services in a Physician Scarcity Area

Section 413a of the Medicare Prescription Drug, Improvement, and Modernization Act of 2003 (MMA) requires that a new five percent bonus payment be established for physicians in designated physician scarcity areas (PSAs). In some cases, a service may be provided in a county that is considered to be a PSA, but the zip code is not considered to be dominant for that area. The bonus payment cannot automatically be made. In order to receive the bonus for those areas, physicians must include the modifier –AR.

–CA   Procedure Payable Only in the Inpatient Setting When Performed Emergently on an Outpatient Who Dies before Admission

On rare occasions, a procedure on the inpatient list must be performed to resuscitate or stabilize a patient with an emergent, life-threatening condition whose status is that of an outpatient and the patient dies before being admitted as an inpatient. The CMS pays claims with an inpatient list procedure code that is appended to modifier –CA.

–CB   Service Ordered by a Renal Dialysis Facility (RDF) Physician As Part of the ESRD Beneficiary's Dialysis Benefit, Is Not Part of the Composite Rate, and Is Separately Reimbursable

In the *Medicare Claims Processing Manual*, Chapter 16, Laboratory Services, section 40.6.2.3, "Skilled Nursing Facility (SNF) Consolidated Billing (CB) and Separately Billable ESRD Laboratory Tests Furnished to Patients of Independent Dialysis Facilities," CMS has identified the diagnostic services as being commonly furnished to ESRD beneficiaries and payable outside the composite rate.

–CD   AMCC Test Has Been Ordered by an ESRD Facility or MCP Physician That Is Part of the Composite Rate and Is Not Separately Billable

–CE   AMCC Test Has Been Ordered by an ESRD Facility or MCP Physician That Is a Composite Rate But Is beyond the Normal Frequency Covered under the Rate and Is Separately Reimbursable Based on Medical Necessity

(Continued on next page)

Exhibit 2.1. (Continued)

–CF AMCC Test Has Been Ordered by an ESRD Facility or MCP Physician That Is Not Part of the Composite Rate and Is Separately Billable

These three pricing modifiers discretely identify the different payment situations for ESRD AMCC (Automated Multi-Channel Chemistry) tests. Medicare policy provides reimbursement for certain routine clinical diagnostic laboratory tests rendered to an ESRD beneficiary within the composite rate payment to the ESRD facility. Separate payment may be made for the clinical diagnostic laboratory test rendered on a particular date of service when 50 percent or more of the covered tests billed for that particular date of service are noncomposite rate tests. Clinical diagnostic laboratory tests included under the composite rate payment are paid through the composite rate paid by the fiscal intermediary (FI).

–CG Innovator Drug Dispensed

No specific guidelines are available from CMS at the time of publication

–E1 Upper left, eyelid
–E2 Lower left, eyelid
–E3 Upper right, eyelid
–E4 Lower right, eyelid

These modifiers are required to add specificity to the reporting of procedures performed on eyelids. The modifiers may be appended to CPT codes and are used to prevent erroneous denials when duplicate HCPCS codes are billed to report separate procedures performed on different anatomical sites or different sides of the body.

–FA Left hand, thumb
–F1 Left hand, second digit
–F2 Left hand, third digit
–F3 Left hand, fourth digit
–F4 Left hand, fifth digit
–F5 Right hand, thumb
–F6 Right hand, second digit
–F7 Right hand, third digit
–F8 Right hand, fourth digit
–F9 Right hand, fifth digit

These modifiers are required to add specificity to the reporting of procedures performed on fingers. They may be appended to CPT codes and are used to prevent erroneous denials when duplicate HCPCS codes are billed to report separate procedures performed on different anatomical sites or different sides of the body.

–GA Waiver of liability statement on file

Modifier -GA indicates that the provider expected the item or service to be denied as not reasonable and necessary and gave an advance beneficiary notice (ABN) to the beneficiary. This modifier is used for the so-called medical necessity denials.

–GF Non-Physician (for example, Nurse Practitioner [NP], Certified Registered Nurse Anesthetist [CRNA], Certified Registered Nurse [CRN], Clinical Nurse Specialist [CNS], Physician Assistant [PA]) services in a critical access hospital

If a professional service is performed by a non physician, modifier –GF is appended next to the HCPCS code for the professional service. The Critical Access Hospital (CAH) will receive 115 percent of 85 percent of the physician fee schedule for these services. (Note: CAHs are excluded from the outpatient PPS because they are paid under a reasonable cost-based system). This modifier is not to be used for CRNA services.

Exhibit 2.1. (Continued)

–GG	Performance and payment of a screening mammogram and diagnostic mammogram on the same patient, same day

Radiologists who interpret screening mammographies are allowed to order and interpret additional films based on the results of the screening mammogram while a beneficiary is still at the facility for the exam. When the radiologist's interpretation results in additional films, Medicare pays for both the screening and the diagnostic mammogram. Modifier –GG should be appended to the diagnostic mammogram code.

–GN   Service delivered personally by a speech–language pathologist or under an outpatient speech language pathology plan of care

–GO   Service delivered personally by an occupational therapist or under an outpatient occupational therapy plan of care

–GP   Service delivered personally by a physical therapist or under an outpatient physical therapy plan of care

These modifiers are used to identify the therapist who provided the therapy service(s).

–GY   Item or service statutorily excluded or does not meet the definition of any Medicare benefit

Modifier –GY is used for the so-called statutory exclusions or categorical exclusions and the technical denials. There are no advance beneficiary notice (ABN) requirements for statutory exclusions or for technical denials except three types of durable medical equipment, prosthetics, orthotics, and supplies (DME-POS) denials.

–GZ   Item or Service Expected to Be Denied as Not Reasonable and Necessary

Modifier –GZ identifies an item or service expected to be denied as not reasonable and necessary when an advance beneficiary notice (ABN) was not signed by the beneficiary. This modifier is used for the so-called medical necessity denials. It is available for providers when they know that an ABN should have been signed but was not and do not want any risk of allegation of fraud or abuse for claiming services that are not medically necessary. By using the –GZ modifier, the provider notifies Medicare that it expects that Medicare will not cover the service and the provider wants to greatly reduce the risk of a mistaken allegation of fraud or abuse.

–KC   Replacement of Special Power Wheelchair Interface

HCPCS Level II codes E2320–E2330 for special power wheelchair interfaces were added to the HCPCS listing effective January 1, 2004. The fee schedule amounts for these codes were calculated based on pricing for the differential cost of furnishing these special interfaces over a standard interface that is paid for as part of the payment for the wheelchair. However, when these items are furnished to replace existing interfaces on wheelchairs that have been in use by the patient for a period of time due to a change in the patient's medical condition or in cases where the existing interface is irreparably damaged or has exceeded its reasonable useful lifetime, the fee schedule payment should reflect payment for the full cost of the replacement special interface. Fee schedule amounts for replacement of special power wheelchair interfaces were established effective January 1, 2005, for use in paying claims for codes E2320–E2330 billed with the –KC modifier.

–KD   Infusion Drugs Furnished Through Implanted DME

In the *Medicare Claims Processing Manual*, Chapter 17, Drugs and Biologicals, section 20.3, "Detailed Procedures for Determining AWPs and the Drug Payment Allowance Limits," CMS provides the 2004 payment limit for drugs when infused through DME.

–KF   Item Designated by FDA as Class III Device

CMS Manual System Pub. 100-20 One-Time Notification, Transmittal 35 (December 24, 2003) provides a listing of the HCPCS codes for DME classified as class III devices by the FDA.

(Continued on next page)

Exhibit 2.1.   (Continued)

–KZ	New Coverage Not Implemented by Managed Care

When Medicare expands coverage of a specific service/procedure, this modifier and/or UB-04 claim form condition code 78 (new coverage not yet implemented by HMO) is used to pay providers on a fee-for-service basis, until the new capitation rates to Medicare+Choice (M+C) organizations are in effect to include the cost of expanded coverage. Contact your fiscal intermediary (FI) for more information.

–LC	Left circumflex coronary artery (for CPT codes 92980–92982, 92995 and 92996)
–LD	Left anterior descending coronary (for CPT codes 92980–92982, 92995 and 92996)

These modifiers are required to add specificity to the reporting of procedures performed on coronary arteries. These modifiers may be appended to CPT codes and are used to prevent erroneous denials when duplicate HCPCS codes are billed to report separate procedures performed on different anatomical sites within the coronary circulation.

–LT	Left side

Modifier –LT is applied to codes that identify procedures that can be performed on contralateral anatomic sites (joints, bones) or paired organs, extremities, and structures (for example, ears, eyes, nasal passages), kidneys, lungs, ureters, and ovaries. It is required when the procedure is performed on only one side to identify the side operated on.

–QM	Ambulance service provided under arrangement by a provider of services

–QN	Ambulance service furnished directly by a provider of services

These modifiers are used to ensure accurate payment under the Medicare ambulance services fee schedule.

–RC	Right coronary artery (for CPT codes 92980–92982, 92995, and 92996)

These modifiers are required to add specificity to the reporting of procedures performed on coronary arteries. These modifiers may be appended to CPT codes and are used to prevent erroneous denials when duplicate HCPCS codes are billed to report separate procedures performed on different anatomical sites within the coronary circulation.

–RT	Right side

Modifier –RT is applied to codes that identify procedures that can be performed on contralateral anatomic sites (joints, bones) or on paired organs, extremities and structures (for example, ears, eyes, nasal passages), kidneys, lungs, ureters, and ovaries. It is required when the procedure is performed on only one side to identify the side operated on.

–SM	Second Surgical Opinion

No specific guidelines are available from CMS at the time of publication.

–SQ	Item Ordered by Home Health

No specific guidelines are available from CMS at the time of publication.

–SW	Services Provided by a Certified Diabetic Educator

No specific guidelines are available from CMS at the time of publication.

–SY	Persons Who Are In Close Contact with Member of High-Risk Population (use only with codes for immunization)

No specific guidelines are available from CMS at the time of publication

–TA	Left foot, great toe

Exhibit 2.1. (Continued)

–T1	Left foot, second digit
–T2	Left foot, third digit
–T3	Left foot, fourth digit
–T4	Left foot, fifth digit
–T5	Right foot, great toe
–T6	Right foot, second digit
–T7	Right foot, third digit
–T8	Right foot, fourth digit
–T9	Right foot, fifth digit

These modifiers are required to add specificity to the reporting of procedures performed on toes. These modifiers may be appended to CPT codes and are used to prevent erroneous denials when duplicate HCPCS codes are billed to report separate procedures performed on different anatomical sites or different sides of the body.

–UF	Services provided in the morning
–UG	Services provided in the afternoon
–UH	Services provided in the evening
–UJ	Services provided at night
–UK	Services provided on behalf of the client to someone other than the client

The CMS has not yet published guidelines for these modifiers.

–UN	Two patients served
–UP	Three patients served
–UQ	Four patients served
–UR	Five patients served
–US	Six or more patients served

These five portable x-ray Level II HCPCS modifiers are for use with only HCPCS code R0075, Transportation of portable x-ray equipment and personnel to home or nursing home, per trip to facility or location, more than one patient seen. One of them must be reported with HCPCS code R0075, and only one may be used at a time.

Only a single transportation payment for each trip the portable x-ray supplier makes to a particular location (for example, nursing home) is allowed. When reporting a transportation service and more than one Medicare patient is x-rayed at the same location, payment for R0075 is prorated among all patients receiving the services.

Exhibit 2.2.   January 2008 Medicare Outpatient Code Editor (OCE) edits

Edit #	OCE Edit	How Edit is Triggered
1	Invalid diagnosis code	
2	Diagnosis and age conflict	Diagnosis code includes an age range, and age is outside that range. The OCE detects inconsistencies between a patient's age and any diagnosis on the claim.
3	Diagnosis and sex conflict	Diagnosis code includes sex designation, and sex does not match. The OCE detects inconsistencies between a patient's sex and any diagnosis on the claim.
4	Medicare Secondary Payer Alert [a, b]	The procedure code has a MSP warning alert indicator.
5	E-code as reason for visit	First letter of the first listed diagnosis code is an E. E-codes are ICD-9 diagnosis codes that begin with an E. They describe the circumstances that caused an injury, not the nature of the injury, and therefore, are not accepted by OCE as a principal diagnosis.
6	Invalid procedure code	HCPCS code is not found in the HCPCS table for the selected OCE version. The OCE checks each HCPCS procedure code against a table of valid HCPCS codes for the time period shown on the claim. If the reported code is not in this table, the code is considered invalid.
7	Procedure and age conflict[c]	Procedure code includes an age range, and age is outside the range. The OCE detects inconsistencies between a patient's age and any HCPCS procedure code on the claim. For example, it is clinically impossible for seventy-eight year old women to deliver a baby. Therefore, either the procedure or age is incorrect.
8	Procedure and sex conflict	Procedure code includes sex designation, and sex does not match. The OCE detects inconsistencies between a patient's sex and any HCPCS procedure code on the claim.
9	Non-covered for reasons other than statute	Non-covered service indicator is on for this procedure code. The OCE identifies services that are never paid under the Medicare program.
10	Service submitted for denial (condition code 21)	The OCE identifies claims billed by a provider for a denial notice and flag the claim for denial.
11	Service submitted for FI/MAC review (condition code 20)	The OCE identifies non-covered claims billed by a provider when a beneficiary requests a Medicare coverage determination, and suspends the claims for FI action.
12	Questionable covered service	The OCE identifies procedures that are only covered by the Medicare program under certain medical circumstances.
13	Separate payment for services is not provided by Medicare (v1.0–v6.30 only)	The OCE detects codes that are not reportable to Medicare, but may be reportable to other insurers. These codes will now pass through the FI claim system, but will not be paid.
14	Code indicates a site of service is not included in OPPS(v1.0–v6.30 only)	The OCE edits for HCPCS codes that describe services not performed in the provider's setting.
15	Service unit out of range for procedure[d,e]	The OCE edits the claim to identify number of units that are clinically impossible or unreasonable for the service billed.
16	Multiple bilateral procedure without modifier 50 (v1.0–v6.30 only)	The OCE identifies HCPCS codes that can be performed bilaterally when the code is billed on more than one line for a single date of service if modifier –50 is not on any of the lines. For example, if the physician performed HCPCS 25066 (Biopsy, soft tissue of forearm and/or wrist; deep) on both the right and left wrist, 25066 should not be on two lines. The correct way to bill the biopsy is on one line with 2506650.

Exhibit 2.2.   (Continued)

Edit #	OCE Edit	How Edit is Triggered
17	Inappropriate specification of bilateral procedure	The OCE identifies HCPCS codes that can be performed bilaterally if the code is billed on more than one line for the same date of service when all or some lines include modifier –50. An example claim might have three lines with HCPCS 29821 (Arthroscopy, shoulder, surgical; synovectomy, complete). 29821 on one line, 2982150 on another line, and 2982150 on a third line. This is incorrect billing and reflects improper use of modifier –50. This edit will also identify when a procedure with "bilateral" in its HCPCS definition is billed on more than one line.
18	Inpatient procedure[f]	Service indicator is C for the procedure code. Note: All line items that occur on the same day as this one, and that do not already have the line item flag set to 1, will have their line item denial flag set to 2. CMS has established a list of procedures that are excluded from OPPS and are paid by Medicare only when performed in an inpatient setting. Performing these procedures in an outpatient setting is considered not reasonable and necessary. OCE identifies these procedures when they are billed on an outpatient claim. Inpatient procedures are listed in Addendum E of the OPPS Final Rule. In addendum B of the OPPS Final Rule, these procedures are assigned status indicator "C."
19	Mutually exclusive procedure that is not allowed by NCCI even if appropriate modifier is present	The OCE uses CCI edits to identify mutually exclusive procedures. Mutually exclusive procedures are those that cannot be performed during the same session. This edit will identify procedures that are always mutually exclusive. These procedures would never be performed on the same day.
20	Code 2 of a code pair that is not allowed by NCCI even if appropriate modifier is present	The OCE uses CCI edits to identify components of a procedure that are billed on the same date of service as the comprehensive procedure. Services that are normally part of a procedure cannot be billed separately, but rather are considered to be included in the code for the more comprehensive procedure. This edit will identify procedures that are always components of the comprehensive procedure and should never be billed with it. This edit is applied to HCPCS code combinations where one of the codes is a component of the more comprehensive code. In this instance, only the comprehensive code is paid.
21	Medical visit on same day as a type T or S procedure without modifier 25	The OCE detects when an evaluation and management (E/M) code is billed on the same day as a type S (significant procedure) or T (surgical service to which multiple procedure payment reduction applies) procedure.
22	Invalid modifier	The OCE checks each modifier against a table of valid modifiers for the time period shown on the claim. If the reported modifier is not in this table, it is considered invalid.
23	Invalid date	The OCE checks the dates on the claim for validity. This edit occurs if there is no date on the claim or if the date is not within the normal calendar range. For example, the date 033200 is invalid since there are not 32 days in March.
24	Date out of OCE range	From date is not within range of any version of the OCE program. The OCE checks the "from" date of the claim and applies this edit if the dates of service are prior to July 1, 1987. The OCE was not established until this date. This edit is used to assist internal FI operations.
25	Invalid age	If the age reported is not between 0 years and 124 years, the OCE assumes the age is in error. If the beneficiary's age is established at over 124, it must be re-entered as 123.

(Continued on next page)

Exhibit 2.2. (Continued)

Edit #	OCE Edit	How Edit is Triggered
26	Invalid sex	The sex code reported must be either "M" for male or "F" for female. If anything else is entered on the claim, it is invalid.
27	Only incidental services reported[g]	The OCE determines if the only items billed on a date of service are incidental services, for example anesthesia or supplies. Under OPPS, these services are packaged and only reimbursed as part of the service/procedure performed. Incidental services are assigned status indicator "N."
28	Code not recognized by Medicare; alternate code for same service available	The OCE identifies codes that are not reportable to Medicare because Medicare requires that an alternate code, usually a HCPCS Level II code, be used.
29	Partial hospitalization service for non-mental health diagnosis	The OCE edits a partial hospitalization claim for a mental health diagnosis. Partial hospitalization claims must include a mental health diagnosis since these programs are for patients who have profound and disabling mental health conditions.
30	Insufficient services on day of partial hospitalization	Partial hospitalization programs are designed to provide individualized, coordinated, comprehensive, and multidisciplinary treatment program. The OCE identifies a date of service on a claim that –Does not have a psychotherapy code. –Contains less than three partial hospitalization HCPCS codes.
31	Partial hospitalization on same day as electroconvulsive therapy or type T procedure (v1.0–v6.30 only)	The OCE identifies dates of service on a claim where the patient has received electroconvulsive therapy (ECT) or a surgical service on the same day as partial hospitalization services.
32	Partial hospitalization claim spans 3 days or less with insufficient services, or electroconvulsive or significant procedure on at least one of the days	This edit combines edits (30) and (31) for partial hospitalization claims with "from" and "through" dates spanning two or three dates of service. The OCE detects that ECT or a procedure is billed on the same day as partial hospitalization services, or that a low intensity of services is billed.
33	Partial hospitalization claim spans more than 3 days with insufficient number of days having mental services.	A claim suspended for medical review (edit 30 or 31) spans more than three days but mental health services were not provided in at least 57% (4/7) of the days. Because partial hospitalization is provided in lieu of inpatient psychiatric care, patients require an intensive treatment program. The OCE determines if a claim with "from" and "through" dates that span more than three days is billed with less than four out of seven days containing partial hospitalization services.
34	Partial hospitalization claim spans more than 3 days with insufficient number of days meeting partial hospitalization criteria	This edit combines edits (30) and (31) for partial hospitalization claims with "from" and "through" dates spanning more than three days. It will determine if the claim as a whole reflects an intensity of services expected in a partial hospitalization program.
35	Only mental health education and training services provided	Occupational therapy (OT) is covered when it is part of an overall active treatment plan for a patient with a diagnosed psychiatric illness. Outpatient psychiatric treatment programs that consist entirely of activity therapy (AT) are not covered. The OCE applies this edit to claims for outpatient hospital psychiatric services when AT or OT are the *only* services billed. The claim will not be selected by this edit if AT or OT is billed on the same day as other outpatient hospital psychiatric services.
36	Extensive mental health services provided on day of electroconvulsive therapy or type T procedure	The OCE identifies dates of service on an outpatient psychiatric services claim where the patient has received ECT or a procedure on the same day they received extensive mental health services. This edit is similar to partial hospitalization edit number (31), but applies to non-partial hospitalization claims.

Exhibit 2.2. (Continued)

Edit #	OCE Edit	How Edit is Triggered
37	Terminated bilateral procedure or terminated procedure with units greater than one	The OCE identifies lines where a terminated procedure contains modifier –50 or has units greater than one. This reflects incorrect billing. When a procedure is terminated, the first procedure that was planned should be reported with the appropriate modifier (73 or 74). Any other procedure is not reported.
38	Inconsistency between implanted device or administrative substance and implantation procedure or associated procedure	The OCE identifies claims where the implanted device does not match the type of procedure performed. Either the procedure or the implant was billed incorrectly.
39	Mutually exclusive procedure that would be allowed by NCCI if appropriate modifier were present	The OCE uses CCI edits to identify procedures that are mutually exclusive unless billed with a modifier to explain the circumstances. This edit applies to HCPCS code combinations where one of the codes is considered to be either impossible or improbable to be performed with the other code. This edit pays the lower priced service.
40	Code 2 of a code pair that would be allowed by NCCI if appropriate modifier were present	The OCE detects components of a procedure that are billed on the same date of service as the comprehensive procedure. This edit identifies procedures that could possibly be billed together if a modifier was present on one of the procedures. This edit is applied to HCPCS code combinations where one of the codes is a component of the more comprehensive code. In this instance, only the comprehensive code is paid.
41	Invalid revenue code	The OCE checks each revenue code against a table of valid revenue codes for the time period shown on the claim. If the reported revenue code is not in this table, it is considered invalid.
42	Multiple medical visits on same day with same revenue code without condition code G0	If multiple medical visits, for example, E/M services, are billed with the same revenue code, condition code G0 is required to indicate that a separate visit was made on the date of service in question.
43	Transfusion or blood product exchange without specification of blood product.	A blood transfusion or exchange is coded, but no blood product is coded.
44	Observation revenue code on line item with non-observation HCPCS code	A 762 (observation) revenue code is used with a HCPCS other than blank or observation code (99217–99220, 99234–99236).
45	Inpatient separate procedures not paid	On the same day, all lines with status indicator C are on the "separate procedure" list, and there is at least one status indicator T line item.
46	Partial hospitalization condition code 41 not approved for type of bill.	Bill type 12x or 14x is present with (partial hospitalization) condition code 41.
47	Service is not separately payable	The claim consists entirely of a combination of line items that: are denied or rejected OR have a status indicator of "N."
48	Revenue center requires HCPCS	The bill type is 13X, 74X, 75X, 76X, or 12X or 14X is present with condition code 41.
49	Service on same day as inpatient procedure[h]	Line item occurs on the same day as a C status indicator.
50	Non-covered based on statutory exclusion[h]	Code is on 'statutory exclusion' list.
51	Multiple observations overlap in time[c]	Not yet applicable.

(Continued on next page)

Exhibit 2.2. (Continued)

Edit #	OCE Edit	How Edit is Triggered
52	Observation does not meet minimum hours, qualifying diagnoses, and/or T procedure conditions (v3.0–v6.30 only)[h]	The observation period is less than 8 hours, or there is not an E/M visit on the same or previous day as the observation, or there is a status indicator T procedure on the same or previous day, or certain clinical criteria are not met.
53	Codes G0378 or G0379 only allowed with bill type 13X or 85X[e]	Code G0378 or G0379 appears on the claim and the bill type is not 13X or 85X.
54	Multiple codes for the same service[h]	Any of the following three pairs of codes appear on the same claim: C1012 and P9033, C1013 and P9031, or C1014 and P9035.
55	Non-reportable for site of service[i]	A HCPCS code beginning with the letter "C" is entered and the bill type is not 12X, 13X or 14X.
56	E/M conditions not met and line item date for OBS code G0244 <u>is not</u> 12/31 or 1/1 (v4.0–v6.30)	There is no E/M visit the day of or the day preceding the observation. AND The date of observation is not 12/31/XX or 01/01/XX.
57	E/M condition not met and line item date for OBS code G0244 is 12/31 or 1/1 (v4.0–6.30 only)	There is no E/M visit the day of or the day preceding the observation. OR AND The date of observation is 12/31/XX or 01/01/XX.
58	G0378 only allowed with G0379[i]	Code G0379 is present without code G0378 for the same line item date OR Code G0378 is present with code G0379 AND Edit 52, 56 or 57 is assigned.
59	Clinical trial requires diagnosis code V707 as other than primary diagnosis[i]	Code G0292, G0293 or G0294 is present AND Diagnosis code V707 is not present as admit or secondary diagnosis.
60	Use of modifier CA with more than one procedure not allowed[i]	Modifier CA is present on more than one line item with status indicator C OR Modifier CA is submitted on a line item with multiple units.
61	Service can only be billed to the Durable Medical Equipment Regional Carrier/DMERC[j]	The procedure code has a "DME only" indicator.
62	Code not recognized by Outpatient Prospective Payment System/OPPS; alternate code for same service may be available[j]	The procedure code has a Not recognized by Medicare for OPPS indicator
63	This occupational therapy/OT code only billed on partial hospitalization claims[j]	Occupational therapy services are present and the bill type is 12X, 13X, or 14X without condition code 41
64	Activity therapy/AT not payable outside the partial hospitalization program[j]	Activity therapy services are present and the bill type is 12X, 13X, or 14X without condition code 41.
65	Revenue code not recognized by Medicare[k]	The revenue code is 100X, 210X, 310X, or 0905–0907; also see edit 48.
66	Code requires manual pricing[k]	The HCPCS code is an unclassified drug code.
67	Service provided prior to FDA approval[k]	The line item date of service of a code is prior to the date of FDA approval.
68	Service provided prior to date of National Coverage Determination (NCD) approval[l]	The line item date of service of a code is prior to the code activation date.
69	Service provided outside approval period[l]	The service was provided outside the period approved by CMS.

Exhibit 2.2.   (Continued)

Edit #	OCE Edit	How Edit is Triggered
70	CA modifier requires patient status code 20	If modifier CA is submitted with an inpatient-only procedure for a patient who did not expire (patient status code is not 20), the claim is returned to the provider.
71	Claim lacks required device code	The use of a device, or multiple devices, is necessary to the performance of certain outpatient procedures. If any of these procedures is submitted without a code for the required device(s), the claim is returned. Discontinued procedures (indicated by the presence of modifier 52, 73 or 74 on the line) are not returned for a missing device code. Conversely, some devices are allowed only with certain procedures, whether or not the specific device is required.
72	Service not billable to the Fiscal Intermediary/Medicare Administrative Contractor	Use of Status Indicator "M" is for services not billable to FI/MAC
73	Incorrect billing of blood and blood products	Return to provider
74	Units greater than one for bilateral procedure billed with modifier 50	Return to provider
75	Incorrect billing of modifier FB or FC	Expand edit 75 to apply to modifier FC in addition to FB—to trigger if modifier FB or FC is appended to a code with status indicator other than S, T, X or V.
76	Trauma response critical care code with revenue code 068x and CPT 99291	Submission of the trauma response critical care code requires that the trauma revenue code (068x) and the critical care E/M code (99291) also be present on the claim for the same date of service. Otherwise, the trauma response critical care code will be rejected.
77	Claim lacks allowed procedure code	Return to provider
78	Claim lacks required radiopharmaceutical	Return to provider

[a] - OCE version 1.0 and version 1.1 only.

[b] - Not applicable for admit diagnosis.

[c] - Not activated.

[d] - Units for all line items with the same HCPCS code are added together when applying this edit. If the total units exceed the code's limits, the procedure edit return buffer is set for all line items that have the HCPCS code. If modifier –91 is present on a line item and the HCPCS code is on a list of codes that are exempt, the unit edits are not applied.

[e] - OCE version 1.0 through version 2.2 only.

[f] - All other line items on the same day as the line with a "C" service indicator are denied (line item/rejection flag = 1, APC return buffer) and edit 49 is assigned. Edit 18 is performed before any other non-fatal edits. No other edits are run on any line(s) with edit 18 or 49.

[g] - Edit 27 is performed immediately following edit 18 if edit 18 has not been triggered. No other edits will be performed on any claim where edit 27 has been assigned.

[h] - Activated version 3.0

[i] - Activated version 3.1

[j] - Activated version 5.0

[k] - Activated version 5.2

[l] - Activated version 6.0

[m] - Activated version 6.3

Part II

Coding under OPPS

Chapter 3

Integumentary System

CPT codes 10040 through 19499 are used to report surgical and related procedures performed on the integumentary system, which includes the skin, subcutaneous and accessory structures, nails, and breast. Common outpatient procedures involving the integumentary system include wound repair, skin grafts, and certain breast procedures such as aspirations, biopsies, implants, and partial mastectomies. See Figure 3.1 for example of structure of the skin.

Figure 3.1.   Structure of skin

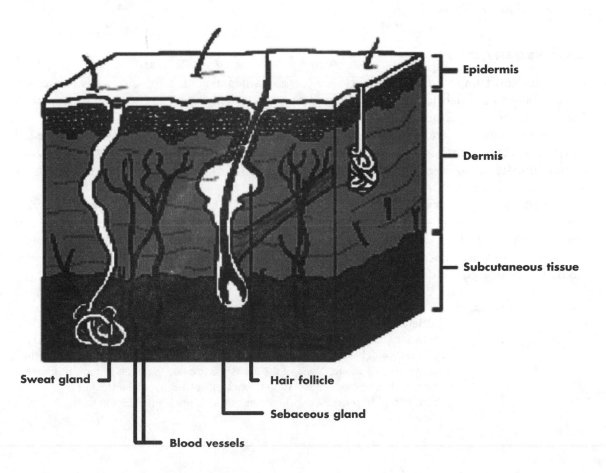

Incision and Drainage

Incision and drainage, or I&D, is a common treatment for skin infections and abscesses. An I&D is performed by first numbing the area with local anesthetic. A scalpel is inserted into the skin overlying the pus, and the pus is drained. I&Ds are commonly performed to treat abscesses and more specifically: carbuncle, suppurative hidradenitis, cutaneous or subcutaneous abscess, cyst, furuncle, paronychia, hematoma, foreign body, and postoperative wound infection.

APC	HCPCS	HCPCS Description	SI	Rel. Wt.	Payment Rate	OPPS OCE
0006			T	1.4066	89.59	
	10060	Drainage of skin abscess				Significant Procedure, Multiple Reduction Applies; Separate APC payment

Coding Guidelines for I&D

Codes for I&D vary based on type of abscess and whether the procedure is simple or single, complicated or multiple. While there is no one specific answer in defining simple vs. complex or complicated in CPT, for I&D procedures, a complicated case may involve the use of drains or packing, as opposed to a simple incision into the abscess itself, with no requirement for further intervention. The most common type of I&D performed is on abscesses of the skin. Codes 10040–10180 are to be reported for I&D procedures.

Debridement

One of the most important determinations necessary when assigning these codes is to ascertain whether a separate debridement code should be reported. In the CPT 2008 manual under the Repair (Closure) guidelines, the following paragraph appears:

"Decontamination and/or debridement: Debridement is considered a separate procedure only when gross contamination requires prolonged cleansing, when appreciable amounts of devitalized or contaminated tissue are removed, or when debridement is carried out separately without immediate primary closure."

A certain amount of debridement is typically included in wound laceration repair services, particularly if the wound edges aren't "clean" and do not lie close together, affording a neat suture line that will easily heal with a good cosmetic outcome. The physician may document that the "wound edges were cleaned, debrided and then closed with sutures," but this type of debridement would be considered included in the wound closure CPT code.

Example: A patient seen in the emergency department (ED) after a ATV accident. The patient has a "road rash" on the arm, which involves multiple small superficial abrasions that are dirty and may contain road gravel and dirt. The physician performs a debridement, removing the superficial skin layer(s), along with the contaminated tissue. None of the abrasions are deep enough to require suture closure. In this case, code 11040 (Debridement; skin, partial thickness) should be reported to reflect a debridement of the skin with partial thickness.

The other critical piece of information necessary to code debridement appropriately is the depth of the debridement procedure. The physician must specify whether it involved partial skin, full-thickness skin, subcutaneous tissue, muscle and/or bone. If this information is not present, the physician should be queried; otherwise, only the most superficial debridement code (11040) may be reported.

Removal of Skin Tags

Skin tags may be associated with seborrheic keratosis, a benign hyperkeratotic lesion of the epidermis. Due to the benign nature of skin tags, they rarely require pathologic examination. In the majority of cases, skin tags are asymptomatic, benign, and require no intervention. In some limited cases, skin tags may be subject to repeated local trauma or irritation resulting in chronic inflammation, pain, bleeding, or localized infection. In these situations intervention may be medically necessary.

Surgical treatment of skin tags includes excision with scissors, cautery, or cryotherapy with liquid nitrogen. Skin tag removal is considered cosmetic in nature and not medically necessary when performed solely to improve appearance or to treat psychological symptomatology or psychosocial complaints.

HCPCS	HCPCS DESCRIPTION
11200	Removal of skin tags, multiple fibro tags, any area, up to and including 15 lesions
11201 (Add on code)	Each additional ten lesions

Use 11201 in conjunction with 11200.

Lesion Excision

A lesion refers to a break in the skin or to any pathological or traumatic structural change in a body part. Lesion excisions are commonly performed to remove tumors, skin cancers, cysts, warts, and recurrent infections.

Coding Guidelines for Lesion Excision

Codes for lesion excision vary according to the size of the lesion. The excision code is determined by the diameter of the actual excision, not by the specimen received in pathology. Measurements must be precise because an error of just one millimeter can result in the selection of an incorrect code. When more than one dimension of a lesion is provided (as when a lesion is asymmetrical or irregular), the largest side must be indicated. For example, when a lesion's dimensions are described as 2 x 1.2 x 0.5 cm, it should be listed as 2 cm. (AMA 1995; 1998b).

Code selection is determined by using the measurement of the greatest clinical diameter of the apparent lesion plus the margin required for complete excision. The margins refer to the narrowest margin required to excise the lesion adequately, based on the physician's judgment. The measurement of lesion plus margin is made *prior to* excision. The excised diameter is the same whether the surgical defect is repaired in a linear fashion or reconstructed (for example, with a skin graft).

For malignant lesions, when frozen-section pathology shows the margins of excision were not adequate, an additional excision may be necessary for complete tumor removal. Only one code is used to report the additional excision and re-excision(s), based on the final widest excised diameter required for complete tumor removal at the same operative session. To report a re-excision procedure performed to widen margins at a subsequent operative session, codes 11600–11646 are used, as appropriate. Modifier –58 should be appended when the re-excision procedure is performed during the postoperative period of the primary excision procedure. For the hospital OPPS, the postoperative period is the same calendar day as the day of the surgery.

> **Example:** A benign lesion of the trunk measures 1.0 cm, and the margin required to adequately excise the lesion is 0.5 cm on both sides, for a total margin of 1.0 cm. The measurement of lesion plus margin is determined as follows: 1.0 cm + 0.5 cm + 0.5 cm = 2.0 cm. In this case, code 11402, Excision, benign lesion including margins, except skin tag (unless listed elsewhere), trunk, arms, or legs; excised diameter 1.1 to 2.0 cm, should be reported to reflect the benign lesion and necessary margin excised from the trunk (AMA 2002f).

Wound Repair

Lacerations are one of the most commonly treated problems in the emergency department. Wound repair techniques range from simple suturing, or stitching, of the wound to debridement and scar revision.

Coding Guidelines for Wound Repair

The integumentary section of the CPT codebook has three categories of wound repair codes: simple, intermediate, and complex. Wound repair codes 12001–13160 classify wound closure utilizing sutures, staples, or tissue adhesives, either singly or in combination with each other or in combination with adhesive strips. A CPT evaluation and management (E/M) code (99201–99499) should be used for wound closure utilizing adhesive strips as the sole repair material.

The lengths of multiple wounds in the same classification (simple, intermediate, complex) should be added together. However, the lengths of different classifications (for example, intermediate and complex repairs) should not be added together. Similarly, the lengths of multiple wounds from all anatomic sites that are grouped together into the same code descriptor should be added together, but the lengths of repairs from different groupings of anatomic sites (for example, face and extremities) should not. When a patient undergoes excision of a benign or malignant lesion, the simple repair of the wound that results from the excision is not coded.

Simple Repair

A simple repair is performed when the wound:

- Is superficial (that is, involves primarily epidermis or dermis, or subcutaneous tissues without significant involvement of deeper structures)
- Requires simple one-layer closure/suturing
- Is not sutured but is treated with chemical or electrocauterization

Excision of benign lesions (11400–11446) and excision of malignant lesions (11600–11646) include simple repair of the wound.

A subcuticular wound closure is a simple repair in which the suture is threaded underneath the skin.

Intermediate Repair

An intermediate repair is performed when the wound requires layered closure of one or more of the deeper subcutaneous tissues and superficial (nonmuscle) fascia, in addition to the skin (epidermal and dermal) closure.

Intermediate repair also includes heavily contaminated wounds that have required extensive cleaning or removal of particulate matter, followed by single-layer closure.

One cannot assume that the term *plastic closure* implies a layer closure and/or an intermediate repair. The type of repair must be verified with the physician. The term *plastic closure* often is used loosely, and the physician may be using it in a different context.

The term *dual-suture wound closure* means that two sutures were used to close a wound. The reason for the dual-suture wound closure must be verified with the physician because an intermediate wound repair code (12031–12057) may or may not be appropriate, as follows:

- When two sutures are used for repair of an irregularly shaped wound (such as an elliptical wound), the closure is in fact a simple repair, not an intermediate one.

- When two sutures are used—and one is an absorbable material such as Vicryl, chromic, gut, or Dexon—an intermediate wound repair is highly probable.

Complex Repair

In complex repair, the wounds require more than layered closure and may involve the following:

- Scar revision
- Debridement, as in traumatic lacerations or avulsions
- Extensive undermining, as in skin grafting
- Stents
- Retention sutures

Necessary preparation for complex repair may include creation of a defect for repairs (for example, excision of a scar requiring a complex repair) or debridement of complicated lacerations or avulsions. Complex repair does not include excision of benign (11400–11446) or malignant (11600–11646) lesions.

Secondary Wound Repair

Codes 12020 and 12021 are assigned for the simple closure or the packing of a simple wound dehiscence, respectively. Code 13160 is required for extensive or complicated secondary closure of a surgical wound or dehiscence.

Skin Grafts

A *skin graft* is a piece of skin transplanted from one part of the body to another to cover an area that is deprived of a covering or protective layer. Skin grafts are identified by size and location of the recipient area and type of graft: free, pedicle flap, or other. Undermining is part of the overall skin grafting procedure and should not be coded separately.

Coding Guidelines for Skin Grafts

The skin graft codes include language that indicates use of the codes according to the total surface area of the repair provided for those body areas addressed by that specific code.

Multiple-site grafting: When multiple sites that are grafted are all identified by the same graft code, the graft code should be used once to identify the complete procedure provided (AMA 2000d).

Repair of graft donor site: A code for repair of the donor site should not be assigned unless skin grafting or local flaps are required to close the donor site.

Preparation of graft recipient site: Codes 15002 and 15004 are used for the excision of open wounds, burn eschar, or scars, and/or the incisional release of scar contractures. Code 15002 applies when these procedures are performed on the trunk, arms, or legs; whereas code 15004, applies to the face, scalp, eyelids, mouth, neck, ears, orbits, genitalia, hands, feet, and/or multiple digits. These codes should be reported for wound site preparation because the purpose of skin grafts is to enhance and promote healing. Therefore, "excisional" preparation of the recipient site is not performed at the time of subsequent graft material placement (AMA 2000a).

Adjacent Tissue Transfer/Rearrangement

Adjacent tissue transfer or rearrangement procedures coded in range 14000–14061 are plastic surgery techniques that use the patient's own tissue and skin for wound repair. These procedures include:

- Z-plasty
- W-plasty
- V-Y plasty
- Rotation flap
- Advancement flap
- Double pedicle

The specific code used is determined by the size (in sq cm) and location of the defect site. Many of the techniques described here are flap procedures. In these procedures, the surgeon lifts a portion of skin and subcutaneous tissue from somewhere on the patient's body (donor site). A portion of this skin and tissue is immediately grafted to a new (recipient) site on the patient's body. The remaining portion of skin and tissue (base) stays partially connected to the donor site until sufficient blood flow and nutrition to the recipient site is established. At that point, the base can be removed and grafted to the recipient site.

Coding Guidelines for Adjacent Tissue Transfer/ Rearrangement

All the adjacent tissue transfer/rearrangement procedures are reported using CPT codes 14000–14350 When a lesion is excised and an adjacent tissue transfer or rearrangement is performed at the same site, excision of the lesion is not reported separately (AMA 1999a, 3). The specific code used is determined by the size and location of the defect site. Codes in the 14000–14350 range require the coder to indicate in square centimeters (sq cm) the size of the defect site to which the adjacent tissue transfer/rearrangement is being applied. To calculate this figure, the coder must multiply the dimensions of the original wound site (for example, a 5 x 4 cm wound is 20 sq cm).

Adjacent tissue transfer actually involves a primary and a secondary "defect," both of which are repaired in the adjacent tissue transfer procedure. By definition, the primary defect is the original defect to be closed and the secondary defect is the defect created by the movement of tissue necessary to close the primary defect.

When another graft or flap is required for closure of the donor site, this is considered an additional procedure and should be reported with a separate CPT code (AMA 1999a, 3).

Destruction of Lesions

The destruction of lesion codes 17000–17004 will be used only for treatment of premalignant lesions. The 17110–17111 codes will be used only for treatment of benign lesions.

For medical necessity coverage of codes 17000–17004, ICD-9-CM code 702.0-Actinic keratosis is required. There is controversy in the academic world regarding actinic keratoses. Some believe they are precancers while others believe they are simply early cancers. All agree they are medically necessary to treat before they become invasive.

For medical necessity coverage of codes 17110–17111, ICD-9-CM codes are reported with the following diagnoses:

216.x	Benign skin lesions
702.1x	Seborrheic keratosis
702.11	Inflamed seborrheic keratosis
078.0	Molluscum contagiosum
078.10	Warts
078.11	Genital warts
706.2	Cyst

In addition to any other benign neoplasm, site-specific codes for the anogenital area and other regions should be used instead if more precise and appropriate. Both ranges of codes 1700x and 1711x are all 10-day global period codes. All can be reported with an E/M, if the E/M is for a separately identifiable service (append Modifier 25), as these codes only describe the destruction of lesions. 1700x and 1711x can be reported on the same patient on the same day when separate diagnoses are appropriate.

Example 1: The physician performed a destruction of two benign lesions at the same session. How is this reported? In this case, code 17110 is used. This same code would cover up to 14 lesions. If the lesions were premalignant, the proper coding would have been 17000 for the first lesion and 17003 for the second.

Example 2: If a very large benign lesion is destroyed, how is it coded? In this case, code 17110 is assigned as size does not matter for these codes.

Example 3: If a patient is treated for 14 actinic keratoses and 9 seborrheic keratoses in the same session, the determination of coding is as follows: Destruction of actinic keratoses would be reported with 17000x1 and 17003x13; the seborrheic keratoses would be reported with; 17110x1.

Under the OPPS, when more than one surgical procedure is performed during a single operative session, the full Medicare payment is made and the beneficiary pays the coinsurance for the procedure having the highest payment rate. Fifty percent payment would be received for the APC with the lowest payment rate.

Moh's Micrographic Surgery

The Moh's process (see Figure 3.2) includes a specific sequence of surgery and pathological investigation. Mohs surgeons examine the removed tissue for evidence of extended cancer roots. Once the visible tumor is removed, Moh's surgeons trace the paths of the tumor using two key tools:

- Map of the surgical site
- Microscope

Once the obvious tumor is removed, the Moh's surgeon:

- Removes an additional, thin layer of tissue from the tumor site
- Creates a "map" or drawing of the removed tissue to be used as a guide to the precise location of any remaining cancer cells
- Microscopically examines the removed tissue thoroughly to check for evidence of remaining cancer cells

If any of the sections contain cancer cells, the Moh's surgeon:

- Returns to the specific area of the tumor site as indicated by the map
- Removes another thin layer of tissue only from the specific area within each section where cancer cells were detected
- Microscopically examines the newly-removed tissue for additional cancer cells

If microscopic analysis still shows evidence of disease, the process continues layer-by-layer until the cancer is completely gone. This selective removal of only diseased tissue allows preservation of much of the surrounding normal tissue. Because this systematic microscopic search reveals the roots of the skin cancer, Moh's surgery offers the highest chance for complete removal of the cancer while sparing the normal tissue. Cure rates exceed 99 percent for new cancers, and 95 percent for recurrent cancers.

Figure 3.2.   Moh's surgery example

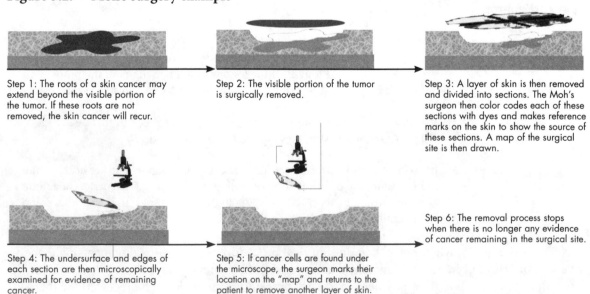

Step 1: The roots of a skin cancer may extend beyond the visible portion of the tumor. If these roots are not removed, the skin cancer will recur.

Step 2: The visible portion of the tumor is surgically removed.

Step 3: A layer of skin is then removed and divided into sections. The Moh's surgeon then color codes each of these sections with dyes and makes reference marks on the skin to show the source of these sections. A map of the surgical site is then drawn.

Step 4: The undersurface and edges of each section are then microscopically examined for evidence of remaining cancer.

Step 5: If cancer cells are found under the microscope, the surgeon marks their location on the "map" and returns to the patient to remove another layer of skin.

Step 6: The removal process stops when there is no longer any evidence of cancer remaining in the surgical site.

(Source: American Medical Association. 2002f (November 14-15)

Reconstruction

The best method of managing the wound resulting from surgery is determined after the cancer is completely removed. When the final defect is known, management is individualized to achieve the best results and to preserve functional capabilities and maximize aesthetics. The Moh's surgeon is also trained in reconstructive procedures and often will perform the reconstructive procedure necessary to repair the wound. A small wound may be allowed to heal on its own, or the wound may be closed with stitches, a skin graft, or a flap. If a tumor is larger than initially anticipated, another surgical specialist with unique skills may complete the reconstruction.

Cost Effectiveness

Besides its high cure rate, Moh's micrographic surgery also has shown to be cost effective. In a study of costs of various types of skin cancer removal, the Mohs process was found to be comparable when compared to the cost of other procedures, such as electrodesiccation and curettage, cryosurgery, excision or radiation therapy. Moh's micrographic surgery preserves the maximum amount of normal skin and results in smaller scars. Repairs are more often simple and involve fewer complicated reconstructive procedures.

With its high cure rate, Moh's surgery minimizes the risk of recurrence and eliminates the costs of larger, more serious surgery for recurrent cancers. Because the Mohs procedure is performed in the surgeon's office and pathological examinations are immediate, the entire process can often be completed in a single day.

Breast Surgery

Surgical procedures are performed on the breast for both diagnostic and treatment purposes. These procedures include aspirations, biopsies, mastectomies, and implants.

- **Puncture aspiration**: Codes 19000 and/or 19001 should be assigned for a puncture aspiration. In this procedure, the physician punctures (pierces) the skin and inserts a needle with a syringe attached into the cyst, which, by definition, is filled with fluid. The fluid contained in the cyst is aspirated (withdrawn) via the needle into a syringe. Pressure is applied to the aspiration site to stop any bleeding.

- **Percutaneous needle core biopsy**: Code 19100 or 19102 should be assigned for a percutaneous needle core biopsy. A stereoscopic x-ray device is used to pinpoint a mass within the breast, and an automated gun is then used to extract the tissue with a large needle. During the procedure, the patient lies face down with one breast protruding through an opening in the examining table. Beneath the table, the x-ray machine and a needle gun, such as a biopsy gun or Bard biopsy gun, are mounted. After a radiologist locates the suspicious mass, the needle gun setting is adjusted, and the large needle is placed slowly into the breast, stopping close to the mass. The gun is fired and a small needle is released to collect tissue for testing.

- **Open incisional biopsy**: Code 19101 is used for an open incisional biopsy. This procedure involves cutting into the lesion areas to obtain a specimen in order to confirm a diagnosis. The entire lesion is not removed.

- **Excisional biopsy**: Code 19120 is assigned for an excisional biopsy, which is designed to remove the entire lesion, whether benign or malignant.

- **Excisional biopsy identified by radiological marker**: Codes 19125, 19126, 19290, and 19291 are used for the removal of an entire lesion(s) that was identified by the preoperative placement of a radiological marker (for example, intravenous dye or needle localization wires).

- **Automated vacuum–assisted or rotating biopsy**: Code 19103 is assigned for an automated vacuum–assisted or rotating biopsy procedure. This is a minimally invasive, image-guided procedure (stereotactic or ultrasound) that helps physicians locate breast abnormalities and obtain tissue samples for diagnosis. The doctor inserts a slender probe into the breast to gently remove questionable tissue, snipping cells off with a tiny rotating blade while the patient lies awake under a local anesthetic.

- **Metallic localization clip**: When a metallic localization clip is placed percutaneously (under image guidance) during the breast biopsy, code 19295 is used in addition to code 19102, Percutaneous needle core biopsy, or code 19101, Automated vacuum assisted/ rotating biopsy.

- **Partial mastectomy/segmental mastectomy**: Code 19301 involves the partial removal of the breast tissue, leaving the breast nearly intact. A wedge of tissue that amounts to approximately one-fourth of the breast (including the overlying skin) is removed. (This procedure is also sometimes called lumpectomy, in which case the coder should confirm that it is, in fact, a partial mastectomy.)

- **Breast implants**: The coding of breast implants varies according to whether the procedure is for the insertion or removal of an implant or implant material.

Coding Guidelines for Breast Surgery

Codes for breast implants include the following:

- Code 19325 for breast augmentation with implant
- Code 19328 for removal of an intact breast implant
- Code 19330 for removal of breast implant material (for example, in the case of a ruptured implant)
- Codes 19340 and 19342 for breast reconstruction with implants

Documentation Requirements for Integumentary System Procedures

The following sections introduce different integumentary system procedures. Each procedure is followed by clinical information that must be documented in the medical record when the procedure is performed.

Excision of Lesions

Excisions of lesions are coded with CPT codes 11300–11313, 11400–11471, 11600–11646.

- The morphology of *each* lesion (for example: benign, premalignant, malignant)
- The dimensions of *each* lesion *plus* the margin required for complete excision of *each* lesion

- The anatomical site of *each* lesion
- The surgical technique used to remove *each* lesion:
  - Excision
  - Shaving
  - Destruction (indicate the method of destruction)
  - Mohs' micrographic surgery (chemosurgery)
- The surgical technique used to close *each* lesion defect site:
  - Adhesive strip application
  - Chemical or electrocauterization
  - Simple repair
  - Layer closure
  - Complex repair
  - Adjacent tissue transfer/rearrangement
  - Split-thickness skin graft
  - Full-thickness skin graft

Wound Repair

Wound repairs are reported with CPT codes 12001–13160.

- The dimensions of *each* wound
- The anatomical site of *each* wound
- The surgical method used to repair *each* wound:
  - Adhesive strip application in combination with other material or as a sole material
  - Chemical or electrocauterization
  - Debridement
  - Simple repair
  - Layer closure
  - Complex repair
  - Secondary wound repair
  - Blood vessel, tendon, nerve repair
  - Ligation and/or exploration of vessels
  - Adjacent tissue transfer/rearrangement
  - Split-thickness skin graft
  - Full-thickness skin graft

Skin Grafts

Skin grafts are reported with CPT codes 15050–15431.

- The type of skin graft (for example, pinch, split-thickness, full-thickness, allograft, xenograft)

- The anatomical site for the donor skin graft
- The surgical technique used to repair the donor site (for example, simple suture, advancement flap, another skin graft)
- The size (in square centimeters) of the defect site (recipient) on which the graft is applied
- The anatomical site (recipient) on which the graft is applied

Breast Biopsy

Breast biopsies are reported with CPT codes 19100–19103, 19120–19272, 19290–19298, 0046T, 0047T, and 0061T.

- Whether or not the biopsy was unilateral or bilateral
- Number of biopsies performed on the breast(s)
- Whether or not imaging guidance was used
- Whether or not radiological marker(s) were used
- Type and number of radiological marker(s) (when used):
  - Needle localization wire
  - Metallic localization clip
  - Other (specify)
- Type of biopsy performed:
  - Catheter lavage of mammary duct (specify number of ducts)
  - Open
  - Percutaneous needle core
  - Percutaneous automated vacuum assisted biopsy
  - Percutaneous rotating biopsy device
  - Excisional (specify number of lesions excised per breast)
  - Microwave phased array thermotherapy

Adjacent Tissue Transfer/Rearrangement

Adjacent tissue transfer/rearrangements are reported with CPT codes 14300–14350.

- The anatomical site of any lesion(s) that is/are excised
- The dimensions in square centimeters of the primary defect (the original defect to be closed)
- The donor site for the adjacent tissue transfer/rearrangement
- The dimensions in square centimeters of the secondary defect (the defect created by the movement of tissue necessary to close the primary defect)
- The type of adjacent tissue transfer/rearrangement performed:
  - Advancement flap
  - V-Y plasty
  - Y-V plasty
  - W plasty
  - Z-plasty

- Rotation flap
- Transpositional flap
- Sliding flap
- Interpolational
- Nasolabial flap
- Other (specify in operative report)
- The technique used to close the donor site for the adjacent tissue transfer/rearrangement

Case Studies

This section contains actual operative reports from real-life cases. All identifiers have been removed or changed for confidentiality and privacy.

Carefully read the clinical documentation in each case study, which may include a procedure report as well as radiology and/or pathology reports, as applicable.

Answer all the review questions at the end of each case study, using a current CPT codebook or HCPCS Level II code listing, as needed.

When appropriate, assign one or more of the following modifiers:

–50	Bilateral Procedure
–59	Distinct Procedural Service
–FA	Left hand, thumb
–F1	Left hand, second digit
–F2	Left hand, third digit
–F3	Left hand, fourth digit
–F4	Left hand, fifth digit
–F5	Right hand, thumb
–F6	Right hand, second digit
–F7	Right hand, third digit
–F8	Right hand, fourth digit
–F9	Right hand, fifth digit
–LT	Left side
–RT	Right side
–TA	Left foot, great toe
–T1	Left foot, second digit
–T2	Left foot, third digit
–T3	Left foot, fourth digit
–T4	Left foot, fifth digit
–T5	Right foot, great toe
–T6	Right foot, second digit
–T7	Right foot, third digit
–T8	Right foot, fourth digit
–T9	Right foot, fifth digit

Do not apply the current version of the Medicare CCI edits to any of these questions; the focus is on the application of the coding guidelines and not on the application of edits that change on a quarterly basis. Of course, when coding in real life, you will need to apply the CCI edits as appropriate for Medicare outpatient cases.

Case Study 3.1

Read the following clinical document and answer the questions for further review.

OPERATIVE REPORT

PREOPERATIVE DIAGNOSIS: Multiple soft tissue masses to the leg

POSTOPERATIVE DIAGNOSIS: Multiple soft tissue masses to the leg

OPERATION: Excision biopsy

ANESTHESIA: Local

ESTIMATED BLOOD LOSS: 5 cc

PROCEDURE/FINDINGS: The patient identified the lesions of concern. Two were on the right leg and one on the left leg. All areas were prepped with sterile DuraPrep and draped in a sterile fashion. Starting on the right area over the greater trochanter, the skin was infiltrated with 0.5% Marcaine with epinephrine. Ultimately, a total of 30 cc was used. Beginning over the right trochanter, a longitudinal incision was made and a 3.5 cm lipomatous mass was removed by blunt dissection. Hemostasis was achieved with electrocautery, and the wound was closed with 3-0 Vicryl, benzoin, and tape closures. On the right anterior thigh, a 3-cm lipomatous mass was removed and the closure was the same as the first. On the left anterior thigh, a 2.5-cm lipomatous mass was removed. This was closed with 4-0 Vicryl, benzoin, and tape closures. There was no evidence of bleeding at the time of closure. Sponge and needle counts correct. The patient tolerated the procedure well and returned to the recovery room awake and in stable condition.

PATHOLOGY REPORT

AGE/SEX: 41/M

STATUS: Reg SDC

SPEC TYPE: Surgical

PREOPERATIVE DIAGNOSIS: Multiple soft tissue masses right and left legs

OPERATION PERFORMED

Procedure: Bilateral excision mass, excisions soft tissue masses

TISSUE REMOVED
A. Rt upper soft tissue mass
B. Rt lower soft tissue mass
C. Lt upper thigh soft tissue mass

OFFICE DESCRIPTION
Part A received labeled right upper soft tissue mass. The specimen consists of a 2.8 x 2.3 x 1 cm pink-to-yellow singly capsulated adipose tissue mass with a yellow lobulated cut surface. Representative sections are submitted in A.

Part B received labeled right lower leg soft tissue. The specimen consists of a 0.6 x 2.3 x 1 cm pink-to-yellow singly capsulated adipose tissue mass with a pink-to-yellow slightly lobulated cut surface. Representative sections are submitted in B.

Part C received labeled left upper thigh, 2.5-cm soft tissue mass. The specimen consists of a 2.3 x 1.2 x 0.8 cm pink-to-yellow semicapsulated adipose tissue mass with pink-to-tan slightly lobulated cut surface. All blocked in C.

PATH PROCEDURES

Procedures: PATH DCPX/3, A1 BLK, B1 BLK, C1 BLK

FINAL DIAGNOSIS: Part A, B C: Soft tissue, upper and lower right leg, upper thigh left leg

BIOPSIES: Mature adipose tissue consistent with lipomas (3)

Questions for Further Review: Case Study 3.1

1. What is the morphology of each lesion (for example, benign, premalignant, malignant)?

2. What are the dimensions of *each* lesion *plus* the margin (if known)?

3. What is the anatomical site of *each* lesion?

4. What surgical technique was used to remove *each* lesion?
   a. Excision
   b. Shaving
   c. Destruction (indicate the method of destruction)
   d. Mohs' micrographic surgery (chemosurgery)

5. What surgical technique was used to close *each* lesion defect site?
   a. Adhesive strip application
   b. Chemical or electrocauterization
   c. Simple repair
   d. Layer closure
   e. Complex repair
   f. Adjacent tissue transfer/rearrangement
   g. Split-thickness skin graft
   h. Full-thickness skin graft

6. CPT surgery code(s) and modifier(s):

Case Study 3.2

Read the following clinical document and answer the questions for further review.

OPERATIVE REPORT

PREOPERATIVE DIAGNOSIS: Enlarging mass in the posterior neck

POSTOPERATIVE DIAGNOSIS: Epidermal inclusion cyst of the posterior neck

ANESTHESIA: IV sedation with local infiltration anesthetic

INDICATIONS: The patient is a 60-year-old man who has noticed an enlarging lump on the back of his neck that has become uncomfortable. Patient requests removal and understands the risks and benefits.

DESCRIPTION OF PROCEDURE: Patient was taken to the operating room, placed in a prone position with oxygen via nasal cannula delivered. When the patient was comfortable, the neck was prepped and draped in a sterile fashion posteriorly. Infiltration of 0.5% Marcaine plain with 2% Xylocaine with epinephrine, mixed 50/50 and using a field block technique, was used to anesthetize the area. A 15 blade was used to create an elliptical excision site over the lump, and radial and deepening dissection was performed, again using the 15 blade to circumscribe the lesion. The lesion was fully excised, and the cavity was noted to be with minimal oozing along the margins of the excision, which were controlled very nicely with the electrocautery. The specimen was examined off to the side and noted to be an epidermal inclusion cyst. The deep layer was closed with 3-0 Vicryl interrupted, and the skin was closed with 4-0 Vicryl subcuticular. The wound was dressed with tape closures. The patient tolerated the procedure well and went to the recovery room in stable condition.

The size of the excision site was 3 cm x 1.5 x 1.0 cm.

SURGICAL PATHOLOGY REPORT

AGE/SEX: 60/M

SPECIMEN(S) RECEIVED: Neck mass

GROSS: Received in formalin is a strip of brown skin measuring 1.4 x 0.4 cm. Present beneath it is a gray-tan cyst measuring 1.3 cm in diameter. It has a thin wall and is filled with grumous brownish-gray debris. ESS bisected.

DIAGNOSIS:
Skin of neck: Epidermal inclusion cyst

Questions for Further Review: Case Study 3.2

1. What is the morphology of *each* lesion (for example, benign, premalignant, malignant)?

2. What are the dimensions of *each* lesion *plus* the margin (if known)?

3. What is the anatomical site of *each* lesion?

4. What surgical technique was used to remove *each* lesion?
   a. Excision
   b. Shaving
   c. Destruction (indicate the method of destruction)
   d. Mohs' micrographic surgery (chemosurgery)

5. What surgical technique was used to close *each* lesion defect site?
   a. Adhesive strip application
   b. Chemical or electrocauterization
   c. Simple repair
   d. Layer closure
   e. Complex repair
   f. Adjacent tissue transfer/rearrangement
   g. Split-thickness skin graft
   h. Full-thickness skin graft

6. CPT surgery code(s) and modifier(s):

Case Study 3.3

Read the following clinical document and answer the questions for further review.

OPERATIVE REPORT

PREOPERATIVE DIAGNOSIS: 2-cm nodular ulcerating lesion tip of nose

POSTOPERATIVE DIAGNOSIS: 2-cm nodular ulcerating lesion tip of nose

OPERATION: Excision and complex closure

BLOOD LOSS: Minimal

ANESTHESIA: Local with sedation

INDICATIONS: This patient presented with the above diagnosis. A malignant lesion was to be ruled out. This was a large nodular elevated lesion with ulceration. It was compatible with squamous carcinoma-keratoacanthoma; however, I saw some element of infiltration at the base of the lesion, which is compatible with basal cell infiltration. Excision was planned. The risk of infection, bleeding, scarring, and need for secondary operation was discussed. No evidence of metastasis was noted. Need of flap or graft and nasal deformity was explained.

DESCRIPTION OF PROCEDURE: After prepping and draping the patient in the usual fashion with Hibiclens solution, markings were made. Anesthesia using a mixture of Xylocaine 1% and 0.25% Marcaine with epinephrine was performed. I proceeded with excising the margins, which were reported to be negative. Then the lesion itself was excised. Hemostasis was assured. A longitudinal direction was selected on the nose. I then closed the incision in three layers of #4-0 Vicryl and #5-0 Prolene suture. A depression at the site of excision was noted, but I felt this would correct as no cartilage was removed and flaps would have left her with more significant scarring. The patient tolerated the procedure well.

COMPLICATIONS: None

PATHOLOGY REPORT

AGE/SEX: 72/F

SPECIMEN(S) RECEIVED:

1. Right margin, nose F.S.
2. Biopsy, left margin, nose F.S.
3. Biopsy, deep margin, nose F.S.
4. Lesion, nose

GROSS:

1. Received in the fresh state for frozen section are two ellipses of gray-white skin. The smaller is 0.3 x 0.1 x 0.1 cm and the larger is 0.8 x 0.3 x 0.3 cm. The specimen is submitted in toto as frozen section control.
   Summary of sections: 1 cassette
   Frozen section diagnosis: No evidence of tumor

2. Received in the fresh state for frozen section is a segment gray-white skin 1.3 x 0.1 x 0.2 cm. The specimen is submitted in toto as a frozen section control.
   Summary of sections: 1 cassette
   Frozen section diagnosis: Actinic changes

3. Received in formalin is fragment of pink-yellow soft tissue 0.5 cm in greatest dimension. The specimen is submitted in toto as a frozen section control.
   Summary of sections: 1 cassette
   Frozen section diagnosis: No evidence of tumor

4. Specimen is received in formalin and consists of an elliptical skin biopsy measuring 1.5 x 1 x 0.8 cm in greatest dimension. The skin surface is tan with a central dome-shaped ulcerated nodule measuring 0.5 cm in greatest dimension. The deep margin is inked and the specimen is serially sectioned and entirely submitted in two cassettes.

DIAGNOSES:

1. Skin of nose, right margin: Negative for carcinoma; moderate solar elastosis
2. Skin of nose, left margin: Negative for carcinoma; moderate solar elastosis
3. Nose, deep margin: Negative for carcinoma; benign fibroadipose tissue
4. Skin of nose, main lesion: Infiltrating, well-differentiated, keratinizing squamous cell carcinoma; Solar elastosis

---

Questions for Further Review: Case Study 3.3

1. What is the morphology of *each* lesion (for example, benign, premalignant, malignant)?

2. What are the dimensions of *each* lesion *plus* the margin (if known)?

3. What is the anatomical site of *each* lesion?

4. What surgical technique was used to remove *each* lesion?
    a. Excision
    b. Shaving
    c. Destruction (indicate the method of destruction)
    d. Mohs' micrographic surgery (chemosurgery)

5. What surgical technique was used to close *each* lesion defect site?
    a. Adhesive strip application
    b. Chemical or electrocauterization
    c. Simple repair
    d. Layer closure
    e. Complex repair
    f. Adjacent tissue transfer/rearrangement
    g. Split-thickness skin graft
    h. Full-thickness skin graft

6. CPT surgery code(s) and modifier(s):

Case Study 3.4

Read the following clinical document and answer the questions for further review.

OPERATIVE RECORD

PREOPERATIVE DIAGNOSIS: Dehiscence right thumb wound

POSTOPERATIVE DIAGNOSIS: Dehiscence right thumb wound

OPERATION: Debridement and closure of dehisced wound, right thumb

ANESTHESIA: Local

INDICATIONS: This 51-year-old diabetic male is several weeks now status post a trigger thumb release. Unfortunately, he developed dehiscence of his wound postoperatively. He has been treated conservatively. The wound is clean right now but has still been open for some time, and fear of infection brings him to the OR now for delayed closure.

PROCEDURE: The patient was taken to the OR and placed in the supine position. The area was infiltrated with 0.5% Marcaine for anesthesia. The arm was elevated for 5 minutes and the tourniquet inflated to 250 mmHg. Total tourniquet time was less than 2 hours.

The open wound, which measured approximately 1.5 cm, was circumferentially incised down to good healthy tissue and then reapproximated with 5-0 nylon suture. Xeroform and a bulky dressing were applied and held with rolled gauze and an elastic wrap.

The estimated blood loss was minimal. The IV fluid replaced was none. Drains and packs were none. Complications were none.

The patient tolerated the procedure well and was taken to the recovery room in a good postoperative condition.

Questions for Further Review: Case Study 3.4

1. What are the dimensions of *each* wound?

2. What are the anatomical sites of *each* wound?

3. What surgical method was used to repair *each* wound?
   a. Adhesive strip application in combination with other material or as a sole material
   b. Chemical or electrocauterization
   c. Debridement
   d. Simple repair
   e. Layer closure
   f. Complex repair
   g. Secondary wound repair
   h. Blood vessel, tendon, nerve repair
   i. Ligation and/or exploration of vessels
   j. Adjacent tissue transfer/rearrangement
   k. Split-thickness skin graft
   l. Full-thickness skin graft.

4. CPT surgery code(s) and modifier(s):

Case Study 3.5

Read the following clinical document and answer the questions for further review.

OPERATIVE REPORT

Age: 70

OPERATION: Split-thickness skin graft to wound of left forearm

PREOPERATIVE DIAGNOSIS: Wound of left forearm

POSTOPERATIVE DIAGNOSIS: Wound of left forearm

OPERATIVE PROCEDURE: The patient was taken to the operating room, placed on the table in the supine position, and prepared and draped in the usual fashion. The patient was noted to have a 6 x 15 cm granulating wound of his left forearm from a previous excision of a large squamous cell carcinoma. He is now to undergo skin grafting of this area. First, the wound was debrided of hypertrophic granulation. Next, a split-thickness skin graft, which measured 14/1000ths of an inch in thickness, was harvested from the left upper thigh area. The skin graft was meshed in a 1:1.5 fashion and placed over the wound. The graft was secured in place with interrupted sutures of #5-0 chromic. Sterile dressings were applied over the graft and a volar plaster splint applied to the left upper extremity for immobilization. Next, the donor area was dressed. The patient was then transferred to the recovery room in stable condition.

ESTIMATED BLOOD LOSS: Minimal

Questions for Further Review: Case Study 3.5

1. What type of skin graft was applied?

2. What was the anatomical site for the donor skin graft?

3. What surgical technique was used to repair the donor site?

4. What was the size (in square centimeters) of the defect site (recipient) on which the graft was applied?

5. On what anatomical site (recipient) was the graft applied?

6. CPT surgery code(s) and modifier(s):

Case Study 3.6

Read the following clinical document and answer the questions for further review.

OPERATIVE REPORT

PREOPERATIVE DIAGNOSIS: Extensive full-thickness skin loss, left axilla status post dehiscent surgical wound

POSTOPERATIVE DIAGNOSIS: Extensive full-thickness skin loss, left axilla status post dehiscent surgical wound

OPERATION PERFORMED: Debridement and split-thickness skin grafting, soft tissue defect, left axilla

ANESTHESIA: General endotracheal anesthesia

ESTIMATED BLOOD LOSS: Minimal

ANTIBIOTICS: Cefotan 2 g IV

SPECIMENS: None

SUMMARY OF PROCEDURE INDICATION: The patient is a 36-year-old white male who has a history of recurrent hidradenitis suppurativa of the axillae. He most recently underwent excision of affected skin in the left axilla on 2/25/XX. This was done on an outpatient basis. In the follow-up, he was noted to have an infection, which progressed, culminating in extensive wound dehiscence of the left axilla. Subsequently, he was treated as an inpatient with IV antibiotics and local wound care and later transferred to an extended care facility where he was continued on IV cephazolin. Because the area of skin loss is greater than 15 x 15 cm, he is now brought for skin grafting for coverage.

PROCEDURE: The patient was brought to the operating room and positioned supine. He was anesthetized and intubated. A roll was placed behind his left shoulder, and the arm was elevated on a blanket. The left anterior leg and thigh were shaved and prepped separately from the wound, which involved the entire left axilla and superior lateral chest wall.

The wound was debrided using the Weck knife and a #10 blade and was also curetted. There was one small sinus opening superiorly, and this was probed, but not widely opened, as it extended into the deep axilla.

Two split-thickness grafts were taken from the anterior and the anterolateral left thigh. These were meshed 1.5:1. The donor site was covered with Xeroform gauze, 4x4s, and ABDs. These were later taped in place.

Now, the arm was extended and the graft applied to completely cover the area. This was done with a total of four pieces. These were secured circumferentially with staples, and seams were approximated and tacked down using #4-0 chromic sutures. Excess graft was trimmed.

The site was dressed with multiple layers of Adaptic, over which mineral oil-soaked cotton batting was applied. Additional layers of Adaptic were placed prior to putting on dry cotton batting, fluffs, and ABDs. These were taped into place and the patient was placed into a sling. He was noted to have a left antecubital PICC line in place.

This completed the procedure, and the patient was extubated and transported to the PACU having tolerated the event well. He will be kept on IV antibiotics for an additional eight days, until the graft dressings are taken down.

Questions for Further Review: Case Study 3.6

1. What type of skin graft was applied?

2. What was the anatomical site for the donor skin graft?

3. What surgical technique was used to repair the donor site?

4. What was the size (in square centimeters) of the defect site (recipient) on which the graft was applied?

5. On what anatomical site (recipient) was the graft applied?

6. CPT surgery code(s) and modifier(s):

Case Study 3.7

Read the following clinical document and answer the questions for further review.

OPERATIVE REPORT

PREOPERATIVE DIAGNOSES:
1. Chronic open wound, left dorsal foot
2. Chronic open wound, left medial foot

POSTOPERATIVE DIAGNOSES:
1. Chronic open wound, left dorsal foot
2. Chronic open wound, left medial foot

OPERATION:
1. Debridement of foot wounds
2. Closure of foot wounds using Apligraf

ANESTHESIA: Local

ESTIMATED BLOOD LOSS: Trace

COMPLICATIONS: None

INDICATIONS: The patient is a 63-year-old, type 2 diabetic male who has chronic wounds of the left foot. This is believed to be secondary to a spider bite. The patient has undergone multiple debridements, as well as IV antibiotic therapy for infection. The wounds are clean, and the infection seems to be clearing. There are exposed tendons on the dorsum of the foot, and, therefore, closure is warranted.

PROCEDURE/FINDINGS: After obtaining informed consent, the patient was taken to the operating room and placed on the table in the supine position. Using 1% lidocaine with 1:100,000 epinephrine, the areas of the wound on the dorsal foot and the medial foot were infiltrated. After waiting an appropriate amount of time for the anesthetic and hemostatic effects to take place, the foot was prepped and draped in the usual sterile fashion. Sharp debridement was used to remove nonviable skin and subcutaneous tissue. The wound on the dorsum of the foot was inspected and measured approximately 7 to 8 cm in greatest dimension. The wound on the medial foot measured approximately 3 cm in greatest dimension. After adequately debriding the wounds, Apligraf was meshed 1-1/2 to 1 and placed in the wound, adequately covering underlying structures. This was affixed to the periphery of the wounds using staples. In total, approximately 40–45 square cm of Apligraf were used.

Next, a dressing consisting of antibiotic ointment, Adaptic, fluffs, and Kerlix was applied, followed by soft roll, Ace bandage, and Coban. The patient tolerated the procedure well and was discharged in stable condition.

Questions for Further Review: Case Study 3.7

1. What type of skin graft was applied?

2. What was the anatomical site for the donor skin graft?

3. What surgical technique was used to repair the donor site?

4. What was the size (in square centimeters) of the defect site (recipient) on which the graft was applied?

5. On what anatomical site (recipient) was the graft applied?

6. CPT surgery code(s) and modifier(s):

Case Study 3.8

Read the following clinical document and answer the questions for further review.

DEPARTMENT OF RADIOLOGY

EXAM: Right breast stereotactic biopsy

INDICATIONS: New lesion

PROCEDURE: Risks and benefits of the procedure were discussed with the patient, including, but not limited to, pain, bleeding, infection, and unsuccessful biopsy, and after questions were answered to her and her daughter's satisfaction, written and verbal consent was obtained.

FINDINGS: Patient was placed prone on stereotactic biopsy table and right breast lesion was approached medially. The inferior portion of the right breast was placed in template with stereotactic views to confirm the lesion seen on previous mammogram, and lesion was targeted. Skin site was topically and locally anesthetized and prepped in sterile fashion. Small dermatotomy was performed, and 11-gauge mammotome device was inserted with satisfactory position confirmed on pre- and postfire images. Sampling was obtained in routine circumferential fashion with satisfactory appearance of the specimen grossly. Cavity was vacuumed and marking clip placed. Clip placement was also confirmed on stereotactic views. Site was dressed in sterile fashion. Patient tolerated the procedure well with no immediate complication. After she received discharge instructions and was informed that biopsy report will go to her doctors as well as myself, she left the department in the company of her daughter.

Upon receipt of biopsy results, as discussed with her daughter, I will attempt to call the patient and notify her doctors as well, with addendum reported with any additional recommendations at that point.

PATHOLOGY DEPARTMENT

PREOP DIAGNOSIS: Right breast mass

OPERATION: Stereotactic right breast biopsy

SPECIMEN SUBMITTED: Right breast mass

GROSS DESCRIPTION: Patient identification agrees on path sheet and container.

The specimen is submitted in formalin labeled right breast mass and consists of multiple cylindrical yellow, red, and gray tissues, ranging in size from .2 x .1 cm. to 3.3 x 0.3 cm. Submitted in toto in three cassettes labeled A through C.

DIAGNOSIS: Right breast mass (stereotactic biopsies). Mucinous (colloid) carcinoma with extensive in-situ component, grade 1

NOTE: The mucinous carcinoma is characterized by clusters of neoplastic cells suspended in lakes of mucin. Ductal carcinoma in-situ accounts for more than 25% of the tumor volume, cribriform, and solid types with mucous production and focal calcifications. Grading of the invasive component is based on the Elston Modification of the Bloom–Richardson grade scheme. Tumor tubule formation score 3, number of mitosis score 1, and nuclear pleomorphism score 1. Total score is 5. DCIS nuclear grade is 1. Tumor involves approximately 10 core fragments. One paraffin block is sent for ERA, PRA, and DNA ploidy.

Slides are submitted for intradepartmental QA activity.
T-04020, M-84803, TR-100

Questions for Further Review: Case Study 3.8

1. Was the biopsy unilateral or bilateral?
   a. Unilateral
   b. Bilateral

2. How many biopsies were performed on the breast(s)?

3. Was imaging guidance used?

4. Was a radiological marker(s) used?
   a. Yes
   b. No

5. If yes, what was the type and number of radiological marker(s)?
   a. Needle localization wire
   b. Metallic localization clip
   c. Other (specify)

6. What type(s) of biopsy was performed?
   a. Catheter lavage of mammary duct (specify number of ducts)
   b. Open percutaneous needle core
   c. Percutaneous automated vacuum-assisted biopsy
   d. Percutaneous rotating biopsy device
   e. Excisional (specify number of lesions excised per breast)
   f. Microwave phased array thermotherapy

7. Was a surgical clip placed?
   a. Yes
   b. No

7. CPT surgery code(s) and modifier(s):

Case Study 3.9

Read the following clinical document and answer the questions for further review.

OPERATIVE REPORT

PREOPERATIVE DIAGNOSIS: Right breast carcinoma

POSTOPERATIVE DIAGNOSIS: Same

OPERATION PERFORMED: Right partial mastectomy, axillary nodal dissection

ANESTHESIA: General

COMPLICATIONS: None

HISTORY: This is a 55-year-old female with an abnormal mammogram and a palpable mass. The abnormal mammography revealed microcalcifications and was followed by stereotactic biopsy and revealed invasive ductal carcinoma. The lesion was small. The patient was counseled and elected to undergo breast-conserving surgery. The above-noted procedure was performed. No complications were encountered.

PROCEDURE: The patient was identified and in the supine position was given general anesthesia with endotracheal intubation. She was placed in the supine position, and the right breast and axillary sites were prepped and draped accordingly. The mass was at the 12 to 10 o'clock area, and there was some post stereotactic induration from a hematoma. A semilinear incision was made over this area, where a partial mastectomy was performed. The skin incision was made and skin flaps developed. The mass was eventually removed by removing almost two segments from the 9 o'clock to the almost 2 o'clock area. The resection was then completed down to the pectoralis fascia and all the blood supply to this area was coagulated. The irrigation was done and hemostasis was complete. When dissection was taking place, at the 8 o'clock position of the mass, there seemed some induration close to the cutting margins. From this area, margin 1 was taken and a deeper margin was labeled as number 2. The pocket was irrigated. Hemostasis was complete. Closure was done in the usual fashion. The incision was made along the skin folds. Skin flaps were developed. The anterior axillary and posterior axillary lines were identified, along with the structures accompanying this location and the axillary vein. The lymphatic bundle, most medial, was labeled as sentinel nodes and sent to pathology separately. Remaining lymph nodes were removed. The irrigation was done. A Jackson-Pratt drain was placed to drain the breast and the axillary sites. Hemostasis was complete, and the closure of the skin took place in the normal fashion. The patient was awakened from anesthesia and, in stable condition, taken to the recovery room for further observation.

SURGICAL PATHOLOGY REPORT

CLINICAL INFORMATION PROVIDED: Invasive ductal carcinoma and ductal carcinoma in situ

DIAGNOSIS: Partial mastectomy; infiltrating and in situ ductal-type mammary adenocarcinoma

SCARFF-BLOOM-RICHARDSON GRADE: 1/3

TUBULAR PATTERN SCORE: 2/3

NUCLEAR GRADE SCORE: 2/3

MITOTIC FREQUENCY SCORE: 1/3

INVASIVE TUMOR SIZE: Less than 1 mm

IN SITU COMPONENT PATTERN AND EXTENT: The tumor is composed predominantly of ductal carcinoma in situ, solid, cribriform, and focal comedo patterns. Margins of excision: Tumor does not appear to involve the margins of resection.
Hormone receptor status: Limited invasive tumor is present to perform hormonal receptors. Original biopsy material may be preferable for performance of such.

LYMPHATIC/VASCULAR INVASION: None identified

OTHER PATHOLOGIC FINDINGS: Previous biopsy site changes:

A. Margin at 8 o'clock #1: Portion of benign mammary tissue with:

   1. Focally florid duct hyperplasia with atypia.

   2. Small fibroadenoma.

   3. Fibrocystic changes.

   4. No invasive or in situ malignancy is identified.

B. Margin at 8 o'clock #2: Portion of benign mammary tissue with fibrocystic changes. No in situ or invasive malignancy is identified.

C. Right axillary sentinel node: One lymph node with reactive changes, no metastatic malignancy is identified either upon H&E staining or by utilizing the cytokeratin immunohistochemical stain.

D. Right axillary node dissection: Eleven lymph nodes, no metastatic carcinoma is identified. (0/11).

Note: In Part A, the residual tumor present is adjacent to the large blood-filled cavity consistent with recent biopsy. The residual tumor present is composed predominantly of ductal carcinoma in situ and measures 1.0 cm in aggregate dimension. The infiltrating part of the tumor is extremely focal and minimal, accounting for less than 1 percent of the tumor and measuring less than 1 mm. The amount of invasive tumor is so little that the performance of estrogen and progesterone receptor markers would be limited. This probably should be done on the original material (if it has not already been done). When the original material is also limited, and estrogen and progesterone receptors are desired upon this material, they can be performed upon request.

SPECIMENS RECEIVED: Gross Description

A. Received in formalin and labeled "Partial mastectomy" is an irregular fragment of yellow-red tissue measuring 8.6 x 7.3 x 3.5 cm. Two sutures mark the superior (12 o'clock) and anterior positions. The margins of excision are inked in black, and the specimen is serially sectioned, revealing a well-delineated area of clotted blood consistent with prior biopsy site, which measures 1.5 x 1.4 x 1.0 cm. No definite tumor is identified. Firm tissue adjacent to the biopsy site is noted abutting on the posterior and inferior (6 o'clock) margin. No definite tumor is grossly identified. All other margins of excision appear free of any lesions suspicious for malignancy. The remainder of the tissue that comprises the specimen appears to be composed of soft yellow tissue. Representative sections, including the entire biopsy area and adjacent tissue, are submitted in ten cassettes labeled 6977, A1–10.

B. Received in formalin and labeled "Margin at 8 o'clock" is one irregular fragment of somewhat firm to rubbery gray-white tissue measuring 2.0 x 1.5 x 0.6 cm. The specimen is inked in black, and entire submitted in a single cassette labeled 6977-B.

C. Received in formalin and labeled "Margin at 8 o'clock #2" is one irregular fragment of rubbery yellow-red tissue with a firm gray-white area focally. The specimen measures 2.0 x 2.0 x 0.7 cm. The margins of excision are inked in black, and the specimen is entirely submitted in a single cassette labeled 6977-C.

D. Received in formalin and labeled "Right axillary sentinel node" is one irregular fragment of lobulated soft yellow tissue measuring 2.7 x 2.5 x 0.5 cm. No structures grossly suggestive of a lymph node are identified. No blue dye is noted either. The entire specimen is submitted in a single cassette labeled 6977-D.

Received in formalin and labeled "Axilla (right) node dissection" is an aggregate of lobulated yellow-red tissue measuring 9.9 x 6.2 x 1.5 cm. Within the aggregate, a number of structures grossly compatible with lymph nodes are identified ranging between 0.2 and 3.4 cm in greatest dimension. Representative sections, including all the apparent lymph nodes, are submitted in five cassettes labeled 6977, E1-5, sections 4 and 5 representing the largest node dissected.

Questions for Further Review: Case Study 3.9

1. Was the procedure unilateral or bilateral?
   a. Unilateral
   b. Bilateral

2. What type of breast excision was performed?
   a. Open excision of malignant breast tumor
   b. Partial mastectomy
   c. Subcutaneous mastectomy

3. What type of lymph node dissection was performed?
   a. Superficial needle biopsy of axillary lymph nodes
   b. Open biopsy of deep axillary lymph nodes

4. Which of the following correctly classifies this case?
   a. 19302–RT
   b. 38525
   c. 19301–RT
   d. 19301–RT and 38525

Explanation:

Case Study 3.10

Read the following clinical document and answer the questions for further review.

OPERATIVE REPORT

OPERATION: Removal of bilateral silicone breast implants and replacement with saline implants

ANESTHESIA: General

PREOPERATIVE DIAGNOSIS: Rupture silicone implant on the right side; suspected rupture on the left side

POSTOPERATIVE DIAGNOSIS: Rupture silicone implant on the right side, suspected rupture on the left side

OPERATIVE INDICATIONS: The patient is a 51-year-old female who underwent bilateral breast augmentation a number of years ago and had subsequent capsule contractures and bilateral gel implant ruptures and needed replacement. She did well for a number of years and suffered an accident while at work; a box fell on her right side. Along the upper medial aspect, she developed a rather large, hard lump that on radiologic examination was revealed to be a probable ruptured implant with silicone granuloma. The recommendations were made for removal of those implants and replacement prosthesis. The procedure was explained to the patient, including its limitations, complications, risks, and alternatives; and she decided to proceed.

OPERATIVE PROCEDURE: Under adequate general endotracheal anesthesia with the patient in the supine position, the chest was prepped and draped in the usual manner. The previous inframammary incisions were opened to the level of the capsule, and careful blunt and sharp dissection on the right side isolated the implant from its submammary position. It was found to be ruptured along the right medial aspect where she had suffered her injury. There was extravasated silicone mixed with fibrosis and breast tissue, and the entire mass was removed and sent to pathology for examination. The pocket was copiously irrigated with saline with 5% Betadine.

Attention was turned to the left side where a similar procedure was carried out, and on this side the implant was found to have a sticky surface to it, but not associated with envelope rupture. The specimen was sent to pathology for examination. The pocket was also irrigated and, using sizers, approximately 400 cc implant was determined to be the correct size, and a saline prosthesis, Mentor style 1600, was selected bilaterally, infused to 40 cc of saline and placed in the same pocket. The incisions were then closed with interrupted 3-0 Monocryl and a subcuticular 3-0 Monocryl. The patient tolerated the entire procedure well and left the operating room in satisfactory condition.

Questions for Further Review: Case Study 3.10

1. The patient had bilateral augmentation performed a number of years ago.
   a. True
   b. False

2. Which of the following procedures was performed?
   a. Removal of right intact mammary implant
   b. Removal of left intact mammary implant
   c. Removal of right mammary implant material
   d. Removal of left mammary implant material

3. Which of the following procedures was performed?
   a. Bilateral mammaplasty augmentation with prosthetic implants
   b. Bilateral immediate insertion of breast prostheses in reconstruction
   c. Bilateral delayed insertion of breast prostheses in reconstruction

4. CPT surgery code(s) and modifier(s): _____

Case Study 3.11

Read the following clinical document and answer the questions for further review.

OPERATIVE REPORT

Preoperative Diagnosis: Basal cell carcinoma, left ear

Postoperative Diagnosis: Same

Operation(s): Wide excision, frozen section, and reconstruction by rotation flap

Description of Operation: Patient was given local infiltration anesthesia of 0.50% Xylocaine with epinephrine. Parts were prepped and draped in the usual fashion. The area of basal cell carcinoma, which was right behind the helical dome, was excised. The total area of excision was about 2 cm x 2 cm. It was given to the pathologist for proper orientation. He who determined that the margins were free, and it was indeed basal cell carcinoma. A superiorly based rotation flap measuring 3 cm x 1.5 cm was then marked, incised, undermined, and transposed into the defect. Closure was done with 5-0 nylon interrupted sutures. Donor site was closed by advancement flaps. At the conclusion of the procedure, the flaps were viable. Hemostasis was satisfactory. A bulky dressing was applied.

The patient left for home in satisfactory condition.

Questions for Further Review: Case Study 3.11

1. What was the anatomical site of any lesion(s) excised?

2. What were the dimensions in sq cm of the primary defect (the original defect to be closed)?

3. What was the donor site for the adjacent tissue transfer/rearrangement?

4. What were the dimensions in sq cm of the secondary defect (the defect created by the movement of tissue necessary to close the primary defect)?

5. What type of adjacent tissue transfer/rearrangement was performed?
   a. Advancement flap
   b. V-Y plasty
   c. Y-V plasty
   d. W plasty
   e. Z-plasty
   f. Rotation flap
   g. Transpositional flap
   h. Sliding flap
   i. Interpolational
   j. Nasolabial flap
   k. Other (specify)

6. What technique was used to close the donor site for the adjacent tissue transfer/rearrangement?

7. CPT surgery code(s) and modifier(s):

Case Study 3.12

Read the following clinical document and answer the questions for further review.

OPERATIVE REPORT

PREOPERATIVE DIAGNOSIS: Squamous cell carcinoma of right ear posteriorly, recurrent

POSTOPERATIVE DIAGNOSIS: Squamous cell carcinoma of right ear posteriorly, recurrent

OPERATIVE PROCEDURE: Multiple frozen sections and excisions of squamous cell carcinoma of the right ear with a large anteriorly based flap reconstruction measuring 5 x 6 cm

DESCRIPTION OF PROCEDURE: The patient was given intravenous sedation. The area, which was basically along the sulcus of the posterior surface of the ear, was marked out with a fine-tip marking pen, and then, skin from the posterior surface of the ear and from the mastoid was taken. The suture was placed at the 12 o'clock position. Dissection was carried down to the perichondrial layer and carried inferiorly in the sulcus down to the lower aspect of the ear. The frozen section margins came back clear on the edges, but there was some tumor on the deep surface. This was adjacent to the cartilage. Therefore, the complete cartilage under this area was excised. This was basically from the helix, all the way back down to the sulcus, for about two-thirds or slightly more of the ear. This was completely resected. Ink was placed on the anterior concave site, and the posterior old, deep margin was completely excised with a specimen down to the site of the head. A further deep margin was taken in the soft tissue part posterior to the cartilaginous component and a completely new deep margin was resected.

This was copiously irrigated with saline and checked for hemostasis with bipolar cautery. A large flap, 5 x 6 cm, was advanced from an anterior-based position to mobilize this tissue and allow closure with interrupted deep 5 and 6-0 Monocryl in the deep layers and 4-0 running chromic on the skin. The ear was packed with moist cotton balls, and light gauze dressing with cling was applied. The patient tolerated the procedure well and left the operating area in good condition. The sponge, needle, and instrument counts were correct. It should be noted that the patient had a blood loss of less than 20 cc.

Questions for Further Review: Case Study 3.12

1. What was the anatomical site of any lesion(s) excised?

2. What were the dimensions in sq cm of the primary defect (the original defect to be closed)?

3. What was the donor site for the adjacent tissue transfer/rearrangement?

4. What were the dimensions in sq cm of the secondary defect (the defect created by the movement of tissue necessary to close the primary defect)?

5. What type of adjacent tissue transfer/rearrangement was performed?
   a. Advancement flap
   b. V-Y plasty
   c. Y-V plasty
   d. W-plasty
   e. Z-plasty
   f. Rotation flap
   g. Transpositional flap
   h. Sliding flap
   i. Interpolational
   j. Nasolabial flap
   k. Other (specify)

6. What technique was used to close the donor site for the adjacent tissue transfer/rearrangement?

7. CPT surgery code(s) and modifier(s):

Case Study 3.13

Read the following clinical document and answer the questions for further review.

OPERATIVE REPORT

PREOPERATIVE DIAGNOSIS: Basal cell carcinoma, left infra-auricular area and keratosis preauricular area left

POSTOPERATIVE DIAGNOSIS: Basal cell carcinoma, left infra-auricular area and keratosis preauricular area left

OPERATION: Excision of basal cell carcinoma measuring 3 x 2 centimeters under frozen section control, and closure with rotation flap. Shave excision keratosis 1 centimeter left preauricular area

ANESTHESIA: Local

BLOOD LOSS: Minimal

COMPLICATIONS: None

INDICATIONS: This 79-year-old patient presented with the above diagnosis, undergoing excision of basal cell carcinoma. This was an infiltrating type. The excision, and pros, cons, and complications were discussed. She had no evidence of metastasis. Risks of infection, bleeding, scarring, need for flap, autograft, and recurrence were discussed, as was the need of secondary operation.

DESCRIPTION OF PROCEDURE: After prepping and draping the patient in the usual fashion with pHisoHex solution, markings were made. Anesthesia was infiltrated. After waiting a few minutes for its effect, elliptical excision was performed. I included a 7-mm margin as this was infiltrating. Hemostasis was assured. Frozen section was submitted, which came back as negative. A rotation flap was needed in order not to distort the earlobe on this patient, as primary closures have resulted in distortion. A superiorly-based flap was outlined, measured about 4 x 2 cm, elevated including skin and subcutaneous tissue, and rotated to the recipient bed. Closure in multiple layers with 4-0 Monocryl and 6-0 Monocryl suture, and 6-0 nylon suture was done. Shave excision of the preauricular lesion was performed. The procedure was tolerated well.

PATHOLOGY REPORT

SURGICAL:

AP Case Type	Surgical
AP Accession No.	S01-12912
AP Result Status	Final
AP Specimen Descr	Biopsy, anterior margin, postauricular left ear, F.S.
	Biopsy, posterior margin, postauricular left ear, F.S.
	Main lesion
	Lesion, face

SPECIMEN:

1. Biopsy, anterior margin, postauricular left ear, F.S.
2. Biopsy, posterior margin, postauricular left ear, F.S.
3. Main lesion
4. Lesion, face

GROSS:

1. Specimen is received fresh and consists of a piece of skin measuring 1.2 x 0.2 cm. The specimen is frozen entirely and subsequently submitted entirely in a single cassette.

   Frozen section diagnosis: No tumor identified

2. Specimen is received fresh and consists of a piece of skin measuring 1.2 x 0.2 cm. The specimen is frozen entirely and subsequently submitted entirely in a single cassette.

   Frozen section diagnosis: No tumor identified

3. Specimen is received in formalin and consists of an ellipse of tan skin with a raised lesion in the center. The skin measure 2.5 x 1.5 cm. The lesion is circular, measures 0.4 cm, and is 0.4 cm away from the surgical cut edge. The specimen is inked. The longitudinal ends are submitted in –1 cassette. The remainder is serially sectioned and submitted entirely in –4 cassettes.

4. Specimen is received in formalin and consists of a shaved biopsy of karatotic-appearing white skin measuring 0.6 x 0.6 x 0.1 cm. The specimen is inked and submitted entirely in a single cassette. ESS –1 cassette.

DIAGNOSIS:

1. Post auricular anterior margin, left ear skin with solar elastosis
   No tumor identified

2. Post auricular posterior margin, left ear
   Skin with sun damage
   No tumor identified

3. Main lesion:
   Basal cell carcinoma
   Scar
   Margins free of tumor

4. Face lesion:
   Seborrheic keratosis

Questions for Further Review: Case Study 3.13

1. What surgical technique was used to remove the basal cell carcinoma, left infra-auricular?
   a. Excision
   b. Shaving
   c. Destruction (indicate the method of destruction)
   d. Mohs' micrographic surgery (chemosurgery)

2. What surgical technique was used to close the basal cell carcinoma, left infra-auricular defect site?
   a. Adhesive strip application
   b. Chemical or electrocauterization
   c. Simple repair
   d. Layer closure
   e. Complex repair
   f. Adjacent tissue transfer/rearrangement
   g. Split-thickness skin graft
   h. Full-thickness skin graft

3. What surgical technique was used to remove the preauricular lesion?
   a. Excision
   b. Shaving
   c. Destruction (indicate the method of destruction)
   d. Mohs' micrographic surgery (chemosurgery)

4. What surgical technique was used to close the preauricular lesion defect site?
   a. Adhesive strip application
   b. Chemical or electrocauterization
   c. Simple repair
   d. Layer closure
   e. Complex repair
   f. Adjacent tissue transfer/rearrangement
   g. Split-thickness skin graft
   h. Full-thickness skin graft
   i. No closure

5. CPT surgery code(s) and modifier(s):

Chapter 4

Musculoskeletal System

CPT codes 20000 through 29999 are used to report surgical and related procedures performed on the musculoskeletal system, which encompasses virtually every part of the human body. Common outpatient procedures involving the musculoskeletal system include trigger point injections, treatment of fractures and dislocations, podiatric surgery, arthroscopic knee surgery, shoulder surgery, and hand surgery.

Trigger Point Injections

A trigger point is a painful area of muscle and surrounding tissue, which may be associated with myofascial pain syndrome. The pain of active trigger points can begin as an acute single muscle syndrome resulting from stress overload or injury to the muscle, or can develop slowly because of chronic or repetitive muscle strain. The pain normally refers distal to the specific hypersensitive trigger point. Trigger point injections are used to alleviate this pain. See Exhibit 4.1 at the end of this chapter for example of trigger finger.

There is no laboratory or imaging test for establishing the diagnosis of trigger points; it depends therefore upon the detailed history and thorough examination. Trigger point injections using local anesthetics alone or with steroids are frequently performed and, for the most part, result in some degree of pain relief. Other myofascial pain treatments include acupuncture, massage therapy, and transcutaneous electrical neural stimulation (TENS). Trigger point injections are intramuscular injections of local anesthetic used to treat chronic pain that does not respond to other treatment.

APC	HCPCS	HCPCS Description	SI	Rel. Wt.	Payment Rate	OPPS OCE
0204			T	2.3213	147.85	
	20552	Injection trigger point, 1 or 2 muscles				Append modifier 59 when multiple occurrences occur on a single day
	20553	Injection trigger point, 3 or more muscles				

APC 0204 has been designated as an exception to the "2 Times Rule." In accordance with section 1833(t)(2) of the Social Security Administration (SSA), subject to certain exceptions, services and items within an APC group cannot be considered comparable with respect to the use of resources if the highest mean cost for an item or service in the APC group is more than two times greater than the lowest median cost for an item or service within the same APC group (referred to as the "2 Times Rule"). In implementing this provision, the median cost of the item or service assigned to an APC group is used.

Coding Guidelines for Trigger Point Injections

Trigger point injection codes 20552–20553 are reported one time per session, regardless of the number of injections or muscles injected (AMA 2003a). To determine the appropriate code, count the number of muscles injected and choose the appropriate code based on the total. Append modifier 59 when multiple occurrences occur on a single day; this is not to be confused with multiple trigger point injections at the same session.

> **Example:** A 51-year-old female patient comes in for a follow-up visit after being previously diagnosed with rheumatoid arthritis (RA). The physician does an examination including a review of systems (ROS), obtains a HPI, and makes a medical decision of moderate complexity.
>
> The physician performs an appropriate level of an E/M visit. During the visit, the patient complains of stiffness and swelling in the hands, elbows, and neck. The clinician also obtains two x-ray views of the patient's left hand and reads them during the visit. Due to the severity of the swelling, the physician decides to give the patient six trigger point injections.

> **Correct coding:** 99213-25, 20553, 73120-LT

> **Incorrect coding:** 99213-25, 20552x6 or 99213-25, 20552, 20553 x 5, 73120

Aspiration/Injection Ganglion Cyst

A ganglion cyst is a small tumor connected to a joint membrane or tendon sheath, usually found on the back of the wrist. Ganglion cysts contain fluid and can cause considerable pain and inflammation at the site. These knotlike masses are noncancerous. Injection into the ganglion cyst is sometimes indicated to provide for relief of pain and to reduce the inflammation in these structures. See Exhibit 4.1 at the end of this chapter for example of ganglion cyst.

Coding Guidelines for Aspiration and/or Injection Ganglion Cyst

Aspiration and/or injections of a ganglion cyst, code 20612, reported multiple times per session, may append modifier –59 (AMA 2008). However, if the patient has a digital nerve block performed prior to the procedure, code 64450 is not reported separately but bundled with the primary procedure code 20612.

Treatment of Fractures/Dislocations

A fracture is a break in a bone. Most commonly, fractures are documented as either "open" or "closed." A closed fracture is one in which skin is intact at the site of fracture. Other terms may be included that also describe closed fractures: comminuted, depressed, elevated, fissured, greenstick, impacted, linear, simple, slipped epiphysis, and spiral. Do not code a fracture that is described as "comminuted" as an open fracture. Comminuted only describes a fracture in which the bone is broken into more than two fragments, but is still closed. An open fracture indicates that the skin is perforated, and there is an open wound communicating with the site of the fracture. Note that the opening in the skin must communicate with the fracture site to be classified as an open fracture.

In some cases the documentation may indicate that the patient has a fracture and also has a laceration at the fracture site. But if the laceration is superficial and doesn't communicate with the fracture, the two should be classified separately, with one code for a closed fracture and another for a laceration. There are other terms associated with open fractures that may appear in the physician documentation. These include: compound, infected, missile, puncture, and with foreign body.

Any fracture that is not described as either open or closed should be classified as a closed fracture.

Example: A patient presents to the emergency room with an open, great toe fracture of the left foot. The orthopedic surgeon determines that the fracture needs debridement to clean the fracture debris and fracture site prior to wound repair and closure. The orthopedic surgeon debrides the tissue, muscle, and exposed bone; determines the fracture to be nondisplaced; then repairs the muscle, fascia, subcutaneous tissue, and closes the wound. The fracture was open, but the treatment was closed, because the surgeon did not surgically open or expose the fracture to the external environment. The debridement was of tissue, muscle, and bone associated with an open fracture.

Therefore, the correct coding for the above scenario would be 28490-LT and 11012-51. The debridement is not considered an "add-on code," for which CPT has specific guidelines. According to CPT guidelines, add-on codes are exempt from multiple procedure concepts if they are commonly carried out in addition to the primary procedure performed. All add-on codes in CPT are readily identified by the specific descriptor, such as "each additional" or "(List separately in addition to primary procedure)." Basically, that means that if a surgeon performs a procedure that can stand alone (or by itself), a –51 modifier would need to be attached to any subsequent procedures. However, if a procedure would or could never be performed alone, that CPT code is exempt from the multiple surgery concepts.

APC	HCPCS	HCPCS Description	SI	Rel. Wt.	Payment Rate	OPPS OCE
0043	28490	Treat big toe fracture	T	1.7682	112.62	50% reduction applies
0019	11012	Debride skin/muscle/bone/fx	T	4.3039	274.13	Significant procedure, multiple reduction applies

A dislocation is a disturbance or disarrangement of the normal relation of the bones entering into the formation of a joint. A reduction or manipulation involves the repositioning or restoration of a bone to its normal anatomical relation by surgical or manipulative procedures.

Coding Guidelines for Treatment of Fracture/Dislocation

The CPT codes for treatment of fractures are listed throughout the musculoskeletal section of the CPT codebook (20000–29999) and include cast and strapping, closed treatment with and without manipulation, open treatment, and percutaneous and external fixation.

Closed Treatment of Fractures

There are three types of treatment for closed fractures: with manipulation, without manipulation, and skeletal traction. An attempted reduction or restoration of a fracture or dislocation to the normal anatomical position is considered a manipulation. An application of a cast, splint, or other immobilization device, without a fracture reduction, is considered to be "without manipulation." Typically the devices applied are to stabilize fractures in long bones or the back/trunk. In some cases, smaller bones in the hands and feet cannot be manipulated. Skeletal traction uses force on a limb through a wire pin, screw, or clamp that will subsequently penetrate the bone. Broken or shattered bones are difficult to reduce and may not be able to be treated with an open procedure.

Open Treatment of Fractures

CPT codes for open treatment classify the procedures used in either of the following situations:

- The fractured bone is surgically opened or exposed to the external environment, with direct visualization of the fracture (bone ends) and use of internal fixation.

- The fractured bone is opened remote from the fracture site in order to insert an intramedullary nail across the fracture site, but the fracture site itself is not directly visualized. Exhibit 4.2 shows an example of a femur fracture before and after surgery.

- Open reduction of a fracture involves manipulative correction of a fracture to anatomical position after incision into the fracture site. Open reduction of a fracture involves deliberate exposure of the bone by the surgeon for the purpose of restoration of the proper anatomy. Open reduction and internal fixation, abbreviated as ORIF, is a very commonly performed procedure for fractures, but the coder should verify that the incision was made to expose the fracture for treatment.

Percutaneous and External Skeletal Fixation

CPT codes for percutaneous skeletal fixation refer to fracture treatment that is neither open nor closed. In these procedures, x-ray imaging is used to place fixation devices such as pins across the fracture site, but the fracture fragments are not visualized. External fixation is a method of immobilizing bones to allow a fracture to heal.

External skeletal fixation is another fracture treatment that may be documented in the medical record. This procedure involves the insertion of percutaneous pins proximal and distal to the fracture and an application of a frame that connects the pins externally. The pins are located internally except for the portion to which the frame is connected. The frame is located external to the body. These devices can be used to hold a reduced fracture or to assist the surgeon in reducing a fracture.

(See CPT codes 20690, 20692, or codes that have "with external fixation system" in their descriptions.)

When assigning CPT codes for fracture treatment, the coder should remember that although the definitions of "open" and "closed" treatment remain the same, CPT describes reduction procedures as "manipulation." Manipulation is defined as the attempted reduction or restoration of a fracture to its normal anatomic alignment by the application of manually applied forces.

Cast and Strapping

Cast and strapping codes (29000–29799) are used to report:

- A replacement cast or strapping procedure during or after the period of normal follow-up care
- An initial service performed without restorative treatment or procedures to stabilize or protect a fracture, injury, or dislocation, and/or to afford pain relief to a patient
- An initial cast or strapping service when no other treatment or procedure (specific to that injury) is performed or expected to be performed by the same physician (for example, when placed by the emergency department physician)

Codes 29000–29799 are *not* used to report an initial cast or strapping service when the restorative treatment (for example, the surgical repair or closed or open reduction of a fracture or joint dislocation) is performed.

Cast, splint, and strap procedures are not consistently performed solely by the physician. These procedures also are performed by nurses, emergency department staff, or orthopedic technicians under supervision of the physician.

In CPT, the splinting, strapping, and casting service is included in any more invasive surgical procedure and is not reported separately. When this type of service is performed in the emergency department setting for comfort and stabilization purposes only, and the patient is to follow-up with another physician for definitive treatment, only the splinting, strapping, or casting service is reported. Do not assign a CPT code for fracture treatment without manipulation. The only time these codes should be assigned is when the entire fracture treatment (meaning no other follow-up is required) is performed on the episode of care in question and no reduction/manipulation service is provided.

If a patient seeks care for a fracture at the physician's office, the following guidelines should be followed for global fracture care.

Codes 29000–29799 are to be used for:

- Replacement casts/strapping during or after follow-up period
- Initial service performed without restorative treatment of a fracture. injury, or dislocation

These services are performed to afford comfort to a patient.

If a cast/strapping/splint is provided as an initial service by the physician rendering the initial care only, the use of casting, strapping, or splinting (29000–29799) and/or supply code (99070) can be billed in addition to an evaluation and management code, as appropriate, if the following rules and guidelines apply:

- No other procedure or treatment is performed or provided
- No other procedure or treatment is expected to be performed

If a physician applies the initial cast, splint, or strapping and also assumes all the subsequent care for the fracture, dislocation, or injury, he/she cannot use CPT codes 29000–29799, because these services are included in the treatment of fracture and/or dislocation codes.

Restorative treatment or procedures rendered by another physician following the application of the initial cast/strapping may be reported with a treatment of fracture and/or dislocation code.

Podiatry Surgery

The human foot contains twenty-six bones, thirty-three joints, and more than one hundred muscles, tendons, and ligaments. Diagnosis and management of foot and ankle disorders depend on whether the problem is extra-articular (involving the tendons, nerves, ligaments, and bones) or articular (involving the joints).

The bones of the feet include:

- Phalanges, or toe bones
- Metatarsals, or long bones of the foot
- Tarsal bones, which form the ankle and heel

The great toe (hallux) has a proximal phalanx and a distal phalanx. Each of the other toes has a proximal phalanx, a middle phalanx, and a distal phalanx.

Surgeons use anatomical reference points as points of origin in locating other anatomical structures or as landmarks from which measurements can be taken. In podiatry surgery, the following anatomical reference points apply to each phalanx, metatarsal, and tarsal bone:

- Base, or proximal end
- Shaft, or body
- Head, or distal end

Joints, or articulations, are the points of connection between the bones of the skeleton. The human foot contains the following joints, among others:

- The interphalangeal (IP) joint is located in the great toe between the base of the distal phalanx and the head of the proximal phalanx.
- The distal interphalangeal (DIP) joint is located in the second through fifth toes between the base of a distal phalanx and the head of a middle phalanx.
- The metatarsophalangeal (MTP) joint is located in the first through fifth toes between the base of a proximal phalanx and the head of a metatarsal.
- The proximal interphalangeal (PIP) joint is located in the second through fifth toes between the base of a middle phalanx and the head of a proximal phalanx.
- The tarsometatarsal joint is located between the base of a metatarsal and the head of a tarsal bone.
- An intertarsal joint is located between two tarsal bones.

Coding Guidelines for Podiatry Surgery

Common types of outpatient podiatry surgery are hammertoe repair, toe amputation, arthrodesis of the great toe, and bunionectomies.

Hammertoe Repair

Common hammertoe correction techniques include arthroplasty, interphalangeal fusion or arthrodesis, partial phalangectomy, and total phalangectomy. Any technique used to repair a toe diagnosed as hammertoe should be coded as 28285. Code 28285 is assigned for each hammertoe that is repaired.

Toe Amputation

The surgical removal of a toe may be required to treat injury, infection, impaired blood supply, or tumor growth. The following codes apply:

- 28810: Assigned when a toe and metatarsal are amputated
- 28820: Used for toe amputation at the level of the metatarsophalangeal joint
- 28825: Assigned for toe amputation at the level of the interphalangeal joint

Example: Code 28285 hammertoe repair is grouped into APC 0055

APC	HCPCS	HCPCS Description	SI	Rel. Wt.	Payment Rate
0055			T	20.8284	1326.64
	28285	Repair of hammertoe			
	28810	Amputation toe and metatarsal			
	28755	Fusion of big toe			

Arthrodesis of Great Toe

Arthrodesis refers to the surgical replacement of a joint by creating a rigid connection, or fusion, between the bones. The bony fusion eliminates motion in the joint. Arthrodesis of the great toe may be performed to relieve pain, restore function and motion, or realign the structures of the foot. The following codes apply:

- 28750: Assigned for arthrodesis of the great toe at the metatarsophalangeal joint
- 28755: Used for arthrodesis of the great toe at the interphalangeal joint
- 28760: Assigned for arthrodesis of the great toe at the interphalangeal joint with extensor hallucis longus tendon transfer to the first metatarsal neck

Example: Codes 28750 and 28760 have similar resources and are grouped into the same APC 0056. Whereas 28755 (arthrodesis of the great toe at the interphalangeal joint) is grouped to APC 0055.

APC	HCPCS	HCPCS Description	SI	Rel. Wt.	Payment Rate
0056			T	44.2687	2819.65
	28750	Fusion of big toe joint			
	28760	Fusion of big toe joint			

Bunionectomies

Hallux valgus is the lateral deviation or subluxation of the great toe. With progressive subluxation of the first metatarsophalangeal joint, footwear exerts pressure on the medial metatarsal head and a thickened bursa, or bunion, develops. Many different procedures can be used to correct the bunion deformity. Common to most procedures is the excision of the exostosis (median eminence) from the medial aspect of the first metatarsal head. Osteotomies, bone resection, and joint replacement, which require prolonged convalescence, may be used in severe bunion cases.

The CPT codes for bunionectomies are found in the range 28110, 28290–28299. These codes represent unilateral procedures.

The complexity of bunion surgeries and the confusing terminology used to describe them make coding of these procedures one of the more difficult challenges for coders. Exhibit 4.3 provides brief descriptions and drawings of the primary bunionectomy procedures.

Example: Codes 28290–28299 have similar resources and are grouped into the same APC 0057. Where as 28110 (partial bunionectomy) is grouped to APC 0055.

APC	HCPCS	HCPCS Description	SI	Rel. Wt.	Payment Rate
0057			T	29.4167	1873.67
	28290–28299	Correction of bunion			

Arthroscopic Knee Surgery

Arthroscopy is used to treat various problems of the knee, including meniscal injuries, ligament injuries, loose bodies within the knee, chondromalacia, and osteoarthritis.

In a knee arthroscopy, a small incision is made in the front of the knee, and the arthroscope is inserted medially or laterally to the patellar tendon. The arthroscope is connected to a light system for viewing, and all parts of the knee are visualized. An irrigating system is set up to flush the joint. Diagnostic arthroscopy permits concurrent surgery or biopsy using triangulation in which instruments are passed through a separate cannula (a tube for insertion into a duct or cavity). After the arthroscope is removed, the incision is closed with a suture. When needed, an adhesive strip and elastic roller bandage are applied.

Coding Guidelines for Arthroscopic Knee Surgery

Common types of outpatient arthroscopic knee surgery include: synovectomy, debridement (chondroplasty), abrasion arthroplasty, arthroscopy with meniscectomy, arthroscopy with meniscus repair, arthroscopic anterior cruciate ligament repair, augmentation or reconstruction, and injections for postoperative pain control.

Synovectomy

The synovium is the thin membrane that lines the inside of freely moving joints. Synovectomy refers to the arthroscopic removal of synovium, using a motorized shaver.

Code 29876 is used for synovectomy, major, from two or more compartments of the knee including:

- The suprapatellar pouch, which is a separate compartment located at the kneecap on the top of the knee
- The medial compartment, which includes the medial femoral condyle, medial tibial plateau, and medial meniscus
- The lateral compartment, which includes the lateral femoral condyle, lateral tibial plateau, and the lateral meniscus
- The intercondylar notch, which is between the medial and lateral compartments

Debridement (Chondroplasty)

Arthroscopic debridement, or chondroplasty, of the knee is a procedure in which a motorized shaver is used to smooth out or resect irregularities of articular cartilage. The articular cartilage is the gristly, white, rubbery cap on the ends of bones where the bones touch each other.

Code 29877 is used for arthroscopic debridement of the articular cartilage of the knee.

For Medicare hospital outpatients, report code G0289 for an arthroscopic knee with removal of loose body or foreign body, or debridement/shaving of articular cartilage (chondroplasty) at the time of other surgical knee arthroscopy in a *different compartment of the same knee*. The documentation must reflect that the physician spent at least fifteen minutes in the compartment where the loose/foreign body removal or chondroplasty was performed.

Abrasion Arthroplasty

Prior to an abrasion arthroplasty, arthroscopic removal of any remnants of articular cartilage left inside the knee is performed to leave a bony surface. Then, an abrader, or bur is used to remove a very thin layer of dead bone to access an area of bleeding bone. Multiple holes may be drilled into the middle of the bone to activate more blood vessels and induce scab formation on the bone. The purpose of scab formation is to patch the articular cartilage of the bone. Without such a patch, the joint fluid would prevent normal bone healing by washing the scab formation away.

Code 29879 includes chondroplasty performed as part of the abrasion arthroplasty, so code 29877 should not be reported separately. When, however, chondroplasty is performed in a separate knee compartment, code 29877 may be reported separately. Distinct procedural service modifier –59 should be appended to indicate that a separate compartment was involved. This code also includes resection of osteophyte and removal of loose or foreign bodies when performed in the same compartment (AMA 2001a).

Arthroscopy with Meniscectomy

Arthroscopy with meniscectomy refers to arthroscopic partial or total resection of the medial and/or lateral meniscus. The medial meniscus is located on the inner side of the knee; the lateral meniscus is located on the outer side of the knee. A basket forceps (used to remove a portion of the meniscus), motorized shaver, scissors, or knives may be used to resect the meniscus.

To separately report arthroscopic debridement/shaving of articular cartilage (29877) and arthroscopic meniscectomy (29880, 29881) performed at the same session, the procedures must be performed in separate compartments of the knee. Appending the –59 modifier to the second procedure communicates that the procedures were performed in separate compartments of the knee (AMA 1999b, 11).

Arthroscopy with Meniscus Repair

Arthroscopic repair of the medial and/or lateral meniscus is performed by making an additional incision on the side of the knee and passing sutures (either from inside the knee outward or outside the knee inward) through the tear in the meniscal cartilage and then tying a knot over it. This stitch holds the torn meniscal cartilage in place. The additional incision is made to allow passage of the needles to insert the sutures through the cartilage in back of the knee, without injury to the blood vessels and nerves in that area. See Exhibit 4.4 for illustration of meniscal cartilage tear.

Codes 29882 and 29883 are used to report arthroscopy with meniscus repair.

Arthroscopic Anterior Cruciate Ligament Repair, Augmentation, or Reconstruction

A ligament is a band or sheet of fibrous tissue that connects two or more bones. One of the main stabilizing ligaments in the knee, the anterior cruciate ligament (ACL) runs from the tibia to the femur through the center of the knee. A rupture or tear of the ACL can be partial or complete and can lead to serious destabilization of the knee.

Code 29888 is used to report arthroscopic ACL repair, augmentation, or reconstruction. The following methods may be used to correct a rupture or tear in the ligament:

- Repair: Sutures or staples are placed into the injured ACL to promote healing. This procedure is performed infrequently (only one to two percent of the time), but most generally for a child or when the ligament is pulled right out of the bone and can be placed back into it.

- Augmentation: The injured ACL is repaired as stated above, and a hamstring tendon is run alongside the injured ligament as a splint.

- Reconstruction: The remains of the injured ACL are removed and replaced with a patellar or hamstring tendon, allograft (donated tissue from a tissue bank), or a synthetic ligament (not frequently used). Reconstruction is the most commonly performed ACL procedure.

From a CPT coding perspective, it would be appropriate to report meniscectomy code 29881 in addition to ACL repair code 29888 because the meniscectomy is not considered an integral component of the ACL repair/reconstruction (AMA 2003b). See Exhibit 4.5 for example of ACL reconstruction.

Example: Codes 28750 and 28760 (fusion big toe joint) have similar resources and are grouped into the same APC 0056; whereas, code 29876 (knee arthroscopy/surgery) and 29877 (chondroplasty) are grouped to APC 0041.

APC	HCPCS	HCPCS Description	SI	Rel. Wt.	Payment Rate
0041		Level I Arthroscopy	T	28.7803	1833.13
	29876	Knee arthroscopy/surgery			
	29877	Chondroplasty			

All the codes in the above section have similar resources and group to APC 0041.

Injections for Postoperative Pain Control

When general anesthesia is administered and pain management injections are performed to provide postoperative analgesia, they are separate and distinct services and are reported in addition to the anesthesia code. Whether the block procedure (insertion of catheter, injection of narcotic or local anesthetic agent) occurs preoperatively, postoperatively, or during the procedure is immaterial.

If, on the other hand, the block procedure is used primarily for the anesthesia itself, the service should be reported using the anesthesia code alone. In a combined epidural/general anesthetic, the block cannot be reported separately (AMA 2008).

Shoulder Surgery

Arthroscopic and open surgical procedures performed on the shoulder in the outpatient setting include arthroscopic subacromial decompression, claviculectomy, open rotator cuff repair, and capsulorrhaphy.

APC	HCPCS	HCPCS Description	SI	Rel. Wt.	Payment Rate	OPPS OCE
0042			T	45.7072	2911.27	Significant Procedure, Multiple Reduction Applies; Separate APC payment
	29827	Arthroscopic rotator cuff repair				

Coding Guidelines for Shoulder Surgery

Common types of outpatient shoulder surgery include arthroscopic subacromial decompression, claviculectomy, open rotator cuff repair, and capsulorrhaphy.

Arthroscopic Subacromial Decompression

Subacromial decompression is a procedure used to treat subacromial impingement syndrome, in which the rotator cuff tendon is pinched between the humeral head and the underside of the acromion. The arthroscopic procedure for subacromial decompression involves the following processes:

- Exposing the subacromial space
- Bursectomy
- Debridement
- Detaching the coracoacromial ligament
- Removing the undersurface of the acromion

When subacromial decompression is performed, a flat undersurface of the acromion and acromioclavicular joint is produced, which enlarges the supraspinatus outlet and prevents impingement.

Code 29826 is used to report arthroscopic subacromial decompression. The partial acromioplasty, arch decompression, excision of bursal tissue, and release of the coracoacromial ligament would not be reported separately because these are considered inclusive components of code 29826 (AMA 2001c).

Claviculectomy

Claviculectomy is the surgical removal of all or part of a clavicle, or collarbone. This procedure can be partial or complete and is performed for the treatment of injuries, osteoarthritis, and, as necessary, to gain access to, or relieve pressure on, underlying tissues and structures.

The following codes are used to report a claviculectomy:

- 29824: Assigned for arthroscopic distal claviculectomy. A distal claviculectomy is also called a Mumford procedure.
- 23120: Used for open partial claviculectomy.
- 23125: The correct code for open total claviculectomy.

Open Rotator Cuff Repair

Rotator cuff injuries are strains or tears of one or more rotator muscles or tendons, the most common site being the supraspinatus muscle. The major muscles of the rotator cuff are the supraspinatus, infraspinatus, and teres minor. An acute tear can result from a fall onto an outstretched hand; an injury incurred in throwing a football, pitching a baseball, or serving in racquetball; or manipulation of a frozen shoulder. Chronic tears originate from overuse or constant stress.

Code 23410 or 23412 is assigned for repairs involving one or two tendons or major muscles of the rotator cuff. Code 23420 is used for repair of a complete shoulder or rotator cuff avulsion, referring to the repair of all three major muscles/tendons of the shoulder cuff (AMA 2008). See Exhibit 4.6 for illustration of rotator cuff repair.

Capsulorrhaphy

The shoulder is the most mobile joint in the body, which makes it especially susceptible to dislocation followed by shoulder instability. Capsulorrhaphy, the suturing of a joint capsule, is used to treat instability of the shoulder, which can cause ongoing pain and increase the risk of recurring dislocations and other problems, such as rotator cuff tear.

The following codes are used to report capsulorrhaphy:

- Codes 23450, 23455, 23460, and 23462 are used for open anterior capsulorrhaphy.
- Codes 23465 and 23466 are used for open glenohumeral joint capsulorrhaphy.
- Code 29806 is used for arthroscopic capsulorrhaphy.

Hand Surgery

Like the human foot, the human hand contains many small bones. The bones of the hand are called carpals, metacarpals, and phalanges.

The thumb has a proximal phalanx and a distal phalanx, and each of the fingers has a proximal phalanx, a middle phalanx, and a distal phalanx.

The anatomical reference points of the hand are similar to those of the foot, with the following terms used to identify the parts of each phalanx, metacarpal, and carpal bone:

- Base, or proximal end
- Shaft, or body
- Head, or distal end

The major joints of the hand are located as follows:

- The interphalangeal (IP) joint is located in the thumb between the base of the distal phalanx and the head of the proximal phalanx.
- The distal interphalangeal (DIP) joint is located in the second through fifth fingers between the base of a distal phalanx and the head of a middle phalanx.
- The metacarpophalangeal (MCP) joint is located in the first through fifth fingers between the base of a proximal phalanx and the head of a metatarsal.
- The proximal interphalangeal (PIP) joint is located in the second through fifth fingers between the base of a middle phalanx and the head of a proximal phalanx.

- The carpometacarpal joint is located between the base of a metacarpal and the head of a carpal bone.
- The intercarpal joint is located between two carpal bones.

Coding Guidelines for Hand Surgery

Common types of outpatient hand surgery include Dupuytren's contracture treatment, carpometacarpal joint interposition arthroplasty, and arthrodesis/fusion.

Dupuytren's Contracture Treatment

Dupuytren's contracture refers to a shortening and thickening of the deep tissue of the palm, or palmar fascia, which creates a flexion deformity of the fingers. The resultant clawing of the hand is treated by surgical incision (fasciotomy) to release the cordlike structures under the skin or by excision (fasciectomy) to remove the diseased fascial tissue in the palm.

The following codes are used to report Dupuytren's contracture:

- Code 26040: Used for percutaneous palmar fasciotomy
- Code 26045: Assigned for open partial palmar fasciotomy
- Code 26121: The correct code for palm only fasciectomy
- Code 26123: Used for partial palmar fasciectomy with release of single digit contracture
- Code 26125: Assigned for fasciectomy release of each additional digit contracture

Carpometacarpal Joint Interposition Arthroplasty

The term *arthroplasty* refers to the surgical reconstruction or replacement of a joint. Carpometacarpal joint interposition arthroplasty is used to treat osteoarthritis of the carpometacarpal (CMC) joint of the thumb. Known as the anchovy procedure, this procedure does not implant an artificial joint or prosthesis but, instead, reroutes tendons to act as a cushion between the thumb and wrist bones. The procedure consists of an excisional arthroplasty combined with a rolled tendon interposition graft. A strip of tendon from the flexor carpi radialis tendon or the palmaris longus tendon is rolled into a ball and placed into the space created by the complete excision of the trapezium.

Although classic carpal tunnel syndrome patients complain of numbness and weakness in their hand(s) with night pain, others present with a myriad of complaints, such as forearm discomfort or shooting pains up the arm, swelling, peculiar hand symptoms, temperature sensitivities and finger soreness.

APC	HCPCS	HCPCS Description	SI	Rel. Wt.	Payment Rate	OPPS OCE
0047			T	35.9040	2286.87	Significant Procedure, Multiple Reduction Applies; Separate APC payment
	25447	Repair wrist joint (s) interposition, intercarpal or carpometacarpal joints				

Code 25447 is assigned for a carpometacarpal joint interposition arthroplasty; an additional CPT code should be assigned for the tendon transfer. See Exhibit 4.7 for an illustration of carpal tunnel.

Arthrodesis/Fusion

Arthrodesis, or fusion, is another procedure used to treat osteoarthritis of the joints of the thumb and fingers. Arthrodesis immobilizes the joints, which helps to eliminate pain and improve the alignment and appearance of the digits.

The following codes are used to report arthrodesis/fusion:

- Code 26820 is used for thumb fusion in opposition with autograft.
- Codes 26841 and 26842 are used for thumb carpometacarpal joint arthrodesis.
- Codes 26843 and 26844 are used for second-, third-, fourth-, or fifth-digit carpometacarpal joint arthrodesis.
- Codes 26850 and 26852 are used for metacarpophalangeal joint arthrodesis.
- Codes 26860, 26861, 26862, and 26863 are used for interphalangeal joint arthrodesis.

Documentation Requirements for Musculoskeletal Procedures

Following each procedure is clinical information that must be documented in the medical record when the procedure is performed.

Injection Procedures

The CPT codebook index should be referred to for codes and code descriptions.

1. Reason for injection:
   - Therapeutic
   - Prophylactic
   - Diagnostic

2. Site of injection:
   - Abscess
   - Anterior segment, eye
   - Aponeurosis (for example, plantar "fascia") (Specify each site.)
   - Bone cyst
   - Bursa
   - Cyst
   - Epidural
   - Flap/graft
   - Ganglion cyst
   - Intra-amniotic
   - Intralesional
   - Intramuscular

- Intrapleural
- Intravenous
- Intravitreal
- Joint
- Ligament (Specify each ligament.)
- Peritoneal cavity
- Retina
- Sentinel node
- Sinus tract
- Subcutaneous
- Subconjunctival
- Tendon sheath (Specify each tendon sheath.)
- Tenon's capsule
- (trans) Tracheal
- Trigger point(s) (Specify site and number of muscles injected.)
- Turbinates
- Ureter
- Urethra
- Vascular
- Vocal cord (through laryngoscope)

3. Substance(s) being injected:
   - Air
   - Alcohol
   - Allergan
   - Anesthetic
   - Antispasmodic
   - Blood or clot patch
   - Chemotherapy
   - Contrast for radiological procedure
   - Gas
   - Gastric stimulant
   - Liquid
   - Lytic solution
   - Medication
   - Neurolytic substance
   - Opioid
   - Pharmacologic agent
   - Sclerosing solution

- Steroid
- Subcutaneous filling material
- Urinary implant material (for example, collagen)
- Vaccine
- Vitreous substitute

4. Dosage of medication/pharmaceutical substance injected

Application of Casts/Strapping

The CPT codes for casts/strapping are in the 20000–29909 range.

1. The patient's diagnosis (for example, sprain, strain, dislocation, fracture)

2. The anatomical site of the disorder. Always specify the anatomical reference point when the fracture or dislocation involves the metacarpals, metatarsals, or phalanges of the fingers or toes:

   - Proximal (base)
   - Shaft/body
   - Distal (head)

3. The type of treatment provided. Document all that apply:

   - Application of cast and/or strapping for stabilization or comfort
   - Restorative treatment—application of cast and/or strapping
   - Restorative treatment—closed manipulation/reduction
   - Restorative treatment—open reduction
   - Restorative treatment—internal fixation
   - Restorative treatment—percutaneous skeletal fixation
   - Restorative treatment—skin or skeletal traction
   - Restorative treatment—external fixation
   - Restorative treatment—soft tissue repair

4. The discharge instructions for the patient, specifically:

   - Will the patient follow up with you or another physician?
   - What is the reason for the follow-up visit?
     - To remove cast/strapping
     - Orthopedic consultation
     - Restorative treatment
     - Other (specify)

Treatment of Fractures/Dislocations

The CPT codebook index should be referred to for codes and code descriptions.

1. The anatomic site of the fracture or dislocation

2. Whether the treatment was open or closed

3. Whether manipulation (reduction) was involved

4. Whether traction was applied

5. Whether percutaneous skeletal fixation was applied

6. Whether internal fixation was applied

7. Whether an external fixation system was applied

8. Whether soft-tissue closure was performed

Arthroscopic Knee Surgery

For arthroscopic knee major synovectomy (CPT code 29876), *each* compartment of the knee in which synovium is removed:

- Suprapatellar pouch
- Intercondylar pouch
- Medial compartment
- Lateral compartment

For arthroscopic knee debridement/chondroplasty (CPT code 29877), *each* compartment of the knee in which debridement/chondroplasty is performed:

- Suprapatellar pouch
- Intercondylar pouch
- Medial compartment
- Lateral compartment

For rotator cuff repair (CPT codes 23130, 23410, 23412, 23415, 23420, 29827):

- Whether the rotator cuff tear is acute or chronic
- Whether the patient has suffered a complete rotator cuff avulsion
- The specific muscles and tendons of the shoulder cuff that were repaired (Note: CPT coding guidelines state that the repair of a complete rotator cuff avulsion refers to the repair of all three major muscles/tendons of the shoulder cuff.)
- Whether an acromioplasty was performed
- Whether each procedure was performed via an open or arthroscopic approach

Case Studies

This section contains actual operative reports from real-life cases. All identifiers have been removed or changed for confidentiality and privacy.

Carefully read the clinical documentation for each case study, which may include a procedure report as well as radiology and/or pathology reports, as applicable.

Answer all the questions for further review that appear at the end of each case study. Use a current CPT codebook or HCPCS Level II code listing, as needed.

When appropriate, assign one or more of the following modifiers:

–50	Bilateral Procedure
–59	Distinct Procedural Service
–FA	Left hand, thumb
–F1	Left hand, second digit
–F2	Left hand, third digit
–F3	Left hand, fourth digit
–F4	Left hand, fifth digit
–F5	Right hand, thumb
–F6	Right hand, second digit
–F7	Right hand, third digit
–F8	Right hand, fourth digit
–F9	Right hand, fifth digit
–LT	Left side
–RT	Right side
–TA	Left foot, great toe
–T1	Left foot, second digit
–T2	Left foot, third digit
–T3	Left foot, fourth digit
–T4	Left foot, fifth digit
–T5	Right foot, great toe
–T6	Right foot, second digit
–T7	Right foot, third digit
–T8	Right foot, fourth digit
–T9	Right foot, fifth digit

Do not apply the current version of the Medicare CCI edits to any of these questions; the focus is on the application of the coding guidelines and not on the application of edits that change on a quarterly basis. When coding in real life, of course, you will need to apply the CCI edits as appropriate for Medicare outpatient cases.

Case Study 4.1

Read the following clinical document and answer the questions for further review.

OPERATIVE REPORT

PREOPERATIVE DIAGNOSIS: Myofascial pain

OPERATION: Trigger point injections

ANESTHESIA: Local

BLOOD LOSS: Minimal

COMPLICATIONS: None

HISTORY: This is a 56-year-old lady with a history of right occipital neuralgia. The pain has greatly diminished, allowing her to reduce her oxycodone; however, she has been experiencing right neck pain that radiates to the right shoulder, right occipital area, and the right temple and right eye. Her pain is currently a 2/10, but intermittently can go as high as a 9/10 sharp, shooting pain. On physical exam, she has full motor strength of the upper extremities, but decreased range of motion with head rotation and trigger points in the right trapezius, right sternocleidomastoid, right splenius cervicis, and capitis muscles.

PROCEDURE: Informed consent and agrees to the risks of bleeding, infection, nerve injury, paralysis, increased pain, failure to relieve pain permanent or temporary, headache, reaction to medications, numbness, and weakness. All questions were answered, options explained. NPO status confirmed. In the supine to right-sided up position, a 1½ inch #25 gauze needle was used to release trigger points using 0.1 cc of 2% lidocaine in two areas of the right trapezius, two areas of the right splenis capitis, two areas of the splenis cervicis, and two areas of the right sternocleidomastoid. She tolerated this well and stretching was done.

ASSESSMENT AND PLAN: The patient suffers from occipital neuralgia with secondary myofascial pain. We will see how trigger point injections work at diminishing the pain in hopes of further diminishing the opioid use. Thank you for this referral.

Questions for Further Review: Case Study 4.1

1. What was the reason for the injection(s)?
   a. Therapeutic
   b. Prophylactic
   c. Diagnostic

2. What was the anatomical site of the injection?
   a. Single trigger point in one muscle
   b. Multiple trigger points in one muscle
   c. Multiple trigger points in multiple muscles

3. What substance(s) was(were) injected?
   a. Anesthetic
   b. Chemotherapy
   c. Steroid

4. What dosage of medication/pharmaceutical substance was injected?

5. CPT surgery code(s) and modifier(s):

Case Study 4.2

Read the following clinical document and answer the questions for further review.

EMERGENCY ROOM REPORT

PROBLEM: Fall

This is a 78-year-old woman who lost her balance while carrying out a bag of garbage. She fell forward, landing on her left wrist on a grass or possibly concrete surface, striking her nose up against her wrist, and breaking her glasses. She experienced a nosebleed. A neighbor helped her to her feet and brought her to the hospital for evaluation. Her nose is no longer bleeding. She has no tenderness or swelling of facial muscles. She has notable ecchymosis about her wrist on the dorsum of her left hand, though she moves this without any notable guarding or tenderness. Her wrist is straight. An x-ray demonstrates that she has a nondisplaced and minor impacted fracture of the distal radius, which is treated today with a short arm splint. Her lungs are clear. Her chest wall is nontender. Her cardiac exam is regular without appreciable gallops or murmurs at a rate of 80. Her abdomen is soft without masses, tenderness, or organomegaly. Her extremities demonstrate no distal edema with good movement of her legs. Her gait is stable.

She is asked to use acetaminophen at 650 mg 3–4 times a day. She will continue to be followed on a routine schedule by Dr. ABC for her tic douloureux, which currently entails use of Neurontin and amitriptyline. I ask that she continue to wear her splint for the next 3–4 weeks.

Questions for Further Review: Case Study 4.2

1. What was the patient's diagnosis?

2. What was the anatomical site of the disorder?

3. What type of treatment was provided?
   a. Application of cast and/or strapping for stabilization or comfort
   b. Restorative treatment: Application of cast and/or strapping
   c. Restorative treatment: Closed manipulation/reduction
   d. Restorative treatment: Open reduction
   e. Restorative treatment: Internal fixation
   f. Restorative treatment: Percutaneous skeletal fixation
   g. Restorative treatment: Skin or skeletal traction
   h. Restorative treatment: External fixation
   i. Restorative treatment: Soft tissue repair

4. What discharge instructions were provided to the patient?
   a. To follow up with this physician
   b. To follow up with another physician for removal of cast/strapping
   c. To follow up with another physician for orthopedic consultation
   d. To follow up with another physician for restorative treatment
   e. To follow up with another physician for other reason (specify)
   f. None of the above

5. CPT surgery code(s) and modifier(s):

Case Study 4.3

Read the following clinical document and answer the questions for further review.

EMERGENCY REPORT

Adm. Date: 8/12/200X   **Age:** 66   **Room #:** ED

CHIEF COMPLAINT: Left wrist pain

HISTORY OF PRESENT ILLNESS: The patient tripped on a curb, fell and extended her hand, and hurt her left wrist.

SOCIAL HISTORY: She is down visiting this area. She used to live here and is visiting family.

PHYSICAL EXAMINATION

GENERAL: She is a pleasant 66-year-old female.

EXTREMITIES: Angulated fracture of the left wrist

RADIOLOGY STUDIES: X-ray reveals a Colles fracture with impaction.

DIAGNOSIS: Colles fracture of the left wrist

PLAN:

1. A long-arm posterior splint
   Tylox (#12) 1 q 4 h. p.r.n. pain
2. Talked over the case with Dr. _____. The patient will need pins and plaster, and she will do that on Monday. He will call her at the location where she is staying on Monday morning.

Questions for Further Review: Case Study 4.3

1. What was the patient's diagnosis?

2. What was the anatomical site of the disorder?

3. What type of treatment was provided?
   a. Application of cast and/or strapping for stabilization or comfort
   b. Restorative treatment: Application of cast and/or strapping
   c. Restorative treatment: Closed manipulation/reduction
   d. Restorative treatment: Open reduction
   e. Restorative treatment: Internal fixation
   f. Restorative treatment: Percutaneous skeletal fixation
   g. Restorative treatment: Skin or skeletal traction
   h. Restorative treatment: External fixation
   i. Restorative treatment: Soft tissue repair

4. What discharge instructions were provided to the patient?
   a. To follow up with this physician
   b. To follow up with another physician for removal of cast/strapping
   c. To follow up with another physician for orthopedic consultation
   d. To follow up with another physician for restorative treatment
   e. To follow up with another physician for other reason (specify)
   f. None of the above

5. CPT surgery code(s) and modifier(s):

Case Study 4.4

Read the following clinical document and answer the questions for further review.

OPERATIVE REPORT

PREOPERATIVE DIAGNOSIS: Left great toe proximal phalanx fracture, interarticular

POSTOPERATIVE DIAGNOSIS: Left great toe proximal phalanx fracture, interarticular

OPERATION: Closed reduction, percutaneous pin fixation, intercondylar left proximal phalanx fracture of the great toe

INDICATIONS: The patient is a 45-year-old female with displaced fracture of the great toe appearing intercondylar with greater than 2-mm displacement of the lateral fragment.

PROCEDURE: The patient was placed under general anesthesia. Fluoroscopic image was used for guidance. The toe was prepped and draped with extremity drapes and Dura-Prep. A tourniquet was placed on the calf but was not used during the case.

The toe underwent closed reduction with a manual adjustment and utilizing a percutaneous clamp. This reduced the articular gap to anatomic.

There was still a small amount of rotational deformity dorsally of the lateral condylar fragment. This was brought down by flexing the toe and using manual adjustment.

With the fragments in place, two 1.6-mm K-wires were passed percutaneously across the condyle and into the shaft. This held the fracture in an anatomically reduced position. The wires were trimmed. The toe was dressed with a gauze dressing and tube gauze.

The patient recovered from anesthesia without complication.

Estimated blood loss was minimal. Fluids instilled were crystalloid.

Questions for Further Review: Case Study 4.4

1. What was the anatomic site of the fracture or dislocation?
2. Was the treatment open or closed?
3. Was manipulation (reduction) involved?
4. Was traction applied?
5. Was percutaneous skeletal fixation applied?
6. Was internal fixation applied?
7. Was an external fixation system applied?
8. Was soft-tissue closure performed?
9. CPT surgery code(s) and modifier(s):

Case Study 4.5

Read the following clinical document and answer the questions for further review.

OPERATIVE REPORT

POSTOPERATIVE DIAGNOSIS: Articular fracture, middle phalanx, right middle finger, with involvement of the proximal interphalangeal joint

OPERATION: Open reduction, fracture distal phalanx, proximal interphalangeal joint, right middle finger

DESCRIPTION OF PROCEDURE: The patient was brought to the operating room, placed in the supine position on the table, and after satisfactory intravenous block anesthesia, the area was prepped and draped in the usual manner. A zig-zag incision was made. Extreme care was taken not to injure the distal nerves. A skin flap was elevated. The C2 pulley area was approached. The flexor tendons were retracted. The fracture fragment, along with the volar plate, was present. The fracture fragment was excised. The tourniquet was released. Hemostasis was secured. A check x-ray showed satisfactory position; hence, no K-wire was inserted to prevent dorsal dislocation. The reduction was found to be stable, and the wound was irrigated with saline. The tourniquet was released after infiltrating the flexor tendons. The skin edges were approximated with #5-0 chromic catgut sutures. The wound was dressed with an Adaptic dressing and dry gauze. A dorsal splint was applied over the middle finger. Circulation to the finger was satisfactory. No complications were encountered during the procedure.

Questions for Further Review: Case Study 4.5

1. What was the anatomic site of the fracture or dislocation?
2. Was the treatment open or closed?
3. Was manipulation (reduction) involved?
4. Was traction applied?
5. Was percutaneous skeletal fixation applied?
6. Was internal fixation applied?
7. Was an external fixation system applied?
8. Was soft-tissue closure performed?
9. CPT surgery code(s) and modifier(s):

Case Study 4.6

Read the following clinical document and answer the questions for further review.

OPERATIVE REPORT

PREOPERATIVE DIAGNOSES:

1. Painful hammertoe deformity, right fourth digit
2. Painful hammertoe deformity, right fifth digit
3. Painful Tailor's bunion, right fifth metatarsal

POSTOPERATIVE DIAGNOSES:

1. Painful hammertoe deformity, right fourth digit
2. Painful hammertoe deformity, right fifth digit
3. Painful Tailor's bunion, right fifth metatarsal

OPERATION:

1. Hammertoe: Correct right fourth digit
2. Hammertoe: Correct right fifth digit
3. Excision Tailor's bunion, right fifth metatarsal

ANESTHESIA:
IV sedation. Local infiltration 10 cc of 1% lidocaine plain, 0.5% Marcaine plain

HEMOSTASIS: Pneumatic ankle tourniquet 250 mmHg

TOURNIQUET TIME: 95 minutes

MATERIALS: 3-0 Vicryl, 4-0 Vicryl, 4-0 nylon

PATHOLOGY: None

PROCEDURE/FINDINGS: The patient was placed on the operating room table in the supine position. A well-padded ankle tourniquet was applied to her right ankle. After aforementioned anesthesia, the tourniquet was inflated to 250 mmHg. The foot was exsanguinated and incisions were planned 4 cm in length over the fifth metatarsal head and neck area. This was made with a #15 scalpel blade. Blunt and sharp tissue dissection took place, denuding the fifth metatarsal of periosteal capsule, the fifth metatarsal having noted to be significantly prominent laterally. Next, utilizing a sagittal saw, the prominence was removed, and the dorsal exostosis was rasped and smoothed. Using large amounts of normal sterile saline, the periosteum was closed with 3-0 Vicryl sutures in superficial fascia, 3-0 Vicryl suture for the skin, 4-0 Vicryl suture running subcuticular stitch. Next the fifth digit was examined. Two semi-elliptical incisions were made obliquely across the fifth digit and sharp dissection took place to the TIPJ and DIPJ. Next, using the sagittal saw, the head of the proximal phalanx was removed. The remaining base was remodeled with a rongeur and flushed with large amounts of normal sterile saline. The digit was then de-rotated and the tendon repaired with a 3-0 Vicryl suture, the skin with 4-0 nylon suture holding the digit in the corrected position.

The fourth digit was then examined and noted to be in significant abducted varus position. Two synovial elliptical incisions were made over the PIPJ. The central ellipse of skin was removed. Blunt and sharp digital dissection took place down to the extensor digitorum lateris tendon. This was incised with a #15 scalpel blade. The head of the middle phalanx was then removed with a sagittal saw and remodeled utilizing a rongeur. This was flushed with large amounts of normal sterile saline, repaired with 3-0 Vicryl suture, de-rotating the toe, and repaired with 4-0 nylon suture. The areas were then injected with 3 cc of 0.5% Marcaine plain. The foot was then dressed with Betadine soaked Adaptic, 4 x 4s, Kerlix, and a conforming bandage. The patient was transferred from the operating room to the recovery room with vital signs stable and neurovascular status to a right foot fully intact. She is to be partial weightbearing and wear a surgical shoe. She was given medications for pain. Percocet one tablet 9.6 h. p.r.n. pain, Motrin 800 mg one tablet t.i.d. She is to return for a postoperative visit in 48 hours.

Questions for Further Review: Case Study 4.6

1. What was the diagnosis for the right fourth and fifth toes?

2. Where was the patient's bunion located?
   a. Right great toe
   b. Left great toe
   c. Right fifth metatarsal
   d. Left fifth metatarsal

3. Which procedure was performed on the fifth metatarsal?
   a. Ostectomy, complete excision
   b. Ostectomy, partial excision
   c. Metatarsectomy

4. Which of the following techniques was used to repair the right fourth and right fifth digits?
   a. Partial phalangectomy
   b. Interphalangeal fusion
   c. Total phalangectomy

5. CPT surgery code(s) and modifier(s):

Case Study 4.7

Read the following clinical document and answer the questions for further review.

OPERATIVE REPORT

PREOPERATIVE DIAGNOSIS: Ischemic necrosis to the second toe of the left foot

POSTOPERATIVE DIAGNOSIS: Ischemic necrosis to the second toe of the left foot

ANESTHESIA: 1% local Xylocaine

OPERATIVE PROCEDURE: Amputation of the second toe of the left foot

The patient was placed in a supine position on the operating room table. Successful local anesthesia was affected with 1% Xylocaine at the base of the second toe. The toe was obviously necrotic. A curvilinear incision was made from the dorsal to plantar in the first webspace around the second toe. The second toe was disarticulated from its articulation at the metatarsophalangeal joint. The bed of the toe was then fairly irrigated; then closure was carried out. The subcutaneous dead space was closed using 2-0 Vicryl and the skin closed using 4-0 nylon. There was ample bleeding during the operation to be optimistic about the viability of the amputation site. The foot was dressed in the sterile dressing and the patient returned to the recovery room in stable condition.

SURGICAL PATHOLOGY REPORT

AGE: 68 **Gender:** F

Specimen(s) Received: Left 2nd toe

Final Diagnosis: Gangrene left 2nd toe; gangrene of skin and subcutaneous tissue

Clinical History: Gangrene left 2nd toe

Gross Description: The specimen is labeled "left second toe."

The specimen is received in formalin and consists of a single toe measuring 5.0 cm from the tip of the toe to the proximal margin. The toe is covered by darkly pigmented skin. The soft tissue at the margin is grossly necrotic. A necrotic area is located at the ventral aspect of the toe. Bone is submitted following decalcification. Representative sections are submitted. Multiple sections/3 cassettes.

Questions for Further Review: Case Study 4.7

1. What procedure was performed on the toe?
   a. Amputation of metatarsal with toe
   b. Amputation toe, metatarsophalangeal joint
   c. Amputation toe, interphalangeal joint

2. On which toe was the procedure performed?

3. CPT surgery code(s) and modifier(s):

Case Study 4.8

Read the following clinical document and answer the questions for further review.

OPERATIVE REPORT

PREOPERATIVE DIAGNOSIS: Severe recurrent hallux valgus deformity of right forefoot

POSTOPERATIVE DIAGNOSIS: Severe recurrent hallux valgus deformity of right forefoot

OPERATIVE PROCEDURE: Right hallux MP arthrodesis

ANESTHESIA: General with supplemental 0.5% plain Marcaine ankle block per surgeon for postoperative analgesia

TOURNIQUET TIME: Slightly over one hour at 300 mmHg

DRAINS: None

COMPLICATIONS: None

IMPRESSION: Percutaneous threaded K-wires

DESCRIPTION OF PROCEDURE: After satisfactory general anesthesia was established with the patient supine on the operating room table, the tourniquet was then placed on the right thigh. Ancef 1 g IV had been administered. After successful anesthesia was established, the right foot and ankle were prepped and draped to a sterile fashion and held elevated for several minutes. The tourniquet was inflated to 300 mmHg.

A dorsal incision was made along the medial border of the extensor hallucis longus tendon. Full-thickness subperiosteal flaps were developed off the base of the proximal phalanx and off the metatarsal head and neck until adequate exposure of the joint surfaces was gained. The articular surfaces were then removed with hand instruments. The subchondral base plate was left in place on the proximal phalangeal side, but perforated multiple times with a K-wire. When adequate bone resection had been gained in order to allow reduction of the deformity, the threaded K-wires were placed on the base of the proximal phalanx out the end of the toe. The hallux was then positioned in proper location for fusion. The K-wires were passed into the metatarsal head. The bone was quite friable, but in spite of this, the fixation appeared to be quite good. The wires were cut off and capped.

The wounds were irrigated and closure was obtained with interrupted 2-0 Vicryl and 4-0 nylon for the skin. A 0.5% plain ankle block was put in place prior to skin closure. The patient was awakened from anesthesia and taken to the recovery room in stable condition. No complications were encountered, and counts were correct.

DISPOSITION: She will be discharged home following recovery from anesthesia with office follow-up next week. She has Tylox, #40, with no refill, for pain. She should keep the dressing dry and foot elevated. She should weight bear on heel only and report any interim problems if they occur.

1. Which of the following procedures was performed?
   a. Hallux valgus correction with resection of joint and insertion of implant
   b. Subtalar arthrodesis
   c. Arthrodesis great toe, interphalangeal joint
   d. Arthrodesis great toe, metatarsophalangeal joint

2. CPT surgery code(s) modifier(s):

Case Study 4.9

Read the following clinical document and answer the questions for further review.

OPERATIVE REPORT

PREOPERATIVE DIAGNOSIS: Hallux valgus bilateral

POSTOPERATIVE DIAGNOSIS: Hallux valgus bilateral

OPERATION PERFORMED: Silver bunionectomy, bilateral

ANESTHESIA: General

PROCEDURE: The patient was placed supine on the operating table, at which time she was put to sleep under general anesthesia. Following this, both feet were prepped with sterile solution and draped in a sterile fashion.

The tourniquet was applied first to the right lower extremity. A dorsally curved incision was made over the metatarsophalangeal joint of the great toe. This was carried down through skin and subcutaneous tissue to the underlying capsule. The capsule was opened longitudinally and the underlying first metatarsal head exposed. Here a large exostosis was removed using an osteotome. This was then smoothed with the rongeurs. The area was then explored, and no other evidence of second pathology could be noted. The area was irrigated with saline solution, following which the capsular layer was closed with interrupted sutures. The skin edges were anesthetized with Marcaine and closed with 5-0 nylon suture. The wound was then dressed in a sterile fashion and the tourniquet released.

Attention was then turned to the left leg, where a tourniquet was applied. A dorsally curved incision was made and carried down through skin and subcutaneous tissue to the underlying capsular layer. Here the capsule was opened. The exostosis was exposed and excised with the use of an osteotome and smoothed with rongeurs. The area was then irrigated with saline solution, following which the capsular layer was closed with 0 Vicryl interrupted sutures. Skin edges were anesthetized with Marcaine and closed with 5-0 Vicryl suture. The wound was dressed in a sterile fashion. The tourniquet was released, and the patient was returned to the recovery room in satisfactory condition.

1. Was the hallux valgus/bunion deformity unilateral or bilateral?
2. What bunion repair technique was used?
3. CPT surgery code(s) and modifier(s):

Case Study 4.10

Read the following clinical document and answer the questions for further review.

OPERATIVE REPORT

PREOPERATIVE DIAGNOSES:
1. Bunion of the right foot
2. Hallux valgus

POSTOPERATIVE DIAGNOSES:
1. Bunion of the right foot
2. Hallux valgus

PROCEDURE PERFORMED: Implant arthroplasty with correction of bunion to the right foot

ANESTHESIA: Local with IV sedation

HEMOSTASIS: Pneumatic ankle tourniquet at 250 mmHg for 69 minutes

PROCEDURE: The 72-year-old patient was brought from the holding area and placed on the operating table in the supine position. After the administration of IV sedation, a local block was achieved using a 0.5% Marcaine plain, approximately 17 cc used in a Mayo block fashion about the right first metatarsal. The foot was prepped and draped, and then an Esmarch bandage was applied for exsanguination, and a pneumatic tourniquet was inflated 250 mmHg.

Attention was directed to the dorsal medial aspect of the right foot in the area of the first metatarsal phalangeal joint. Just medial to the extensor tendon, a 5-m curvilinear incision was made. The incision was deepened via sharp and blunt dissection, taking care to preserve and protect all neurovascular structures. Those structures encountered were retracted to the side or bovied as required. The incision was carried down to the level of the joint capsule, about the first metatarsal phalangeal joint. Here a T-shaped capsulotomy was performed extending from the base of the distal phalanx onto the neck of the first metatarsal and also down along the medial aspect of the joint. All soft tissue was then dissected free from the head of the first metatarsal and the base of the proximal phalanx. Quite a few erosions were noted to the joint cartilage, a lot of gouty tophi was present that was imbedded into the joint cartilage and pocketed into the joint capsule. The capsule was quite thick around the head of the first metatarsal. As much as possible, this was cleaned up and removed.

I then used a power oscillating saw to resect the cartilaginous head of the first metatarsal and the cartilaginous surface of the base of the proximal phalanx. I used a Shannon-type bur to ream out both the first metatarsal distal portion and the proximal portion of the proximal phalanx of the great toe. In doing this, I was able to create a channel for acceptance of the implant stems. I went ahead and irrigated the wound and used sizers to measure the appropriate implant. I decided on a total flexible hinged implant, size #3, and we used the grommets. I went ahead and placed this in the normal manner and reevaluated the joint. We found that the implant was the right size for the patient. There was good range of motion at the first metatarsal phalangeal joint, with no impingement of bone. We did a final irrigation of the wound and then began to close the soft tissues using 3-0 and 2-0 Vicryl for the periosteal tissues and joint capsule. I performed a capsulorrhaphy along the medial aspect of the head of the first metatarsal and then closed subcutaneous tissues and skin using 4-0 Vicryl in a running subdermal suture fashion. I augmented the closure with tape closures and then injected 1 cc of dexamethasone phosphate for his postoperative anti-inflammatory effect. We dressed the wound with Adaptic, sterile 4x4 gauze, 3-inch Kling, and a mildly compressive Coban wrap. Pneumatic tourniquet was released to reveal an instantaneous reflex hyperemia to digits 1 to 5 of the right foot. Estimated blood loss for this procedure was less than 5 cc. There were no specimens for pathology. The patient tolerated the surgery and anesthesia without complication and left the operating room for recovery with vital signs stable and neurovascular status intact.

Questions for Further Review: Case Study. 4.10

1. Was the hallux valgus/bunion deformity unilateral or bilateral?
2. What bunion repair technique was used?
3. CPT surgery code(s) and modifier(s):

Case Study 4.11

Read the following clinical document and answer the questions for further review.

OPERATIVE REPORT

ANESTHESIA: 20 cc of a 50–50 mixture of 1% lidocaine plain and 0.5% Marcaine plain with intravenous sedation, monitored anesthesia care

PREOPERATIVE DIAGNOSES:

1. Painful bunion deformity, right foot
2. Painful, contracted hammertoe deformity, proximal interphalangeal joint and distal interphalangeal joint, right second digit
3. Metatarsophalangeal joint contracture with extensor digitorum longus contracture, right second digit

POSTOPERATIVE DIAGNOSES:

1. Painful bunion deformity, right foot
2. Painful contracted hammertoe deformity, proximal interphalangeal joint and distal interphalangeal joint, right second digit
3. Metatarsophalangeal joint contracture with extensor digitorum longus contracture, right second digit

OPERATIONS:

1. Austin osteotomy, modified McBride bunionectomy, with 0.062 Kirschner wire fixation, right foot
2. Proximal interphalangeal joint and distal interphalangeal joint arthroplasties, right second toe, with 0.042 Kirschner wire fixation
3. Metatarsophalangeal joint capsulotomy and extensor digitorum longus tendon lengthening, second metatarsophalangeal joint, right foot

HEMOSTASIS: Pneumatic ankle tourniquet at 250 mmHg for a tourniquet time of 105 minutes

MATERIALS: 2-0 Vicryl, 3-0 Vicryl, 4-0 nylon, 0.042 Kirschner wire, 0.062 Kirschner wire

INJECTABLES: 1 cc of dexamethasone phosphate and 0.5% Marcaine 5 cc plain

INDICATIONS: This 47-year-old female presents to the facility requesting a surgical intervention of her painful bunion deformity of the right foot, contracted metatarsophalangeal joint, and hammertoe deformity of the right second digit. The patient relates that conservative therapy has failed to alleviate her symptomatology. She understands her risks and the possible complications of the proposed surgery as well as the postoperative course.

She has had medical clearance provided, and she has signed a consent form. No guarantees as to the outcome of the surgery were given.

PROCEDURE/FINDINGS: The patient was brought to the operating room and placed on the operating room table in the normal supine position. A well-padded ankle tourniquet was applied to her right ankle, but it was not inflated at this time. After suitable anesthesia had been obtained utilizing a 50/50 mixture of 1% lidocaine plain with 0.5% Marcaine plain for 20 cc in a posterior tibial block and Mayo block fashion, the foot was prepared in the usual sterile manner. The foot was then exsanguinated and the tourniquet inflated to 250 mmHg.

Attention was then directed over the dorsal aspect of the second digit. A linear incision was made from the distal interphalangeal joint over the proximal interphalangeal joint and metatarsophalangeal joint. The incision was deepened with blunt and sharp tissue dissection down to the level of the joint capsule. The joint capsule at the proximal interphalangeal joint was then incised, incising the extensor digitorum longus tendon. The medial and lateral collateral ligaments were dissected free from the proximal phalanx head, denuding it. The distal interphalangeal joint was also incised with a #15 scalpel blade. The head of the middle phalanx was also denuded. Both the middle phalanx head and the proximal phalanx head were then removed using a sagittal saw.

Next, a 0.042 Kirschner wire was retrograded through the middle phalanx, crossing the distal interphalangeal joint, holding the distal phalanx in a corrected fashion. The Kirschner wire was then retrograded through the proximal phalanx shaft down to its base. Care was taken to leave space between the proximal phalanx, middle phalanx, and distal phalanx. The tendon was then repaired with a 4–0 Vicryl suture.

The metatarsophalangeal joint was dissected free of soft tissue, and the extensor digitorum longus tendon was lengthened in a sagittal plane in Z fashion. The metatarsophalangeal joint capsule was then incised with a 115 scalpel blade. The toe was noted to relocate without tension.

The superficial fascia was repaired with 3–0 Vicryl suture, and the skin was reapproximated with 4–0 nylon suture.

Attention was then directed to the first metatarsophalangeal joint, where a linear incision was made approximately 4 cm in length over the dorsal medial aspect. Blunt and sharp tissue dissection took place down to the level of the joint capsule. The superficial fascia was then dissected free from the joint capsule of the dorsal medial exostoses. The first interspace was entered with a pair of Metzenbaum scissors, and the superficial and deep fibers of the deep transverse metatarsal ligament were sharply incised. Next, a #15 scalpel blade was used to incise the fibular sesamoidal ligament. The fibular sesamoid was noted to be freed of its lateral attachments. The adductor hallucis tendon was then isolated and grasped with a straight hemostat. This was dissected free from the fibular sesamoid, and a section of the tendon was removed.

Next, a linear capsulotomy was made over the dorsal medial aspect of the first metatarsophalangeal joint. The joint capsule was dissected free of the dorsal medial exostosis, which was exposed into the wound. This dorsal medial exostosis was removed with a sagittal saw, taking care to leave the plantar sagittal groove intact.

Next, a chevron osteotomy was planned with the apex at the center of the first metatarsophalangeal joint. The chevron osteotomy was performed from medial to lateral with the use of a sagittal saw. The capital fragment was shifted over approximately 0.5 cm. This was then impacted into the shaft of the metatarsal. A 0.062 Kirschner wire was retrograded from distal plantar lateral through proximal medial dorsal. This was retrograded down past the subchondral bone plate with the capital fragment in the corrected position. The remaining exostoses on the shaft of the first metatarsal were removed with a sagittal saw, and the area was rasped smooth.

Next, a medial capsulorrhaphy was performed. This was repaired with 2–0 Vicryl suture, holding the hallux in a rectus position. The wound was copiously lavaged with large amounts of normal sterile saline. The capsule was then repaired with 2–0 Vicryl suture, holding the hallux in a corrected position. The superficial fascia was repaired with 3–0 Vicryl suture. The skin was reapproximated with a 4–0 nylon suture running subcuticular stitch reinforced with tape closures. Then 1 cc of dexamethasone phosphate was injected into the second toe in the metatarsophalangeal joint. The wound was dressed with large amounts of Kerlix, Kling, and 4 x 4s after it had been blocked with 0.5% Marcaine plain, 5 cc.

At this time, the tourniquet was released for a total tourniquet time of 105 minutes. The patient was noted to have immediate capillary refill from digits one through five. The foot was then dressed with 4 x 4s, Kerlix, Kling, and an Ace bandage. The patient was transferred from the operating room to the recovery room with vital signs stable and neurovascular status to her right foot fully intact.

She was given postoperative instructions as to ice and elevation 15 minutes per hour and to elevate as much as possible for the first 72 hours. Prescriptions for Motrin 800 mg one tablet t.i.d. p.c., Keflex 500 mg one tablet t.i.d. for 5 days, and Percocet one tablet q. 4–6h. p.r.n. pain. Should the patient have any postoperative complications, concerns, or questions, she was instructed to call Dr. Martin at the answering service. A follow-up appointment was made for Monday, April 28.

Questions for Further Review: Case Study 4.11

1. Which of the following techniques was used to repair the right second hammertoe?
    a. Partial phalangectomy
    b. Interphalangeal fusion
    c. Total phalangectomy

2. Which of the following techniques was used to repair the right second metatarsophalangeal joint contracture?
    a. Capsulotomy
    b. Capsulotomy with tendon lengthening

3. What bunion repair technique was used?

4. CPT surgery code(s) and modifier(s):

Case Study 4.12

Read the following clinical document and answer the questions for further review.

OPERATIVE REPORT

OPERATIVE INDICATIONS: The patient is a 23-year-old male with a history of left knee injury and subsequent left anterior cruciate ligament disruption. The patient lives an active lifestyle and is now indicated for a left ACL reconstruction.

OPERATIVE PROCEDURE: The patient was brought to the operating room and after successful placement of an epidural catheter, the patient's left lower extremity was prepped and draped in the usual sterile fashion, after a tourniquet had been placed on his left upper thigh. Two transverse incisions were marked below the distal pole of the patella, approximately 4.5 cm distal and slightly medial to the tibial tubercle. Each incision was approximately 5 cm in length. These incisions were then infiltrated subcutaneously with a mixture of 0.25% Marcaine and 1% lidocaine with 1:100,000 epinephrine. Prior to making the incisions, the knee was examined under anesthesia. There was evidence of a 2+ Lachman with approximately 7-mm excursion, with no end point. In addition, there was a positive pivot shift. Range of motion was from +10-1/2 of extension to 130-1/2 of flexion. There was no evidence of a posterior drawer or posterolateral rotary instability. In addition, there was no varus or valgus instability at both 0 and 30-1/2 of flexion.

At this point, the incisions were opened through the subcutaneous tissue and down to the level of the patellar tendon paratenon. This was then cleared. Any obvious bleeding was stopped with electrocautery. The paratenon was incised to expose the underlying patellar tendon. Similarly, the distal incision was opened down to the level of the paratenon, which was also opened. The paratenon was then opened between the two incisions underneath the tissue bridge. At this point, the paratenon was opened up over the patella. The medial and lateral edges of the patellar tendon were exposed. A 10-mm ACL blade was used to make a cut in the central third of the patellar tendon. This was taken down to the level of the tibial tubercle, where a 2.5 x 1 cm bone block was measured out. An oscillating saw was used to make cuts in the bone, and the bone plug was removed. Similarly, a patellar bone plug was measured out, approximately 2 x 1 cm, and again, an oscillating saw was used to remove the patellar bone block. The graft was then taken to the back table and fashioned so that each bone plug would be able to go through a 10-mm sizer. Sutures were placed on either end of the bone plug. The overall length of the graft was 81 mm.

At this point, attention was turned to the knee. Two portals were made medially and laterally in the inferior position through the proximal defect. The scope was then introduced into the anterolateral portal, the knee was inflated with saline, and examination of the knee was begun. The patellofemoral joint was found to be without evidence of the articular damage. The medial femoral condyle had no evidence of damage. In the medial compartment, there was evidence of a tear of the medial meniscus at the inferior edge, which was approximately 6 mm in length. This tear was probed and found to be stable, and was not in need of excision or repair. Attention was now turned to the intercondylar notch. There was evidence of a stenotic notch, as well as a disrupted anterior cruciate ligament, with a few remaining fibers intact. The PCL was found to be normal throughout.

Examination of the lateral compartment now revealed a peripheral tear in the posterior horn, extending posterolaterally for approximately 1.5 cm. The tear was at the periphery, and there was a small margin of meniscus remaining. The tear could be easily subluxed into the joint and reduced. At this point, meniscal repair was carried out. The meniscus was subluxed into the joint, and the peripheral tissue was rasped using an end-cutting shaver. The meniscus was then reduced. Four suture anchors were placed into the meniscus, approximately 1 cm apart in the midsubstance of the meniscus. With the meniscus reduced, each end was tied down with secure knots. The meniscus at this point was reprobed and found to be stable and reduced along the periphery. There was no evidence of articular damage, of either the lateral or medial femoral condyles.

At this point, a notchplasty was performed in the intercondylar notch using a 5.5-mm bur. After the soft tissue had been removed, the over-the-top position was established approximately 7 cm from the posterior ridge in the one o'clock position. This point was then marked with the bur. The tibial drill guide was placed into the knee and on the tibial eminence, just slightly medial to the tibial spine, just anterior to the PCL insertion. At this point, the drill guide was connected and the drill bit placed through the tibia and arthroscopically visualized. The drill guide then was overreamed using a 10-mm reamer. The chamfer was used to chamfer out the tibia hole and remove any remaining soft tissue. With the knee in hyperflexion, the intercondylar notch was visualized. A guide wire was placed into the previously marked hole in the isometric position in the femoral intercondylar notch. A series of dilators was used to dilate the femoral tunnel, starting with 4 mm and up to 10 mm. When this had been done, the femoral tunnel was inspected and found to have a good posterior wall. The tunnel was then rasped.

At this point, the graft was brought to the table. A Beeth needle was placed through the tibial bony canal, into the femoral canal, and out through the skin of the thigh, with the knee approximately 90-1/2 of flexion. The graft was then passed intra-articularly through the knee with the cancellous bone surface facing anteriorly. This was visualized arthroscopically, and the bone plug in the femur was found to be well seated.

At this point, a guide wire was placed superiorly into the femoral canal, and a 7 x 20 Kurosaka screw was placed over the guide wire, which securely fastened the femoral bone plug. At this point, the knee was brought through a range of motion and visualized arthroscopically. At full extension, there was no evidence of impingement of the graft. In addition, there was no evidence of excursion of the graft at the tibial side.

With the graft under tension and the knee in slight flexion, attention was now turned to the tibial bone plug. Again, the cancellous surface was facing anteriorly, and a guide wire was placed into the tibial bone plug. At this point, with tension on the graft, a 9 x 20 Kurosaka screw was placed into the tibial bone plug. Again, the knee was taken through a range of motion and the Lachman test was found to be negative. At this point, the sutures were removed from both the femoral and tibial ends. The wounds were irrigated copiously and closed in an interrupted fashion using #2-0 Vicryl sutures for the sub-cutaneous tissue and then a running #3-0 Prolene subcuticular suture. An intra-articular drain was placed into the knee prior to closure. At this point, tape closures were placed over the wound, which had been cleaned and dried. A dry sterile dressing and an ice pack were placed on the knee. Postoperatively, the patient will be placed on protocol #3, which requires six weeks of crutches and toe-touch weightbearing. The patient had the epidural removed and was brought to the recovery room in stable condition.

DRAINS: One soft Hemovac

ESTIMATED BLOOD LOSS: Approximately 100 cc

SPECIMENS: None

COMPLICATIONS: None

Questions for Further Review: Case Study 4.12

1. The patellar bone graft was harvested to repair which condition?
    a. Left anterior cruciate ligament disruption
    b. Lateral posterior horn meniscal tear

2. Which technique was used to repair the lateral compartment posterior horn tear?
    a. Open meniscectomy
    b. Arthroscopic meniscectomy
    c. Arthroscopic meniscal repair
    d. Open meniscal repair

3. Which of the following procedures was/were performed to correct the left anterior cruciate ligament disruption?
    a. Notchplasty
    b. Use of the drill to chamfer out the tibia hole
    c. Placement of the patellar bone plug graft
    d. All of the above

4. CPT surgery code(s) and modifier(s):

Case Study 4.13

Read the following clinical document and answer the questions for further review.

OPERATIVE REPORT

PREOPERATIVE DIAGNOSIS: Meniscus tear, right knee

POSTOPERATIVE DIAGNOSIS:
1. Tear of right medial meniscus
2. Grade 2 to 3 chondromalacia of the medial and lateral femoral condyles

OPERATION: Arthroscopic partial right medial meniscectomy and chondroplasty, medial and lateral femoral condyle

PROCEDURE/FINDINGS: Under satisfactory general anesthesia, with the tourniquet high on the right leg, the leg was prepped and draped in the usual sterile manner.

The arthroscope was introduced anterolaterally, a Veress needle in the suprapatellar pouch medially, and the knee was distended with Ringer's and inspected.

The suprapatellar pouch and patellofemoral joint were normal. Medially, however, there was noted to be tearing of the posterior horn of the medial meniscus. Using a basket and motorized shaver, a partial medial meniscectomy was carried out. There was also grade 2 to 3 chondromalacia of the medial and lateral femoral condyles. Using a turbo whisker, these were debrided as well. The gutters were normal. The anterior and posterior cruciate ligaments were intact.

The knee was copiously irrigated with Ringer's, followed by Marcaine with epinephrine. The wounds were closed with 5-0 nylon sutures. Sterile dressings were applied.

The patient left the operating room in satisfactory condition.

Questions for Further Review: Case Study 4.13

1. Which technique was used to repair the meniscal tear?
   a. Arthroscopic medial meniscectomy
   b. Arthroscopic lateral meniscectomy
   c. Arthroscopic medial and lateral meniscectomy

2. In which of the following compartments of the knee was the chondromalacia debridement performed?
   a. Suprapatellar pouch
   b. Intercondylar pouch
   c. Medial compartment
   d. Lateral compartment

3. CPT surgery code(s) and modifier(s):

Case Study 4.14

Read the following clinical document and answer the questions for further review.

OPERATIVE REPORT

PREOPERATIVE DIAGNOSES:
1. Synovitis of the right knee
2. Arthrosis of patellofemoral joint of the right knee
3. Tear of the posterior horn of the medial meniscus of the right knee
4. Tear of the middle one third of the lateral meniscus of the right knee

POSTOPERATIVE DIAGNOSIS:
1. Synovitis of the right knee
2. Arthrosis of patellofemoral joint of the right knee
3. Tear of the posterior horn of the medial meniscus of the right knee
4. Tear of the middle one third of the lateral meniscus of the right knee

OPERATION: Right knee arthroscopy, with:
1. Extensive synovectomy of the mediolateral compartment of the right knee
2. Partial medial meniscectomy
3. Partial lateral meniscectomy
4. Abrasion arthroplasty of the patellofemoral articulation

ANESTHESIA: Epidural with sedation

TOURNIQUET: None used

ESTIMATED BLOOD LOSS: Minimal blood loss

DESCRIPTION OF PROCEDURE: The patient was taken to the operating room and after induction of an epidural anesthetic, he was given perioperative antibiotics. The right knee and lower extremity were prepped and draped in a sterile fashion, and three portals were created: one superomedially for outflow, one inferolaterally for the arthroscope, and one inferomedially for instrumentation. At this time, the joint was distended with saline solution, utilizing arthroscopic pump, and initially attention was turned to the patellofemoral articulation. There was extensive synovitis noted, which precluded adequate visualization of the articular surfaces, and a synovectomy was performed with a 4-mm aggressive meniscal resector, with hemostasis obtained with the Arthrocare wand.

With this completed, there was noted to be significant loss of articular cartilage of the medial femoral condyle superiorly, as well as the lateral facet of the patella, with grade 4 changes. There was also fibrillation with grade 3 changes in the marginal articular regions of the patellofemoral joint. Utilizing the 4-mm aggressive resector in high-speed mode, an abrasion arthroplasty was performed on the eburnated subchondral bone to stimulate punctate bleeding, and chondroplasty was utilized from the articular margins to remove any fibrillated articular fragments. With this completed, attention was turned to the lateral compartment of the knee, where, again, extensive synovitis was noted, which precluded appropriate visualization of the anterior horn of the meniscus. A synovectomy was once again performed, with a 4-mm aggressive meniscal resector, and hemostasis was obtained with an Arthrocare wand. At this point, the lateral meniscus was identified and probed. There was noted to be a radial tear in the middle one third of the lateral meniscus, and a 4-mm aggressive meniscal resector was used to perform a partial lateral meniscectomy. The meniscus was then sealed with the Arthrocare wand, and probing of the lateral meniscus upon completion of the partial lateral meniscectomy revealed no further tears or subluxation into the joint. At this point, the arthroscope was placed in the intercondylar region where the anterior and posterior cruciate ligaments were identified and probed. There was no evidence of acute hemorrhage. There was some slight laxity of the ACL noted with a firm end point. At this time, attention was directed to the medial compartment of the knee, where, again, profound synovitis was noted. Synovectomy was performed with a 4-mm aggressive meniscal resector, and hemostasis was obtained with the Arthrocare wand. The medial meniscus was then identified and probed. There was noted to be a complex tear of the posterior horn of the medial meniscus, with both vertical and horizontal cleavage components. Utilizing a combination of biting basket scissors, as well as the 4-mm aggressive meniscal resector and Arthrocare wand, a partial meniscectomy was performed. With this completed, the remaining medial meniscus was probed and showed no evidence of further tears or subluxation to the joint. There were some grade 2–3 chondral changes of the medial femoral condyle noted.

At this time, the joint was copiously irrigated and drained. The three portal sites were closed with a simple 3-0 Prolene suture and 20 cc of 0.25 percent Marcaine with epinephrine, as well as 10 mg of morphine were instilled intra-articularly for postoperative analgesia. A bulky, dry, sterile dressing was applied.

The patient tolerated the procedure well and was taken to the recovery room without complications.

COMPLICATIONS: None

Questions for Further Review: Case Study 4.14

1. What procedures were performed on the eburnated subchondral bone?
   a. Arthroscopic microfracture
   b. Arthroscopic abrasion arthroplasty
   c. Arthroscopic chondroplasty

2. From which compartment of the knee was synovium removed?
   a. Suprapatellar pouch
   b. Intercondylar pouch
   c. Medial compartment
   d. Lateral compartment

3. Which technique was used to repair the meniscal tear?
   a. Arthroscopic medial meniscectomy
   b. Arthroscopic lateral meniscectomy
   c. Arthroscopic medial and lateral meniscectomy

4. What procedure was performed for postop pain control?
   a. Intra-articular/joint injection of medication
   b. Peripheral nerve injection of medication

5. CPT surgery code(s) and modifier(s):

Case Study 4.15

Read the following clinical document and answer the questions for further review.

OPERATIVE REPORT

PREOPERATIVE DIAGNOSES:
1. Acromioclavicular joint arthritis, right shoulder
2. Possible superior labrum anterior and posterior lesion or labrum tear, right shoulder

POSTOPERATIVE DIAGNOSES:
1. Osteoarthritis right acromioclavicular joint
2. Anterior superior labrum anterior and posterior lesion, right shoulder

TITLE OF THE OPERATION:
1. Arthroscopic superior labrum anterior and posterior lesion repair with one 3.0-mm Bio FasTac suture anchor
2. Arthroscopic distal clavicle excision, right shoulder

ANESTHESIA: General

PREOPERATIVE NOTE: The patient is a 57-year-old gentleman with a long history of right shoulder pain. Preoperative evaluation indicated pain emanating from an arthritic AC joint, and we suspected a SLAP lesion as well. We did not suspect the rotator cuff or impingement. Therefore, the above procedure was recommended.

DETAILS OF THE PROCEDURE: Under general anesthetic, the patient was placed supine in the semi-sitting position with the head on a Mayfield headrest. The right shoulder was scrubbed, prepped, and draped in the usual manner. The posterior viewing portals were established through the glenohumeral joint. The articular cartilage in the glenoid and humeral sides was normal. The posterior labrum and direct superior labrum were normal. However, the anterior superior labrum was detached. There was a SLAP lesion under the biceps anchored anteriorly coming down to the approximately 1 o'clock. We probed this through an anterior portal in the rotator interval and found this to be true. The biceps tendon anchor was normal except for the anterior portion of the anterior superior labrum. The biceps tendon exited the joint normally. The rotator cuff was normal.

We prepared the anterior superior glenoid neck with a shaver and a bur after using the periosteal elevator to mobilize the soft tissue. Next, we placed a single 3.0 Bio FasTac suture anchor at approximately 12:30 on the anterior superior glenoid rim. We used standard arthroscopic knot-tying techniques to tie down the anterior superior labrum with the anterior portion of the biceps anchor. Fortunately, the majority of the biceps anchor was intact. We had established this using a peel-back sign intraoperatively. When the labrum was repaired, we probed it and found it to be stable.

Next, the subacromial space was entered. A lateral working portal was established. We excised enough of the subacromial bursa to visualize the anterior acromion. We denuded the anterior acromion across to the AC joint, removing the inferior AC joint ligaments. The distal clavicle was clearly identified. We removed the osteophyte on the medial end of the anterior acromion, which was in part partial of the AC joint osteophyte. We then did approximately an 8-mm distal clavicle excision through the same anterior portal that we used for the labrum repair by redirecting it directly into the AC joint. We removed all the clavicle up to, but not including, the superior AC joint ligaments.

Next, the arthroscopic instruments were removed. The portals were closed with 4-0 nylon. A sterile dressing was applied followed by a shoulder immobilizer. Sponge and instrument counts are correct. The patient tolerated the procedure well and was transferred to the recovery room in satisfactory condition.

POSTOPERATIVE PLAN: The patient will be discharged home today and I will see him in the office in a few days time for follow-up.

Questions for Further Review: Case Study 4.15

1. Which of the following techniques was used to repair the SLAP lesion?
   a. Arthroscopic distal clavicle excision
   b. Arthroscopic excision of subacromial bursa
   c. Arthroscopic placement of a suture anchor on the anterior superior glenoid rim

2. Arthroscopic subacromial decompression is supported by which of the following operative report excerpts?
   a. "subacromial space was entered"
   b. "excised enough of the subacromial bursa"
   c. "removing inferior AC joint ligaments"
   d. "removed the osteophyte. . . acromion"

3. Which of the following procedures was performed on the clavicle?
   a. Open total claviculectomy
   b. Open partial claviculectomy
   c. Arthroscopic distal claviculectomy

4. CPT surgery code(s) and modifier(s):

Case Study 4.16

Read the following clinical document and answer the questions for further review.

OPERATIVE NOTE

ANESTHESIA: General, with interscalene block augmentation, right shoulder

PREOPERATIVE DIAGNOSIS: Torn rotator cuff

POSTOPERATIVE DIAGNOSIS:

1. Massive tear, rotator cuff
2. AC joint arthritis
3. Dislocated biceps tendon anteriorly

OPERATIVE PROCEDURES:

1. Open repair of massive and chronic rotator cuff tear with acromioplasty and CA ligament resection
2. Open Mumford procedure (AC joint resection)
3. Biceps tenodesis

PROCEDURE: Under a good general anesthetic, augmented by interscalene block, the patient's right shoulder is examined. The patient has no abnormalities on inspection. The patient is put through a massive range of motion. With the arm abducted to 90 degrees, he can externally rotate to about 70, internal rotation is about 50, and forward elevation is to about 160–170. There is no evidence of instability.

At this point, the patient is placed in the beach chair position and the sandbag placed underneath the operative scapula. The right shoulder and neck are prepped and draped in the usual fashion for right shoulder surgery. A modified anterolateral approach is made to the shoulder. A 2-inch incision starts under the palpable AC joint and extends distally and laterally for a couple of inches. The incision is taken through skin and subcutaneous tissues, down to the deltoid. The deltoid is split along the raphe, separating the anterior and middle deltoid fibers. The deltoid is subperiosteally dissected from the anterolateral border of the acromion. The CA ligament is identified and resected. The humeral head is depressed with a cloverleaf retractor, and an anterior inferior acromioplasty is performed.

The undersurface of the acromion is smoothed out with a rasp. We are very happy with our decompression. The AC joint is identified. There is inferior spurring and arthritic changes in the AC joint, so a Mumford is performed. An oblique osteotomy is performed, removing the distal 1 cm of the clavicle, maintaining the superior AC ligaments. Thorough irrigation of this area is performed. Again, the undersurface is rasped to a smooth surface. We are very happy with our decompression of the subacromial arch area.

Attention is now paid to the cuff. There is an obvious massive tear involving the supraspinatus, infraspinatus, and teres minor. There is also a rotator interval split. The biceps tendon is dislocated anteriorly. The hypertrophic bursa is resected. The biceps tendon is relocated into its bicipital groove and tenodesed with #1 Ethibond. The free edges of the rotator cuff are identified, and 0 Vicryl is used for stay sutures. The cuff is mobilized. We are very happy with the mobilization. A trough is made into the greater tuberosity. The cuff is then repaired tendon-to-bone into the trough with #1 Ethibond.

We are very happy with our repair. The rotator interval is then closed with #1 Ethibond as well. There is no undue tension with the cuff at the neutral position. Thorough irrigation is performed. Hemostasis is achieved, where necessary, and closure started. The deltoid is reattached to the anterior acromion with #1 Ethibond. The deltoid split is closed with #1 Ethibond. The subcutaneous tissues are closed with 2-0 Vicryl and the skin with staples. The wounds are cleaned and dried. A sterile compression dressing is applied. The patient is put into an abductor pillow. There were no intraoperative complications. The patient tolerated the procedure well and went to the recovery room in good condition.

Questions for Further Review: Case Study 4.16

1. Removal of the distal clavicle is also called a:
   a. Mumford procedure
   b. SLAP repair
   c. Bankhart repair

2. The massive rotator cuff tear involved which of the following muscles and tendons?
   a. Supraspinatus
   b. Infraspinatus
   c. Teres minor
   d. All of the above

3. What procedure was performed on the biceps tendon?
   a. Tenodesis
   b. Resection
   c. Transplantation

4. Code 23420 includes an acromioplasty.
   a. True
   b. False

5. CPT surgery code(s) and modifier(s):

Case Study 4.17

Read the following clinical document and answer the questions for further review.

OPERATIVE REPORT

PREOPERATIVE DIAGNOSIS: Recurrent anterior shoulder dislocation, left

POSTOPERATIVE DIAGNOSIS: Recurrent anterior shoulder dislocation, left

OPERATION: Open capsular shift reconstruction, left shoulder

ANESTHESIA: General anesthesia

ESTIMATED BLOOD LOSS: Less than 100 cc

DRAINS: None

INDICATIONS FOR SURGERY: This is a 24-year-old gentleman who is status post open Bankart reconstruction, left shoulder. He had done excellent until he had a work-related injury June 26, 2000. His shoulder slipped out of joint, and he has had a couple of other episodes of dislocations of the shoulder that required reduction in the emergency room, so he was admitted for elective reconstruction.

His exam under general anesthesia revealed significant anterior instability, some subluxation posteriorly. Negative sulcus sign.

PROCEDURE/FINDINGS: The skin was prepped and draped in a sterile fashion. The original surgical incision over the anterior left shoulder was excised. The deltopectoral interval was developed. The cephalic vein was not encountered; I would probably say it had been previously ligated. There was significant scar tissue adjacent to the conjoined tendon. It was carefully separated. The underlying subscapularis muscle was identified. The subscapularis muscle was transected 1 cm medial to its insertion on the humerus and then carefully dissected free of the capsule and retracted so that the capsule could be identified. The previously placed capsular stitches were still in place and identified. The capsule was split longitudinally to the glenoid at the junction of the proximal two-thirds and lower third of the capsule and a Bankart lesion encountered. The labrum was excised additionally inferiorly, and the glenoid rim and neck were roughened with a rasp. Mitek SuperAnchors were placed, one at about 5:30 and the other at approximately 8:30 on the glenoid. Then these anchors and attached stitches were used to reattach the inferior capsule and labrum to the glenoid, pulling it superiorly. Then, using previously placed #2 Ethibond sutures, the inferior capsule was pulled and reefed superiorly underneath the superior capsule. Stitches were placed, but not tied, and then with the arm in the neutral position and some slight abduction, the stitches were tied. This gave excellent stability to the shoulder. The superior capsule was then pulled inferiorly further reinforcing the repair.

At this point, soft tissues were injected with 25% Marcaine with epinephrine, and the subscapularis muscle was reattached to the humerus with #2 Ethibond and some #1 Vicryl sutures. Subcutaneous tissue was closed with 2-0 Vicryl and the skin with skin clips. Sling and swathe were applied and the patient returned to the recovery room in satisfactory condition.

Questions for Further Review: Case Study 4.17

1. The patient had an anterior shoulder dislocation.
   a. True
   b. False

2. Which of the following codes classifies the procedure performed?
   a. 23450: Capsulorrhaphy, anterior; Putti-Platt procedure or Magnuson type operation
   b. 23455: Capsulorrhaphy, anterior; with labral repair (for example, Bankart procedure)

Case Study 4.18

Read the following clinical document and answer the questions for further review.

OPERATIVE REPORT

PREOPERATIVE DIAGNOSIS: Dupuytren disease, right hand

POSTOPERATIVE DIAGNOSIS: Dupuytren disease, right hand

OPERATION: Excision of Dupuytren disease, right hand, from right thumb, right middle finger, and right palm

ANESTHESIA: General

INDICATIONS: This is a 56-year-old female with painful and large Dupuytren nodules at the aspect of the first webbed space by the thumb, at the PIP joint of the middle finger with approximately 30% contracture, and at the A1 pulley area in line with the ring finger. She desires definitive treatment and presents for excision.

PROCEDURE: The patient was taken to the operating room and placed in the supine position. After general anesthesia was obtained, a tourniquet was placed high on the right upper extremity, and the right upper extremity was prepped and draped in the usual sterile fashion. First, the arm was exsanguinated and the tourniquet inflated to 250 mmHg. The total tourniquet time was less than 2 hours.

Infiltration of 0.5% Marcaine was performed at each of the sites where the Dupuytren disease was present for postoperative anesthesia.

First, attention was directed to the palmar area in line with the ring finger. A transverse incision was made at the distal/palmar crease where the disease was present. The skin was sharply dissected away from the disease. Circumferential dissection of the disease was completed. It was cut distally and dissected proximally. Careful attention was paid to protect the underlying neurovascular bundles and flexor tendon.

The disease was completely excised and sent to Pathology. The wound was copiously irrigated. Hemostasis was obtained with electrocautery. The skin was gently approximated with 5-0 nylon.

Next, attention was paid to the PIP joint of the middle finger, where, again, a transverse incision was made at the PIP crease. Circumferential dissection was carried out around the ulnar aspect of the digit. The ulnar neurovascular bundle was first identified and then dissection carried out and completed around the disease. It was also released proximally and dissected distally. It was taken off of the middle phalanx, and this helped correct the 30% contracture of the PIP joint.

Next, attention was paid to the first webbed space just below the thumb. A transverse incision was made over longitudinal disease. And again, circumferential dissection was carried out around the disease protecting underlying neurovascular structures.

The disease was able to be excised in toto. This wound was also gently approximated with 5-0 nylon after copious irrigation and hemostasis being obtained with electrocautery. All wounds were dressed with Xeroform and dressing sponges. This was held with Kerlix and then an Ace wrap.

Estimated blood loss was minimal. The IV fluids replaced were less than 2,000 cc of crystalloid. Drains and packs were none. Complications were none.

The patient tolerated the procedure well and was taken to the recovery room in a good postoperative condition.

SURGICAL PATHOLOGY REPORT

Age: 56 **Sex**: F

CLINICAL DIAGNOSIS: Dupuytren's disease, right thumb, middle, and ring fingers

TISSUE SUBMITTED: Fascia, right thumb, middle, and ring fingers

GROSS: Fascia, right thumb, middle, ring finger

The specimen is received in formalin and consists of three fragments of firm, rubbery whitish-yellow, partially friable tissue, ranging in size from 1.0 x 0.8 x 0.5 cm up to 1.5 x 1.0 x 1.0 cm. Representative sections will be submitted in one cassette.

DIAGNOSIS: Tissue from right hand, fragments of adipose tissue with fibrovascular tissue and fibrotendinous components showing fibroblastic cellular proliferative changes compatible with a fibromatosis of Dupuytren's contracture

---

Questions for Further Review: Case Study 4.18

1. Which of the following procedures was performed?
   a. Percutaneous palmar fasciotomy
   b. Open partial palmar fasciotomy
   c. Palm-only fasciectomy
   d. Partial palmar fasciectomy with release of single digit
   e. Partial palmar fasciectomy with release of multiple digits

2. Which digits were released?
   a. Right thumb
   b. Right middle finger
   c. Right ring finger

3. CPT surgery code(s) and modifier(s):

Case Study 4.19

Read the following clinical document and answer the questions for further review.

OPERATIVE REPORT

PREOPERATIVE DIAGNOSIS: Right thumb pan trapezial arthritis

POSTOPERATIVE DIAGNOSIS: Same

OPERATION PERFORMED: Right thumb trapeziectomy and ligament reconstruction tendon interposition (LRTI)

ANESTHESIA: Axillary block

INDICATIONS FOR OPERATION: The patient is a 69-year-old gentleman with a long history of bilateral thumb pain. He's been treated nonoperatively for pan trapezial arthritis with splints and anti-inflammatory drugs and has been unresponsive. He now is scheduled for surgical intervention.

DESCRIPTION OF OPERATION: The patient was brought to the operating room, and axillary block anesthesia was performed. After adequate anesthesia, the right upper extremity was prepped and draped in the usual sterile manner. The limb was exsanguinated with an Ace wrap, tourniquet brought to 275 mm of mercury. Longitudinal incision was made over the base of the thumb, metacarpal, carried sharply down through the skin and subcutaneous tissue. Superficial radial nerve was identified and protected. The capsule over the trapeziometacarpal joint was then sharply incised. The radial nerve was identified and retracted approximately, and perforators were cauterized. Subperiosteal dissection was then carried around the trapezium. It was split with a sagittal saw and removed piecemeal. A flexor carpi radialis tendon was then harvested in the proximal forearm and pulled through the defect left by the trapezium. The base of the metacarpal was then removed using the oscillating saw. A 4-mm bur was then used to make a tunnel through the metacarpal at the base. The tendon was then passed up through this hole and folded down on itself and held in place with 4-0 Ti-Cron incorporating the lower capsule. The remaining tendon was then woven in an anchovy type fashion and placed in the defect.

The capsule was then closed using 4-0 Ti-Cron. Tendon interval closed with 4-0 Vicryl. Tendon interval closed with 4-0 Vicryl. Skin closed with 4-0 Vicryl and 4-0 nylon. The patient was placed in a standard postoperative bulky dressing with a splint. He tolerated the procedure well and was brought to the recovery room in stable condition.

Questions for Further Review: Case Study 4.19

1. The trapezium is a:
    a. Carpal bone
    b. Metacarpal bone
    c. Phalanx

2. The flexor carpi radialis tendon was harvested from which site?
    a. Wrist
    b. Hand
    c. Proximal forearm

3. The operative report states: "The tendon was then passed up through this hole and folded down on itself." What type of arthroplasty is this?
    a. Interposition
    b. Intermission

4. CPT surgery code(s) and modifier(s):

Case Study 4.20

Read the following clinical document and answer the questions for further review.

OPERATIVE RECORD

PREOPERATIVE DIAGNOSES:
1. Chronic painful mallet deformity, left little finger
2. Distal interphalangeal joint arthritis, left little finger

OPERATION: Distal interphalangeal joint fusion, left little finger, with autograft

ANESTHESIA: Local

INDICATIONS: This is a 46-year-old female who suffered an injury to her little finger DIP joint and has had pain, redness, and irritation in that joint since July of this year.

On physical exam, she had a chronic mallet deformity, but on exam she also had pain at the DIP joint consistent with possible early osteoarthritis. She presented for definitive treatment.

PROCEDURE: The patient was taken to the operating room and placed in the supine position. A digital block was performed with 0.5% Marcaine plain. A tourniquet was placed high on the left upper extremity. The left upper extremity was prepped and draped in the usual sterile fashion. The arm was exsanguinated. The tourniquet was inflated to 250 mmHg. The total tourniquet time was less than 2 hours.

First, an S-shaped incision was made on the dorsum of the DIP joint, taken down to the level of the extensor mechanisms, where flaps were raised. The previous disruption of the extensor mechanism was identified. The DIP joint was entered, and there was significant loss of cartilage off the middle phalanx, as well as the distal phalanx. Because of these findings, it was elected to perform a DIP joint fusion.

Using a rongeur, a lot of bone was removed from the ends of the middle phalanx, as well as from the proximal end of the distal tufts, down to good cancellous bleeding bone. Local bone graft was also harvested from the middle phalanx.

Next, using Acutrak fusion set, the distal phalanx and middle phalanx were prepared. A 24-mm screw was placed with our graft interposed between the two ends. Good compression of the distal tuft on the middle phalanx was noted. Good placement of the hardware and alignment of the digit were noted on AP and lateral views of the C-arm.

This being the case, the wound was copiously irrigated. Hemostasis was obtained with bipolar electrocautery. Using vertical mattress sutures over the extensor mechanism using full-thickness sutures, the wound was repaired. This was supplemented with horizontal mattress sutures medially and laterally for the skin edges.

The blood loss was minimal. The IV fluid replaced was none. Drains and packs were none. Complications were none.

The patient tolerated the procedure well and was taken to the recovery room after nonadherent gauze and a bulky dressing were placed and held with tube gauze.

Questions for Further Review: Case Study 4.20

1. Which joint was repaired in the little finger?
   a. Proximal interphalangeal (PIP) joint
   b. Distal interphalangeal (DIP) joint

2. Which of the following procedures was performed?
   a. Arthrodesis interphalangeal joint with autograft
   b. Arthrodesis interphalangeal joint with internal fixation
   c. Arthrodesis interphalangeal joint without internal fixation

3. CPT surgery code(s) and modifier(s):

Exhibit 4.1. Trigger Finger and Ganglion Cyst Example

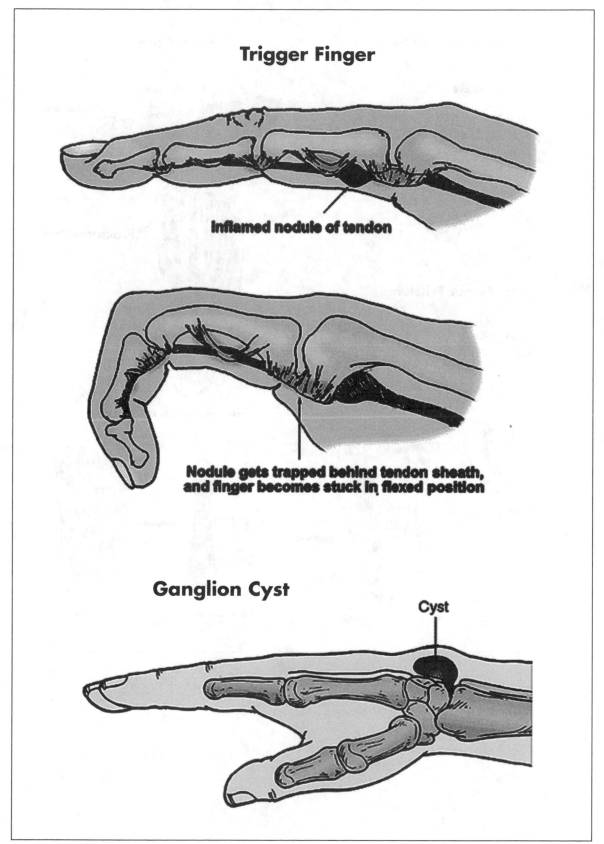

Trigger Finger

Inflamed nodule of tendon

Nodule gets trapped behind tendon sheath,
and finger becomes stuck in flexed position

Ganglion Cyst

Cyst

Exhibit 4.2. Fracture examples

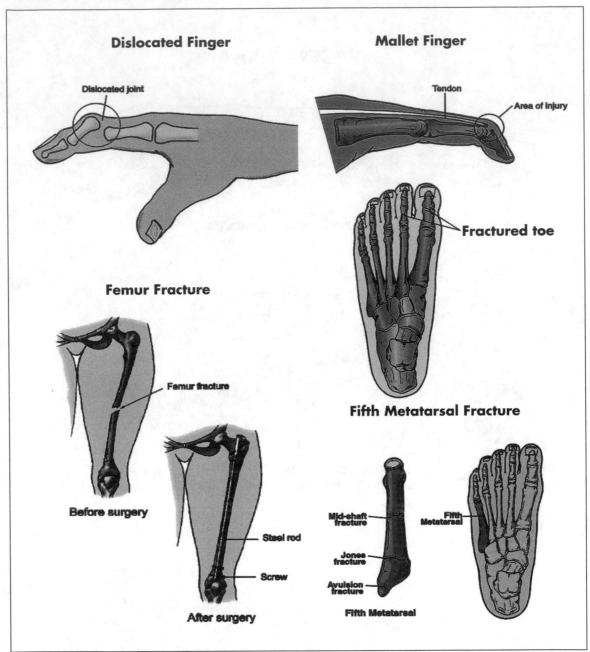

Exhibit 4.3. Primary Bunionectomy Procedures

Clinical Notes: The Bane of the Bunion

Bunionectomies are performed to relieve pain, restore impaired function, and improve appearance of the feet. This procedure is not limited to one age group or specific segment of the population.

Bunions, or hallux abducto valgus deformities, are not isolated problems but are commonly accompanied by deformities of the lesser toes.

The procedure for treatment of the bunion includes the removal of the bump from the medial side of the great toe. It may also include removing a wedge of the bone and soft tissue repair.

Following are brief descriptions and drawings of the primary bunionectomy procedures.

Figure 4a.1. Silver procedure (28290)

This is the simplest bunion procedure in which the bunion is removed. Surgeons may refer to this as removal of the medial eminence.

An incision is made into the medial side of the toe and on the side of the joint capsule. The bony exostosis is removed from the first metatarsal head. This procedure should include the following type of information:

- An incision is made over the bunion from proximal phalanx to metatarsal shaft.
- A capsulotomy is performed and exposes the medial eminence.
- The eminence is removed with a sharp osteotome.
- Closure of the capsule follows and suture of the skin.

(See figure at right)

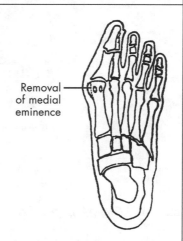

Removal of medial eminence

Figure 4a.2. McBride procedure; Keller procedure; Keller-Mayo procedure (28293)

The procedure includes all elements of the Silver procedure (removal of the medial eminence) plus removal or release of the lateral sesmoid bone. (See figure at right)

Keller Procedure

The Keller procedure includes removal of the medial eminence plus a resection of the base of the proximal phalanx of the great toe. A hemi-implant is optional with this procedure. However, if implant is used, code 28293 is assigned. (See figure at right)

Keller-Mayo Procedure

This procedure includes all the elements of the Keller procedure plus there is partial resection of the first metatarsal head. A total double stem implant is usually used when this procedure is performed. (See figure at right)

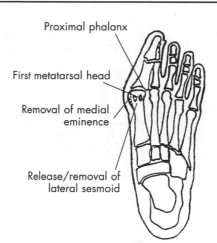

Proximal phalanx

First metatarsal head

Removal of medial eminence

Release/removal of lateral sesmoid

Joplin Procedure

The Joplin procedure entails removal of the medial eminence plus fusion of the hallux interphalangeal joint of the great toe. The extensor tendon of the great toe is transferred to the head or neck of the first metatarsal. (See figure at right)

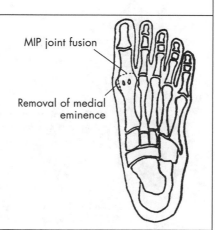

MIP joint fusion

Removal of medial eminence

Exhibit 4.4. Runner's knee and Meniscal cartilage tear example

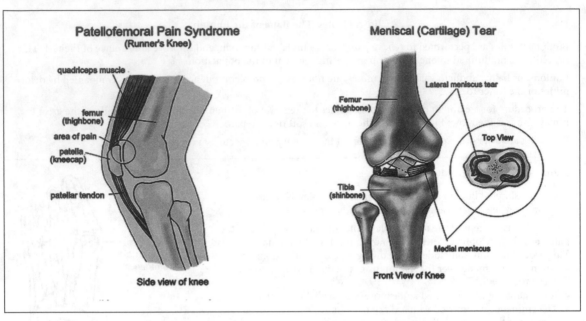

Exhibit 4.5. ACL Reconstruction example

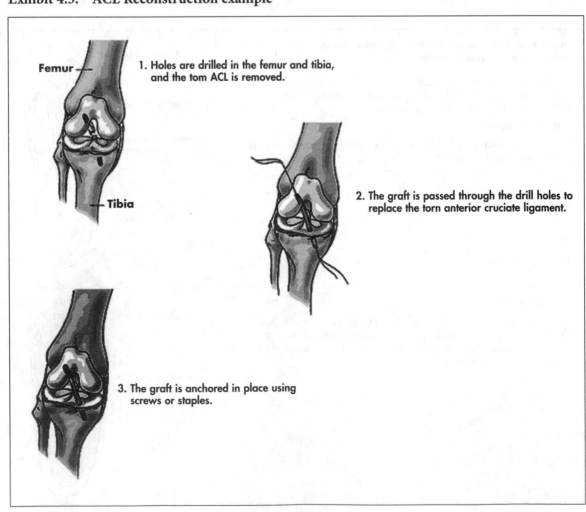

Exhibit 4.6. Rotator cuff injury example

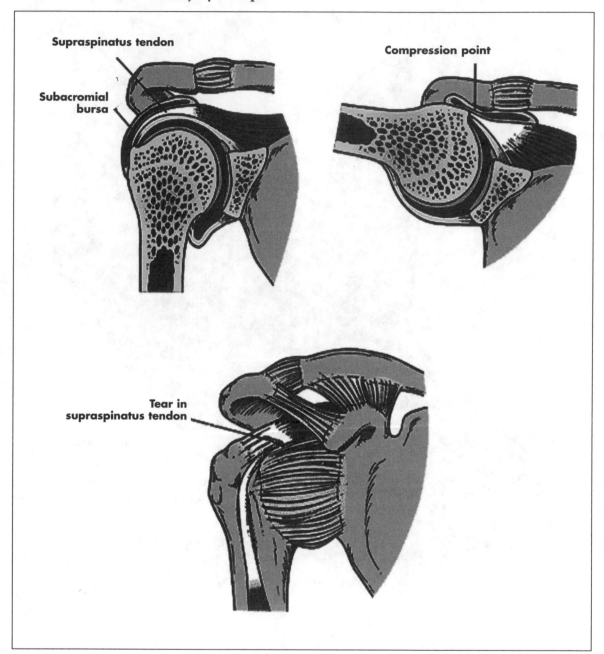

Exhibit 4.7. Carpal tunnel sydrome example

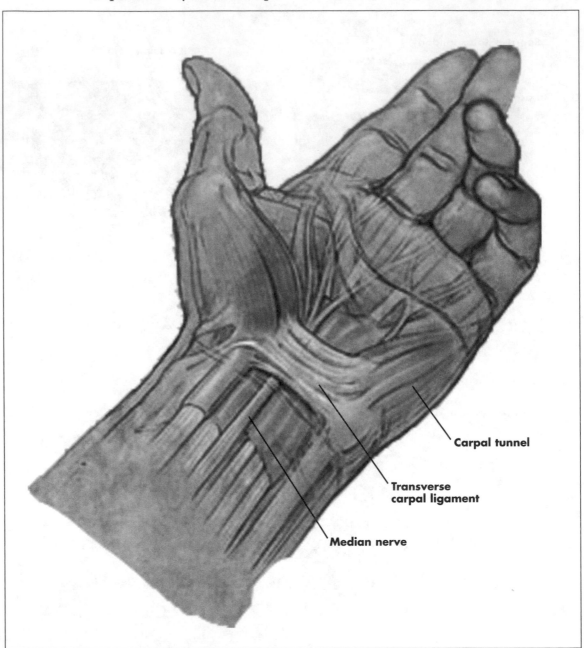

Carpal tunnel

Transverse
carpal ligament

Median nerve

Chapter 5

Respiratory System

Codes 30000 through 32999 are used to report surgical procedures performed on the respiratory system, which includes the nose, accessory sinuses, larynx, trachea and bronchi, lungs, and pleura. Outpatient procedures involving the respiratory system include turbinate resection, bronchoscopy, laryngoscopy, functional endoscopic sinus surgery, septoplasty, and rhinoplasty.

Turbinate Resection

Much of the space inside the nose is taken up by the turbinates, which warm and humidify air as it is inhaled and passed through the nose. Turbinate resection (removal) is performed when these structures become blocked for any of a number of reasons.

The turbinates are bony plates covered by spongy mucosa with curved margins, also called concha. Three turbinates are on each side of the nasal vestibule: inferior, middle, and superior.

The *inferior turbinate* is a bony plate generally covered with relatively thick mucosa on the lateral wall of the nasal cavity, separating the middle from the inferior meatus, and articulating with the ethmoid, lacrimal, maxilla, and palate bones. It is large and fills the lower portion of the nasal airway, extending from the front to the rear of the nose. This turbinate is very important in determining nasal airway patency. The *middle turbinate* is a part of the ethmoidal labyrinth (bone), projecting from the lateral wall of the nasal cavity and separating the superior meatus from the middle meatus. The *superior turbinate* is also part of the ethmoidal labyrinth, projecting from the lateral wall of the nasal cavity and separating the superior meatus from the sphenoethmoidal recess. It is the smallest turbinate and uncommonly associated with significant nasal/sinus disease.

APC	HCPCS	HCPCS Description	SI	Rel. Wt.	Payment Rate	OPPS OCE
0254			T	23.9765	1527.16	
	30140	Resection inferior turbinate				Significant Procedure, Multiple Reduction Applies; Separate APC payment

Coding Guidelines for Turbinate Resection

Prior to CY 2006, the codes for 30130 and 30140 did not specify the specific turbinate site. They are now referred to as "inferior" turbinate. On the rare occasion when the middle or superior turbinate is removed for therapeutic reasons, use code 30999, Unlisted procedure, nose.

Because there are three separate turbinates, questions often arise as to the reporting of excision/resection of the turbinates, particularly the inferior and middle turbinates (AMA 2003a).

The following guidelines apply to the coding of turbinate resection:

- It is not always correct to routinely include all turbinate excisions into the nasal endoscopic ethmoid procedures (AMA 2003a).

- The middle turbinate is part of the ethmoid bone; therefore, if the middle turbinate is removed when performing endoscopic ethmoidectomy (codes 31254, 31255) or endoscopic polypectomy (code 31237), removal of the middle turbinate (codes 30130, 30140) would not be reported separately (AMA 2003a).

- It is important that the documentation reflect inferior turbinate when procedure codes 30130 and 30140 are being reported. These codes can be reported separately with surgical procedures such as sphenoid, maxillary, or frontal sinus procedures, and septoplasty (AMA 2003a).

- When reporting code 30140, documentation in the operative report should reflect that the physician entered/incised the mucosa and, for the most part, preserved it. The simple statement, "excised the turbinate(s)" is often not enough documentation to reflect that the submucous resection of the inferior turbinate was performed. Coders may need to ask the physician for the specific technique performed (AMA 2003a).

- It also is important to include the appropriate diagnosis for performing the turbinate procedure, such as hypertrophy with airway obstruction (AMA 2003a).

- If the turbinate procedure was performed to gain access to the ethmoid bone, codes 30130 and 30140 would not typically be reported, nor would code 31240. However, if a separate diagnosis indicates medical necessity with supporting documentation, the appropriate turbinate code (30130, 30140) may be reported by appending modifier –59 to the code (AMA 2003a).

- Occasionally, the middle turbinate has a bubble formed in its interior portion. This is called a concha bullosa and is a common anatomic variation. Large concha bullosa can contribute to sinus congestion and sinus pain. The very front portion is removed to show the interior of the concha bullosa (AAO-HNS 2007).

- If the patient has a concha bullosa and the middle turbinate is removed for therapeutic reasons, code 31240 would be appropriate.

When reporting codes 30130 and 30140, it should be noted that these codes are unilateral because three turbinates are in each right and left nasal cavity (AMA 2003a).

CPT code 30930, Fracture nasal turbinate(s), therapeutic, is intended to apply to the inferior turbinates, typically for airway improvement, and is independent of the sinus procedure code 31255, Nasal/sinus endoscopy, surgical; with ethmoidectomy, total. However, if the surgeon merely fractures the middle turbinates medially to facilitate the sinus procedure (31255), it is considered part of that service and should not be reported separately. Do not report code 30801, 30802, or 30930, in conjunction with 30130 or 30140 (AMA 2007a). The procedures performed should be clearly documented in the patient's medical record (AMA 2002b).

Excision inferior turbinate code 30130 is considered a unilateral procedure. If the procedure is performed on both sides of the nose, it is appropriate to append the –50 modifier to the code to indicate that a bilateral procedure was performed (AMA 1998a, 11).

Code 30140 is considered unilateral. If partial or complete submucous inferior turbinate resection is performed bilaterally, modifier –50 should be appended to code 30140 (AMA 2002b; 2003c).

Code 30930 is unilateral. Therefore, if therapeutic fracture of nasal inferior turbinates is performed bilaterally, modifier –50 should be appended (AMA 2001d).

A turbinectomy is not considered an integral component of a dacryocystorhinostomy. Therefore, when a dacryocystorhinostomy and turbinectomy are performed at the same session by the same provider, code 30130, Excision of turbinate, partial or complete, any method, should be reported in addition to code 68720 (AMA 2001e).

Sinus Procedures

Caldwell-Luc Procedure

Caldwell-Luc is used for treatment of chronic sinusitis, removal of polyps, cysts or foreign bodies, reduction of facial fractures, closure of dental fistulas into the maxillary sinus, and as a route to the ethmoid and sphenoid sinuses. This means opening the maxillary sinus (the largest sinus in the cheek) and removing the diseased lining. Under a general anesthetic, a small cut is made in the upper jaw and a small amount of bone is removed to open the sinus. The diseased tissue lining the sinus is cleared away. The natural opening of the sinus into the nasal cavity is often enlarged at the same time to improve drainage of normal secretions and reduce the chance of recurrent disease (NYEE 2008).

APC	HCPCS	HCPCS Description	SI	Rel. Wt.	Payment Rate	OPPS OCE
0256			T	39.8776	2539.96	
	30130	Caldwell-Luc exploration, maxillary sinus				Significant Procedure, Multiple Reduction Applies; Separate APC payment
	31032	Caldwell-Luc exploration with removal of polyps				Significant Procedure, Multiple Reduction Applies; Separate APC payment

Coding Guidelines for Caldwell-Luc Procedures

When reporting code 31030 versus 31032, documentation in the operative report should reflect sinusotomy, radical without removal of antrochoanal polyps. Use code 31032 to reflect with removal of antrochoanal polyps.

Sinus Endoscopy

A surgical sinus endoscopy includes a sinusotomy and diagnostic endoscopy. Codes 31231–31294 are used to report unilateral procedures unless otherwise specified.

Coding Guidelines for Sinus Endoscopy

The following guidelines apply to the coding of sinus endoscopy:

Codes 31231–31235 for diagnostic evaluation refer to employing a nasal/sinus endoscope to inspect the interior of the nasal cavity and the middle and superior meatus, the turbinates, and the spheno-ethmoid recess. Any time a diagnostic evaluation is performed all these areas would be inspected, and a separate code is not reported for each area (AMA 2007b).

Functional Endoscopic Sinus Surgery

Functional endoscopic sinus surgery (FESS) involves the use of an endoscope to perform diagnostic or therapeutic procedures to restore sinus ventilation and normal function. FESS is considered a minimally invasive procedure that requires local anesthesia and may be performed in the physician's office.

The following structures in the nose may be involved:

- Nasal cavity
- Meatus
- Turbinates
- Ethmoids
- Sphenoids
- Frontal sinuses

Coding Guidelines for Functional Endoscopic Sinus Surgery

- Codes 31233–31294 are used to report unilateral procedures unless otherwise specified.
- Codes 31254, 31255, 31256, and 31267 include uncinate process removal (AMA 1997a).

The reference to "tissue" in code 31267 can include (AMA 1997a):

- Polyps
- Mucous membrane
- Bony partitions
- Massive fungal concretions and debris

Code 61795, for computer-assisted planning for stereotactic surgery, must be reported in addition to the code for the primary procedure when it is performed in conjunction with any ear, nose, throat, head, and neck procedures, including FESS. Examples would include those procedures described by codes 31254–31256, 31267, 31276, 31287, 31288, 31290–31294, and 61548 (AMA 2001b). Such planning may take approximately one to two hours and includes determination of the coordinates for the target measurement of the anterior commissure and posterior commissure line (AC–PC line) and angle calculation. Using a computer, various trajectories are determined to assist the physician in choosing the specific trajectory and calculating the entry point through the skull (AMA 2000a).

Bronchoscopy

A bronchoscopy is an examination of the interior bronchial tree using a lighted endoscope called a bronchoscope. The examination is generally for diagnostic purposes, such as obtaining specimens for culture or biopsy, but it also can be used for therapeutic maneuvers, such as removing foreign bodies. The bronchoscopy CPT codes are in the code range 31622–31656.

Coding Guidelines for Bronchoscopy

The following guidelines apply to the coding of bronchoscopy:

- Surgical bronchoscopy always includes diagnostic bronchoscopy when both are performed by the same physician (AMA 2000b, 10).

- The series of bronchoscopy codes 31623 through 31656 is used to describe unilateral procedures. To indicate that a procedure from this series was performed bilaterally, modifier –50 should be appended to the appropriate code. Therefore, modifier –50 should be appended to code 31624 when bronchial alveolar lavage (BAL) is performed bilaterally. Please note that code 31622, Bronchoscopy (rigid or flexible); with or without fluoroscopic guidance; diagnostic, with or without cell washing (separate procedure), is inherently bilateral, so it would not be appropriate to append modifier –50 (AMA 2002c).

Laryngoscopy

Laryngoscopy is a procedure that is performed to allow visualization and examination of vocal chords to see if they are functioning normally. Laryngoscopies also are done to remove foreign objects or lesions or to perform biopsies.

Coding Guidelines for Laryngoscopy

Laryngoscopies can be performed by indirect, direct, and operative direct methods as follows:

- Codes 31505–31513 classify indirect laryngoscopies. When an indirect laryngoscopy is performed, the visualization of the larynx is accomplished using a warm laryngeal mirror positioned at the back of the patient's throat, a head mirror held in front of the mouth, and a light source. The patient sits erect in a chair and sticks his or her tongue out as far as possible with a tongue depressor, and the larynx is observed while the patient is at rest and as the patient speaks.

- Codes 31515–31529 are assigned for direct laryngoscopies. These codes classify the visualization of the larynx by passage of a rigid or fiberoptic endoscope through the mouth and pharynx to the larynx. When a direct laryngoscopy is performed, the correct code depends on whether the procedure was accomplished with an operating microscope (microsurgery) or a flexible fiberoptic scope.

- Codes 31536–31571 are used for operative direct laryngoscopic procedures, in which examination of the larynx is performed with the patient under general anesthesia by passing a rigid or fiberoptic endoscope through the mouth and pharynx to the larynx.

APC	HCPCS	HCPCS Description	SI	Rel. Wt.	Payment Rate	OPPS OCE
0074			T	17.0160	1083.82	
	31505	Diagnostic Laryngoscopy				Significant Procedure, Multiple Reduction Applies; Separate APC payment
	31510	Laryngoscopy with biopsy				Significant Procedure, Multiple Reduction Applies; Separate APC payment

Septoplasty

A septoplasty is an operation to correct defects or deformities of the nasal septum, often by alteration or partial removal of supporting structures. The nasal septum is the wall dividing the nasal cavity in half.

Coding Guidelines for Septoplasty

- Code 30520 is used for a major septal repair or septoplasty with cartilage. This code would be assigned for a primary or secondary septoplasty or submucosal resection.

- A septoplasty with a cartilage graft is included in code 30520 if a secondary incision is not made to obtain the graft. Generally, septal cartilage is available for grafting in the immediate surgical area; therefore, an additional code would not be assigned. This code also includes a septal bone graft provided the bone is repositioned within the septum.

- Code 20912 is reported when the cartilage graft is obtained for use outside the septum.

- Code 20900 is used when bone is transferred to a second site outside the septum.

Rhinoplasty

Rhinoplasty is one of the most common forms of plastic surgery. Often referred to as a "nose job," rhinoplasty techniques are used to alter the shape, size, or overall look of the nose.

Primary rhinoplasty refers to an operation in which excess bone and cartilage are removed or cartilage grafts are added to reshape the nose. Secondary rhinoplasty refers to a repeat surgery, which is performed to correct or prevent problems that develop after a previous rhinoplasty. Secondary rhinoplasties can be the most difficult because the normal anatomy of the nose has been altered and scar tissue may be present.

Rhinoplasty also is performed for cleft lip and palate reconstruction in children and adults.

Coding Guidelines for Rhinoplasty

Codes used to classify rhinoplasties include:

- 30400, 30410, and 30420 for primary rhinoplasty
- 30430, 30435, and 30450 for secondary rhinoplasty
- 30460 and 30462 for rhinoplasty due to cleft lip or cleft palate

Documentation Requirements for Respiratory System Procedures

Each procedure is followed by clinical information that must be documented in the medical record when the procedure is performed.

Turbinate Surgery

CPT codes 30130, 30140, 30801, 30802, and 30930 are used to report turbinate surgery.

1. The disease process for *each* turbinate (for example, hypertrophy)

2. The type of procedure performed on *each* turbinate:

   - Excision
   - Submucous resection (Specify that the mucosa was entered and/or incised and preserved.)
   - Superficial cauterization/ablation
   - Intramural cauterization/ablation
   - Therapeutic fracture
   - Reduction

3. Whether *each* procedure is unilateral or bilateral

4. The surgical approach used for the turbinate surgery:

   - Open
   - Endoscopic

Laryngoscopy

CPT codes 31505–31579 are used to report laryngoscopies.

1. Whether the laryngoscope is rigid or flexible fiberoptic (brand name of scope does not indicate to coders whether the scope is rigid or flexible)

2. Whether the laryngoscopy is indirect or direct

3. The type of anesthesia administered

4. Whether an operating microscope was utilized

Bronchoscopy

CPT codes 31622–31656 are used to report bronchoscopies.

1. The type of bronchoscopy performed

   - Diagnostic
   - Therapeutic

2. Whether or not an endoscopic ultrasound was performed.

3. The laterality of *each* therapeutic procedure performed

   - Unilateral
   - Bilateral

4. *Each* therapeutic procedure performed

- Brushing
- Protected brushing
- Bronchial alveolar lavage (BAL)
- Biopsy (See 4 below.)
- Dilation: Tracheal or bronchial
- Closed reduction of fracture
- Stent placement—tracheal or bronchial
- Revision of stent (inserted at previous session)
- Foreign body removal
- Tumor excision
- Tumor destruction
- Stenosis relief using other than excision (for example, laser therapy, cryotherapy)
- Catheter(s) placement for intracavitary radioelement application
- Initial aspiration of tracheobronchial tree
- Subsequent aspiration of tracheobronchial tree
- Contrast injection for segmental bronchography

5. Each biopsy technique performed.

- Bronchial/endobronchial biopsy
- Transbronchial lung biopsy (Specify each lobe)
- Transbronchial needle aspiration biopsy (Specify each lobe)

FESS

CPT codes 31233–31294 are used to report FESS. Whether a nasal/sinus endoscopy report is used or an operative report is dictated, the surgeon must document the following clinical elements in the medical record:

1. Whether each nasal/sinus procedure was performed endoscopically (FESS) or via open technique

2. All FESS procedures performed

3. Whether each FESS procedure was unilateral or bilateral

4. Whether the ethmoidectomy was anterior (partial) or anterior and posterior (total)

5. Whether the patient had a maxillary antrostomy only or a maxillary antrostomy with removal of tissue (for example, polyps, mucous membrane, bony partitions, or massive fungal concretions/debris)

6. Whether the patient had a sphenoidotomy only or a sphenoidotomy with removal of tissue from the sphenoid sinus

Case Studies

This section contains actual operative reports from real-life cases. All identifiers have been removed or changed for confidentiality and privacy.

Carefully read the clinical documentation for each case study, which may include a procedure report as well as radiology and/or pathology reports, as applicable.

Answer all the questions for further review at the end of each case study. Use a current CPT codebook or HCPCS Level II code listing, as needed.

When appropriate, assign one or more of the following modifiers:

−50	Bilateral Procedure
−59	Distinct Procedural Service
−FA	Left hand, thumb
−F1	Left hand, second digit
−F2	Left hand, third digit
−F3	Left hand, fourth digit
−F4	Left hand, fifth digit
−F5	Right hand, thumb
−F6	Right hand, second digit
−F7	Right hand, third digit
−F8	Right hand, fourth digit
−F9	Right hand, fifth digit
−LT	Left side
−RT	Right side
−TA	Left foot, great toe
−T1	Left foot, second digit
−T2	Left foot, third digit
−T3	Left foot, fourth digit
−T4	Left foot, fifth digit
−T5	Right foot, great toe
−T6	Right foot, second digit
−T7	Right foot, third digit
−T8	Right foot, fourth digit
−T9	Right foot, fifth digit

Do not apply the current version of the Medicare CCI edits to any of these questions; the focus is on the application of the coding guidelines and not on the application of edits that change on a quarterly basis. When coding in real life, of course, you will need to apply the CCI edits as appropriate for Medicare outpatient cases.

Case Study 5.1

Read the following clinical document and answer the questions for further review.

OPERATIVE REPORT

PREOPERATIVE DIAGNOSIS: Hypertrophy of bilateral turbinates

POSTOPERATIVE DIAGNOSIS: Hypertrophy of bilateral turbinates

OPERATIVE PROCEDURE: Submucous resection bilateral inferior turbinates

ANESTHESIA: General

INDICATIONS FOR SURGERY: Patient is a 43-year-old male who underwent a septoplasty in the remote past. He continues to have nasal obstruction bilaterally despite adequate medical therapy.

OPERATIVE FINDINGS: Hypertrophy of the inferior turbinates was present with minimal response to vasoconstriction. Bony component was large. Nasal septum was fairly midline.

DESCRIPTION OF PROCEDURE: Patient was brought to the operative suite and placed in the supine position on the operating table. General endotracheal anesthesia was induced without difficulty. The patient was carefully padded and positioned. The face was draped in the usual sterile fashion. The inferior turbinates were infiltrated with 1% Xylocaine with 100,000 epinephrine, using a control syringe.

After waiting an adequate time for vasoconstriction, an incision was made along the inferior border of the right inferior turbinate with a #15 blade. The turbinate mucosa and medial and lateral turbinate bone was elevated with a freer elevator. A portion of the anterior turbinate bone was then removed with the ethmoid forceps. The medial and lateral turbinate mucosal flaps were reapproximated and closed with interrupted 4-0 Chromic suture. A submucous resection of the left inferior turbinate was performed in precisely the same fashion. The nose was then thoroughly suctioned and loosely packed along the floor of the nose with a rolled Telfa gauze soaked in Bacitracin ointment. Anesthesia was then reversed without difficulty. The patient tolerated the procedure well.

Questions for Further Review: Case Study 5.1

1. What was the disease process for *each* turbinate?

2. What type of procedure was performed on *each* turbinate?
   a. Excision
   b. Submucous resection
   c. Superficial cauterization/ablation
   d. Intramural cauterization/ablation
   e. Therapeutic fracture
   f. Reduction

3. Was each turbinate procedure unilateral or bilateral?
   a. Unilateral
   b. Bilateral

4. What was the surgical approach used for the turbinate surgery?
   a. Open
   b. Endoscopic

5. CPT surgery code(s) and modifier(s):

Case Study 5.2

Read the following clinical document and answer the questions for further review.

OPERATIVE REPORT

PREOPERATIVE DIAGNOSIS: Cough, bronchiectasis

POSTOPERATIVE DIAGNOSIS: Cough, smooth pink endobronchial lesion

OPERATION: Flexible fiberoptic bronchoscopy

DESCRIPTION OF PROCEDURE: The patient was made aware of the risks and benefits of the procedure and agreed to commence.

The patient was prepared with 0.45% tetracaine instilled through the right naris and the posterior pharynx. The patient was given conscious sedation with 3 mg of Versed and 75 mcg of fentanyl.

The scope was then inserted through the right naris without difficulty. The larynx and vocal cords were well visualized. There was some mild erythema on the vocal cords, but they are otherwise intact. There are no lesions, no obstruction, normal appearing vocal cord function. Additional tetracaine was instilled on the vocal cords. The scope was then passed into the proximal trachea. The tracheal mucosa was clear and sharp. There were no lesions, no obstructions, no pathology. The carina was noted to be sharp. The right upper lobe, right middle lobe, and right lower lobe were also fully patent. There was mild erythema. There were minimal secretions. The anatomy was all completely normal. The left upper lobe and left lower lobe were also well visualized with normal appearing anatomy, no lesions or obstructions. In the right lower lobe, in the medial basilar subsegment, there appeared to be a small, smooth, pinkish, rounded, raised endobronchial area. BAL was performed of the right middle lobe and sent for cultures and cytology. A BAL was also performed of the left lower lobe and sent for cultures and cytology. Finally, endobronchial biopsy was performed on the right lower lobe basilar bronchial obstruction. One solid piece of tissue was taken. The patient had significant bleeding, however, from this single biopsy requiring copious saline lavage. The patient did report after the biopsy was taken that she has always been a "bleeder." The patient otherwise tolerated the procedure well. The bleeding had stopped by the time the procedure had finished.

SURGICAL PATHOLOGY REPORT

AGE/SEX: 57/F

SPECIMEN(S) RECEIVED: Right lower lobe basilar subsegment endobronchial biopsy

GROSS: Specimen is received in formalin and consists of small fragments of tan-white tissue measuring 0.1 cm in aggregate. ESS, 1 cassette

DIAGNOSIS: Endobronchial biopsy, right lower, basilar segment
   A. Benign respiratory mucosa with mild chronic inflammation and a small focus of squamous metaplasia
   B. See C.04-112 and 113

Questions for Further Review: Case Study 5.2

1.   What type of bronchoscopy was performed?
     a.   Diagnostic
     b.   Therapeutic

2.   What was the laterality of *each* therapeutic procedure performed?

3.   Identify *each* therapeutic procedure performed.
     a.   Brushing
     b.   Protected brushing
     c.   Bronchial alveolar lavage (BAL)
     d.   Biopsy
     e.   Dilation: Tracheal or bronchial
     f.   Closed reduction of fracture
     g.   Tracheal stent placement
     h.   Foreign body removal
     i.   Tumor excision
     j.   Tumor destruction
     k.   Stenosis relief using other than excision (for example, laser therapy, cryotherapy)
     l.   Catheter(s) placement for intracavitary radioelement application

m.   Initial aspiration of tracheobronchial tree
n.   Subsequent aspiration of tracheobronchial tree
o.   Contrast injection for segmental bronchography

4.   Identify *each* biopsy technique performed.
     a.   Bronchial/endobronchial biopsy
     b.   Transbronchial lung biopsy (specify *each* lobe)
     c.   Transbronchial needle aspiration biopsy (specify *each* lobe)

5.   CPT surgery code(s) and modifier(s):

Case Study 5.3

Read the following clinical document and answer the questions for further review.

OPERATIVE REPORT

PREOPERATIVE DIAGNOSIS: Laryngeal papillomatosis

POSTOPERATIVE DIAGNOSIS: Laryngeal papillomatosis

OPERATIVE PROCEDURE: Microlaryngoscopy and laser excision of laryngeal papillomata and cidofovir injection

FINDINGS: A 79-year-old with recurrent papillomatosis

ESTIMATED BLOOD LOSS: 1 cc

SPECIMEN: None

DESCRIPTION OF PROCEDURE: With the patient in the supine position under general anesthesia, the Jako adult laryngoscope was inserted and held with a Lewy laryngoscope holder. The cords were visualized under the binocular operating microscope. Papillomata were limited to the two lesions on the left and true cord. There was one lesion at the junction of the anterior middle third of the right cord and a lesion just above that on the false cord. The cords were treated with adrenaline on each side for hemostasis, and then each lesion site was infiltrated with cidofovir. The laser was used to debulk the gross lesions at each site. He tolerated the procedure well and left the operating room in good condition.

Questions for Further Review: Case Study 5.3

1.   Was the laryngoscope rigid or flexible fiberoptic?
2.   Was the laryngoscopy indirect or direct?
3.   What type of anesthesia was administered?
4.   Was an operating microscope used?
5.   CPT surgery code(s) and modifier(s):

Case Study 5.4

Read the following clinical document and answer the questions for further review.

OPERATIVE REPORT

PREOPERATIVE DIAGNOSIS: Chronic paranasal sinusitis, deviated septum

POSTOPERATIVE DIAGNOSIS: Chronic paranasal sinusitis, deviated septum

OPERATIVE PROCEDURE: Right endoscopic anterior and posterior ethmoidectomy, left endoscopic anterior and posterior ethmoidectomy, a right endoscopic frontal recess dissection, left endoscopic frontal sinus dissection, a right endoscopic sphenoidotomy without removal of tissue, left endoscopic sphenoidotomy without removal of tissue, and septoplasty

ANESTHESIA: General

INDICATIONS: This patient is a 50-year-old female with a significant history of nasal congestion, rhinorrhea, and postnasal drainage. There is a long-standing chronic paranasal sinus disease along with aspirin sensitivity and asthma. She has previously undergone endoscopic sinus surgery in 1999, with recurrent disease occurring. CT scan reveals pansinusitis despite aggressive medical treatment.

OPERATIVE FINDINGS: Significant deviation of the perpendicular plate of the ethmoid to the right was present with a high degree of obstruction. A left maxillary crest spur was noted. Both middle turbinates are extremely lateralized. There are dense adhesions between the lateral nasal wall and the lateral portion of the middle turbinate. Dense polypoid material filling the ethmoid sinuses is present. Thick mucoid material in the sphenoid and sinuses is present. Thick mucoid material in the sphenoid and frontal sinuses was evacuated. The maxillary sinuses were clear.

DESCRIPTION OF PROCEDURE: The patient was brought to the operative suite and placed in the supine position on the operating table. General endotracheal anesthesia was induced without difficulty. The patient was carefully padded and positioned. The face was draped in the usual sterile fashion with the eyes lubricated and untaped so that they could be inspected during the procedure. Because the patient has a high degree of nasal obstruction due to a deviated septum, septoplasty was performed first.

The nasal septum and inferior turbinates were infiltrated with 1% Xylocaine with 1:100,000 epinephrine using a controlled syringe. After waiting an adequate time for vasoconstriction, a left hemitransfixion incision was made. A left submucous perichondrial tunnel was elevated. The cartilaginous septum was sharply disarticulated from the bony septum, and bilateral submucous periosteal tunnels were elevated. The maxillary crest spur on the left was removed with ethmoid forceps. The deviated portion of the perpendicular plate of the ethmoid was removed by first making a relaxing incision in it with septal scissors. The deviated portion was removed with the ethmoid forceps and a portion trimmed with the Jansen-Middleton forceps. The cartilaginous septum was allowed to swing back to the midline. The posterior septal pocket was reconstructed with morcellized bone and cartilage. The septal flaps were reapproximated using a 4-0 plain-gut mattress suture. Hemitransfixion incision was closed with a 4-0 Chromic interrupted suture.

Rigid nasal endoscopy was then performed with the 0–degree telescope with the above findings noted. The middle turbinates and lateral nasal walls were infiltrated with 1% Xylocaine with 1:100,000 epinephrine in a standard fashion. Cocaine 4% on O-tips was then placed in the middle meatus bilaterally. After waiting an adequate time for vasoconstriction, the left nasal cavity was approached with the 0-degree telescope. Abundant polypoid material within the middle meatus was removed with the shaver. The middle turbinate was markedly lateralized along its inferior portion. Anterior and inferior portion of the middle turbinate was resected using the straight-biting forceps and shaver. The superior and posterior portions of the middle turbinate were preserved. The shaver was then used to dissect within the ethmoid cavity, carrying dissection back to the face of the sphenoid. Dissection along the face of the sphenoid allowed opening of the natural ostium of the sphenoid sinus with the shaver, and thick mucoid material was suctioned from the sinus. The 25-degree telescope and the shaver were then used to dissect polypoid material on the roof of the ethmoid cavity in a posterior-to-anterior direction. Several small bony elements were removed with a curette and the shaver. Dissection was then carried out with the 25-degree telescope in the region of the frontal recess using the shaver and the frontal sinus punch. The natural ostium was easily identified. The mucosa in this region was not disturbed. Thick mucus within the frontal sinus was evacuated. The frontal sinus was then easily transilluminated. The 25-degree telescope was used to visualize the natural ostium of the maxillary sinus, which was noted to be clear with normal mucosa within the sinus.

An anterior and posterior ethmoidectomy along with the frontal recess dissection and an endoscopic sphenoidotomy was performed in the right side in precisely the same fashion. A small bony element in the region of the anterior ethmoid artery was not disturbed on the right. The mucosa of the frontal recess was also not disturbed. Thick mucus was evacuated from the sphenoid and frontal sinus. The nose was then thoroughly suctioned. Bacitracin ointment was placed in the ethmoid cavities bilaterally along with the small sinus pack.

The nose was thoroughly suctioned, and a rolled Telfa gauze soaked in Bacitracin ointment was placed on the inferior portion of the nasal cavity. The anesthesia was then reversed without difficulty. The patient tolerated the procedure well.

Questions for Further Review: Case Study 5.4

1. What procedure was performed to correct the deviated septum?
   a. Primary rhinoplasty
   b. Septal dermatoplasty
   c. Septoplasty

2. What type of bilateral sphenoidotomy was performed?
   a. Endoscopic sphenoidotomy
   b. Endoscopic sphenoidotomy with removal of tissue from the sphenoid sinus

3. What type of bilateral ethmoidectomy was performed?
   a. Open partial (anterior only)
   b. Open total (anterior and posterior)
   c. Endoscopic partial (anterior only)
   d. Endoscopic total (anterior and posterior)

4. How was the endoscopic frontal sinus exploration with removal of tissue from frontal sinus performed?
   a. Unilaterally
   b. Bilaterally

5. CPT surgery code(s) and modifier(s):

Case Study 5.5

Read the following clinical document and answer the questions for further review.

Operative Report

PREOPERATIVE DIAGNOSES:

1. Deviated nasal septum
2. Bilateral chronic pansinusitis

POSTOPERATIVE DIAGNOSES:

1. Deviated nasal septum
2. Bilateral chronic pansinusitis

OPERATIONS:

1. Septoplasty
2. Bilateral endoscopic anterior ethmoidectomy
3. Bilateral endoscopic maxillary sinusotomy

ANESTHESIA: LMAC

DESCRIPTION OF PROCEDURE: With the patient in supine position with elevated head, and under adequate IV sedation by anesthesiologist, the nose and face were prepped and draped in sterile fashion. A mixture of topical Pontocaine with epinephrine was sprayed into the nasal cavity. After removing the nasal packs, examination revealed grossly deviated septum to the right side. Using 0-degree endoscope, examination revealed polypoid and inflamed mucosa of the middle meatus bilaterally. Xylocaine 1% with epinephrine was injected into the septum, the turbinates, and both middle and inferior meatus.

First, the septoplasty was done as follows: A routine Cottle incision was made, and mucoperichondrial flaps were elevated on both sides. The septum was incised close to the floor. Soft tissue was elevated from the maxillary crest and its deflected part removed using a chisel and a hammer. Then part of the septum in its midsection was removed, which brought the septum into the midline.

Next, attention was diverted for endoscopic sinus surgery using 0-degree endoscope. First, uncinectomy and infundibulotomy were done on the left side and the anterior ethmoid cells were exenterated. Tissue was polypoid and inflamed. Bleeding was controlled with half-inch gauze soaked with Neo-Synephrine. Likewise, a right ethmoidectomy was done with similar findings.

Then, through the left inferior meatus, intranasal antrostomy was done. Mucosa was somewhat hypertrophic, but there were no polyps or cysts. Likewise, a right maxillary sinusotomy was done with similar findings.

Next, the incision was closed with interrupted catgut sutures. An 18-French catheter was placed along the floor of the nose, and nasal packing was done using petroleum jelly gauze mixed with an antibiotic ointment. A routine nasal and lip dressing was applied. The patient remained stable during the surgery and left the OR in satisfactory condition.

Surgical Pathology Report

AGE/SEX: 45/M

SPECIMEN(S) RECEIVED:

1. Left ethmoid sinus
2. Nasal septum
3. Right ethmoid sinus

GROSS:

1. Specimen is received in formalin and consists of fragments of tan-pink soft tissue measuring in aggregate 1 cm. ESS—1 cassette
2. Specimen is received in formalin and consists of fragments of cartilaginous and bony tissue measuring in aggregate 3 x 1.5 x 0.5 cm; RSS—1 cassette after decalcification.
3. Specimen is received in formalin and consists of soft tan small amount of bony tissue measuring in aggregate 1.5 x 0.5 cm. ESS—1 cassette after decalcification

DIAGNOSES:

1. Left ethmoid sinus tissue: Chronically inflamed respiratory mucosa and admixed bone fragments
2. Nasal septal tissue: Benign bone and cartilage
3. Right ethmoid sinus tissue: Chronically inflamed respiratory mucosa and admixed bone fragments

---

Questions for Further Review: Case Study 5.5

1. What procedure was performed to correct the deviated septum?
   a. Primary rhinoplasty
   b. Septal dermatoplasty
   c. Septoplasty

2. What type of bilateral ethmoidectomy was performed?
   a. Open partial (anterior only)
   b. Open total (anterior and posterior)
   c. Endoscopic partial (anterior only)
   d. Endoscopic total (anterior and posterior)

3. What type of bilateral maxillary antrostomy was performed?
   a. Endoscopic maxillary antrostomy
   b. Endoscopic maxillary antrostomy with removal of tissue from the maxillary sinus
   c. Open maxillary antrostomy

4. CPT surgery code(s) and modifier(s):

Case Study 5.6

Read the following clinical document and answer the questions for further review.

Operative Report

PREOPERATIVE DIAGNOSIS: Bilateral chronic paranasal sinusitis

POSTOPERATIVE DIAGNOSIS: Bilateral chronic paranasal sinusitis

OPERATIVE PROCEDURES:

1. Right endoscopic anterior and posterior ethmoidectomy
2. Left endoscopic anterior and posterior ethmoidectomy
3. Right endoscopic maxillary antrostomy without removal of tissue
4. Left endoscopic maxillary antrostomy without removal of tissue
5. Right endoscopic frontal recess dissection
6. Left endoscopic frontal recess dissection

ANESTHESIA: General

ESTIMATED BLOOD LOSS: The estimated blood loss was 16 ml.

INDICATIONS: This patient is a 56-year-old white female with a significant history of nasal obstruction and recurrent paranasal sinusitis. CT scan reveals chronic pansinusitis with anterior posterior ethmoid disease and maxillary sinus disease. Minimum mucosal thickening of the sphenoid sinus was noted. There is disease within the frontal recess bilaterally.

OPERATIVE FINDINGS: Polypoid degeneration of the mucosa of the ethmoid sinuses bilaterally is present. An extreme paradoxical curvature of the right middle turbinate necessitated partial excision of the anterior and inferior portion of this turbinate. The posterior and superior attachment was preserved. Moderate thickening of the mucosa of the maxillary sinuses is noted. Multiple bony elements were obstructing the frontal recess. The face of the sphenoid was clear.

DESCRIPTION OF PROCEDURE: The patient was brought to the operating suite and placed in the supine position on the operating table. General endotracheal anesthesia was induced without difficulty. The patient was carefully padded in position. The face was draped in the usual sterile fashion with the eyes lubricated and untaped so that they could be inspected during the procedure.

A rigid nasal endoscopy was performed with the 0-degree telescope with the above findings noted. The middle turbinate and lateral nasal wall were infiltrated with Xylocaine 1% with 1:100,000 epinephrine using a control syringe. After waiting an adequate time for vasoconstriction, the right nasal cavity was approached with the 0-degree telescope. The extreme paradoxical curvature of the right middle turbinate was trimmed anteriorly and inferiorly with the straight-biting forceps and the shaver. The uncinate process was then fractured anteriorly with curved probe and incised in its midportion with the pediatric backbiting forceps. The superior and inferior portions of the uncinate process were then removed with the shaver. The anterior wall of the bulla was followed up into the frontal recess with the 25- and 45-degree telescope, where suction with a curette and various upbiting forceps allowed removal of bony elements in the frontal recess and open access to the frontal sinus. The normal mucosa in this region was not disturbed. A large polyp was removed from just inferior to the frontal recess. The 25-degree telescope was then used to identify the natural ostium of the maxillary sinus. It was quite small. It was enlarged through the posterior fontanelle with the straight-biting forceps and the shaver. The 0-degree telescope and the shaver were then used to dissect into the ethmoid bulla inferiorly and medially. Dissection was carried back through the ground lamella into the posterior ethmoid system. The dissection was then carried back to the face of the sphenoid. The 25-degree telescope and the curette along with the shaver were then used to dissect along the roof of the ethmoid cavity in a posterior-to-anterior direction. In this fashion, a complete ethmoidectomy was performed.

A complete ethmoidectomy, along with maxillary antrostomy and frontal recess dissection, was performed on the left and precisely in the same fashion with the exception of preserving the middle turbinate completely. A Bolger maneuver was then performed medially on both sides.

Bacitracin ointment was used to fill the ethmoid cavity along with small sinus packs. The nose was thoroughly suctioned. The anesthesia was reversed without difficulty. The patient tolerated the procedure well.

Questions for Further Review: Case Study 5.6

1. What type of ethmoidectomy was performed?
   a. Endoscopic unilateral partial (anterior only)
   b. Endoscopic unilateral total (anterior and posterior)
   c. Endoscopic bilateral partial (anterior only)
   d. Endoscopic bilateral total (anterior and posterior)

2. What type of maxillary antrostomy was performed?
   a. Endoscopic unilateral maxillary antrostomy
   b. Endoscopic unilateral maxillary antrostomy with removal of tissue from the maxillary sinus
   c. Endoscopic bilateral maxillary antrostomy
   d. Endoscopic bilateral maxillary antrostomy with removal of tissue from the maxillary sinus

3. How was the endoscopic frontal sinus surgery performed?
   a. Unilaterally
   b. Bilaterally

4. CPT surgery code(s) and modifier(s):

Case Study 5.7

Read the following clinical document and answer the questions for further review.

Operative Report

PREOPERATIVE DIAGNOSIS: Chronic right maxillary, ethmoid, and frontal sinusitis

POSTOPERATIVE DIAGNOSIS: Chronic right maxillary, ethmoid, and frontal sinusitis

PROCEDURES:

1. Nasal endoscopy
2. Right maxillary sinusotomy
3. Right anterior ethmoidectomy and right frontal recess exposure

PROCEDURE IN DETAIL: After informed verbal and written consent was obtained, the patient was brought to the operating room and placed in the supine position. General anesthesia was induced. The external nose was injected with lidocaine and epinephrine. Cocaine-soaked pledgets were inserted into the nose for decongestion. The ENT Insta-Trak image-guided system was affixed onto the head. Tracking was initiated and corresponded nicely to anatomical markers. Initially, I started with a zero-degree endoscope. She had a small, somewhat thin middle turbinate. I medialized this, visualizing the uncinate process. The uncinate had somewhat of an anterior curve to it. I used the microdebrider to remove the entire uncinate. Despite being injected with local, the tissue was incredibly hyperemic, it bled very easily, and was friable. After removing portions of the uncinates, I encountered white purulent material filling what I presume was the maxillary ostium. I did culture this. Following this purulent material with the backbiter, I made several cuts. There was a moderate amount of bleeding obscuring easy landmarks. After more microdebriding around this site, and using a backbiter, I was finally able to enter the maxillary sinus ostium. Once again, the tissue was incredibly edematous, incredibly swollen, and the sinus cavity itself was filled with purulent material. I suctioned this out and copiously flushed out the nose. Next, I proceeded to perform an anterior ethmoidectomy. I did this, revealing very hyperemic tissue anteriorly. As I entered the large ethmoid cavity, there was no significant polypoid material or purulent material. I did follow the bulla superiorly and I identified using the ENT Insta-Trak, the frontal sinus recess. This was not located underneath the uncinate process, but it was located posterior to the ethmoid bulla. I cleaned this out with the microdebrider. A polypoid mass that seemed to be narrowing somewhat the lumen of this frontal recess was clearly visible on the CAT scan. I removed this with a 45-degree Blakesley. I took out the anterior wall of this, trying to create as best as I could a nice opening into the frontal sinus. On her CAT scan, this area was opacified as well. I used a very minimal suction Bovie to try to dry up some key places, and I suctioned out the whole area and irrigated it. I did place a Merocel pack into the whole entire ostiomeatal complex, and it was taped onto the side of her face. Overall blood loss was minimal. She tolerated this extremely well.

Questions for Further Review: Case Study 5.7

1. The ENT Insta-Trak image-guided system is a stereotactic computer-assisted volumetric device.
    a. True
    b. False

2. What type of maxillary antrostomy was performed?
    a. Endoscopic unilateral maxillary antrostomy
    b. Endoscopic unilateral maxillary antrostomy with removal of tissue from the maxillary sinus
    c. Endoscopic bilateral maxillary antrostomy
    d. Endoscopic bilateral maxillary antrostomy with removal of tissue from the maxillary sinus

3. What type of ethmoidectomy was performed?
    a. Endoscopic unilateral partial (anterior only)
    b. Endoscopic unilateral total (anterior and posterior)
    c. Endoscopic bilateral partial (anterior only)
    d. Endoscopic bilateral total (anterior and posterior)

4. How was the endoscopic frontal sinus surgery performed?
    a. Unilaterally
    b. Bilaterally

5. CPT surgery code(s) and modifier(s):

Case Study 5.8

Read the following clinical document and answer the questions for further review.

OPERATIVE REPORT

PREOPERATIVE DIAGNOSIS: Cleft nasal deformity

OPERATION: Cleft tip rhinoplasty with auricular cartilage graft

POSTOPERATIVE DIAGNOSIS: Cleft nasal deformity

ANESTHESIA: General endotracheal

COMPLICATIONS: None

INDICATIONS FOR PROCEDURE: Patient has a history of a complete cleft lip and palate and presents at this time for secondary cleft nasal correction. There is significant collapse of the alar rim and caudal displacement of the lower lateral cartilages. We will plan a cleft rhinoplasty and will most likely require a columellar strut graft from the ear. Risks of the procedure, including bleeding, infection, asymmetry, and need for further revisions, were reviewed.

DESCRIPTION OF PROCEDURE: After obtaining informed consent, the patient was taken to the operating room and placed in supine position. Patient underwent induction of general endotracheal anesthesia without complication. Patient was administered IV antibiotics.

The entire face and bilateral ears were prepped and draped in the usual sterile fashion. I began by making markings using gentian violet of the midline of the nose and the proposed placement of the lower lateral cartilages. The nasal tip, columella, and dorsum of the nose were infiltrated with 0.5% lidocaine with 1:200,000 epinephrine. Following this, a stairstep columellar incision was made. Dissection was carried up the medial crura, up to the level of the nasal tip. Bilateral rim incisions were used for additional cartilage exposure. A significant amount of scarring was encountered in the left lower lateral cartilage, and a small amount of scarred subcutaneous tissue was resected using super sharp scissors. Following complete mobilization up to the nasal bony region, the lower lateral cartilages were placed in proper alignment and an intercrural stitch was used for movement of bifid tip cartilage to the midline. Following this, the lateral portion of the lower lateral cartilage was suspended to the upper lateral cartilage using interrupted 4-0 clear nylon suture. This left a nice contour; however, the tip still lacked in tip projection.

Therefore, from the right ear, the right postauricular sulcus area was designed for ear cartilage strut graft. The incision was made in the postauricular sulcus and the cartilage was harvested using a 15C scalpel blade with special care to avoid injury to the cartilage graft. A portion of the cartilage graft was used as a columellar strut and the other portion was made into an umbrella-type tip graft, of which both were secured with 4-0 clear nylon suture. The skin was returned to its normal position, and there was excellent tip projection and left alar support in symmetry. Therefore, the wounds were closed using interrupted 6-0 fast-absorbing gut suture on the nasal columella and, intranasally, the rim incisions were closed using interrupted 5-0 chromic suture. The right postauricular sulcus was closed using a running 5-0 chromic suture. A bolstered ear dressing for compression and dorsal nasal tape closures were applied.

Questions for Further Review: Case Study 5.8

1. Which of the following correctly classifies the procedure performed?
   a. Code 30400, Rhinoplasty, primary; lateral and alar cartilages and/or elevation of nasal tip
   b. Code 30430, Rhinoplasty, secondary; minor revision (small amount of nasal tip work)
   c. Code 30460, Rhinoplasty for nasal deformity secondary to congenital cleft lip and/or palate, including columellar lengthening; tip only
   d. Code 30462, Rhinoplasty for nasal deformity secondary to congenital cleft lip and/or palate, including columellar lengthening; tip, septum, osteotomies
   e. Code 21235, Graft; ear cartilage, autogenous, to nose or ear (includes obtaining graft)

Case Study 5.9

Read the following clinical document and answer the questions for further review.

OPERATIVE REPORT

PREOPERATIVE DIAGNOSIS: Cleft nasal deformity

OPERATION: Septorhinoplasty

POSTOPERATIVE DIAGNOSIS: Cleft nasal deformity

ANESTHESIA: General endotracheal

ESTIMATED BLOOD LOSS: Minimal

SPECIMENS: None

DRAINS: None

COMPLICATIONS: None

OPERATION: A Medpor implant was placed into the nasal tip.

INDICATIONS: The patient had a history of left unilateral cleft lip and palate and had a residual cleft nasal deformity. Patient complained of difficulty breathing through the nose. On exam, patient was found to have a left nasal stenosis and a septal deviation to the right nostril.

PROCEDURE: The patient was taken to the operating room and placed on the operating room table in supine position. Patient was given general endotracheal anesthesia, after which the face was prepped and draped in the usual sterile fashion.

We began by placing pledgets soaked with 4% cocaine solution into both nares. We then injected with 1% lidocaine with epinephrine. We made an incision with a #15 blade in the right septal mucosa. A Freer elevator was then used to free up the mucosa from off the underlying septal cartilage. The Freer elevator was then used to cut through the septal cartilage to the other side, leaving the mucosa intact in the left nostril. A Freer elevator was then used to free the mucosa from off the septal cartilage on the left side. When this was completed, a swivel knife was inserted and a 2 x 3 cm piece of septal cartilage was removed.

At this point, we inserted a nasal speculum and could see that the right nostril was now open. We then made rim incisions bilaterally. A tenotomy scissors was used to free the dorsal skin and subcutaneous tissue from off the underlying cartilage and bone. This was continued up to the nasal bone and across the tip to completely free the soft tissue from the cartilage tip. We then used a rasp to file the nasal bone at the right portion of the dorsum. The implant was used in place of a cartilage graft to support the nasal tip and prevent left nostril collapse. When this was completed, we then used a Medpor implant, which was sculpted and then inserted into the tip and dorsum. When the Medpor implant was placed, we noted that the left nostril was now open by a significant degree.

The incisions were then closed with 5-0 chromic suture. A Doyle nasal splint was placed into the left nostril, and Steri-Strips were applied to the dorsum of the nose.

ADDENDUM: As part of the operation, we thinned the submucosal tissue from out of the left naris, thus helping to create a larger nostril opening.

Questions for Further Review: Case Study 5.9

1. Which of the following correctly classifies the procedure performed?
   a. Code 30400, Rhinoplasty, primary; lateral and alar cartilages and/or elevation of nasal tip
   b. Code 30430, Rhinoplasty, secondary; minor revision (small amount of nasal tip work)
   c. Code 30460, Rhinoplasty for nasal deformity secondary to congenital cleft lip and/or palate, including columellar lengthening; tip only
   d. Code 30462, Rhinoplasty for nasal deformity secondary to congenital cleft lip and/or palate, including columellar lengthening; tip, septum, osteotomies
   e. Code 21235, Graft; ear cartilage, autogenous, to nose or ear (includes obtaining graft)

Chapter 6

Cardiovascular, Hemic and Lymphatic Systems

CPT codes 33010 through 37799 are used to report surgical procedures on the cardiovascular system, which includes the heart and pericardium, arteries, and veins. Nonsurgical procedures on the cardiovascular system are classified in the medicine section of CPT.

CPT codes 38100 through 38999 are used to report surgical procedures on the hemic and lymphatic systems, which include the spleen, lymph nodes, and lymphatic channels.

Common outpatient procedures involving the cardiovascular system and the hemic and lymphatic systems include cardiac catheterizations, percutaneous transluminal coronary angioplasties (PTCAs), creation of arteriovenous fistulas and grafts, implantation of vascular access devices (VADs), and lymphatic biopsies and excisions.

Pacemaker or Pacing Cardioverter-Defibrillator Procedures

A pacemaker/implantable cardioverter defibrillator (ICD) insertion is a procedure in which a pacemaker and/or an ICD is inserted to assist in regulating problems with the heart rate (pacemaker) or heart rhythm (ICD).

When a problem develops with the heart's rhythm, such as a slow rhythm, a pacemaker may be selected for treatment. A pacemaker is a small electronic device composed of three parts: a generator, one or more leads, and an electrode on each lead. A pacemaker signals the heart to beat when the heartbeat is too slow.

A generator is the "brain" of the pacemaker device. It is a small metal case that contains electronic circuitry and a battery. The lead (or leads) is an insulated wire that is connected to the generator on one end, with the other end placed inside one of the heart's chambers. The electrode on the end of the lead touches the heart wall. In most pacemakers, the lead senses the heart's electrical activity. This information is relayed to the generator by the lead. If the heart's rate is slower than the programmed limit, an electrical impulse is sent through the lead to the electrode and the pacemaker's electrical impulse causes the heart to beat at a faster rate.

When the heart is beating at a rate faster than the programmed limit, the pacemaker will monitor the heart rate, but will not pace. No electrical impulses will be sent to the heart unless the heart's natural rate falls below the pacemaker's low limit.

Pacemaker leads may be positioned in the atrium or ventricle or both, depending on the condition requiring the pacemaker to be inserted. An atrial dysrhythmia/arrhythmia (an abnormal heart rhythm caused by a dysfunction of the sinus node or the development of another atrial pacemaker within the heart tissue that takes over the function of the sinus node) may be treated with an atrial pacemaker.

A new type of pacemaker, called a biventricular pacemaker, is currently used in the treatment of congestive heart failure. Sometimes in heart failure, the two ventricles (lower heart chambers) do not pump together in a normal manner. When this happens, less blood is pumped by the heart. A biventricular pacemaker paces both ventricles at the same time, increasing the amount of blood pumped by the heart. This type of treatment is called cardiac resynchronization therapy.

A pacemaker system includes a pulse generator containing electronics, a battery, and one or more electronics (lead). Pulse generators are placed in a subcutaneous "pocket" created in either a subclavicular site or underneath the abdominal muscles just below the ribcage. Electrodes may be inserted through a vein (transvenous) or they may be placed on the surface of the heart (epicardial). The epicardial location of electrodes requires a thoracotomy for the electrode insertion (AMA 2008).

A single-chamber pacemaker system includes a pulse generator and one electrode inserted in either the atrium or ventricle. A dual chamber pacemaker system includes a pulse generator and one electrode inserted in the right atrium and one electrode inserted in the right ventricle. In certain circumstances, an additional electrode may be required to achieve pacing of the left ventricle (biventricular pacing). Separately report codes 33224 or 33225 for transvenous placement of the electrode. Separately report codes 33202–33203 for epicardial placement of the electrode.

Codes 33202–33203 were established to separate the services of lead placement from generator placement. When a cardiologist places the generator and one or more of the electrodes by a transvenous route, for cases of biventricular generator placement, and left ventricular lead placement performed by another physician at a different session, these codes will allow reporting of the separate services of lead placement from the generator placement.

Pacemaker procedures include the following:

The electrodes of a pacing cardioverter-defibrillator system are positioned in the heart via the venous system (transvenously), in most circumstances. In certain circumstances, an additional electrode may be required to achieve pacing of the left ventricle (biventricle pacing). Electrode positioning on the epicardial surface of the heart requires a thoracotomy, or thoracoscopic placement of the leads.

APC	HCPCS	HCPCS Description	SI	Rel. Wt.	Payment Rate	OPPS OCE
0089			T	121.6508	7748.43	
	33206	Insertion of heart pacemaker				Significant Procedure, Multiple Reduction Applies; Separate APC payment.

Insertion, Removal, and Repositioning of Cardiac-Defibrillator System

An implantable cardioverter defibrillator (ICD) looks very similar to a pacemaker, except that it is slightly larger. It has a generator, one or more leads, and an electrode for each lead. These components work very much like a pacemaker. However, the ICD is designed to deliver an electrical shock to the heart when the heart rate becomes dangerously fast, or "fibrillates."

An ICD senses when the heart is beating too fast and delivers an electrical shock to convert the fast rhythm to a normal rhythm. Some devices combine a pacemaker and ICD in one unit for persons who need both functions.

The ICD has another type of treatment for certain fast rhythms called antitachycardia pacing (ATP). When ATP is used, a fast pacing impulse is sent to correct the rhythm. After the shock is delivered, a "back-up" pacing mode is used if needed for a short while.

The procedure for inserting a pacemaker or an ICD is the same. The procedure generally is performed in an electrophysiology (EP) lab or a cardiac catheterization lab.

Pacing cardioverter-defibrillator pulse generators may be implanted in a subcutaneous infraclavicular pocket or in an abdominal pocket. Removal of a pacing cardioverter-defibrillator pulse generator requires opening of the existing subcutaneous pocket and disconnection of the pulse generator from its electrodes.

Repositioning of a pacemaker electrode, pacing cardioverter-defibrillator electrode(s), or a left ventricular pacing electrode is reported using 33215 or 33226, as appropriate.

Replacement of a pacemaker electrode, pacing cardioverter-defibrillator electrode(s), or a left ventricular pacing electrode is reported using 33206–33208, 33210–33213, or 33224, as appropriate.

Cardiac Catheterization

Cardiac catheterization involves the passage of a tubular instrument, or catheter, into the heart through a vein or artery. The catheter may be used to inject contrast media and/or to measure pressures within the heart's chambers or great vessels. Cardiac catheterization is used mainly in the diagnosis and evaluation of congenital, rheumatic, and coronary artery lesions.

Catheterization procedures include the following:

- Right heart cardiac catheterization, which includes the study of the right atrium and ventricle, the tricuspid and pulmonic valves, the main pulmonary artery and its branches, and the superior and inferior vena cava

- Left heart cardiac catheterization, which includes the study of the left atrium and ventricle, the mitral and aortic valves, the ascending left aorta, and possibly the pulmonary veins

- Combined right and left heart cardiac catheterization, which is a single procedure with study and evaluation of both the right and left sides of the heart

Coding Guidelines for Cardiac Catheterization

Cardiac catheterization procedures are classified in the medicine section of CPT in the code range 93501–93572.

- Cardiac catheterization procedure codes include the following components:
  - Introduction, positioning, and repositioning of catheter
  - Recording of intracardiac and intravascular pressure
  - Obtaining blood samples for measurement of blood gases, dye dilution, or other dilution curves
  - Cardiac output measurements, such as dye dilution, Fick, or other method, with or without rest and case study, and/or other studies
  - Electrode catheter placement
  - Final evaluation and report
- Codes 93501–93533 are used to report the introduction of the cardiac catheter.
- Codes 93539–93545 are assigned for the angiography injection procedures performed in con-

junction with cardiac catheterization. These codes should be reported only once per cardiac catheterization, although multiple codes from this section may be applied, depending on the number of different structures visualized during the procedure (AMA, 1997b; AMA 2002).

- Codes 93555 and/or 93556 are used to report the technical details of angiography imaging supervision, interpretation, and report. Codes 93555 and 93556 should be reported only once, even though multiple angiographic procedures may have been performed (AMA 1997b).

The term *conduits* as used in code 93539, whether native or used for bypass, refers to arterial bypass vessels (AMA 2001b).

Percutaneous Transluminal Coronary Angioplasty

Angioplasty is a reparative procedure performed on a blood vessel. Used to open up arteries blocked by plaque, coronary angioplasty is frequently performed as a percutaneous transluminal coronary artery (PTCA) balloon dilatation. For balloon angioplasty to be effective, the tiny balloon must tear and crack the cholesterol and plaque deposits on the inner wall of the artery that block the supply of blood to the heart muscle. When this is accomplished, the blood vessel begins an effort to heal itself. Because the healing of the dilated, atherosclerotic artery is less than perfect, reocclusion of a balloon angioplasty site is relatively frequent.

Coding Guidelines for PTCA

PTCAs are assigned to codes 92982 and 92984, as appropriate:

- Code 92982 is assigned for single-vessel PTCA.
- Code 99284 is used for each additional vessel PTCA.

Codes 92980 and 92981 are used to report coronary artery stenting. Coronary angioplasty (92982, 92984) or atherectomy (92995, 92996), in the same artery, is considered part of the stenting procedure and is not reported separately. Codes 92973 (percutaneous transluminal coronary thrombectomy), 92974 (coronary brachytherapy), and 92978, 92979 (intravascular ultrasound) are add-on codes for reporting procedures performed in addition to coronary stenting, atherectomy, and angioplasty, and are not included in the "therapeutic interventions" in 92980.

Arteriovenous Fistulas and Grafts

An arteriovenous (AV) fistula is an abnormal passage or communication between two blood vessels. Fistulas can be surgically acquired, traumatic, or congenital, as follows:

- A surgically acquired fistula refers to the surgical joining of an artery and a vein under the skin for purposes of hemodialysis. Such fistulas are created to allow repeated access to the arterial or venous system, with access to the blood circulation through the fistula rather than through the patient's normal arterial or venous anatomy. Fistulas are commonly created in an extremity, usually in the arm. Grafts are often required to create a conduit between the blood vessels. The fistula/graft material may be natural (from the patient's own body) or synthetic (such as Dacron, polytetrafluoroethylene [PTFE], or a bovine graft).

- Traumatic fistulas are caused when a trauma, such as a knife wound, creates a small opening between two vessels that lie in close proximity. When the wound heals, the opening between the vessels remains, causing a short circuit of blood between the arterial and venous circulations. Traumatic fistulas commonly occur in the femoral arteries and veins in the lower extremities and in the upper extremities around the wrist.

- A congenital fistula is an abnormal opening or a complex plexus of vessels between the arterial and venous systems. One of the most common congenital AV fistulas occurs in the head in a condition known as intracranial arterial venous malformation.

Coding Guidelines for AV Fistulas and Grafts

The following guidelines apply to the coding of fistulas and grafts (AMA 1999d; 2001c; 2001f; 2003d):

- Code 36821, Arteriovenous anastomosis, open; direct, any site, involves connecting the vein directly to the artery without an interposing graft (two adjacent vessels are connected). This is usually possible when the artery and the vein are very close to each other.

- Code 36825, Creation of arteriovenous fistula by other than direct arteriovenous anastomosis, autogenous graft, involves creating an arteriovenous anastomosis between two vessels using an interposing graft made of the patient's natural vein (autogenous). For chronic hemodialysis, vascular access usually requires the surgical construction of an AV fistula between the patient's artery and vein, most often in the forearm. The fistula "matures" in four to six weeks, and increased blood flow causes the venous site to become enlarged.

- Code 36830, Creation of arteriovenous fistula by other than direct arteriovenous anastomosis, nonautogenous graft, involves creating an arteriovenous anastomosis between two vessels using a synthetic material as an interposing graft (nonautogenous). A nonautogenous AV fistula/graft is a tube made from Gortex, PTFE, or similar biocompatible material. The tube is surgically tunneled under the skin in a loop that connects an artery to a vein.

- Code 36831, Open AV graft thrombectomy without revision, involves opening the fistula/graft, inserting a catheter (for example, Fogarty) into the fistula, and extracting the clots.

- Code 36832, Open AV graft revision without thrombectomy, involves opening the fistula/graft, straightening a kink, and re-anastomosing the graft. Usually, a long synthetic patch is sewn as a "patch angioplasty" along the length of the arteriotomy, using ocular loupe magnification.

- Code 36833, Open AV graft thrombectomy with revision, involves opening the fistula/graft, inserting a catheter into the fistula, and extracting the clots. After this thrombectomy is performed, a long synthetic patch is sewn as a "patch angioplasty", along the length of the arteriotomy, using ocular loupe magnification.

- Code 36870, Percutaneous AV graft thrombectomy, can involve removing the thrombus from the graft in a variety of methods. Heparin may be given systemically; thrombolytic drugs may be given into the graft, either as a bolus, as an infusion, or using a pulsed-spray technique. A limited dose of thrombolytic agent may be instilled into the thrombus for initiation of thrombolysis. The thrombus also may be removed mechanically with a variety of specially-designed devices or with Fogarty-type angioplasty balloons. The thrombus is then macerated and the shunt cleared.

When these accesses thrombose, most develop what is termed an "arterial plug," or a small, densely fibrotic clot, at the arterial anastomosis, that typically will not dissolve and usually sticks in the graft, narrowing or occluding the arterial inflow. These codes also describe removal of this portion of the thrombus, which usually requires an additional step for removal separate from the rest of the procedure to declot the graft.

Do not report code 36593 in conjunction with code 36870. Code 36593 classifies thrombolytic agent declotting of implanted VAD or catheter.

- Puncture into the graft to allow access to both anastomoses is coded with 36145 and should be coded twice (36145, 36145–59) when two separate punctures are performed.

- Code 75790 is reported for diagnostic fistulogram imaging. This code would be reported once for all imaging services directly related to the initial procedure. Follow-up imaging studies performed either at a different session on the same day or on a separate day are separately reportable (AMA 2000a).

- Codes 35476 and 75978 are assigned for a venous anastomotic stenosis treated with balloon angioplasty to restore patency and flow.

A single-venous angioplasty code is assigned when there is treatment of multiple venous stenoses clumped in the same vessel.

When a separate vessel from the initially treated stenotic vessel is involved, such as the subclavian vein, percutaneous transluminal angioplasty (PTA) of that lesion should be coded as a second venous angioplasty (for example, 35476, 75978, 35476–59, 75978–59). Modifier –59 is used to delineate the treatment of a separate vessel.

- Services not included in code 36870 that should be reported separately when performed additionally are: catheterization (36145); angioplasty of the graft/fistula, venous, or arterial anastomoses (35473–35476, 75962, 75964, 75978); stenting (37205, 37206, 75960); fistulography (75790); and thrombolytic infusion over one hour in length (37201, 75896).

APC	HCPCS	HCPCS Description	SI	Rel. Wt.	Payment Rate	OPPS OCE
0088			T	38.7673	2469.24	
	36821	Arteriovenous anastomosis, open; direct any site				Significant Procedure, Multiple Reduction Applies; Separate APC payment.

Code 37607, Ligation or banding of AV graft/fistula, refers to:

- Ligation, which is occlusion of the lumen of a vessel by application of a suture ligature that cuts off the flow in the vessel and causes it to clot

- Banding, which is wrapping of an AV fistula, usually with synthetic material, to reduce blood flow from any outside source

Vascular Access Devices

Vascular access devices (VADs) are sterile catheter systems implanted subcutaneously, typically under local anesthesia, for various purposes such as the following:

- Infusion of total parenteral nutrition (TPN)
- Administration of antibiotics
- Administration of chemotherapy
- Administration of blood and blood products
- Aspiration of blood samples for laboratory analysis
- Bolus injections of medication (relatively large volumes of a drug administered rapidly to hasten or magnify a response)

These systems are designed to provide repeated access to the vascular system without the trauma or complications of multiple venipunctures. When not in use, VADs are flushed with a heparinized solution to maintain patency.

Coding Guidelines for Vascular Access Devices

Codes for reporting the placement and maintenance of VADs are found in the CPT code range 36555–36597.

- To qualify as a central venous access catheter or device, the tip of the catheter/device must terminate in the subclavian, brachiocephalic (innominate), or iliac veins; the superior or inferior vena cava; or the right atrium.
- The venous access device may be peripherally inserted, as when the basilic or cephalic vein is the catheter entry site.
- The venous access device may be centrally inserted, as when the jugular, subclavian, femoral vein, or inferior vena cava is the catheter entry site.
- Tunneling is the process of passing the catheter under the skin through a subcutaneous tract. Typically, the dictation will state, "the catheter was passed through a subcutaneous tunnel" or "a subcutaneous tunnel was formed." Technically, this is done by creating two incision sites in the skin, then passing a "tunneler" under the skin so that the two holes are connected.
- The work required for removal of a nontunneled central venous access catheter is considered to be inherent in the evaluation and management visit in which it is performed (AMA 2003d).

For CPT coding, insertion involves placement of catheter through a newly- established venous access.

For CPT coding of device replacement, if an existing central venous access device is removed and a new one placed via a separate venous access site, appropriate codes for both procedures (removal of old, if code exists, and insertion of new device) should be reported.

For CPT coding, repair involves fixing a device without replacement of either the catheter or the port/pump other than pharmacologic or mechanical correction of intracatheter or pericatheter occlusion (code 36595 or 36596).

For CPT coding, for repair, partial (catheter only) replacement, complete replacement, or removal of both catheters (placed from separate venous access sites) of a multicatheter device, with or without subcutaneous ports/pumps, use the appropriate code describing the service with a frequency of two.

- Code 36595 is for mechanical removal of pericatheter obstructive material, such as a fibrin sheath from a central venous device via separate venous access. This procedure involves stripping the fibrin sheath from or about the existing catheter by use of either a transcatheter snare or a balloon under imaging guidance.

- Code 36596 is for mechanical removal of intraluminal (intracatheter) obstructive material from a central venous device through the device lumen. This procedure involves clearing the intraluminal obstructive material with a guide wire, brush, or other mechanical device under imaging guidance.

- Code 36593 is for declotting by thrombolytic agent of an implanted VAD or catheter. This procedure involves introducing a thrombolytic agent through a syringe and then slowly instilling it into the device or catheter.

Exhibit 6.1, at the end of this chapter, offers more information on the coding of VADs.

APC	HCPCS	HCPCS Description	SI	Rel. Wt.	Payment Rate	OPPS OCE
0676			T	2.4824	158.11	
	36593	Declot vascular device				Significant Procedure, Multiple Reduction Applies; Separate APC payment.

Lymphatic Biopsy or Excision

Lymphatic biopsy or excision refers to the removal of a lymph node for examination, usually to determine whether it is cancerous.

Coding Guidelines for Lymphatic Biopsy or Excision

CPT codes 38500 through 38530 are used to indicate the excision or biopsy of one or more lymph nodes.

- The level of biopsy or excision (superficial or deep) of a lymph node must be known before a correct code can be selected.

- The site of the lymph node must be known to select a biopsy, excision, or lymphadenectomy code.

Documentation Requirements for Cardiovascular, Hemic, and Lymphatic System Procedures

Each procedure is followed by clinical information that must be documented in the medical record when the procedure is performed.

Cardiac Catheterization

CPT Codes 93501–93572 are used to report cardiac catheterizations.

1. Whether the patient has a congenital cardiac anomaly

2. The side(s) of the heart that was catheterized.

   - Left side
   - Right side
   - Right and left sides

3. If left heart catheterization, the method that was used to access the left side of the heart.

   - Percutaneous retrograde from the brachial artery, axillary artery, or femoral artery
   - Retrograde
   - Transseptal through intact septum
   - Left ventricular puncture (with or without retrograde left heart catheterization)

4. Whether an angiography was performed. If yes, on which site(s).

   - Pulmonary
   - Right ventricular
   - Right atrial
   - Left ventricular
   - Left atrial
   - Selective coronary (injection of radiopaque material may be by hand)
   - Aortic root
   - All sites listed above

5. Whether selective visualization/opacification of bypass graft(s) was performed. If yes, list the site(s).

   - Arterial conduits (for example, internal mammary)
   - Aortocoronary venous bypass grafts

6. Whether additional code(s) should be assigned to classify the imaging supervision, interpretation, and report for the injection procedure(s) performed during the cardiac catheterization.

- 93555
- 93555 and 93556

Venous Access Device

CPT codes 36555–36597 are used to report venous access devices.

1. Age of patient

2. Each device involved

   - Single catheter
   - Multicatheter device (Tesio)
   - Subcutaneous port
   - Subcutaneous pump

3. Type of procedure

   - Insertion
   - Replacement (Specify if same or different venous access site is being used.)
   - Repair
   - Removal of device(s)
   - Removal of obstructive material (Specify pericatheter or intraluminal.)
   - Repositioning under fluoroscopic guidance

4. Catheter entry site

   - Jugular
   - Subclavian
   - Femoral vein
   - Inferior vena cava
   - Basilic vein
   - Cephalic vein
   - Other (specify)

5. Whether the catheter was tunneled

Case Studies

This section contains actual operative reports from real-life cases. All identifiers have been removed or changed for confidentiality and privacy.

Carefully read the clinical documentation for each case study, which may include a procedure report as well as radiology and/or pathology reports, as applicable.

Answer all the questions for further review at the end of each case study. Use a current CPT codebook or HCPCS Level II code listing, as needed.

When appropriate, assign one or more of the following modifiers:

–50	Bilateral Procedure
–59	Distinct Procedural Service
–FA	Left hand, thumb
–F1	Left hand, second digit
–F2	Left hand, third digit
–F3	Left hand, fourth digit
–F4	Left hand, fifth digit
–F5	Right hand, thumb
–F6	Right hand, second digit
–F7	Right hand, third digit
–F8	Right hand, fourth digit
–F9	Right hand, fifth digit
–LC	Left circumflex, coronary artery (For Medicare, hospitals use with codes 92980–92984, 92995, 92996)
–LD	Left anterior descending coronary artery (For Medicare, hospitals use with codes 92980–92984, 92995, 92996)
–RC	Right coronary artery (For Medicare, hospitals use with codes 92980–92984, 92995, 92996)
–LT	Left side
–RT	Right side
–TA	Left foot, great toe
–T1	Left foot, second digit
–T2	Left foot, third digit
–T3	Left foot, fourth digit
–T4	Left foot, fifth digit
–T5	Right foot, great toe
–T6	Right foot, second digit
–T7	Right foot, third digit
–T8	Right foot, fourth digit
–T9	Right foot, fifth digit

Do not apply the current version of the Medicare CCI edits to any of these questions; the focus is on the application of the coding guidelines and not on the application of edits that change on a quarterly basis. When coding in real life, of course, you will need to apply the CCI edits as appropriate for Medicare outpatient cases.

Case Study 6.1

Read the following clinical document and answer the questions for further review.

OPERATIVE REPORT

PREOPERATIVE DIAGNOSIS: Advanced ovarian carcinoma, planned chemotherapy

POSTOPERATIVE DIAGNOSIS: The same

OPERATION PERFORMED: Placement of a permanent venous access catheter

COMPLICATIONS: None

HISTORY: This is a 69-year-old female with advanced ovarian carcinoma. She was prepped for placement of venous catheter. It was done without any complications.

PROCEDURE: The patient was identified in the supine position, given sedation, and monitored by anesthesia staff. The upper chest was prepped and draped accordingly. The left subclavian side was then infiltrated with 1% Xylocaine. The venous entrance was successful on the first attempt. The guidewire was advanced, and subsequently the skin incision was made and the trocar introduced. With removal of the guide wire and the trocar, but the sleeve in place, we were able to advance the catheter. Its distal tip was adjusted to be in the distal superior vena cava. The internal wire was advanced, and the catheter was then tunneled into the left anterior chest wall subcutaneous pocket. The length was cut accordingly, and we attached nipples to port with locking mechanism slipped over it. The port was fixed to the chest wall fascia. Hemostasis was complete. The port was accessed and flushed, and free blood flow was confirmed. The closure of the skin took place in the usual fashion.

The patient was awakened and taken to the recovery room in stable condition for further observation.

Questions for Further Review: Case Study 6.1

1. What is the age of the patient?

2. Identify each device involved in this case.
   a. Single catheter
   b. Multicatheter device (Tesio)
   c. Subcutaneous port
   d. Subcutaneous pump

3. What type of procedure(s) was performed?
   a. Insertion
   b. Replacement (specify whether same or different venous access site is being used)
   c. Repair
   d. Removal of device(s)
   e. Removal of obstructive material—pericatheter
   f. Removal of obstructive material—intraluminal
   g. Repositioning under fluoroscopic guidance

4. What was the catheter entry site?
   a. Jugular
   b. Subclavian
   c. Femoral vein
   d. Inferior vena cava
   e. Basilic vein
   f. Cephalic vein
   g. Other (specify)

5. Was the catheter tunneled?
   a. Yes
   b. No

6. CPT surgery code(s) and modifier(s):

Case Study 6.2

Read the following clinical document and answer the questions for further review.

RADIOLOGY DEPARTMENT

EXAM DATE: 11/09/XX   **AGE:** 46

PROCEDURE: Tesio catheter placement

CLINICAL HISTORY: Patient with left groin Tesio catheters, which had been inadvertently withdrawn

Patient was informed of the risks of the procedure and written consent obtained. Conscious sedation was administered with monitoring of heart rate, blood pressure, and respiratory rate.

The patient was placed in a supine position on the fluoroscopy table, and the left groin Tesio catheter was prepped and draped in a sterile fashion. 1% lidocaine was injected into the subcutaneous tissues for anesthesia. Arterial and venous Tesio catheters were dissected free at the entrance site in the groin and exchanged over a guide wire for new arterial and venous Tesio catheters. The catheters were placed at the junction of the left common iliac vein and IVC. Each catheter was then tunneled to a new exit site in the left thigh. The catheters functioned appropriately at the conclusion of the procedure.

IMPRESSION: Successful Tesio change

Questions for Further Review: Case Study 6.2

1. What is the age of the patient?

2. Identify each device involved in this case.
   a. Single catheter
   b. Multicatheter device (Tesio)
   c. Subcutaneous port
   d. Subcutaneous pump

3. What type of procedure(s) was performed?
   a. Insertion
   b. Replacement: Same access site is being used.
   c. Replacement: Different venous access site is being used.
   d. Repair
   e. Removal of device(s)
   f. Removal of obstructive material—pericatheter
   g. Removal of obstructive material—intraluminal
   h. Repositioning under fluoroscopic guidance

4. What was the catheter entry site?
   a. Jugular
   b. Subclavian
   c. Femoral vein
   d. Inferior vena cava
   e. Basilic vein
   f. Cephalic vein
   g. Other (specify)
   h. Not applicable

5. Was the catheter tunneled?
   a. Yes
   b. No

6. CPT surgery code(s) and modifier(s):

Case Study 6.3

Read the following clinical document and answer the questions for further review.

DEPARTMENT OF RADIOLOGY

AGE: 49

EXAM: Removal of a tunneled dialysis catheter

INDICATIONS: Patient had a tunneled catheter inserted in December 200X and has a fistula that is working properly.

TECHNIQUE: The skin was prepped and draped in the usual sterile fashion. Local anesthesia was administered. Using dissection, the cuff of the catheter was released from the subcutaneous tissues and the catheter was removed. Hemostasis was achieved. A sterile dressing was placed.

IMPRESSION: Removal of a tunneled dialysis catheter with dissection as described

---

Questions for Further Review: Case Study 6.3

1. What is the age of the patient?

2. Identify each device involved in this case.
   a. Single catheter
   b. Multicatheter device (Tesio)
   c. Subcutaneous port
   d. Subcutaneous pump

3. What type of procedure(s) was performed?
   a. Insertion
   b. Replacement: Same access site is being used.
   c. Replacement: Different venous access site is being used.
   d. Repair
   e. Removal of device(s)
   f. Removal of obstructive material—pericatheter
   g. Removal of obstructive material—intraluminal
   h. Repositioning under fluoroscopic guidance

4. What was the catheter entry site?
   a. Jugular
   b. Subclavian
   c. Femoral vein
   d. Inferior vena cava
   e. Basilic vein
   f. Cephalic vein
   g. Other (specify)
   h. Not applicable

5. Was the catheter tunneled?
   a. Yes
   b. No

6. CPT surgery code(s) and modifier(s):

Case Study 6.4

Read the following clinical document and answer the questions for further review.

OPERATIVE REPORT

PREOPERATIVE DIAGNOSIS: Left defected port-a-cath, advanced ovarian carcinoma

POSTOPERATIVE DIAGNOSIS: Same

OPERATION PERFORMED: Removal of defected port-a-cath and placement of a new port-a-cath

ANESTHESIA: Local/monitor

COMPLICATIONS: None

HISTORY: This is a 73-year-old female with a long history of ovarian carcinoma, treated successfully, but remains with disease. She was found with a defected port-a-cath on recent portogram. Its removal was advised along with placement of new one. These were performed and no complications were encountered.

PROCEDURE: The patient was identified, and in the supine position was given sedation and monitored by anesthesia staff. She was prepped and draped accordingly. The left anterior chest wall port was noted. The previous scar was anesthetized with 1% Xylocaine. Incision was made and the port was identified. The stay sutures were cut and the port was removed along with full length of the catheter. Then the patient was repositioned into Trendelenburg. She is very petite, and thus much attention was paid for venous puncture to avoid the pneumothorax. After appropriate preparation of right subclavian site, vena puncture was attempted and was successful on the third attempt. Eventually, the guide wire was advanced and then the trocar, after skin incision was made. Then the catheter's tip was adjusted to be in the distal SVC. Subsequently, the catheter was tunneled to the previous port site. The catheter was then attached to the reservoir, and this was placed in its pocket and final confirmation of free flow of blood was made. The port was flushed with concentrated heparinized saline solution. The skin closure took place in the usual fashion. The patient was awake in stable condition and taken to the recovery room for further observation.

Questions for Further Review: Case Study 6.4

1. What is the age of the patient?

2. Identify each device involved in this case.
    a. Single catheter
    b. Multicatheter device (Tesio)
    c. Subcutaneous port
    d. Subcutaneous pump

3. What type of procedure(s) was performed?
    a. Insertion
    b. Replacement: Same access site is being used.
    c. Replacement: Different venous access site is being used.
    d. Repair
    e. Removal of device(s)
    f. Removal of obstructive material—pericatheter
    g. Removal of obstructive material—intraluminal
    h. Repositioning under fluoroscopic guidance

4. What was the catheter entry site?
    a. Jugular
    b. Subclavian
    c. Femoral vein
    d. Inferior vena cava
    e. Basilic vein
    f. Cephalic vein
    g. Other (specify)
    h. Not applicable

5. Was the catheter tunneled?
    a. Yes
    b. No

6. CPT surgery code(s) and modifier(s):

Case Study 6.5

Read the following clinical document and answer the questions for further review.

RADIOLOGY REPORT

EXAMINATION: IR, REV IMPLANT VEN ACC PORT

EXAMINATION:
1. Contrast injection through two separate lumens of dialysis catheter
2. Dialysis catheter exchange over guide wires

CONTRAST: 20 cc

COMPLICATIONS: None

MEDICATIONS: Local anesthesia

PROCEDURE: Risks and benefits of the procedure were explained to the patient and informed consent was obtained. The 74-year-old patient was prepped and draped in the usual sterile fashion. Contrast was injected separately into the two lumens of the dialysis catheter. Images were obtained. A guide wire was then placed through both lumens of the catheters. Existing catheter was removed with blunt dissection over the guide wires. A new catheter was then inserted over the guide wires with the distal tips in the right atrium.

The catheter was secured in position. The patient tolerated the procedure well without acute complication.

FINDINGS: Initial dye study revealed small amount of intraluminal thrombus in the distal tips of both the red and blue lumens of the catheters. The catheters were then exchanged using intermittent fluoroscopic guidance.

IMPRESSION: Successful revision of hemodialysis catheter with exchange over guide wires. Existing catheters had intraluminal fibrin sheath.

Questions for Further Review: Case Study 6.5

1. What is the age of the patient?

2. Identify each device involved in this case.
   a. Single catheter
   b. Multicatheter device (Tesio)
   c. Subcutaneous port
   d. Subcutaneous pump

3. What type of procedure(s) was performed?
   a. Insertion
   b. Replacement: Same access site is being used.
   c. Replacement: Different venous access site is being used.
   d. Repair
   e. Removal of device(s)
   f. Removal of obstructive material—pericatheter
   g. Removal of obstructive material—intraluminal
   h. Repositioning under fluoroscopic guidance

4. What was the catheter entry site?
   a. Jugular
   b. Subclavian
   c. Femoral vein
   d. Inferior vena cava
   e. Basilic vein
   f. Cephalic vein
   g. Other (specify)
   h. Not applicable (not documented)

5. Was the catheter tunneled?
   a. Yes
   b. No

6. CPT surgery code(s) and modifier(s):

Case Study 6.6

Read the following clinical document and answer the questions for further review.

CARDIAC CATHETERIZATION REPORT

INDICATIONS: The patient is a 72-year-old gentleman with progressive aortic insufficiency and evidence of left ventricular dilatation. He is scheduled for right and left heart catheterization to assess the degree of valvular heart disease prior to planned valve surgery.

PROCEDURE: Right and left heart catheterization via the right femoral artery and vein using 6 French introducers and catheters for the left heart catheterization and a 6 French Bard catheter for the right heart catheterization.

HEMODYNAMICS: Please see accompanying report. Right heart pressures were moderately elevated. The mean pulmonary capillary wedge pressure was 25 mmHg with prominent V waves.

COMPLICATIONS: None

LEFT VENTRICULOGRAPHY: The left ventricle is mildly dilated. There is mild anterior hypokinesis. The estimated left ventricular ejection fraction is 50%.

AORTOGRAPHY: The aortic root is dilated. The focal aneurysm involves the take-off of the left main coronary artery. Severe aortic insufficiency is present.

CORONARY ANGIOGRAPHY: Right coronary: The right coronary artery is dominant and free of obvious disease. Left coronary: The left coronary artery could not be cannulated due to a focal aneurysm involving the take-off of the left main coronary artery.

CONCLUSIONS:

1. Severe aortic insufficiency
2. Dilated left ventricle with an estimated ejection fraction of 50%
3. Mild mitral insufficiency
4. Nonobstructive right coronary arteries
5. Moderate pulmonary hypertension
6. Unable to assess left coronary artery

Questions for Further Review: Case Study 6.6

1. Does the patient have a congenital cardiac anomaly?
    a. Yes
    b. No

2. What side(s) of the heart was catheterized?
    a. Left side
    b. Right side
    c. Right and left sides

3. If left heart catheterization, what method was used to access the left side of the heart?
    a. Percutaneous retrograde from the brachial artery, axillary artery, or femoral artery
    b. Retrograde
    c. Transseptal through intact septum
    d. Left ventricular puncture (with or without retrograde left heart catheterization)
    e. Not applicable

4. Was angiography performed? If yes, on which site(s)?
    a. Pulmonary
    b. Right ventricular
    c. Right atrial
    d. Left ventricular
    e. Left atrial
    f. Selective coronary (Injection of radiopaque material may be by hand.)
    g. Aortic root
    h. All sites listed above

5. Was selective visualization/opacification of bypass graft(s) performed?
   a. Yes
   b. No

   If yes, on which site(s)?
   a. Arterial conduits (for example, internal mammary)
   b. Aortocoronary venous bypass grafts

6. Which additional code(s) should be assigned to classify the imaging supervision, interpretation, and report for the injection procedure(s) performed during the cardiac catheterization?
   a. 93555
   b. 93555 and 93556

7. CPT surgery code(s) and modifier(s):

Case Study 6.7

Read the following clinical document and answer the questions for further review.

CARDIAC CATHETERIZATION REPORT

INDICATIONS: The patient is a 69-year-old male with a history of hypertension and a family history of early coronary artery disease, who presents now with chest pain syndrome.

PROCEDURE: The right groin was prepped and draped in the usual sterile fashion with use of 1% lidocaine. Left heart catheterization was performed percutaneously via the right femoral artery using 5 French catheters. Left ventriculography was performed in the 30-degree RAO projection using a pigtail catheter. Coronary angiography was performed in multiple projections using the standard Judkins technique. The left coronary was cannulated using a 5 French Judkins 5 left catheter. At the conclusion of the procedure, the sheath was removed, hemostasis achieved, and a pressure dressing applied. The patient was transferred to the ambulatory care unit in stable condition.

MEDICATIONS: None

HEMODYNAMICS: Of note, the left ventricular end diastolic pressure is within normal limits.

COMPLICATIONS: None

LEFT VENTRICULOGRAPHY: Left ventricular systolic function is within normal limits. There are no evident wall motion abnormalities. The overall ejection fraction is estimated to be 60%. There is no evidence of mitral regurgitation or mitral valve prolapse.

CORONARY ANGIOGRAPHY:

Right coronary: The right coronary artery is the dominant vessel giving rise to the posterior descending artery. There is a 30% stenosis of the proximal right coronary artery, a 35% stenosis in the mid-right coronary artery, and a 20% stenosis in the distal right coronary artery.

Left coronary: The left main coronary artery is widely patent and free of stenosis. The left anterior descending artery extends to the apex of the left ventricle. There was a 90% stenosis in the mid-left anterior descending artery between the origins of the first and second diagonal branches. The left circumflex artery gives rise to one large obtuse marginal obtuse branch. The left circumflex artery and its branches are free of stenosis.

CONCLUSIONS:
1. Normal left heart pressures
2. Normal left ventricular systolic function. The ejection fraction is estimated to be 60%.
3. No evidence of mitral regurgitation or mitral valve prolapse
4. Right dominant coronary circulation
5. Mild disease in the proximal, mid-, distal right coronary artery
6. Severe stenosis in the mid-left anterior descending artery

Questions for Further Review: Case Study 6.7

1. Does the patient have a congenital cardiac anomaly?
   a. Yes
   b. No

2. What side(s) of the heart was catheterized?
   a. Left side
   b. Right side
   c. Right and left sides

3. If left heart catheterization, what method was used to access the left side of the heart?
   a. Percutaneous retrograde from the brachial artery, axillary artery, or femoral artery
   b. Retrograde
   c. Transseptal through intact septum
   d. Left ventricular puncture (with or without retrograde left heart catheterization)

4. Was angiography performed?
   a. Yes
   b. No

   If yes, on which site(s)?
   a. Pulmonary
   b. Right ventricular
   c. Right atrial
   d. Left ventricular
   e. Left atrial
   f. Selective coronary (injection of radiopaque material may be by hand)
   g. Aortic root
   h. All sites listed above

5. Was selective visualization/opacification of bypass graft(s) performed?
   a. Yes
   b. No

   If yes, on which site(s)?
   a. Arterial conduits (for example, internal mammary)
   b. Aortocoronary venous bypass grafts

6. Which additional code(s) should be assigned to classify the imaging supervision, interpretation, and report for the injection procedure(s) performed during the cardiac catheterization?
   a. 93555
   b. 93555 and 93556

7. CPT surgery code(s) and modifier(s):

Case Study 6.8

Read the following clinical document and answer the questions for further review.

CARDIAC CATHETERIZATION REPORT

PROCEDURES:

1. Coronary angiography
2. Left heart catheterization
3. Bypass graft study
4. Coronary angioplasty

HISTORY: Patient is a 56-year-old woman. She has hypertension. The patient has a history of smoking. She has hypercholesterolemia and diabetes. She also has a history of chest pain and a prior history of coronary artery disease.

TECHNIQUE: A 6 Fr sheath was inserted in the right femoral artery utilizing the Seldinger technique. The left coronary artery was injected utilizing a 6 Fr FR4 catheter. A 6 Fr FR4 catheter was used to inject the right coronary artery. The arterial graft was injected utilizing a 6 Fr FR4 catheter. Coronary angioplasty was performed, and the equipment utilized is described in the intervention summary section. 10,000 units of heparin were administered. Intracoronary nitroglycerin was given during this case. 240 cc of nonionic contrast were administered.

HEMODYNAMICS:
Left Heart Pressures
Resting:

	Systolic	Diastolic	EDP	a	v	m
Ao	140	76				100
LV	140		13			

Coronary Angiography
Dominance: Right

Left Main
The left main was normal.

Left Anterior Descending
There was moderate diffuse disease of the proximal segment of the left anterior descending artery (LAD). The midsegment of the LAD had a single discrete 99% stenosis. Distal flow was via a bypass graft. There also was a 40% single discrete stenosis of the distal segment of the LAD.

There was an 85% diffuse stenosis of the proximal segment of the first diagonal branch (Diag 1) of the LAD. The Diag 1 was small. The midsegment of the Diag 1 had a diffuse 85% stenosis.

There was mild diffuse disease of the proximal segment of the left circumflex artery (LCX).

There was moderate diffuse disease of the entire vessel segment of the first obtuse marginal branch (OMI) of the LCX. The OMI was small.

There was a single discrete total occlusion of the proximal segment of the second obtuse marginal branch (OM2) of the LCX. The OM2 was small. There was an 85% single discrete stenosis of the proximal segment of the first left posterolateral branch (LPL1) of the LCX. Distal flow was via a bypass graft.

Right Coronary Artery
There was a single discrete total occlusion of the proximal segment of the right coronary artery (RCA).

Bypass Grafts
Three bypass grafts were evaluated during this procedure:

1. Left internal mammary artery graft to the LAD

   There was a left internal mammary artery graft with a single anastomosis to the left anterior descending artery (LAD).

   There was no evidence of obstruction in this graft.

2. Saphenous vein graft to the LPL1

There was a saphenous vein graft with a single anastomosis to the first left posterolateral branch (LPL1) of the LCX.

There was no evidence of obstruction in this graft. Distal flow was normal.

This graft is a free radial artery graft, not a saphenous vein graft.

3. Saphenous vein graft to the RCA

There was a saphenous vein graft with a single anastomosis to the right coronary artery (RCA).

There was no evidence of obstruction in this graft. Distal flow was normal.

Indication for Intervention
Coronary intervention was indicated for treatment of stable angina.

Intervention Summary
First Diagonal Branch of the LAD
Proximal 85%

Angioplasty was performed on the 85% stenosis in the proximal segment of the Diag 1.

According to the ACC/AHA classification system, this lesion was a type B1 lesion.

Angioplasty was accomplished through a 6 Fr CLS 3 5 guide utilizing a Maverick 20-mm balloon with a maximum size of 2.0 mm and a maximum inflation pressure of 12 atmospheres.

The final outcome was defined as successful. The residual stenosis following this intervention was 20%. Distal flow was normal.

Mid 85%

Angioplasty was performed on the stenosis in the midsegment of the Diag 1. This lesion was designated a type B1 lesion based on ACC/AHA classification system.

Angioplasty was accomplished through a 6 Fr CLS 3 5 guide utilizing a Maverick 20-mm balloon with a maximum size of 2.0 mm and a maximum inflation pressure of 12 atmospheres.

The final outcome was defined as successful. The residual stenosis following this intervention was 20%. Distal flow was normal.

Conclusions
Three-vessel coronary artery disease (LAD, LCX and RCA)
Patent left internal mammary artery graft to the LAD
Patent saphenous vein graft to the LPL1
Patent saphenous vein graft to the RCA
Successful angioplasty of the proximal D1 lesion
Successful angioplasty of the mid-D1 lesion

Recommendations: The patient's medical regimen was changed as follows: Complete Integrelin infusion.

Complications/Events: The patient had no complications during these procedures.

Questions for Further Review: Case Study 6.8

1. Does the patient have a congenital cardiac anomaly?
   a. Yes
   b. No

2. What side(s) of the heart was catheterized?
   a. Left side
   b. Right side
   c. Right and left sides

3. If left heart catheterization, what method was used to access the left side of the heart?
   a. Percutaneous retrograde from the brachial artery, axillary artery, or femoral artery
   b. Retrograde
   c. Transseptal through intact septum
   d. Left ventricular puncture (with or without retrograde left heart catheterization)

4. Was angiography performed?
    a.   Yes
    b.   No

    If yes, on which site(s)?
    a.   Pulmonary
    b.   Right ventricular
    c.   Right atrial
    d.   Left ventricular
    e.   Left atrial
    f.   Selective coronary (injection of radiopaque material may be by hand)
    g.   Aortic root
    h.   All sites listed above

5. Was selective visualization/opacification of bypass graft(s) performed?
    a.   Yes
    b.   No

    If yes, on which site(s)?
    a.   Arterial conduits (for example, internal mammary)
    b.   Aortocoronary venous bypass grafts

6. Which additional code(s) should be assigned to classify the imaging supervision, interpretation, and report for the injection procedure(s) performed during the cardiac catheterization?
    a.   93555
    b.   93556
    c.   93555 and 93556

7. What type of angioplasty was performed?
    a.   Percutaneous transluminal pulmonary artery balloon angioplasty
    b.   Open transluminal balloon angioplasty, aortic
    c.   Open transluminal balloon angioplasty, venous
    d.   Percutaneous transluminal coronary balloon angioplasty
    e.   Percutaneous transluminal balloon angioplasty, aortic
    f.   Percutaneous transluminal balloon angioplasty, venous

8. On how many vessels was the angioplasty performed?
    a.   One vessel
    b.   Two vessels

9. CPT surgery code(s) and modifier(s):

Case Study 6.9

Read the following clinical document and answer the questions for further review.

CARDIAC CATHETERIZATION REPORT

PROCEDURES: Aortic root aortogram; coronary angioplasty

HISTORY: Patient is a 71-year-old man with hypertension and diabetes. He also has a history of chest pain and a prior history of coronary artery disease.

TECHNIQUE: A 6 Fr sheath was inserted into the right femoral artery utilizing the Seldinger technique. The aortic root was injected utilizing a 6 Fr 155 Pigtail catheter. Coronary angioplasty was performed, and the equipment utilized is described in the intervention summary section. 10,000 units of heparin were administered. Intracoronary nitroglycerin was given during this case. 170 cc of nonionic contrast were administered.

HEMODYNAMICS
Left Heart Pressures
Resting:

	Systolic	Diastolic	EDP	a	v	m
Ao	96	56				74

Aortography
Normal

Aortic Regurgitation
None

Comments
There were three aortic cusps.
Unable to visualize a SVG to diagonal.

Coronary Angiography
Dominance: Right

Left Main
This vessel was not injected.

Left Anterior Descending
This vessel was not injected.

Left Circumflex
This vessel was not injected.

Right Coronary Artery
This vessel was not injected. There was a 99% long segmental stenosis of the midsegment of the right posterior descending branch (RPDA) of the right coronary artery (RCA) at the anastomosis site of the bypass graft. The RPDA was small. Distal flow was decreased.

Indication for Intervention
Coronary intervention was indicated for treatment of a critical lesion in an asymptomatic patient status post a myocardial infarction.

Intervention Summary
Right Posterior Descending Branch of the RCA
   Mid 99%

      Angioplasty was performed on the 99% stenosis in the midsegment of the RPDA at anastomosis site of bypass graft. According to the ACC/AHA classification system, this lesion was a type B2 lesion.

      Angioplasty was accomplished through a 6 Fr RCB guide utilizing a Maverick® 15-mm balloon with a maximum size of 2.0 mm and a maximum inflation pressure of 10 atmospheres.

      The final outcome was defined as successful. There was no residual stenosis following this intervention. Distal flow was normal.

      The SVG to RPDA was engaged with RCB guide. It is widely patent. Unable to cross with luge or whisper wire. The Cross It wire was then successfully advanced to the distal RPDA.

CONCLUSIONS
No evidence of aortic regurgitation
Successful angioplasty of the mid-RPDA lesion

COMPLICATIONS/EVENTS: The patient had no complications during these procedures.

Questions for Further Review: Case Study 6.9

1. Does the patient have a congenital cardiac anomaly?
    a. Yes
    b. No

2. What side(s) of the heart was catheterized?
    a. Left side
    b. Right side
    c. Right and left sides
    d. Not done

3. Was angiography performed?
    a. Yes
    b. No

    If yes, on which site(s)?
    a. Pulmonary
    b. Right ventricular
    c. Right atrial
    d. Left ventricular
    e. Left atrial
    f. Selective coronary (injection of radiopaque material may be by hand)
    g. Aortic root
    h. All sites listed above

4. Was selective visualization/opacification of bypass graft(s) performed?
    a. Yes
    b. No

    If yes, on which site(s)?
    a. Arterial conduits (for example, internal mammary)
    b. Aortocoronary venous bypass grafts

5. Which additional code(s) should be assigned to classify the imaging supervision, interpretation, and report for the injection procedure(s) performed during the cardiac catheterization?
    a. 93555
    b. 93556
    c. 93555 and 93556

6. What type of angioplasty was performed?
    a. Percutaneous transluminal pulmonary artery balloon angioplasty
    b. Open transluminal balloon angioplasty, aortic
    c. Open transluminal balloon angioplasty, venous
    d. Percutaneous transluminal coronary balloon angioplasty
    e. Percutaneous transluminal balloon angioplasty, aortic
    f. Percutaneous transluminal balloon angioplasty, venous

7. On how many vessels was the angioplasty performed?
    a. One vessel
    b. Two vessels

8. CPT surgery code(s) and modifier(s):

Case Study 6.10

Read the following clinical document and answer the questions for further review.

OPERATIVE REPORT

PREOPERATIVE DIAGNOSIS: Left supraclavicular deep cervical node

POSTOPERATIVE DIAGNOSIS: Left supraclavicular deep cervical node

PROCEDURE: Incisional biopsy under intravenous analgesia

WHAT WAS FOUND: The patient was found to have a deep cervical chain lymph node on the left side of the neck that was clinically suspicious for malignancy. The patient has a history of left breast cancer.

WHAT WAS DONE: With the patient in the supine position and under IV analgesia of Versed and Demerol, 1% Xylocaine with epinephrine was infiltrated into the area in the supraclavicular fossa. Using sharp and blunt dissection, the node was identified lying beneath the sternocleidomastoid muscle. No attempt was made to do a complete dissection in this area. The node was retracted by placing a 2-0 chromic stitch through it and brought into the field. Using sharp and blunt dissection, the node was divided and bleeding controlled with the cautery unit. The wound was reapproximated by using 2-0 chromic to reapproximate the muscular layers and subcuticular 4-0 Vicryl for skin. The patient tolerated this well and was discharged to recovery in satisfactory condition.

SURGICAL PATHOLOGY REPORT

AGE/SEX: 45/F
STATUS: REG CLI
SP TYPE: SURGICAL P

Left supraclavicular lymph node: Metastatic poorly differentiated adenocarcinoma with focal mucin production

Left lymph node

Supraclavicular node, left
Excision of left supraclavicular node

The specimen is received in formalin, labeled "left lymph node" and consists of a fragment of irregularly shaped, beige-to-yellow, lobulated tissue measuring 2 x 1.5 x 1 cm. Sectioning through the specimen reveals a granular beige-to-yellow cut surface. The specimen is submitted in its entirety in Cassettes A-1 and A-2.

Questions for Further Review: Case Study 6.10

1. What procedure was performed?
   a. Needle biopsy
   b. Excisional biopsy—superficial
   c. Excisional biopsy—deep

2. On which lymph node(s) was the procedure performed?

3. CPT surgery code(s) and modifier(s):

Case Study 6.11

Read the following clinical document and answer the questions for further review.

OPERATIVE REPORT

PREOPERATIVE DIAGNOSIS: Chronic renal failure

POSTOPERATIVE DIAGNOSIS: Chronic renal failure

OPERATION: Left radial artery cephalic vein primary arteriovenous fistula

ANESTHESIA: Local with intravenous sedation

INDICATIONS: This is a 66-year-old woman who was very recently started on hemodialysis and at this time has chronic hemodialysis catheter in the right jugular vein. She was brought to the operating room today to create a peripheral access. Her preoperative evaluation revealed that the cephalic vein on the right side, which was her nondominant side, was discontinuous, and I felt that it would be less likely to succeed as an A-V fistula. On the left side, she had a very nice cephalic vein, which had two side branches that eventually we ligated.

PROCEDURE/FINDINGS: The patient was sedated and place in the supine position. The left upper extremity was prepped with DuraPrep solution and appropriate drapes were applied. Local anesthesia was instilled.

A vertical incision was made overlying the distal left radial artery just above the wrist. The radial artery was dissected free and controlled with vessel loops. We then dissected subcutaneously and dissected the cephalic vein free for a length of about 2 cm. It was followed distally and ligated with 5-0 Vicryl and divided. It was cannulated. A Fogarty catheter was passed up the vein without any difficulty. As it was withdrawn, the vein was just mildly dilated. After that, an end-to-side anastomosis was created suturing the end of the vein to the side of the distal left radial artery, which did have some mild diabetic-related vascular disease. Finally, after the anastomosis was completed with 6-0 Prolene suture, the tourniquets were released from the vessels, and there was a good pulse and thrill in the newly created fistula. The side branches were then ligated through two small incisions, and 9-0 Vicryl ties were used for that purpose.

At the conclusion of the operation, she had a strong pulse in the fistula going well up almost to the antecubital area. The wound was closed with 3-0 Vicryl and staples. Dry sterile dressings were applied. The patient was taken to the recovery area in fair general condition.

Questions for Further Review: Case Study 6.11

1. What type of arteriovenous fistula was surgically created?
   a. Open arteriovenous anastomosis by upper basilic vein transposition
   b. Open arteriovenous anastomosis direct from an artery to a vein
   c. Creation of arteriovenous fistula by autogenous graft
   d. Creation of arteriovenous fistula by nonautogenous graft

2. CPT surgery code(s) and modifier(s):

Case Study 6.12

Read the following clinical document and answer the questions for further review.

OPERATIVE REPORT

PREOPERATIVE DIAGNOSIS: 56-year-old male with end-stage renal disease

POSTOPERATIVE DIAGNOSIS: End-stage renal disease

PROCEDURE PERFORMED: Right arm arteriovenous graft

ANESTHESIA: Intravenous sedation with local

Fluids: 500 cc

ESTIMATED BLOOD LOSS: Minimal

SPECIMENS: None

DESCRIPTION OF PROCEDURE: Patient came to the operating room and was placed on the operating table. After IV was placed and patient was given IV sedation, the right arm from the axilla down to the wrist was prepped and draped in the standard surgical fashion. Attention was turned to the veins in the forearm. Dissection was made at the patient's antecubital fossa, at which time the brachial artery was located. The cephalic vein was also located, and another incision was made 2 cm proximal to the patient's wrist. When these vessels were isolated, a tunnel was placed in the subcutaneous tissue from the antecubital fossa to the wrist in a circular fashion. At this point, the PTFE graft was brought on to the table. Approximately 6 mm diameter of PTFE graft was used. The graft was sutured into the vein, and then the graft was brought through the subcutaneous tunnel ensuring that there was enough skin to cover the distal portion of the graft as it made its turn in the subcutaneous tissue. The graft was then sutured to the artery. Upon release of the vessel clamp, a bruit was appreciated, and a thrill was felt in the graft. Patient tolerated the procedure well.

DISPOSITION: To the PACU and then to be discharged home in stable condition

---

Questions for Further Review: Case Study 6.12

1. What type of arteriovenous fistula was surgically created?
   a. Open arteriovenous anastomosis by upper basilic vein transposition
   b. Open arteriovenous anastomosis direct from an artery to a vein
   c. Creation of arteriovenous fistula by autogenous graft
   d. Creation of arteriovenous fistula by nonautogenous graft

2. CPT surgery code(s) and modifier(s):

Case Study 6.13

Read the following clinical document and answer the questions for further review.

OPERATIVE REPORT

OPERATION: Thrombectomy and revision of left brachial artery to axillary vein PTFE arteriovenous fistula

ANESTHESIA: Local, 1% Xylocaine plus sedation

PREOPERATIVE DIAGNOSIS: Chronic renal failure secondary to polycystic kidney disease

POSTOPERATIVE DIAGNOSIS: Chronic renal failure secondary to polycystic kidney disease

OPERATIVE INDICATIONS: The patient is a 58-year-old female with chronic renal insufficiency supported on hemodialysis. She previously had a functioning left brachial artery to axillary vein PTFE fistula. This fistula clotted approximately three weeks prior to this procedure. She is brought to the operating room at this time for an attempt at thrombectomy and revision of her fistula.

OPERATIVE PROCEDURE: The patient was brought to the operating room and placed in the supine position, and the left arm was prepped and draped in the usual manner. The scar at the axillary area was infiltrated with 1% Xylocaine. A longitudinal incision was made in the prior scar. Dissection was carried through the soft tissue to identify PTFE graft. The graft was dissected free from surrounding soft tissue down to its anastomosis to the axillary vein. Dissection was carried more proximally along the axillary vein about 3 cm more proximal to the prior anastomosis. The vein was mobilized circumferentially over a distance of about 3 cm. The patient was then heparinized systemically with 3,000 units of heparin. The PTFE graft was divided just proximal to the venous anastomosis. The end of the graft attached to the vein was oversewn with a 5-0 Prolene suture. A #3 Fogarty catheter was then passed into the PTFE graft distally. The graft contained mostly liquid thrombus. An occluding thrombus at the arterial anastomosis was left undisturbed for the time being. A segment of tapered 4 to 7 mm PTFE graft, 15 cm in length, was obtained. The axillary vein was controlled with a vessel loop distally and a baby renal clamp proximally. A linear venotomy was made. The axillary vein was found to contain a well-organized thrombus. This thrombus was removed using an endarterectomy dissector and a #3 Fogarty catheter. The thrombus was about 4 cm in length and easily removed. There was good antegrade and retrograde bleeding from the axillary vein.

The Fogarty catheter would not pass beyond about 20 cm; however, there may be a more central obstruction to the subclavian vein, but it was elected to proceed with construction of a new venous anastomosis. The 7-mm segment of the PTFE graft was cut on a bevel and an end-to-side anastomosis was constructed between the PTFE and the axillary vein using running suture of 6-0 Prolene. When this anastomosis was completed, the graft was measured to the appropriate length to reach the old PTFE graft. Both of these grafts were cut transversely. An end-to-end, graft-to-graft anastomosis was then constructed using a running suture of 6-0 Prolene. The graft-to-graft anastomosis was left open and a #4 Fogarty was used to dislodge the occluding thrombus at the arterial anastomosis. This short thrombus came out intact with the meniscus present. The graft had good inflow. The graft-to-graft anastomosis was completed and blood flow was established through the fistula. There was a soft thrill present over the fistula. Heparin was not reversed. The axillary incision was closed in two layers with interrupted simple sutures of 3-0 Vicryl in the subcutaneous tissue and a running subcuticular suture of 4-0

Monocryl in the skin. A few tape closures were applied. The procedure was completed and an occlusive dressing was applied. The patient was returned to the outpatient area in stable condition.

ESTIMATED BLOOD LOSS: 20 cc

BLOOD REPLACEMENT: None

DRAINS: None

PATHOLOGY REPORT

FINAL DIAGNOSIS: Fistula contents: left brachial excision, blood clot

SPECIMEN(S) SUBMITTED: Fistula contents, left brachial

CLINICAL DATA: ESRD secondary PCKD

GROSS DESCRIPTION: Received fresh is a red-brown tubular-shaped segment of soft tissue measuring 7.0 x 0.6 x 0.5 cm. The specimen was sectioned to reveal a laminated cut surface. Representative sections are submitted in one cassette.

Questions for Further Review: Case Study 6.13

1. What type of arteriovenous (AV) fistula did this patient have at the beginning of this procedure?
   a. Congenital fistula
   b. Traumatic fistula
   c. Surgically created fistula

2. What type of procedure was performed?
   a. Percutaneous thrombectomy
   b. Open thrombectomy
   c. Open revision of AV fistula with thrombectomy
   d. Open revision of AV fistula without thrombectomy

3. What devices were used to perform this procedure?
   a. Endarterectomy dissector
   b. Foley catheter
   c. Fogarty catheter
   d. Balloon catheter

4. CPT surgery code(s) and modifier(s):

Case Study 6.14

Read the following clinical document and answer the questions for further review.

OPERATIVE REPORT

PREOPERATIVE DIAGNOSIS: Thrombosed AV fistula

POSTOPERATIVE DIAGNOSIS: Same

OPERATION(S): Lysis and balloon angioplasty of AV fistula

DESCRIPTION OF OPERATION: This patient has chronic renal failure and had a new fistula placed in the right arm approximately a month ago. It is now clotted. The patient was brought to the angio suite, where she was placed in the supine position. The patient was then monitored with an EKG monitor and blood pressure device. Following this, the right arm was prepped with Betadine and draped aseptically. Utilizing a Seldinger technique, the graft was entered, placing a sheath facing the arterial and the venous anastomosis. This was done with fluoroscopic guidance. Following this, the patient received 250,000 units of urokinase and 5,000 units of heparin divided equally into each sheath. We could not get a good pulse. Therefore, a percutaneous embolectomy was performed successfully. An excellent pulse was felt. Following this, a fistulogram was performed, which demonstrated stenosis in the area of the venous anastomosis with a good subclavian vein. This was then dilated utilizing a 6-mm balloon catheter. Following balloon dilatation, an excellent thrill was palpated throughout the fistula and a good radial pulse palpated distally. Subsequent fistulogram demonstrated successful dilatation of the region of stenosis; however, there was an area of residual stenosis. At this time, we elected to stop the procedure and remove the catheter. Because of the residual stenosis, the patient will be brought back for a fistulogram in about a month. The patient was then transferred to the floor with an excellent thrill in her graft.

Questions for Further Review: Case Study 6.14

1. What type of arteriovenous (AV) fistula did this patient have at the beginning of this procedure?
   a. Congenital fistula
   b. Traumatic fistula
   c. Surgically created fistula

2. What types of procedures were performed?
   a. Percutaneous thrombectomy
   b. Open thrombectomy
   c. Open revision of AV fistula with thrombectomy
   d. Open revision of AV fistula without thrombectomy
   e. Percutaneous transluminal balloon venous angioplasty

3. How many times was an AV fistulogram performed?

4. CPT surgery code(s) and modifier(s):

Exhibit 6.1. Coding resource: CPT VAD coding

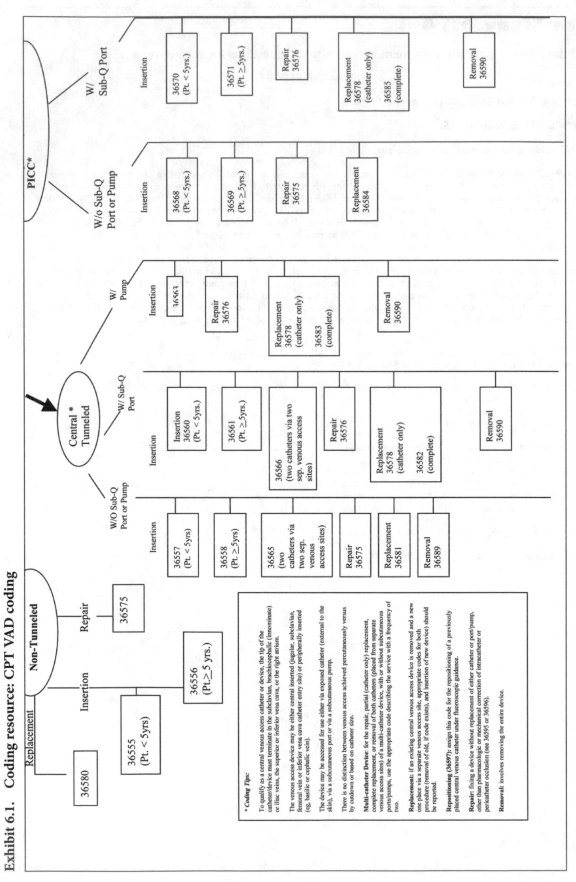

Chapter 7

Digestive System

CPT codes 40490 through 49999 are used to report surgical and related procedures performed on the digestive system, which includes the mouth and associated structures, esophagus, stomach, intestines, rectum, anus, liver, and pancreas. Common outpatient procedures involving the digestive system include gastrointestinal endoscopies, echoendoscopies, capsule enteroscopies, esophageal dilation, hernia repair, treatment and repair of anal fistulas, and hemorrhoid surgery.

Gastrointestinal Endoscopies

An endoscopy is the examination of a body tube or cavity with a lighted instrument specifically designed for that purpose. The instrument may be a rigid metal tube or a flexible fiberoptic endoscope.

Endoscopic techniques and procedures commonly performed on the digestive system include the following:

- Esophagoscopy is limited to study of the esophagus.

- In an esophagogastroduodenoscopy (EGD), the endoscope traverses the pyloric channel.

- Proctosigmoidoscopy is the examination of the rectum and the sigmoid colon.

- Sigmoidoscopy involves examining the entire rectum and the sigmoid colon and may include examining a portion of the descending colon.

- In a colonoscopy, the entire colon, from the rectum to the sigmoid colon, descending colon, transverse colon, ascending colon, and cecum, is examined. The examination must include the proximal colon to the splenic flexure, and it may include the terminal ileum.

- The hot-biopsy forceps technique uses an electrical current that simultaneously excises and fulgurates polyps, avoids the bleeding associated with cold-forceps biopsy, and preserves the specimen for histological examination.

- A cold biopsy is similar to a hot biopsy except that the forceps are not hooked up to a fulgurator, and a cold biopsy is used for smaller specimens.

- Ablation involves the elimination or hemorrhage control of a tumor or mucosal lesion, usually sessile polyps that are smooth and located on the wall of the intestine.

- Snare technique involves placing an electrical conducting pad on the patient's buttock. A loop is slipped out of a long, thin plastic tube and over the lesion, and the snare is closed down onto the lesion. Electrical current is then used to coagulate and cut the lesion.

- Bipolar cautery is electrosurgery using a pair of electrodes. Tissue between them is coagulated by flow of current from one to the other. Bipolar current, unlike hot biopsy forceps, does not require a grounding plate; a current simply runs from one portion of the tip of the device to another. Examples include the bipolar electrocautery capsule (BICAP) and the BiLAP bipolar probe. The latter is a bipolar unit with cutting and coagulation functions.

Coding Guidelines for Gastrointestinal Endoscopies

When multiple techniques are used on different lesions or polyps, the procedure report should specifically describe the technique, the type of lesion, and the location of the lesion. The CPT code descriptors for each specific technique include language to indicate that each code should be reported only once, even when multiple sites are treated with the same technique. When different techniques are used on separate sites, the code with the highest value should be listed first on the claim. Other codes should be listed with distinct procedural service modifier –59 to identify that the service was performed at a separate site (AMA 2004a).

Snare devices also may be used without electrocautery to "decapitate" small polyps. Most often, the colonoscopy report will specify that a snare technique was used. The report also may include the phrase "hot snare," "monopolar snare," "cold snare," or "bipolar snare," all of which should be reported using a code for endoscopy with snare technique removal.

Example: Code 45385, Colonoscopy with removal of tumor, polyp, or other lesion by snare technique.

APC	HCPCS	HCPCS Description	SI	Rel. Wt.	Payment Rate	OPPS OCE
0143			T	8.8486	563.60	
	45385	Lesion removal colonscopy				Significant Procedure, Multiple Reduction Applies; Separate APC payment

The ablation of the tissue (tumor, polyp, or other lesion) can be performed with many different types of devices (heater probe, bipolar cautery probe, argon laser, and so on) regardless of whether a sample was obtained with a biopsy forceps before the ablative device is applied.

In unusual cases, the procedure report may indicate that a polyp was injected with saline or "lifted" prior to removal by another technique. In other cases, injection will be performed to "tattoo" an area with India ink for later identification during a subsequent procedure or during surgery. In both cases, a code for endoscopy with submucosal injection should be reported as an additional service to any other therapeutic procedure.

Reports also may describe injection in conjunction with attempts to control spontaneous bleeding resulting from causes including diverticulosis, angiodysplasia, or prior-session interventions. This procedure is then correctly reported with a code for endoscopy with control of bleeding, rather than a code for endoscopy with submucosal injection.

Bleeding that starts as a result of a therapeutic intervention, such as snare removal or biopsy, and is controlled by any method is considered part of the initial therapeutic procedure and should not be reported separately with codes for endoscopy with control of bleeding or endoscopy with submucosal injection.

The term "biopsy, single or multiple" found in endoscopy codes such as 45380, Colonoscopy with biopsy, single or multiple, is accepted and understood by colonoscopists to mean the use of a forceps to grasp and remove a small piece of tissue without the application of cautery. Colonoscopy reports may describe the biopsy of a lesion or polyp using a cold forceps or may describe the biopsy without mentioning the specific device. The biopsy may be from an obvious lesion that is too large to remove, from a suspicious area of abnormal mucosa, or from a lesion or polyp so small that it can be removed completely during the performance of the biopsy, which is often demonstrated with the cold-biopsy forceps technique. The technique is the same, and the service is reported with code 45380 regardless of the final histology of the piece of tissue removed. Code 45385 should not be used for a report describing the removal of a small polyp by biopsy or cold forceps technique. Code 45385 should be used for removal of tumors or polyps, or other lesions by snare technique.

CMS Rules for Reporting Endoscopic Biopsy

According to the AMA and the official coding guidelines for CPT, when a lesion is biopsied and subsequently removed during the same operative session, only the code for the removal of the lesion is reported. However, when one lesion is biopsied and a separate lesion is removed during the same operative session, a code for the biopsy of one lesion and an additional code for the removal of the separate lesion should be reported with modifier –59 appended to the code reported for the biopsy procedure (AMA 1999e, 11).

The CMS has developed more specific rules for reporting endoscopic biopsies for Medicare outpatients. It is important to note that the term **excision**, as used in these rules, includes the variety of terms in the CPT manual that describe the excision or destruction of a lesion (for example, resection, removal, or fulguration). The CMS reporting rules for Medicare reimbursement are as follows (CMS 1999):

1. When a single lesion is biopsied, but not excised, use only the biopsy code.

   Example: A colonoscopy with biopsy of a sigmoid colon polyp is performed. The remaining portion of the polyp is not excised. This situation would require CPT code 45380 for a colonoscopy with biopsy.

2. When a biopsy of a lesion is obtained and the remaining portion of the same lesion is then excised, code only for the excision.

   Example: A colonoscopy with biopsy and cauterization of a sigmoid colon polyp is performed. CPT code 45383 for a colonoscopy with ablation of polyp is reported.

3. When multiple biopsies are obtained (from the same or different lesions) and none of the lesions are excised, use only the biopsy code and list it once.

   Example: A colonoscopy with two biopsies of a single sigmoid colon polyp is performed. CPT code 45380 for a colonoscopy with single or multiple biopsy is assigned.

   Example: A colonoscopy with biopsy of a sigmoid colon polyp and biopsy of a transverse colon polyp is performed. CPT code 45380 for a colonoscopy with single or multiple biopsy is reported.

4. When a biopsy and an excision are performed, use both codes when the biopsy is taken from a different lesion than that which is excised and the code for the excision does not include the phrase "with or without biopsy." If such a phrase is included, do not use a separate biopsy code.

> **Example:** A colonoscopy with biopsy of a sigmoid colon polyp and snare removal of a transverse colon polyp is performed. This situation would require CPT code 45380 for a colonoscopy with single or multiple biopsy and CPT code 45385 for a colonoscopy with snare removal of polyp.

Echoendoscopies

As mentioned previously, an endoscopy involves examination of the interior of a canal or hollow viscus by means of a special instrument. The rigid metal tube has a fiberoptic light source attached to it for illuminating the tissues during examination.

Ultrasound is a diagnostic imaging technique that uses high-frequency sound waves and a computer to create images of blood vessels, tissues, and organs. Ultrasounds are used to view internal organs as they function and to assess bloodflow through various vessels.

Echoendoscopy, or endoscopic ultrasonography, combines endoscopy with ultrasound to permit high-resolution imaging of the gastrointestinal system.

Coding Guidelines for Echoendoscopies

Code selection for procedures using endoscopic ultrasonography is based on the following guidelines:

- Codes 43231, 43237, 43259, and 45341 are used for endoscopic ultrasound examination.
- Codes 43232, 43238, 43242, and 45342 are used for transendoscopic ultrasound-guided intramural or transmural fine needle aspiration and/or biopsies.
- Code 43241 is used for transendoscopic intraluminal tube or catheter placement.
- Codes 43256, 45327, 45345, and 45387 are used for transendoscopic stent placement.

APC	HCPCS	HCPCS Description	SI	Rel. Wt.	Payment Rate	OPPS OCE
0141			T	8.5030	541.59	
	43241	Upper GI endoscopy with tube				Significant Procedure, Multiple Reduction Applies; Separate APC payment

Capsule Enteroscopies

Capsule enteroscopy is a noninvasive, painless, diagnostic procedure that yields color video images of the small intestine to assist the physician in identifying and treating gastrointestinal disorders.

M2A (mouth-to-anus) capsule endoscopy, approved by the Food and Drug Administration in August 2001, has been heralded as a revolution in endoscopic imaging of the small intestine. Traditional endoscopic procedures are invasive. None of them, except for surgical placement of the endoscope (intraoperative enteroscopy), are as good as M2A has proved to be at providing physicians with diagnostic information.

In this procedure, the patient swallows a capsule that is about the size of a large vitamin pill and contains a color camera, battery, light source, and transmitter. The camera takes two pictures every second for eight hours, transmitting images to a recording device about the size of a portable CD player that the patient wears around the waist.

The camera moves naturally through the digestive tract while the patient goes about his or her normal activities. About eight hours after ingesting the camera, the patient returns the recording device to the doctor so the images can be downloaded to a computer and evaluated. The camera is naturally excreted and not retrieved.

Coding Guidelines for Capsule Enteroscopies

Following are coding guidelines for capsule enteroscopies:

- Code 91110 is assigned for a capsule endoscopy that includes the esophagus through the ileum. Code 91111 is assigned for a capsule endoscopy with esophagus only (AMA 2008).

- Modifier 52–Reduced services would be assigned when a capsule endoscopy is performed and extends past the esophagus, however does not proceed to the ileum. Code 91110–52 would be reported.

- Visualization of the colon is not reported separately with an additional CPT code.

Esophageal Dilation

Dilation involves the stretching or enlarging of an opening, or lumen, of a hollow structure. Balloon dilation of the esophagus is a procedure performed to treat anatomical or functional narrowing (stricture) of the esophagus caused by a variety of conditions. A balloon catheter is inserted at the narrowed area of the esophagus and inflated for dilation under direct endoscopic observation. In endoscopic balloon dilation, the endoscope remains in place as the balloon-tipped catheter is passed through the scope's instrument channel. Through-the-scope (TTS) balloon dilators are utilized during endoscopic balloon dilation.

Endoscopic guide wire dilation is a procedure in which a small wire is passed endoscopically through the stenotic area of the esophagus to guide a dilating device. The endoscope is first passed down the patient's esophagus. Then a flexible-tipped guide wire is passed though the endoscope into the stomach, after which the endoscope is withdrawn, leaving the guide wire in place. A series of dilators, called bougies or sounds, each with a small central lumen created to accommodate the guide wire, is then passed over the guide wire. After the largest desired dilator has been used, the guide wire and the dilators are removed.

Bougies are metal or rubber devices with two compartments: a soft, tapered tip that is inserted into an orifice or organ cavity to facilitate passage into the stricture; and a reservoir containing a weighted substance (usually mercury) that pulls the bougie through the narrowed area.

Guided bougies (for example, Savary or American) involve the use of a guide wire, whereas unguided bougies, or sounds, advance through the patient's esophagus without a guide wire. The unguided bougie is generally used to calibrate an orifice in the gastrointestinal tract and may or may not be placed with endoscopic guidance. Hurst and Maloney bougies are two examples of unguided bougies that use neither guide wire nor endoscopic guidance.

Coding Guidelines for Esophageal Dilation

Surgical endoscopy always includes diagnostic endoscopy. It is appropriate to report two separate codes for endoscopy with dilation. For example:

- Code 43200, Esophagoscopy, rigid or flexible; diagnostic, with or without collection of specimen(s) by brushing or washing (separate procedure).

- Code 43450, Dilation of esophagus, by unguided sound or bougie, single or multiple passes

Code 43450 does not include the endoscopy. Therefore, code 43200 can be reported along with the dilation procedure. The −59 modifier should be appended to code 43200 to denote that a separately distinct procedure has been performed (AMA 2001j).

APC	HCPCS	HCPCS Description	SI	Rel. Wt.	Payment Rate	OPPS OCE
0140			T	5.8431	372.17	
	43450	Dilate esophagus				Significant Procedure, Multiple Reduction Applies; Separate APC payment

Gastroenterologic tests included in CPT codes 91000–91299 are frequently complementary to endoscopic procedures. Esophageal and gastric washings for cytology are described as part of an upper endoscopy (CPT code 43235) and, therefore, CPT codes 91000 (esophageal intubation) and 91055 (gastric intubation) should not be separately reported when performed as part of an upper endoscopic procedure. Provocative testing (CPT code 91052) can be expedited during gastrointestinal endoscopy (procurement of gastric specimens); when performed at the same time as GI endoscopy, CPT code 91052 should be coded with modifier −52 indicating a reduced level of service was performed (NCCI April 2007).

Hernia Repair

A hernia is a protrusion of a part or structure through the tissues that contain it. CPT hernia repair codes are categorized primarily by the type of hernia (inguinal, femoral, incisional, and so on). Some types of hernia are further categorized as "initial" or "recurrent," based on whether the hernia has required previous repair. Additional variables accounted for by some of the codes include patient age and clinical presentation (reducible versus incarcerated or strangulated).

CPT codes for recurrent hernia repairs are not assigned for hernias that have only been treated in the past using "manual reduction." According to the AMA, the recurrent hernia repair codes should only be assigned for hernias that were surgically treated in the past.

If a hernia repair is performed at the site of an incision for an open abdominal procedure, the hernia repair is not separately reportable. The hernia repair is separately reportable if it is performed at a site other than the incision and is medically reasonable and necessary. An incidental hernia repair is not medically reasonable and necessary and should not be reported separately.

When a recurrent hernia requires repair, the appropriate recurrent hernia repair code is reported. A code for incisional hernia repair is not to be reported in addition to the recurrent hernia repair unless a medically necessary incisional hernia repair is performed at a different site. In this case, modifier −59 should be attached to the incisional hernia repair code (NCCI April 2007).

Coding Guidelines for Hernia Repair

Codes 49491–49521, Repair of inguinal hernia, are based on age of the patient and whether the procedure was reducible or incarcerated/strangulated. A hernia can often be pushed gently back into place. This is called a reducible hernia. When a hernia cannot be pushed back into place, it means a piece of the intestine has become trapped, or incarcerated, in the inguinal canal. Symptoms include pain, nausea, vomiting, inability to have a bowel movement, and a bulge that remains even when lying down. When a portion of the intestine is incarcerated, its blood supply can be cut off, which means the intestinal tissue will die. This condition is called a strangulated hernia. Inguinal hernias usually increase in size with time and can occur on both sides of the body.

Code 49525, Repair inguinal hernia, sliding, is a form of an inguinal hernia in which a retroperitoneal structure "slides" down the posterior abdominal wall and herniates directly or indirectly into the inguinal canal, dragging overlying peritoneum with it. Thus, sliding hernias lie behind and outside the peritoneal sac.

Incisional hernias are caused by thinning or stretching of scar tissue that forms after surgery. This weakened scar tissue then creates a weakness in the abdominal wall. Excessive weight gain, physical activity that places pressure on the abdomen, pregnancy, straining during bowel movements because of constipation, severe vomiting, or chronic and intense coughing causes the scar tissue to thin or stretch. Because the abdominal wall is weak, the hernia occurs during abdominal strain.

The following codes are used for incisional hernia repairs:

- 49560   Repair initial incisional or ventral hernia; reducible

- 49561   Repair initial incisional or ventral hernia; incarcerated or strangulated require surgical intervention.

- 49565   (Reducible) and 49566 (incarcerated or strangulated) should be used for recurrent incisional or ventral hernia.

APC	HCPCS	HCPCS Description	SI	Rel. Wt.	Payment Rate	OPPS OCE
0154			T	30.6788	1954.06	
	49560	Repair ventral hernia initial, reducible				Significant Procedure, Multiple Reduction Applies; Separate APC payment
	49561	Repair ventral hernia initial, block				Significant Procedure, Multiple Reduction Applies; Separate APC payment

Surgical Laparoscopy

Surgical laparoscopy always includes diagnostic laparoscopy. To report a diagnostic laparoscopy, use code 49320.

Use codes 49650–49569 for laparoscopic repair of incisional or ventral hernias. Code 49659 is for an unlisted laparoscopy procedure, such as hernioplasty, herniorrhaphy, or herniotomy.

Mesh and other Prosthesis

Code 49568, Implantation of mesh or other prosthesis for incisional or ventral hernia repair, should be assigned separately in addition to codes 49560, 49561, 49565, and 49566 when mesh is used for incisional or ventral hernia repair.

CPT code 49568 should not be reported with these other hernia repair codes. If an incisional or ventral hernia repair with mesh/prosthesis implantation is performed, as well as another type of hernia repair at the same patient encounter, CPT code 49568 may be reported with modifier –59 to bypass edits bundling CPT code 49568 into all hernia repair codes other than the incisional or ventral hernia repair codes.

All codes for bilateral procedures in hernia repair have been deleted from the CPT coding system. For Medicare hospital outpatient reporting, the bilateral procedure –50 must be appended to the appropriate hernia code to indicate that it was performed bilaterally.

Anal Fistulas

An anal fistula is an abnormal passage leading from the anal canal to the skin around or near the anus. Surgical treatment is usually required for drainage and to prevent recurrent infections.

Coding Guidelines for Anal Fistulas

The following codes are used to classify anal fistula procedures:

- Codes 46270 and 46275 are used for surgical treatment (fistulectomy/fistulotomy) of anal fistula.
- Code 46280 is used for complex or multiple surgical treatment (fistulectomy/fistulotomy) with or without placement of anal seton. Code 46020 (placement of seton) should not be reported in addition to code 46280.
- Code 46030 is used for removal of anal seton, other marker.
- Code 46285 is used for second-stage treatment.
- Code 46288 is used for closure of anal fistula with rectal advancement flap.
- Code 46706 is used for repair with fibrin glue.
- Code 46604 is used for endoscopy anal dilation.
- Code 45905 is used for dilation of anal sphincter.

APC	HCPCS	HCPCS Description	SI	Rel. Wt.	Payment Rate	OPPS OCE
0147			T	8.7031	554.34	
	49560	Anoscopy and dilation				Significant Procedure, Multiple Reduction Applies; Separate APC payment

Hemorrhoid Surgery

Hemorrhoids are dilated veins that supply the anal and rectal regions of the body. When these dilated veins become inflamed and enlarged, they can cause painful swelling, itching, and bleeding. The surgical procedure to remove enlarged veins around the anus is called a hemorrhoidectomy.

Coding Guidelines for Hemorrhoid Surgery

The following codes are used to report hemorrhoid surgery:

- Codes 46255–46258 classify a simple hemorrhoidectomy.

- Codes 46260–46262 classify a complex or extensive hemorrhoidectomy, generally indicated when three or more columns of hemorrhoids are present, representing extensive disease and requiring an extensive operation for removal. For example, when the documentation in the health record states three- or four-column hemorrhoidectomy with subsequent closure to avoid stenosis and leakage, these procedures should be reported with codes 46260–46262 (complex or extensive), as appropriate.

- Code 46947 classifies hemorrhoidopexy. This procedure is also known as the prolapse and hemorrhoids (PPH) procedure, stapled hemorrhoidectomy, stapled hemorrhoidopexy, and circumferential mucosectomy.

- PPH is a technique developed in the early 1990s that reduces the prolapse of hemorrhoidal tissue by excising a band of the prolapsed anal mucosa membrane with the use of a circular stapling device. In PPH, the prolapsed tissue is pulled into a device that allows the excess tissue to be removed while the remaining hemorrhoidal tissue is stapled. This restores the hemorrhoidal tissue back to its original anatomical position.

Documentation Requirements for Digestive Procedures

Each procedure is followed by clinical information that must be documented in the medical record when the procedure is performed.

Gastroenterology Endoscopy

Gastroenterology endoscopy is reported with CPT codes 43200–43259, 44360–44397, 45300–45392, 46600–46615.

1. *Each* anatomical site examined with the endoscope, for example:

   - Esophagus
   - Stomach
   - Descending colon
   - Transverse colon
   - Small intestine

2. Whether an endoscopic ultrasound examination was performed. If so, each anatomical site is examined with the echoendoscope.

3. Whether a transendoscopic device was placed:

- Catheter placement
- Intraluminal tube placement
- Stent placement (including predilation)

4. The type of surgical procedure performed on *each* lesion (for example, polyp, tumor, cyst) present:

- Biopsy of specimen
- Bipolar cautery removal
- Snare technique removal
- Hot-biopsy removal
- Destruction/ablation/fulguration
- Submucosal injection (for example, India ink, saline, corticosteroids, Botox)

5. The type of instrument/approach used on *each* lesion (if applicable).

- Cold-biopsy forceps
- Hot-biopsy forceps
- Transendoscopic ultrasound-guided intramural fine needle aspiration/biopsy(s)
- Transendoscopic ultrasound-guided transmural fine needle aspiration/biopsy(s)

Esophageal Dilation

Esophageal dilation is reported with CPT codes 43220, 43226, 43248, 43249, and 43450–43458.

1. Whether the patient has a current diagnosis of achalasia
2. Whether an endoscopy was performed
3. Each anatomical site examined with the endoscopy:

- Esophagus
- Stomach
- Duodenum

4. The method of dilation utilized:

- Balloon (either less than 30 mm in diameter or larger than 30 mm in diameter)
- Insertion of guide wire followed by dilation over guide wire
- Unguided sound
- Bougie
- Retrograde dilators

Hernia Repair

Hernia repair is reported with CPT codes 49491–49590 and 49650–49659.

1. The patient's past history of hernia repair surgery on the left and/or right sides (the documentation should clearly indicate whether the current hernia is initial or recurrent)

2. The patient's age

3. If patient is less than one year old, specify the patient's gestational age at birth.

4. The type of unilateral or bilateral hernia(s) currently being repaired:

   - Inguinal
   - Sliding inguinal
   - Lumbar
   - Femoral
   - Incisional (ventral)
   - Epigastric
   - Umbilical
   - Spigelian

5. The clinical presentation of *each* hernia:

   - Reducible
   - Incarcerated
   - Strangulated

6. The surgical repair method(s) utilized:

   - Open
   - Laparoscopic
   - Mesh application

Hemorrhoidectomy

Hemorrhoidectomy is reported with CPT codes 46083, 46221–46262, 46500, 46934–46936, 46945, and 46946.

1. The type of hemorrhoid(s) present:

   - Tag
   - Internal
   - External
   - Internal and external
   - Prolapsed
   - Thrombotic

2. The location of *each* hemorrhoid plexus, such as the following examples:

   - There were internal hemorrhoids at 1, 2, 3, and 4 o'clock.
   - There were four columns of internal hemorrhoids.
   - Internal hemorrhoids were in all four quadrants.

3. The surgical technique used to repair *each* hemorrhoid:

   - Incision
   - Excision (hemorrhoidectomy)
   - Enucleation
   - Injection of sclerosing agent
   - Destruction (for example, laser, electrocauterization)
   - Simple ligation (for example, rubber band)
   - Ligation (surgical)
   - Fissurectomy
   - Fistulectomy
   - Hemorrhoid stapling/hemorrhoidopexy

Anal Fistula Repair

Anal fistula repair is reported with CPT codes 46020, 46030, 46270, 46275, 46280, 46285, 46288, and 46706.

1. The type of fistula:

   - Single
   - Multiple
   - Complex

2. The level of the fistula:

   - Subcutaneous
   - Submuscular

3. The type of repair:

   - Fistulectomy
   - Fistulotomy
   - Placement of anal seton
   - Instillation of fibrin glue
   - Closure with rectal advancement flap
   - Second-stage repair

Case Studies

Answer all the questions for further review at the end of each case study. Use a current CPT code-book or HCPCS Level II code listing, as needed.

When appropriate, assign one or more of the following modifiers:

–50	Bilateral Procedure
–59	Distinct Procedural Service
–FA	Left hand, thumb
–F1	Left hand, second digit
–F2	Left hand, third digit
–F3	Left hand, fourth digit
–F4	Left hand, fifth digit
–F5	Right hand, thumb
–F6	Right hand, second digit
–F7	Right hand, third digit
–F8	Right hand, fourth digit
–F9	Right hand, fifth digit
–LT	Left side
–RT	Right side
–TA	Left foot, great toe
–T1	Left foot, second digit
–T2	Left foot, third digit
–T3	Left foot, fourth digit
–T4	Left foot, fifth digit
–T5	Right foot, great toe
–T6	Right foot, second digit
–T7	Right foot, third digit
–T8	Right foot, fourth digit
–T9	Right foot, fifth digit

Do not apply the current version of the Medicare CCI edits to any of these exercises; the focus is on the application of the coding guidelines and not on the application of edits that change on a quarterly basis. When coding in real life, of course, you will need to apply the CCI edits as appropriate for Medicare outpatient cases.

Case Study 7.1

Read the following clinical document and answer the questions for further review.

OPERATIVE NOTE

AGE: 80 **DATE:** 11/21/200X

PROCEDURE: Colonoscopy

PREMEDICATIONS: Sublimaze 75 mcg, Versed 1.75 mg IV

INDICATIONS FOR PROCEDURE: Colonic polyp follow-up

PROCEDURE FINDINGS: The colonoscope was passed to the cecum. Multiple diminutive polyps were seen, and three were removed from the transverse colon and one from the ascending colon. Two were removed with snare cautery technique and two were removed with hot-biopsy forceps. The patient tolerated the procedure well. The remainder of the colon was unremarkable without other mass lesions or inflammatory changes. No diverticula encountered.

IMPRESSION: Multiple diminutive colonic polyps (4) submitted to Pathology

DEPARTMENT OF PATHOLOGY
SURGICAL PATHOLOGY RESULT REPORT

CLINICAL HISTORY: Colon polyp, follow-up

OPERATION: Biopsy

GROSS DESCRIPTION: Received in four parts:

Specimen #1: In formalin labeled "biopsy ascending" are two fragments of pink-tan soft tissue, ranging from 0.1 to 0.2 cm in greatest dimension. The specimen is entirely submitted labeled 1A with multiple levels prepared.

Specimen #2: In formalin labeled "transverse polyp #1" is a single, irregular fragment of pink-tan soft tissue measuring 0.3 cm in greatest dimension. The specimen is entirely submitted labeled 2A with multiple levels prepared.

Specimen #3: In formalin labeled "transverse polyp #2" are two fragments of pink-tan soft tissue, ranging from 0.1 to 0.3 cm in greatest dimension. The specimen is entirely submitted labeled 3A with multiple levels prepared.

Specimen #4: In formalin labeled "polyp transverse colon #3" is a single, irregular fragment of pink-tan soft tissue measuring 0.2 cm in greatest dimension. The specimen is entirely submitted labeled 4A with multiple levels prepared.

FINAL DIAGNOSIS:

Biopsy, ascending colon: Fragments of colonic mucosa showing a focus of adenomatous glands

Transverse colon polyp #1: Tubular adenoma

Transverse colon polyp #2: Tubular adenoma

Transverse colon polyp #3: Tubular adenoma

Questions for Further Review: Case Study 7.1

1. Identify *each* anatomical site examined with the endoscope:
   a. Esophagus
   b. Stomach
   c. Duodenum
   d. Small intestine
   e. Anus
   f. Rectum
   g. Sigmoid colon
   h. Descending colon
   i. Transverse colon
   j. Ascending colon
   k. Cecum

2. Was an endoscopic ultrasound examination performed?
   a. Yes
   b. No

   If yes, list each anatomical site examined with the echoendoscope.

3. Was a transendoscopic device placed?
   a. Yes
   b. No

   If yes, what type of placement?
   a. Catheter placement
   b. Intraluminal tube placement
   c. Stent placement (including predilation)

4. Identify the surgical procedure performed on *each* lesion present.
   a. Biopsy of specimen
   b. Bipolar cautery removal
   c. Hot-biopsy removal
   d. Snare technique removal
   e. Destruction/ablation/fulguration
   f. Submucosal injection (India ink, saline, corticosteroids, Botox)
   g. Other (specify)

5. Identify the type of instrument/approach used on *each* lesion (if applicable)
   a. Cold-biopsy forceps
   b. Hot-biopsy forceps
   c. Transendoscopic ultrasound-guided intramural fine needle aspiration/biopsy(s)
   d. Transendoscopic ultrasound-guided transmural fine needle aspiration/biopsy(s)
   e. Not documented/applicable

6. CPT surgery code(s) and modifier:

Case Study 7.2

Read the following clinical document and answer the questions for further review.

COLONOSCOPY REPORT

PROCEDURE: Total colonoscopy with hot-biopsy destruction of sessile 3-mm midsigmoid colon polyp and multiple cold biopsies taken randomly throughout the colon

PREOPERATIVE DIAGNOSIS: Fecal incontinence, diarrhea, constipation

BOWEL PREPARATION: The bowel preparation with GoLytely was good.

ANESTHETIC: Demerol 50 mg and Versed 3 mg, both given intravenously

PROCEDURE: The digital examination revealed no masses. The pediatric variable flexion Olympus colonoscope was introduced into the rectum and advanced to the cecum. A picture was taken of the appendiceal orifice and the ileocecal valve. The scope was then carefully extubated. The mucosa looked normal. Random biopsies were taken from the ascending colon, the transverse colon, the descending colon, sigmoid colon, and rectum. There was a 3-mm sessile polyp in the midsigmoid colon, which was destroyed by hot biopsy.

IMPRESSION: Sigmoid colon polyp destroyed by hot biopsy

RECOMMENDATION: I have asked the patient to call my office in a week to get the results of the pathology. Cold biopsies taken because of history of diarrhea.

Questions for Further Review: Case Study 7.2

1. Identify *each* anatomical site examined with the endoscope:
   a. Esophagus
   b. Stomach
   c. Duodenum
   d. Small intestine
   e. Anus
   f. Rectum
   g. Sigmoid colon
   h. Descending colon
   i. Transverse colon
   j. Ascending colon
   k. Cecum

2. Was an endoscopic ultrasound examination performed?
   a. Yes
   b. No

   If yes, list each anatomical site examined with the echoendoscope.

3. Was a transendoscopic device placed?
   a. Yes
   b. No

   If yes, what type of placement?
   a. Catheter placement
   b. Intraluminal tube placement
   c. Stent placement (including predilation)

4. Identify the surgical procedure performed on *each* lesion present.
   a. Biopsy of specimen
   b. Bipolar cautery removal
   c. Hot-biopsy removal
   d. Snare technique removal
   e. Destruction/ablation/fulguration
   f. Submucosal injection (India ink, saline, corticosteroids, Botox)
   g. Other (specify)

5. Identify the type of instrument/approach used on *each* lesion (if applicable)
   a. Cold-biopsy forceps
   b. Hot-biopsy forceps
   c. Transendoscopic ultrasound-guided intramural fine needle aspiration/biopsy(s)
   d. Transendoscopic ultrasound-guided transmural fine needle aspiration/biopsy(s)
   e. Not documented/applicable

6. CPT surgery code(s) and modifier(s):

Case Study 7.3

Read the following clinical document and answer the questions for further review.

OPERATIVE REPORT

PREOPERATIVE DIAGNOSIS: History of polyps

POSTOPERATIVE DIAGNOSIS: Polyps in ascending colon, right transverse colon, and rectum

OPERATION: Colonoscopy

ANESTHESIA: Versed 3 mg, fentanyl 100 mcg IV

DESCRIPTION OF PROCEDURE: The patient was placed in the left lateral position. The colonoscope was guided into the cecum. The ileocecal valve and the appendiceal lumen were visualized and photographed. The colon was circumferentially inspected in its entire length. At the level of the mid-ascending colon, a small sessile polyp was found and removed using cold-biopsy forceps. Also, in the transverse colon, a small sessile polyp was found and removed with cold-biopsy forceps. No signs of bleeding. No signs of acute inflammation or diverticulosis was seen in the sigmoid colon. At the level of 10 cm, a small, flat lesion was found, and multiple biopsies were taken. No other mucosal lesions were seen throughout the exam. Air was aspirated, the colonoscope removed, the procedure was terminated. The patient was taken to the outpatient department in stable condition.

SURGICAL PATHOLOGY REPORT

AGE/SEX: 68/M

SPECIMEN(S) RECEIVED:

1. Colon, hepatic flexure biopsy
2. Ascending colon biopsy
3. Colon biopsy at 30 cm

GROSS:

1. Specimen is received in formalin and consists of a single fragment of tan tissue measuring 0.2 cm in greatest dimension. ESS: 1 cassette
2. Specimen is received in formalin and consists of a single fragment of tan tissue measuring 0.2 cm in greatest dimension. ESS: 1 cassette
3. Specimen is received in formalin and consists of two fragments of tan tissue each measuring 0.2 cm in greatest dimension. ESS: 1 cassette

DIAGNOSIS:

1. Adenomatous polyp, hepatic flexure
2. Adenomatous polyp, ascending colon
3. Biopsies of colon at 30 cm
4. Benign colonic mucosa including an occasional small lymphoid aggregate

---

Questions for Further Review: Case Study 7.3

1. Identify _each_ anatomical site examined with the endoscope.
   a. Esophagus
   b. Stomach
   c. Duodenum
   d. Small intestine
   e. Anus
   f. Rectum
   g. Sigmoid colon
   h. Descending colon
   i. Transverse colon
   j. Ascending colon
   k. Cecum

2. Was an endoscopic ultrasound examination performed?
   a. Yes
   b. No

   If yes, list each anatomical site examined with the echoendoscope.

3. Was a transendoscopic device placed?
   a. Catheter placement
   b. Intraluminal tube placement
   c. Stent placement (including predilation)
   d. No

4. Identify the surgical procedure performed on _each_ lesion present.
   a. Biopsy of specimen
   b. Bipolar cautery removal
   c. Hot-biopsy removal
   d. Snare technique removal
   e. Destruction/ablation/fulguration
   f. Submucosal injection (India ink, saline, corticosteroids, Botox)
   g. Other (specify)

5. Identify the type of instrument/approach used on *each* lesion (if applicable)
   a. Cold-biopsy forceps
   b. Hot-biopsy forceps
   c. Transendoscopic ultrasound-guided intramural fine needle aspiration/biopsy(s)
   d. Transendoscopic ultrasound-guided transmural fine needle aspiration/biopsy(s)
   e. Not documented/applicable

6. CPT surgery code(s) and modifier(s):

Case Study 7.4

Read the following clinical document and answer the questions for further review.

OPERATIVE REPORT

PREOPERATIVE DIAGNOSIS: Crohn's disease with a known sigmoid stricture. The patient has had symptomatic marked improvement on medical management, limited at this time to Asacol 800 mg t.i.d.

POSTOPERATIVE DIAGNOSIS: Active Crohn's disease, limited to the sigmoid colon with scarring and pseudopolyp formation. Biopsies were obtained. Sigmoid stricture negotiated with difficulty with the colonoscope. Subsequent dilation accomplished with an 18-mm TTS balloon dilator.

OPERATION: Colonoscopy, biopsy, and balloon dilation of colon stricture

SEDATION: Versed 3 mg of Demerol 50 mg IV

PROCEDURE/FINDINGS: A digital examination showed scarring from a previous perirectal abscess. No mass was identified. There was no active rectal disease at this time. The Pentax video colonoscope was introduced and passed to the terminal ileum, which appeared normal. No pathology was seen in the proximal colon. A segment of approximately 15 cm was in the midsigmoid with marked deformity, active inflammation, and some ulceration consistent with active Crohn's disease. Diverticula also were in this area. It was quite difficult to negotiate with the colonoscope, but this was eventually accomplished, taking care not to risk perforation. Following the inspection of the more proximal colon, this area was multiply biopsied and dilated with an 18-mm TTS balloon in the usual fashion without complications. Photographic documentation was obtained. The procedure was well tolerated.

Questions for Further Review: Case Study 7.4

1. Identify *each* anatomical site examined with the endoscope.
   a. Esophagus
   b. Stomach
   c. Duodenum
   d. Small intestine
   e. Anus
   f. Rectum
   g. Sigmoid colon
   h. Descending colon
   i. Transverse colon
   j. Ascending colon
   k. Cecum

2. Was an endoscopic ultrasound examination performed?
   a. Yes
   b. No

   If yes, list each anatomical site examined with the echoendoscope.

3. Was a transendoscopic device placed?
   a. Yes
   b. No

   If yes, what type of placement?
   a. Catheter placement
   b. Intraluminal tube placement
   c. Stent placement (including predilation)

4. Identify the surgical procedure performed on *each* lesion present.
   a. Biopsy of specimen
   b. Bipolar cautery removal
   c. Hot-biopsy removal
   d. Snare technique removal
   e. Destruction/ablation/fulguration
   f. Submucosal injection (India ink, saline, corticosteroids, Botox)
   g. Other (specify)

5. Identify the type of instrument/approach used on *each* lesion (if applicable)
   a. Cold-biopsy forceps
   b. Hot-biopsy forceps
   c. Transendoscopic ultrasound-guided intramural fine needle aspiration/biopsy(s)
   d. Transendoscopic ultrasound-guided transmural fine needle aspiration/biopsy(s)
   e. Not documented/applicable

6. CPT surgery code(s) and modifier(s):

Case Study 7.5

Read the following clinical document and answer the questions for further review.

OPERATIVE REPORT

OPERATION: Sigmoidoscopy and rectal ultrasound

INDICATIONS: Rectal cancer

PROCEDURE: After informed consent was obtained, the patient was brought to the endoscopy suite. Adequate sedation and monitoring were achieved with 25 mg of Demerol and 2 mg of Versed.

The video colonoscope was placed gently into the patient's rectum and advanced approximately 20 cm from the anal verge. On the first fold was a 2-cm flat polypoid lesion with an adjacent ulceration indicating the area that was previously removed. Thereafter, the GFUM-20 echo endoscope was placed gently into the patient's rectum and advanced until approximately 25 cm from the anal verge. The echo endoscope was withdrawn. The lesion was clearly identified after the patient was turned and water was placed in the lumen using about 7.5 and 12 megahertz. The lesion itself was interrogated. The lesion itself was consistent with a T1 lesion. There was no adjacent lymphadenopathy. Echo endoscope was withdrawn.

The patient tolerated the procedure well. There were no immediate complications.

IMPRESSION: Sigmoidoscopy and endosonography of rectal cancer, endosonographic findings consistent with a T1 lesion.

RECOMMENDATIONS: Transanal excision

Questions for Further Review: Case Study 7.5

1. What type of endoscopy was performed?
   a. Colonoscopy
   b. Sigmoidoscopy
   c. Esophagogastroduodenoscopy

2. Was an endoscopic ultrasound examination performed?
   a. Yes
   b. No

3. Was a transendoscopic device placed?
   a. Yes
   b. No

   If yes, what type of placement?
   a. Catheter placement
   b. Intraluminal tube placement
   c. Stent placement (including predilation)

4. Identify the surgical procedure performed on *each* lesion present.
   a. Biopsy of specimen
   b. Bipolar cautery removal
   c. Hot-biopsy removal
   d. Snare technique removal
   e. Destruction/ablation/fulguration
   f. Submucosal injection (India ink, saline, corticosteroids, Botox)
   g. Other (specify)
   h None

5. CPT surgery code(s) and modifier(s):

Case Study 7.6

Read the following clinical document and answer the questions for further review.

OPERATIVE REPORT

PREOPERATIVE DIAGNOSIS: Possible pancreatic mass and abdominal discomfort

OPERATIVE PROCEDURE: Esophagogastroduodenoscopy and endoscopic ultrasound with fine needle aspiration

PROCEDURE: Today, after informed consent was obtained, the patient was brought to the endoscopy suite. Adequate sedation and monitoring was achieved by the anesthesiologist. The video gastroscope was placed gently into the patient's mouth, posterior pharynx, and, ultimately, into the second portion of the duodenum. There was mild antral gastritis. The previously placed biliary stent was clearly identified. Thereafter, the GSUM-20 echoendoscope was placed gently into the patient's mouth, posterior pharynx, and, ultimately, into the second portion of the duodenum. Multiple views of the duodenum were obtained as well as the retroperitoneal area. There was a 2.5 x 2.5 centimeter mass within the head of the pancreas that appeared to invade the portal splenic confluence. In addition, a 1.3 x 0.75 centimeter lymph node was adjacent to the duodenum. The superior mesenteric artery was identified and did not appear to be invaded. Thereafter, the linear-array echoendoscope was placed gently into the patient's mouth, posterior pharynx, and duodenum. Several passes were made and tissue was obtained. The echoendoscope was withdrawn. The patient tolerated the procedure well. There were no immediate complications.

IMPRESSION:

1. Gastroscopy to the second portion of the duodenum, antral gastritis, stent in place
2. Endosonography revealed a 2.5 x 2.5 centimeter mass with a 1.3 x 0.75 centimeter lymph node suspicious for pancreatic carcinoma
3. Fine needle aspiration performed with multiple passes via the linear-array echoendoscope

Note: There were several views of the mass; however, several of the best views were obstructed by intervening vessels and thus long views with placement of needle deep through normal pancreatic tissue was necessary to obtain tissue.

I await the results of the fine needle aspiration.

Questions for Further Review: Case Study 7.6

1. Identify *each* anatomical site examined with the endoscope.
   a. Esophagus
   b. Stomach
   c. Duodenum
   d. Small intestine
   e. Anus
   f. Rectum
   g. Sigmoid colon
   h. Descending colon
   i. Transverse colon
   j. Ascending colon
   k. Cecum

2. Was an endoscopic ultrasound examination performed?
   a. Yes
   b. No

   If yes, list each anatomical site examined with the echoendoscope.

3.   Was a transendoscopic device placed?
     a.   Yes
     b.   No

     If yes, what type of placement?
     a.   Catheter placement
     b.   Intraluminal tube placement
     c.   Stent placement (including predilation)

4.   Identify the surgical procedure performed on *each* lesion present.
     a.   Biopsy of specimen
     b.   Bipolar cautery removal
     c.   Hot-biopsy removal
     d.   Snare technique removal
     e.   Destruction/ablation/fulguration
     f.   Submucosal injection (India ink, saline, corticosteroids, Botox)
     g.   Other (specify)

5.   Identify the type of instrument/approach used on *each* lesion (if applicable)
     a.   Cold-biopsy forceps
     b.   Hot-biopsy forceps
     c.   Transendoscopic ultrasound fine needle aspiration/biopsy(s)
     d.   Not documented/applicable

6.   CPT surgery code(s) and modifier(s):

Case Study 7.7

Read the following clinical document and answer the questions for further review.

PROCEDURE NOTE

PROCEDURE: EGD endoscopy and esophageal dilation

CLINICAL NOTE: This is a 53-year-old white male with dysphagia.

PREOPERATIVE PREP: The patient received Fentanyl 0.125 mg and Versed 5 mg intravenously immediately prior to the procedure.

ENDOSCOPIC FINDINGS: An Olympus video gastroscope was passed readily into the esophagus. Approximately a 4-cm hiatal hernia was noted. At the esophagogastric junction, a Schatzki's ring was clearly noted. The scope could pass readily through it. Small erosions were seen above the Schatzki's ring. Biopsies were taken from the distal esophagus.

The stomach was carefully inspected throughout and appeared normal. The duodenal bulb and second portion of duodenum appeared normal.

A 20-mm TTS balloon was inflated at the Schatzki's ring and held for a minute. The scope and balloon were then removed.

IMPRESSION:

1. Erosive esophagitis
2. Schatzki's ring
3. Hiatal hernia

RECOMMENDATIONS: Aciphex 20 mg p.o. b.i.d. and follow-up in the next 1–2 months

SURGICAL PATHOLOGY RESULT REPORT

CLINICAL HISTORY: Dysphagia

OPERATION: Esophagogastroduodenoscopy: Esophageal erosions

GROSS DESCRIPTION: In formalin labeled "biopsy distal esophagus" are two fragments of pink-tan soft tissue, ranging from 0.1 to 0.2 cm in greatest dimension. The specimen is entirely submitted labeled 1A with multiple levels prepared.

FINAL DIAGNOSIS:
Biopsy, distal esophagus

Fragment of squamous epithelium with no significant histologic abnormalities, and a separate fragment of ulcerated tissue showing acute inflammatory exudate.

GMS stain is negative for fungus.

No viral cytopathic changes are noted.

Questions for Further Review: Case Study 7.7

1. Does the patient have a current diagnosis of achalasia?
   a. Yes
   b. No

2. Was an endoscopy performed?
   a. Yes
   b. No

3. Identify *each* anatomical site examined with the endoscope.
   a. Esophagus
   b. Stomach
   c. Duodenum
   d. All of the above

4. Identify the method of dilation utilized.
   a. Balloon (less than 30 mm in diameter)
   b. Balloon (larger than 30 mm in diameter)
   c. Insertion of guide wire followed by dilation over guide wire
   d. Unguided sound
   e. Bougie
   f. Retrograde dilators.

5. CPT surgery code(s) and modifier(s):

Case Study 7.8

Read the following clinical document and answer the questions for further review.

OPERATIVE REPORT

PREOPERATIVE DIAGNOSIS: Dysphagia, atypical chest symptoms

PROCEDURE: Upper endoscopy with balloon and Maloney dilation

POSTOPERATIVE DIAGNOSIS: Status post dilation, no obvious strictures seen; otherwise normal exam

ANESTHESIA: Cetacaine spray p.o., Versed 5, Sublimaze 0.075 IV pus

INDICATIONS: This 51-year-old woman was referred for swallowing difficulties and complaints of abdominal pain refractory to Protonix therapy.

PROCEDURE: With the patient in the left decubitus position, the Olympus video endoscope was inserted easily into the esophagus, which appeared entirely normal proximally. There was a possibility of fusiform narrowing of the GE junction, but no signs of erosions, hiatal hernia, rings, or Barrett's mucosa. The gastric folds were unremarkable. Retroflex exam of the GE junction was normal. There were no signs of ulcers. The pylorus and duodenum were patent to the fourth portion. The GE junction was then dilated with the 15- and then the 18-mm-diameter TTS-CRE balloon with no obvious effects. There was minimal spasm. The balloon and instrument were then removed and the esophagus empirically dilated with the 54-French Maloney dilator with no significant resistance. No heme was obtained. The patient tolerated the procedure very well.

RECOMMENDATIONS:

1. Barium swallow if symptoms persist
2. Would avoid NSAID agents, discontinue Protonix otherwise

Questions for Further Review: Case Study 7.8

1. Does the patient have a current diagnosis of achalasia?
   a. Yes
   b. No

2. Was an endoscopy performed?
   a. Yes
   b. No

3. Identify *each* anatomical site examined with the endoscope.
   a. Esophagus
   b. Stomach
   c. Duodenum
   d. All of the above

4. Identify the method of dilation utilized.
   a. Balloon (less than 30 mm in diameter)
   b. Balloon (larger than 30 mm in diameter)
   c. Insertion of guide wire followed by dilation over guide wire
   d. Unguided sound
   e. Bougie
   f. Retrograde dilators.

5. CPT surgery code(s) and modifier(s):

Case Study 7.9

Read the following clinical document and answer the questions for further review.

OPERATIVE REPORT

AGE: 58

OPERATION: Mesh repair of recurrent incisional hernia

ANESTHESIA: Local standby

PREOPERATIVE DIAGNOSIS: Recurrent incisional hernia

POSTOPERATIVE DIAGNOSIS: Recurrent incisional hernia

OPERATIVE INDICATIONS: This patient had a previous incisional hernia repair twenty-six years ago and developed a recurrence 5 finger breadths below and 2 finger breadths to the right of the midline. Repair was advised.

OPERATIVE PROCEDURE: The patient was brought to the operating room, and after satisfactory general endotracheal anesthesia was obtained, was prepared and draped in the usual fashion. A horizontal incision over the area of the hernia defect was made through the skin and subcutaneous tissue. The bleeding points were controlled with the Bovie cautery and #3-0 Vicryl ties throughout. The hernia sac was identified, opened, and noted to contain omentum. The omentum was dissected free from the hernia sac and replaced intraperitoneally. A segment of polypropylene mesh was placed under the dissected fascial edges of the defect and anchored in place with #4-0 Prolene sutures placed in a horizontal mattress fashion. The defect itself was then closed with interrupted figure eight #0 Prolene sutures. The wound was irrigated with dilute antibiotic solution and with local anesthetic as well. Subcutaneous tissue was closed with interrupted #3-0 Vicryl, and the skin was closed with a running #4-0 Vicryl subcuticular suture. Steri-Strips and a sterile occlusive dressing were positioned. The patient tolerated the procedure well and left the operating room in satisfactory condition.

ESTIMATED BLOOD LOSS: 5 cc, no replacement

DRAINS: None

Questions for Further Review: Case Study 7.9

1. Does the patient have a past history of hernia repair surgery on the left and/or right side(s)?
   a. Yes
   b. No

2. What is the patient's age?

3. If patient is less than one year old, specify the patient's gestational age at birth.

4. Identify the type of unilateral or bilateral hernia(s) currently being repaired.
   a. Inguinal
   b. Sliding inguinal
   c. Lumbar
   d. Femoral
   e. Incisional (ventral)
   f. Epigastric
   g. Umbilical
   h. Spigelian

5. What is the clinical presentation of *each* hernia?
   a. Reducible
   b. Incarcerated
   c. Strangulated

6. What surgical repair method(s) was utilized?
   a. Open
   b. Laparoscopic
   c. Mesh application

7. CPT surgery code(s) and modifier(s):

Case Study 7.10

Read the following clinical document and answer the questions for further review.

OPERATIVE REPORT

PREOPERATIVE DIAGNOSIS: Bilateral inguinal hernias

OPERATION: Bilateral inguinal herniorrhaphies

POSTOPERATIVE DIAGNOSIS: Bilateral inguinal hernias

ANESTHESIA: General

ESTIMATED BLOOD LOSS: Minimal

INDICATIONS: This case is about a 5-week-old baby born at 38 weeks' gestation who presents with a large right inguinal hernia and a small left inguinal hernia. He is taken now to the operating room for repair.

PROCEDURE: After successful induction of general endotracheal anesthesia, the patient was placed in the supine position and prepped and draped in the usual sterile fashion. A curved incision was made in a skin fold in the right groin. The subcutaneous tissue was opened with cautery. The external oblique was opened sharply in the direction of its fibers down through the external ring. The cremasteric fibers were dissected away from the cord, and the cord was elevated into the wound. Anteromedially in the cord was a large hernia sac, and this was dissected away from the vas and the vessels. The sac was dissected up to the level of the internal ring where it was doubly ligated with 4-0 PDS. The excess sac was excised. The floor of the canal was repaired by suturing the conjoined tendon to Poupart ligament with 4-0 PDS. The testicle was returned to the scrotum, and the external oblique was closed over the cord with running 4-0 PDS. The subcutaneous tissue was closed with Vicryl, and the skin was closed with subcuticular Vicryl and Steri-Strips.

A matching incision was made in the left groin. The subcutaneous tissue was again opened with cautery. The external oblique was opened in the direction of its fibers down through the external ring. The cremasteric fibers were dissected away from the cord. Anteromedially in the cord was a small hernia sac, and this was dissected away from the vas and vessels. The sac was dissected to the level of the internal ring where it was doubly ligated with 4-0 PDS. The excess sac was excised. The testicle was returned to the scrotum. The external oblique was closed over the cord with running 4-0 PDS. The subcutaneous tissue was closed with Vicryl, and the skin was closed with subcuticular Vicryl and Steri-Strips. Occlusive dressings were applied to the wound. Both testes were in the scrotum at the completion of the case. The sponge count was correct. The patient tolerated the procedure well and went to the recovery room in stable condition.

Questions for Further Review: Case Study 7.10

1. Does the patient have a past history of hernia repair surgery on the left and/or right side(s)?
   a. Yes
   b. No

2. What is the patient's age?

3. If patient is less than one year old, specify the patient's gestational age at birth.

4. Identify the type of unilateral or bilateral hernia(s) currently being repaired.
   a. Inguinal
   b. Sliding inguinal
   c. Lumbar
   d. Femoral
   e. Incisional (ventral)
   f. Epigastric
   g. Umbilical
   h. Spigelian

5. What is the clinical presentation of *each* hernia(s)?
   a. Reducible
   b. Incarcerated
   c. Strangulated

6. What surgical repair method(s) was utilized?
   a. Open
   b. Laparoscopic
   c. Mesh application

7. CPT surgery code(s) and modifier(s):

Case Study 7.11

Read the following clinical document and answer the questions for further review.

OPERATIVE REPORT

PREOPERATIVE DIAGNOSIS: Umbilical hernia

OPERATION: Primary umbilical herniorrhaphy

POSTOPERATIVE DIAGNOSIS: Small incarcerated umbilical hernia

ANESTHESIA: General

INDICATIONS: The patient is a 50-year-old gentleman who noted one month ago that he had a small painful mass at his umbilicus. He thinks that the mass has not grown in size in the interim. He is unable to completely reduce it.

DESCRIPTION OF PROCEDURE: The patient was brought to the operating room and placed supine on the operating room table. After the induction of general anesthesia, the patient's abdomen was prepped and draped in the usual sterile fashion. 0.25% bupivacaine was injected into the umbilicus for local anesthesia. A 1.5-cm incision was made supraumbilically. Bovie electrocautery was used to delineate the umbilical fascial defect. Fat was herniated through the small hole and incarcerated. When the edges of the fascial defect were identified and cleaned, four 0 Tycron sutures were used to close the defect. A 2-0 Vicryl suture was used to tack the umbilicus down to the anterior fascia. Two 4-0 silk sutures were used as deep stitches, and the skin was closed using a 4-0 running subcuticular stitch. Steri-Strips were applied. A cotton ball was inserted into the umbilicus. A clean, dry dressing was applied. Dr. Smith was present and scrubbed for the entire procedure. All sponge, needle, and instrument counts were correct at the end of the case. The patient was awakened from anesthesia and taken to the recovery room in stable condition.

Questions for Further Review: Case Study 7.11

1. Does the patient have a past history of hernia repair surgery on the left and/or right side(s)?
   a. Yes
   b. No

2. What is the patient's age?

3. If patient is less than one year old, specify the patient's gestational age at birth.

4. Identify the type of unilateral or bilateral hernia(s) currently being repaired.
   a. Inguinal
   b. Sliding inguinal
   c. Lumbar
   d. Femoral
   e. Incisional (ventral)
   f. Epigastric
   g. Umbilical
   h. Spigelian

5. What is the clinical presentation of *each* hernia(s)?
   a. Reducible
   b. Incarcerated
   c. Strangulated

6. What surgical repair method(s) was utilized?
   a. Open
   b. Laparoscopic
   c. Mesh application

7. CPT surgery code(s) and modifier(s):

Case Study 7.12

Read the following clinical document and answer the questions for further review.

OPERATIVE REPORT

PREOPERATIVE DIAGNOSIS: Recurrent abdominal pain

POSTOPERATIVE DIAGNOSIS: Normal enteroscopy with jejunal diverticula

OPERATION: Given capsule, M2RA, enteroscopy

DESCRIPTION OF PROCEDURE: Following appropriate discussion of the risks, indications, alternatives to capsule enteroscopy, informed consent was obtained.

The patient was placed in recumbent position, the template placed on the abdomen and eight antenna markers delineated. The antennae were then located by adhesive tape in this region. The patient easily swallowed the M2RA capsule endoscope and proceeded to record events for the next 8 hours.

Review of the data shows a basically normal enteroscopy. At one hour and 55 minutes, the capsule endoscope passes through the pylorus into a normal-appearing duodenal bulb and postbulbar duodenum. Villi appear entirely normal throughout the small bowel. There was no obstruction, no scarring, no evidence of luminal narrowing. Two small, few millimeter diverticula were noted in the jejunum. At four hours and 27 minutes, the capsule then passes through the ileocecal valve into the ileum, which is visualized in its proximal extent with some degree of liquid fecal debris, some degree of small amounts of effervescent bubbles noted. No masses were seen, no evidence of inflammatory bowel disease. The procedure was well tolerated.

COMPLICATIONS: None

Questions for Further Review: Case Study 7.12

1. What type if endoscopy was performed?
   a. Capsule endoscopy
   b. Flexible fiberoptic endoscopy
   c. Echoendoscopy
   d. Rigid endoscopy

2. Was the esophagus through ileum examined?
   a. Yes
   b. No

3. CPT surgery code(s) and modifier(s):

Case Study 7.13

Read the following clinical document and answer the questions for further review.

OPERATIVE REPORT

PREOPERATIVE DIAGNOSIS: Right rectal abscess

POSTOPERATIVE DIAGNOSIS: Right anterior fistula

OPERATION PERFORMED: Fissurectomy

ANESTHESIA: Local/monitor

PROCEDURE: With patient in a jackknife position, the anus was appropriately prepped and draped. Local anesthesia was given in the usual fashion. The patient had a prominent right anterior crypt that probed deeply. Superficial cutting over the mucosa and submucosa revealed the opening of a crypt that was inflamed. No secondary opening was noted, but in the area of the previous incision, the drainage tract was opened, revealing entry into a chronic cavity. It appeared deep, and a primary fissurectomy would not appear to be in the patient's best interest, so the external and internal sphincter were looped with a Seton, which was tied with 3 interrupted #2 Silks. The patient will have this removed in approximately 6 weeks if there is no flare-up of the wound. This was discussed with both the patient and family.

Questions for Further Review: Case Study 7.13

1. What type of anal fistula procedure was performed?
   a. Fistulectomy
   b. Fistulotomy
   c. Placement of anal seton
   d. Instillation of fibrin glue
   e. Closure with rectal advancement flap
   f. Second-stage repair
   g. Removal of anal seton

2. CPT surgery code(s) and modifier(s):

Case Study 7.14

Read the following clinical document and answer the questions for further review.

OPERATIVE REPORT

AGE: 56

OPERATION: Anal advancement flap

ANESTHESIA: General endotracheal

PREOPERATIVE DIAGNOSIS: Recurrent posterior midline fistula

POSTOPERATIVE DIAGNOSIS: Recurrent posterior midline fistula

OPERATIVE INDICATIONS: This is a gentleman who was referred to me with a recurrent post–anal space abscess and fistula. The patient underwent previous surgery for treatment of a unilateral horseshoe fistula. This included a cutting Seton for the remaining posterior midline fistula. The patient was doing well but then still noticed some purulent drainage from the left buttock. Examination under anesthesia revealed a small recurrent posterior midline fistula. This did encompass some of the external sphincter complex. A seton was placed previously. The patient was seen in the office. Although the fistulous tract appeared to be relatively superficial, the patient was quite concerned about incontinence because he had seepage from his previous fistulotomies. The patient, therefore, presents at this time for anal advancement flap treatment of this disease. The patient has no sequelae or indications of Crohn's disease.

OPERATIVE PROCEDURE: Following adequate general anesthesia, the patient was placed in the lithotomy position. The perineum and the rectum were prepped with Betadine and draped in the usual fashion. The proctoscope was used to remove the remaining effluence from the rectum. The fistulous opening in the posterior midline was identified. The seton was in place. The seton was removed. Next, a semicircular advancement flap was created. This fistulous opening was relatively low, and a house flap would not be necessary for adequate closure of this. We raised a core of mucosa and internal sphincter fibers. This was up into the anal canal. We came across the base of the fistulous tract. The flap was raised easily. The blood supply to this was excellent. The flap was completely raised so that the midportion of the flap could be brought down below the fistulous opening without difficulty. A probe was placed through the external fistulous communication through the muscle. A curet was used to remove any remaining necrotic tissue in the tract. There was very little. We closed the internal opening at the muscular layer with multiple, interrupted sutures of 2-0 Vicryl. This completely obliterated the internal opening. Next, we excised the mucosal fistulous opening. We then reapproximated the mucosa to the skin using multiple interrupted sutures of 2-0 Vicryl. Prior to closure of the flap, we ensured that there was excellent hemostasis of the undersurface. The flap could be brought down without tension as the sutures were secured. A 10 French mushroom catheter was placed into the external fistulous opening and secured to the skin with a 3-0 Prolene. A dry, sterile dressing was applied. The patient tolerated the procedure well. The specimen was forwarded to pathology for final analysis.

PATHOLOGY REPORT

FINAL DIAGNOSIS: Perianal region, partial excision, consistent with fistula

SPECIMEN (S) SUBMITTED: Fistula tract

CLINICAL DATA: Perianal fistula

GROSS DESCRIPTION: Received fresh are two yellow-red, irregular-shaped segments aggregating to 2.2 x 0.6 x 0.5 cm. The specimen is totally submitted in Hollande's in cassette A1.

AGE: 56 **SEX:** M

Questions for Further Review: Case Study 7.14

1. What types of repairs were performed?
    a. Fistulectomy
    b. Fistulotomy
    c. Placement of anal seton
    d. Instillation of fibrin glue
    e. Closure with rectal advancement flap
    f. Second-stage repair
    g. Removal of anal seton

2. CPT surgery code(s) and modifier(s):

Case Study 7.15

Read the following clinical document and answer the questions for further review.

OPERATIVE REPORT

PREOPERATIVE DIAGNOSIS: Left lateral internal and external hemorrhoids with marked prolapse

POSTEROPERATIVE DIAGNOSIS: Same

OPERATION PERFORMED: Hemorrhoidectomy

ANESTHESIA: Local with conscious sedation

PROCEDURE: With patient in the jackknife position, the anus was prepped and draped. Local anesthesia was given in the usual fashion. The hemorrhoid was outlined with a scalpel, dissected off the internal and external sphincter. The hemorrhoidal base went down, as this was a substantial prolapse. Due to the enormity of the hemorrhoid complex, this was transfixed with a 3-0 Vicryl and tied. The base was hemostatic after amputation of the hemorrhoidal complex. The area of defect was closed to the dentate line with continuous 3-0 Vicryl. This was then tied. 5-0 was used to close the skin. The patient tolerated the procedure well and went on to the recovery room uneventfully. The family was informed of the findings.

Questions for Further Review: Case Study 7.15

1. What type of hemorrhoid(s) was present?
   a. Tag
   b. Internal
   c. External
   d. Internal and external
   e. Prolapsed
   f. Thrombotic

2. What surgical technique was used to repair *each* hemorrhoid?
   a. Incision
   b. Excision (hemorrhoidectomy)
   c. Enucleation
   d. Injection of sclerosing agent
   e. Destruction (for example, laser, electrocauterization)
   f. Simple ligation (for example, rubber band)
   g. Ligation (surgical)
   h. Fissurectomy
   i. Fistulectomy

3. CPT surgery code(s) and modifier(s):

Case Study 7.16

Read the following clinical document and answer the questions for further review.

OPERATIVE NOTE

AGE: 50

PREOPERATIVE DIAGNOSIS: Complex internal and external hemorrhoids with Grade 4 prolapse and internal component

Chronic posterior midline anal fissure, sphincter spasm

PROCEDURE: Complex hemorrhoidectomy and fissurectomy

Lateral sphincterotomy

POSTOPERATIVE DIAGNOSIS: Same

ANESTHESIA: Local with IV sedation

INDICATIONS FOR PROCEDURE: Rectal bleeding, prolapse of hemorrhoids and pain

PROCEDURE: The patient was placed in the jackknife position. Monitoring of vital signs and intravenous sedation was in the care of the anesthesiologist. The skin of the perianal was prepped and draped in the usual sterile fashion. A local anesthetic consisting of 30 cc of 1% Lidocaine with epinephrine and sodium bicarbonate and 60 mg of Toradol was infiltrated in the skin of the perianal area and anal canal. The anal canal was then gently dilated and inspected. The hemorrhoids were located in three major quadrants: left lateral, right anterolateral, and right posterior lateral. The fissure was in the posterior midline.

The hemorrhoidal group to be excised first was the one in the left lateral quadrant. The V-shaped incision was made over the skin of the perianal area. The two arms of the incision were extended into the anal canal in a parallel fashion and then narrowed at the apex of the hemorrhoidal pedicle. This island of skin and anodermal mucosa was then excised altogether with underlying hemorrhoidal vessels. The hemorrhoidal vessels were sharply dissected from the sphincter complex, keeping the fibers of the sphincter muscle under direct vision and never causing any injury. Flaps were then raised and excised, and more hemorrhoidal tissue was excised sparing the overlying skin and abnormal mucosa.

A lateral sphincterotomy was then performed in the left lateral quadrant after dissecting the internal anal sphincter from the external anal sphincter. The sphincterotomy was limited to the distal 8 mm of the internal anal sphincter. The wound was then closed primarily with #3–0 chromic continuous interlocking suture.

The hemorrhoid group to be removed second was the one in the right anterolateral quadrant, and it was removed following exactly the same technique that has been just described for the hemorrhoid in the left lateral quadrant, with the exception that no sphincterotomy was performed in this sector. The hemorrhoid in the right posterior lateral quadrant was also excised in a similar fashion, with the difference that the anal fissure was also excised in a similar fashion. Once again, no sphincterotomy was performed at this level.

The anal fissure in the posterior midline was then excised and primarily repaired with #3–0 chromic continuous interlocking suture and sent for pathology together with the rest of the hemorrhoidal tissue.

At the completion of the procedure, the anal canal was inspected with large and small retractors. The suture line was individually inspected and irrigated. There was no evidence of ongoing bleeding. The external part of the incisions was covered with Bacitracin ointment. The large piece of Surgicel was left in the anal canal for postoperative hemostasis. The patient tolerated the procedure well and was transferred to the recovery room in good condition.

Estimated blood loss was about 50 cc. There was no evidence of intraoperative complication.

SURGICAL PATHOLOGY RESULT REPORT

AGE: 48 **SEX:** F

CLINICAL HISTORY: Hemorrhoids per computer

GROSS DESCRIPTION: In formalin labeled "hemorrhoids and tissue" are irregular fragments of soft tissue up to 3 cm. in greatest dimension. They are partially covered by wrinkled grey-tan mucosa. Sectioning shows numerous dilated blood-filled vessels. Representative sections labeled 1A and 1B.

HEMORRHOIDS AND TISSUE: Anorectal mucosa with hemorrhoids and reactive surface epithelial changes.

Questions for Further Review: Case Study 7.16

1. What type of hemorrhoid(s) was present?
    a. Tag
    b. Internal
    c. External
    d. Internal and external
    e. Prolapsed
    f. Thrombotic

2. What was the location of *each* hemorrhoid plexus?

3. What surgical technique was used to repair *each* hemorrhoid?
    a. Incision
    b. Excision (hemorrhoidectomy)
    c. Enucleation
    d. Injection of sclerosing agent
    e. Destruction (for example, laser, electrocauterization)
    f. Simple ligation (for example, rubber band)
    g. Ligation (surgical)
    h. Fissurectomy
    i. Fistulectomy

4. CPT surgery code(s) and modifier(s):

Chapter 8

Urinary and Male Genital Systems, Reproductive System, and Intersex Surgery

CPT codes 50010–55899 are used to report surgical and related procedures performed on the urinary and male genital systems. Common outpatient procedures involving the urinary and male genital systems include urinary endoscopies, retrograde pyelograms, ureteral stents, orchiectomy, and penile prostheses. One code is included in the Reproductive System Procedures (55920) and two in Intersex Surgery (55970, 55980).

Urinary Endoscopies

A urinary endoscopy is performed when a visual examination of specific components of the urinary system is warranted. Endoscopies can be diagnostic or surgical. A surgical endoscopy always includes a diagnostic endoscopy. The diagnostic endoscopy should be coded only if a surgical procedure was not performed.

Coding Guidelines for Urinary Endoscopies

Urinary endoscopies involve the insertion of a scope into anatomical sites, such as the urethra (cystourethroscopy), ureter (ureteroscopy), and renal pelvis (pyeloscopy). Diagnostic examinations can be performed through the scope, as well as therapeutic procedures such as: biopsy, lesion removal/destruction, catheterization, and dilation.

The descriptions of cystoscopy codes must be applied with care. Regardless of the number of tumors or clots treated, each code is reported only once. Also, the descriptions include information on size of tumors biopsied or removed, as well as additional related services performed.

- Code 52204, Cystourethroscopy, with biopsy(s), should be reported only one time, regardless of the number of biopsies performed. For example, multiple biopsies may be performed in different areas of the bladder, but the procedure is coded as one event (AMA 2003e).

- When multiple bladder tumors are fulgurated or resected using a cystourethroscope, the tumor sizes should not be added together for a cumulative total size. Each tumor should be measured individually to determine the appropriate category—small, medium, large.

- Code 52234, which is cystoscopy for treatment of small (0.5 up to 2.0 cm) bladder tumor(s), should be reported once for single or multiple tumors that individually measure 0.5 up to 2.0 cm.

- Code 52235 should be reported once for medium-sized, single or multiple tumors that individually measure 2.0–5.0 cm.

- Tumors larger than 5.0 cm would be considered large tumors and would be reported once using code 52240 (AMA 2002d).

- Cystoscopy with multiple obstructing clots, code 52001, has been revised and clarified. This code is used for evaluation of large clots obstructing the bladder neck and causing urinary retention (AMA 2002e). Do not report code 52001 in conjunction with 52000 (Cystoscopy).

- Codes 52344–52355 are used to classify cystoscopy with ureteroscopy.

- Codes 52351–52355 are used for cystoscopy with ureteroscopy and pyeloscopy.

- Code 52353 is applied for cystoscopy and ureteroscopy with lithotripsy.

- Codes 52317 and 52318 pertain to bladder calculus litholapaxy.

APC	HCPCS	HCPCS Description	SI	Rel. Wt.	Payment Rate	OPPS OCE
0161			T	17.9420	1142.80	
	52204	Cystoscopy w/biopsy				Significant Procedure, Multiple Reduction Applies; Separate APC payment
	52001	Cystoscopy, removal of clots				Significant Procedure, Multiple Reduction Applies; Separate APC payment

Lithotripsy

Code 50590 is used for extracorporeal shock wave lithotripsy (ESWL). Lithotripsy is a technique used to break up stones that form in the kidney, bladder, ureters, or gallbladder. There are several ways of doing this, although the most common is extracorporeal (outside the body) shock wave lithotripsy. The shock waves are focused on the kidney stone and break the stone into tiny pieces, which are passed out of the body naturally during urination.

The official coding guidelines for CPT state that when the same lesion is biopsied and subsequently removed during the same operative session, only the code for the removal of the lesion should be reported. However, if one lesion is biopsied and a separate lesion is removed during the same operative session, it would be appropriate to report a code for the biopsy of one lesion and an additional code for the removal of the separate lesion, with modifier –59 appended to the code reported for the biopsy procedure (AMA 1999e).

CMS has developed rules for reporting endoscopic biopsies for Medicare outpatients that are more specific than the official coding guidelines for CPT. It is important to note that the term *excision*, as used in these rules, includes the variety of terms in the CPT manual that describe the excision or destruction of a lesion, for example, by resection, removal or fulguration. The CMS rules for Medicare reimbursement are as follows (CMS 1991):

1. When a single lesion is biopsied, but not excised, use only the biopsy code.

2. When a biopsy of a lesion is obtained and the remaining portion of the same lesion is then excised, code only for the excision.

3. When multiple biopsies are obtained from the same or different lesions and none of the lesions is excised, use only the biopsy code and list it once.

4. When a biopsy and an excision are performed, use both codes when the biopsy is taken from a different lesion than that which is excised and the code for the excision does not include the phrase "with or without biopsy." If such a phrase is included, do not use a separate biopsy code.

The following examples illustrate how to report the official guidelines listed above.

- A cystoscopy with biopsy of a 0.5-cm bladder dome tumor is performed; the remaining portion of the tumor is not excised: Code 52204, Cystourethroscopy, with biopsy.

- A cystoscopy with biopsy and fulguration of a 0.5-cm bladder dome tumor is performed: Code 52234, Cystourethroscopy with fulguration of small bladder tumor(s).

- A cystoscopy with two biopsies of a single bladder dome tumor is performed: Code 52204, Cystourethroscopy, with biopsy.

- A cystoscopy with biopsy of a bladder dome tumor and biopsy of a trigone bladder tumor is performed: Code 52204, Cystourethroscopy, with biopsy.

- A cystoscopy with biopsy of a 0.3-cm urethral polyp and fulguration of a 0.4-cm trigone bladder lesion is performed: Code 52224, Cystourethroscopy, with fulguration (including cryosurgery or laser surgery) or treatment of minor (less than 0.5 cm) lesion(s) with or without biopsy. (Note: Although in this example, two separate procedures—biopsy and fulguration—are performed on two separate lesions, assign only code 52224, which classifies "with or without biopsy" for lesions of this size.)

Endoscopic injections are coded by anatomical area targeted. Code 51715 is assigned for endoscopic injection of implant material, such as Teflon or collagen, into the urethra and/or bladder neck. Code 52327 is used to classify endoscopic injection of implant material into the subureteral area.

Retrograde Pyelograms

Retrograde pyelography involves the injection of contrast material via ureteral catheterization to allow radiological imaging of the renal pelvis. Such imaging is typically used to diagnose renal calculi/stones.

Coding Guidelines for Retrograde Pyelograms

The following guidelines apply to the coding of retrograde pyelograms:

- When a retrograde pyelogram or ureteropyelography is performed by ureteral catheterization through a cystoscope, code 52005 is assigned. To perform the retrograde pyelogram, the physician must inject contrast into the renal pelvis, which can only be done after the ureter has been catheterized.

- Ureteral catheterization is included in codes 52320–52330, 52352, and 52353. Code 52005, Cystourethroscopy with ureteral catheterization, should not be reported with any of these codes.

- Code 52332 is reported in addition to 52005 when an indwelling stent is placed in addition to a diagnostic cystourethroscopy.

- According to the CCI edits, provided the services described by codes 52332 and 52005 are performed, both codes may be reported with a modifier, as appropriate (AMA 2001g).

Ureteral Stents

Placement of a ureteral stent has many applications in urological surgery. This procedure is performed to maintain urine drainage and to relieve obstruction caused by tumors, strictures, and urinary calculi.

Coding Guidelines for Ureteral Stents

The following guidelines apply to the coding of ureteral stents:

- Placement and removal of a temporary ureteral stent is an integral component of codes 52320–52355 and is not reported separately.

- An additional code is reported for self-retaining, indwelling ureteral stents intended to remain in the ureter beyond the intraoperative period.

- Code 50393 is used for percutaneous ureteral stent placement.

- Code 50605 applies to ureteral stent placement via ureterotomy.

- Code 52332 is reported for cystoscopic ureteral stent placement.

- Code 52332 should be listed twice (or with bilateral procedure modifier -50) for cystourethroscopic bilateral ureteral stent placement (for example, placement of self-retaining ureteral stents in both ureters through the same cystoscope at the same cystourethroscopic diagnostic and/or therapeutic intervention).

- Code 52310 or 52315 is used for cystourethroscopic removal of a self-retaining, indwelling ureteral stent, planned or staged during the associated normal postoperative follow-up period of the original procedure.

- No additional reporting is warranted for the noncystourethroscopic removal of a self-retaining ureteral stent when the stent is removed during the normal postoperative follow-up period associated with its insertion (for example, inserted via ureterotomy or percutaneously).

- CPT code 52332 (Cystourethroscopy, with insertion of indwelling ureteral stent) should not be reported to describe insertion and removal of a temporary ureteral stent during diagnostic or therapeutic cystourethroscopy (CPT codes 52320–52355). The insertion and removal of a temporary ureteral stent during these procedures is not separately reportable and should not be reported with CPT codes 52005 or 52007. Similarly, the insertion and removal of a temporary ureteral catheter (CPT codes 52005, 52007) during cystourethroscopic procedures coded as CPT codes 52320–52355 is not separately reportable (NCCI 2007).

- The code pertaining to the appropriate level of service evaluation and management (E/M) should be used if a noncystourethroscopic removal of a self-retaining ureteral stent is performed beyond the normal postoperative follow-up period associated with its insertion (for example, inserted via ureterotomy or percutaneously) (AMA 1996a).

APC	HCPCS	HCPCS Description	SI	Rel. Wt.	Payment Rate	OPPS OCE
0162			T	24.7749	1578.01	
	52204	Cystoscopy and treatment				Significant Procedure, Multiple Reduction Applies; Separate APC payment

Orchiectomy

Laparoscopic orchiectomy (code 54690) is a unilateral procedure. The modifier –50 should be appended for a bilateral procedure (AMA 1997c, 21).

Coding Guidelines for Orchiectomy

The following guidelines apply to the coding of an orchiectomy:

- Codes 54520, 54522, 54530, and 54535 are used for open orchiectomy procedures.

- Partial orchiectomy code 54522 was added to describe the conservative removal of a benign epidermoid intratesticular cyst or other benign intratesticular tumor or cyst, such as a hamartoma or squamous epithelial cyst. Testicular epidermoid cysts are very rare, benign lesions that usually occur in early adult life. The procedure involves opening the testis tunica and carefully removing the lesion from the surrounding germinal substance. The pathologic tissue is sent to pathology to confirm its benign nature before the tunica is closed and the testis is replaced in the scrotum. This procedure enables testicular preservation.

- Code 54520 describes a complete removal of the testis performed for orchitis, prostatic cancer, chronic pain (orchalgia), trauma, or iatrogenic injury. Removal of malignant tumors is described by codes 54530 and 54535 (AMA 2000a).

Penile Prostheses

A penile prosthesis, or implant, is a device that is surgically placed into a man's body and is designed to help him achieve an erection.

Following are three types of penile prosthesis:

- Noninflatable semirigid implants are flexible rods implanted into the penis, one in each corpora cavernosa, or chamber. The rods are malleable so the penis is rigid enough for penetration, yet flexible enough that it can be moved into a position for concealment. The flexible rod is simply bent upward for intercourse and downward for concealment.

- Inflatable self-contained implants have no parts outside the penis. One cylinder is in each corporeal body, with no pump or reservoir outside the penis. The implant comprises two cylinders in one functional unit.

- Inflatable multicomponent implants contain at least two penile cylinders, one in each corporeal body and a pump placed in the scrotum. A reservoir also may be placed behind the muscles of the lower abdomen.

Coding Guidelines for Penile Prostheses

The following guidelines apply to the coding of penile prostheses:

- Code 54400, 54415, 54416, or 54417 is used for noninflatable (semirigid) implant or removal procedures.

- Codes 54401, 54415, 54416, and 54417 are applicable to inflatable (self-contained) implant or removal procedures.

- Codes 54405, 54406, 54408, 54410, and 54411 are assigned for multicomponent inflatable implant removal and repair procedures.

Laterality Status of Urinary CPT Codes

Several urinary CPT codes are considered either unilateral or bilateral. For unilateral codes, the modifier –50 may be required (AMA 2001c; 2001e; 2001b).

- Modifier –50 should not be appended to the following codes, which are considered to be inherently bilateral procedures: 52000, 52010, 52204–52285, 52305–52318.

- The following codes contain the language "unilateral or bilateral" in the code descriptor, so modifier –50 should not be appended: 52290, 52300, and 52301.

- Code 52005 identifies a singular, unilateral ureteral catheterization by use of the language "with ureteral catheterization." Thus, modifier –50 should be reported with this code when a cystoscopy with bilateral ureteral catheterization is performed.

- When bilateral ureteral stents are placed, bilateral procedure modifier –50 should be appended to code 52332.

- Codes 52005, 52007, and 52320–52355 are most often performed unilaterally. To identify the additional work required when the procedure is performed bilaterally, modifier –50 should be appended.

- When endoscopic visualization of the urinary system involves several regions (for example, kidney, renal pelvis, calyx, and ureter), the appropriate CPT code is defined by the approach (for example, nephrostomy, pyelostomy, ureterostomy, and so on) as indicated in the CPT descriptor. When multiple endoscopic approaches are simultaneously necessary to accomplish a medically necessary service (for example, renal endoscopy through a nephrostomy and cystourethroscopy performed at the same session), they may be separately coded with the multiple procedure modifier –51 on the less extensive codes. When multiple endoscopic approaches are necessary to accomplish the same procedure, the successful endoscopic approach should be reported (NCCI 2007).

The following CPT codes would be appropriate to use with modifier –50 when performing a bilateral procedure.

50020–50290	Kidney (incision and excision categories)
50390–50405	Kidney (introduction and repair categories)
50541–50548	Kidney (laparoscopy)
50551–50580	Kidney (endoscopy)
50590	Kidney (lithotripsy)
50605–50630	Ureter (incision)
50740–50760	Ureter (repair)
50780–50840	Ureter (repair)
50860–50940	Ureter (repair)
50945–50980	Ureter (laparoscopic and endoscopic categories)
52005–52010	Endoscopy—Cystoscopy, Urethroscopy, and Cystourethroscopy
52320–52355	Ureter and Pelvis
54500–54560	Testes (excision)
54640–54680	Testes (repair)
54690–54692	Testes (laparoscopy)
54700–54840	Epididymis (incision)
55400	Vas Deferens (repair)
55500–55550	Spermatic cord (excision and laparoscopy categories)

Case Studies

This section contains actual operative reports from real-life cases. All identifiers have been removed or changed for confidentiality and privacy.

Carefully read the clinical documentation for each case study, which may include a procedure report as well as radiology and/or pathology reports, as applicable.

Answer all the questions for further review at the end of each case study. Use a current CPT codebook or HCPCS Level II code listing, as needed.

When appropriate, assign one or more of the following modifiers:

–50	Bilateral Procedure
–59	Distinct Procedural Service
–FA	Left hand, thumb
–F1	Left hand, second digit
–F2	Left hand, third digit
–F3	Left hand, fourth digit
–F4	Left hand, fifth digit
–F5	Right hand, thumb
–F6	Right hand, second digit
–F7	Right hand, third digit
–F8	Right hand, fourth digit
–F9	Right hand, fifth digit
–LT	Left side
–RT	Right side
–TA	Left foot, great toe
–T1	Left foot, second digit
–T2	Left foot, third digit
–T3	Left foot, fourth digit
–T4	Left foot, fifth digit
–T5	Right foot, great toe
–T6	Right foot, second digit
–T7	Right foot, third digit
–T8	Right foot, fourth digit
–T9	Right foot, fifth digit

Do not apply the current version of the Medicare CCI edits to any of these exercises; the focus is on the application of the coding guidelines and not on the application of edits that change on a quarterly basis. When coding in real life, of course, you will need to apply the CCI edits as appropriate for Medicare outpatient cases.

Case Study 8.1

Read the following clinical document and answer the questions for further review.

OPERATIVE REPORT

ASSISTANT: None

PREOPERATIVE DIAGNOSIS: Bilateral ureteral obstruction

POSTOPERATIVE DIAGNOSIS: Bilateral ureteral obstruction

OPERATION: Cystoscopy and bilateral stent change

PROCEDURE/FINDINGS: Under general anesthesia, the patient was placed in the lithotomy position and prepped and draped in the usual fashion. The cystoscopy was remarkable for bladder erythema. The right stent was grasped and brought through the metal opening. An attempt was made to pass a guide wire, but this was not possible. A stent was placed over the guide wire to the midureter. Contrast was injected. After numerous manipulations, the guide wire was finally manipulated into the renal pelvis. A #620 double-J stent was placed with good position by fluoroscopy. The left stent was removed. The guide wire was placed. A #822 double-J stent was placed without difficulty with good position by fluoroscopy.

The procedure was tolerated well. The patient was given Zyvox® preoperatively.

Questions for Further Review: Case Study 8.1

1. What type of endoscopy was performed?
   a. Cystoscopy
   b. Ureteroscopy
   c. Both of the above

2. What type of procedure was performed?

3. Was the procedure unilateral or bilateral?
   a. Unilateral
   b. Bilateral

4. CPT surgery code(s) and modifier(s):

Case Study 8.2

Read the following clinical document and answer the questions for further review.

OPERATIVE REPORT

PREOPERATIVE DIAGNOSIS: Bladder lesion in an HIV-positive patient

POSTOPERATIVE DIAGNOSIS: Bladder lesion in an HIV-positive patient

OPERATION: Transurethral resection of bladder tumor, small

PROCEDURE/FINDINGS: The patient was placed on the operating table in the dorsal lithotomy position. The genitalia were prepped and draped in the standard sterile surgical fashion. The lesion was noted on the floor of the bladder inferior to the left intereureteric ridge and had an appearance of basal cell carcinoma of the skin, although a little bit more translucent and was about 6 mm in diameter and raised about 5 mm. No other lesions were present. With the resectoscope and one deep swipe, this was resected off. The tissue underneath looked fairly normal as far as musculature. I did not feel like doing a further resection because it just did not appear to be an invasive neoplasm in this setting. If indeed it is, I will have to go back and do a much more thorough job, but the problem is that the intramural ureter sits right next to it.

We produced satisfactory coagulation. No untoward problems. The bladder was emptied. I did not feel that I needed a catheter.

The patient returned to the recovery room in satisfactory condition with no untoward problems.

SURGICAL PATHOLOGY RESULT REPORT

AGE/SEX: 33/M

SPEC TYPE: Surgical P

PREOPERATIVE DIAGNOSIS: Small bladder tumor

OPERATIVE PROCEDURE: Transurethral resection, bladder

DATE: XXXX

GROSS DESCRIPTION: Received labeled bladder tumor. The specimen consists of a nodule of a rubbery, firm, pink-tan tissue measuring 0.5 x 0.3 x 0.2 cm in greatest dimensions. All blocked.

PATHOLOGY PROCEDURES: Path DLG, ABXX3

FINAL DIAGNOSIS: Bladder, TUR: Chronic cystitis with overlying urothelial hyperplasia with reactive atypia. No definitive evidence of neoplasm identified.

Questions for Further Review: Case Study 8.2

1. What type of endoscopy was performed?
   a. Cystoscopy
   b. Ureteroscopy
   c. Both of the above

2. What type of procedure was performed?

3. What was the size of the bladder lesion in centimeters?

4. CPT surgery code(s) and modifier(s):

Case Study 8.3

Read the following clinical document and answer the questions for further review.

OPERATIVE REPORT

PREOPERATIVE DIAGNOSIS: Right ureteral obstruction

POSTOPERATIVE DIAGNOSIS: Same secondary to right ureteral calculus

OPERATION: Cystoscopy, right retrograde pyelogram; ureteroscopy; insertion of JJ stent

PROCEDURE: The patient was placed on the operating table and after successful induction of general anesthesia was prepped and draped in the usual sterile fashion. Cystoscopy was done first, and a right ureteral catheter was inserted in the right ureter. Through the right ureteral catheter, contrast was inserted and an obstruction of the right ureter just above the sacrum was seen. An attempt to pass guide wire was made with some difficulty, and the guide wire was passed beyond the obstruction, which appeared to be that of a calculus. Having passed the guide wire, it was then possible to dilate the ureteral orifice, and a ureteroscope was put in place after the ureteral orifice was dilated. The ureteroscope could only be passed into the distal ureter. The diameter of the ureter was narrow, and it was not felt warranted or possible to insert the ureter beyond the distal ureter safely, so further attempts at ureteroscopy were deferred. Instead of 5 French, a 24-cm JJ ureteral catheter was put over the guide wire into the renal pelvis and brought out into the bladder. The bladder was drained, and the patient was taken to the recovery room in good condition.

Questions for Further Review: Case Study 8.3

1. What type of endoscopy was performed?
   a. Cystoscopy
   b. Ureteroscopy
   c. Both of the above
   d. Pyeloscopy

2. What type of procedure was performed?

3. Was the procedure(s) unilateral or bilateral?
   a. Unilateral
   b. Bilateral

4. CPT surgery code(s) and modifier(s):

Case Study 8.4

Read the following clinical document and answer the questions for further review.

OPERATIVE REPORT

AGE: 51

OPERATION: Cystoscopy, retrograde pyelogram, ureteroscopy, insertion of double-J stent, and extracorporeal shock wave lithotripsy

ANESTHESIA: General

PREOPERATIVE DIAGNOSIS: Right caliceal diverticulum with six calculi and distal right ureteral calculus

POSTOPERATIVE DIAGNOSIS: Caliceal diverticulum with six calculi

OPERATIVE INDICATIONS: This female presented with a history of right-sided flank pain. Investigations, including an IVP and CT scan, demonstrated presence of a cystic cavity of a caliceal diverticulum or a focal caliectasis, with six calculi and presence of a possible distal right ureteral calculus. The risks and benefits to the above procedures were explained, and the patient elected to proceed.

OPERATIVE PROCEDURE: Under adequate general anesthesia with endotracheal intubation and appropriate lines and monitoring devices, the patient was initially placed in the lithotomy position and prepped and draped in the usual manner. Intravenous ampicillin and gentamicin were administered. Cystoscopy was performed, which failed to identify any bladder pathology. The right ureteral orifice was slightly gaping but appeared otherwise unremarkable. The right retrograde pyelography was performed under fluoroscopy, which failed to confirm one way or another whether there was a distal ureteral calculus. For this reason, ureteroscopy was performed with the semirigid scope. The ureteroscopy was performed to the level of the pelvic brim using the 6/7.5 French semirigid Wolf ureteroscope. Following that, the disposable ureteroscopic sheath was advanced under fluoroscopic control up to the edge of the kidney, and flexible nephroscopy was performed in an attempt to identify the opening between the caliceal diverticulum or the focal caliectasis. Despite excellent visualization within the kidney, the connection to the cavity containing the stones could not be visualized. The ureteroscope was removed, leaving a 0.38 wire in its place followed by removal of the working sheath. A 7 French, 26-cm double-J stent was placed under fluoroscopic control, and the position was confirmed fluoroscopically within the kidney and in the bladder. This completed the cystoscopic portion. The bladder was drained, and the patient was repositioned for extracorporeal shock wave lithotripsy. The head of the Storz lithotripter was positioned, and the position of the stone was confirmed in two planes. The lithotripsy was then commenced using a setting of 17 kilovolts. A total of 3,000 shocks were delivered to the kidney. There were no complications from the procedure. The patient tolerated the procedure extremely well and was transferred to the recovery room in stable and satisfactory condition.

Questions for Further Review: Case Study 8.4

1. What type of endoscopy was performed?
   a. Cystoscopy
   b. Ureteroscopy
   c. Pyeloscopy
   d. All of the above

2. Which of the following procedures was performed?
   a. Removal of ureteral calculus
   b. Removal of urethral calculus
   c. Fragmentation of ureteral calculus
   d. Fragmentation of urethral calculus
   e. Treatment of ureteral stricture
   f. Treatment of ureteropelvic junction stricture
   g. Treatment of intrarenal stricture
   h. Lithotripsy
   i. Electroshock wave lithotripsy
   j. Biopsy of lesion
   k. Resection of lesion

3. Ureteral catheterization was performed.
   a. True
   b. False

4. Insertion of ureteral stent was performed.
   a. True
   b. False

5. CPT surgery code(s) and modifier(s):

Case Study 8.5

Read the following clinical document and answer the questions for further review.

OPERATIVE REPORT

PREOPERATIVE DIAGNOSIS: Question recurrent ureteropelvic junction obstruction

OPERATION: Cystoscopy, retrograde ureteroscopy, balloon dilation of ureteropelvic junction obstruction following prior incisional treatment and placement of stent

POSTOPERATIVE DIAGNOSIS: Recurrent ureteropelvic junction obstruction

INDICATIONS: This is an 86-year-old female who had symptomatic left ureteropelvic junction obstruction. After discussing all the options, she elected retrograde endopyelotomy for six months or so. She has had an excellent result but has redeveloped symptoms. Lasix diuretic scan does reveal equivocal obstruction of the left side. Her symptoms have improved, but we elected to assess this and possibly assess the ureteropelvic junction.

PROCEDURE: After sterile prep and drape, the cystoscopy was performed in the dorsal lithotomy position. A left-sided retrograde pyelogram was performed after a guide wire passed easily into the left kidney. There was some mild narrowing and dilation of the left collecting system. The 7.5-French flexible ureteroscope passed easily into the kidney, however. There was some mild narrowing at the ureteropelvic junction and a large hydronephrotic left kidney. There might have been a small amount of narrowing, but fundamentally there was a clear opening at the ureteropelvic junction. We decided at this point to balloon dilate with a 7-mm balloon of a total of 10 minutes. Follow-up ureteroscopy revealed the UPJ to be patent.

Contrast did drain well from the kidney when we were completed. We will see her in follow-up. She tolerated the procedure well.

Questions for Further Review: Case Study 8.5

1. What type(s) of endoscopy was performed?
   a. Cystoscopy
   b. Ureteroscopy
   c. Pyeloscopy
   d. All of the above

2. Which of the following procedures was performed?
   a. Removal of ureteral calculus
   b. Removal of urethral calculus
   c. Fragmentation of ureteral calculus
   d. Fragmentation of urethral calculus
   e. Treatment of ureteral stricture
   f. Treatment of ureteropelvic junction stricture
   g. Treatment of intrarenal stricture
   h. Lithotripsy
   i. Electroshock wave lithotripsy
   j. Biopsy of lesion
   k. Resection of lesion

3. Ureteral catheterization was performed.
   a. True
   b. False

4. Insertion of ureteral stent was performed.
   a. True
   b. False

5. CPT surgery code(s) and modifier(s):

Case Study 8.6

Read the following clinical document and answer the questions for further review.

OPERATIVE REPORT

PREOPERATIVE DIAGNOSIS: Right vesicoureteral reflux

OPERATION: Cystoscopy and coaptite injection

POSTOPERATIVE DIAGNOSIS: Right vesicoureteral reflux

ANESTHESIA: General endotracheal

COMPLICATIONS: None

INDICATIONS: The patient is a 7-year-old girl with a history of right grade 3 vesicoureteral reflux. The diagnosis, potential sequelae, treatment options, risks, and complications were discussed with her parents, and the decision was made to proceed with coaptite injection.

PROCEDURE: The patient underwent smooth induction of general anesthesia and was placed in low dorsal lithotomy position. The genitalia were prepped and draped in sterile fashion. The genitalia were normal in appearance. Cystoscopy was performed with a 14-French sheath using the 0-degree lens. The urethra was patent. Bilateral ureteral orifices were slightly displaced laterally with slight patulous right orifice. Bladder mucosa was smooth without brachial remnant. The Williams needle was advanced into the sumacs under the right ureteral orifice and 0.4 cc were injected with nice elevation of the mucosa, creating a mound under the orifice. There was urinary efflux from the orifice after the procedure. An intraoperative cryptogram showed no evidence of reflux. The patient tolerated the procedure without complications and returned to recovery in good condition. Sponge and instrument counts were correct.

Questions for Further Review: Case Study 8.6

1. What type of endoscopy was performed?
   a. Cystoscopy
   b. Ureteroscopy
   c. Pyeloscopy
   d. All of the above

2. Which of the following procedures was performed?
   a. Endoscopic injection of implant material into the submucosal tissues of the urethra and/or bladder neck
   b. Endoscopic subureteric injection of implant material

3. How should the surgical component of the intraoperative cystogram be coded?
   a. Code 51600, Injection procedure for cystography or voiding urethrocystography
   b. Code 51610, Injection procedure for retrograde urethrocystography
   4. CPT surgery code(s) and modifier(s):

Case Study 8.7

Read the following clinical document and answer the questions for further review.

OPERATIVE REPORT

PREOPERATIVE DIAGNOSIS: History of microhematuria and right ureteral stricture

OPERATION: Right ureteroscopy with ureteral dilation and right ureteral stent placement

POSTOPERATIVE DIAGNOSIS: History of microhematuria and right ureteral stricture

ANESTHESIA: General anesthesia

ESTIMATED BLOOD LOSS: Minimal

COMPLICATIONS: None

FINDINGS: Circumferential distal right ureteral stricture. No mucosal abnormalities were apparent at the time of operation. Anterior and posterior urethra were within normal limits. Bladder neck was high. The right and left ureteral orifices were normal in appearance and location. There was 1+ bladder trabeculation.

INDICATIONS: A 70-year-old male with a history of microhematuria. IVP was performed, which revealed a right distal ureteral stricture. Cystoscopy was performed, which revealed prostatic enlargement. Procedure involving right ureteroscopy, possibly biopsy, and stricture dilatation was fully explained to the patient. The patient is aware of risks and alternatives, and desires to proceed.

TECHNICAL DESCRIPTION: The patient was brought to the operating room, where general anesthesia was induced. The patient was placed in the dorsal lithotomy position and prepped and draped in the normal sterile fashion. A 21-French rigid cystoscope sheath with a 25-degree lens was inserted per urethra into the patient's bladder. A cone-tipped catheter could not be passed up the right ureteral orifice. A 6-French access catheter could not be advanced up the ureteral orifice as well. A 0.035-guide wire was advanced through the right ureteral orifice. This was performed under fluoroscopic guidance. The 6-French access catheter was placed over the wire, and this was quite tight. The guide wire was placed up to the renal pelvis, confirmed by fluoroscopy. The access catheter was removed. The cystoscope was removed from the patient's bladder. The guidewire was secured as our safety wire. We decided to dilate the right distal ureter. A UroMax ureteral dilating balloon was placed at the right ureteral orifice under direct vision with the cystoscope. The distal ureter was dilated to 18 atmospheres of pressure. This was held for approximately two to three minutes. The UroMax dilating balloon was deflated and removed. The cystoscope was removed.

A MICRO-6 semirigid ureteroscope was advanced along the guide wire to the right ureteral orifice. We quickly encountered a circumferential ureteral stricture. There were no obvious mucosal abnormalities at this point. We decided to reinsert the UroMax ureteral dilating balloon to dilate the stricture. The MICRO-6 ureteroscope was removed from the patient's bladder. The UroMax dilating balloon was passed over the guide wire to the point where the stricture was encountered. The stricture was dilated. A waste was seen on the fluoroscopic images, and this was seen to pop open.

Pressure was held for approximately two to three minutes, and then the balloon was deflated and the UroMax was withdrawn. The MICRO-6 was reinserted per urethra up the right ureteral orifice. At this point, we encountered a through-and-through ureteral tear. Periureteric fat was seen. We attempted to place a 7.5-French flexible ureteroscope over the wire, which could not be accomplished. Therefore, we decided to place a right ureteral stent. The guide wire was backloaded onto the cystoscope. The cystoscope was reinserted into the patient's bladder, visualizing the right ureteral orifice. A 7-French by 26-cm right ureteral stent was advanced up the guide wire to the renal pelvis under fluoroscopic guidance. The wire was removed. Good curl was seen proximally in the renal pelvis. Good curl was also seen distally in the bladder. All instrumentation was removed at this point. A 16-French Foley catheter was inserted into the patient's bladder without difficulty. This irrigated well. This was hooked to dependent drainage. The patient's urinary output at the end of the case was pink in color. The patient tolerated the procedure well and was awakened from anesthesia. He was transferred to the PACU in good condition. Dr. B. was present, participating, and available for postoperative questioning.

Questions for Further Review: Case Study 8.7

1. What type(s) of endoscopy was performed?
   a. Cystoscopy
   b. Ureteroscopy
   c. Pyeloscopy
   d. All of the above

2. Which of the following procedures was performed?
   a. Removal of ureteral calculus
   b. Removal of urethral calculus
   c. Fragmentation of ureteral calculus
   d. Fragmentation of urethral calculus
   e. Treatment of ureteral stricture
   f. Treatment of ureteropelvic junction stricture
   g. Treatment of intrarenal stricture
   h. Lithotripsy
   i. Electroshock wave lithotripsy
   j. Biopsy of lesion
   k. Resection of lesion

3. Ureteral catheterization was performed.
   a. True
   b. False

4. Insertion of ureteral stent was performed.
   a. True
   b. False

5. CPT surgery code(s) and modifier(s):

Case Study 8.8

Read the following clinical document and answer the questions for further review.

OPERATIVE NOTE

AGE/SEX: 46/M

PREOPERATIVE DIAGNOSIS: Right testicular mass

OPERATION:

1. Testicular ultrasound
2. Partial orchiectomy

POSTOPERATIVE DIAGNOSIS: Right testicular mass

ANESTHESIA: General

COMPLICATIONS: None

INDICATIONS: This is a white male with azoospermia. During his evaluation, he was found to have a hypoechoic area in his right testicle. He also has a significant amount of microlithiasis. There is concern this is a testicular tumor. It does have blood flow. After consenting the patient for partial or possible total orchiectomy and agreeing to a scrotal approach, we took the patient to the operating room.

PROCEDURE: He was placed in the supine position and prepped and draped in the usual sterile fashion. Palpation of the testicle when the patient relaxed demonstrated no obvious firmness or masses. A small midline raphe incision was made. This was carried down to the right testicle, and the right testicle was delivered. It was noted to be only 4 x 3 mm in size. Intraoperative ultrasound was then used to localize the mass. A marker was used to delineate the edges of the lesion. It was not noted to be close to the testicular vessels. We then performed a partial orchiectomy excising this lesion. I sent two frozen sections of this lesion off to Pathology. Examination there revealed a number of atrophic seminiferous tubules with no evidence of testicular cancer. Approximately half the specimen was sampled by frozen analysis, the other half sent for permanent analysis. Given these results and the fact it was nonpalpable, as well as negative markers, we then elected to close. This ultrasound lesion was excised. Hemostasis was checked. The tunica was closed with a 3-0 running Vicryl. The dartos was then closed with a 3-0 running chromic. Several 4-0 interrupted chromic stitches were placed in the skin. The patient tolerated the procedure without complications. He was awakened and returned to the recovery room in stable condition.

SURGIGAL PATH REPORT

AGE/SEX: 46/M

SOURCE OF TISSUE:

1. Testicular biopsy (1FS-1)
2. Right testicular biopsy (2FS-1)
3. Right testicular mass

GROSS: Specimen 1 labeled "testicular biopsy" consists of a 0.7 x 0.6 x 0.3 cm, rubbery, tan piece of tissue. All tissue is submitted for frozen section as 1FS-1.

Specimen 2 labeled "right testicular biopsy" consists of a 0.6 x 0.4 x 0.3 cm, rubbery, tan piece of tissue. All tissue is submitted for frozen section as 2FS-1.

Specimen 3 labeled "right testicular mass" consists of three rubbery, pink-to-purple, glistening irregular fragments of tissue varying from 0.5–1.0 cm in maximum dimension. All tissue is submitted in one cassette.

FROZEN SECTION DIAGNOSIS:

1FS-1 negative for carcinoma

2FS-1 atrophied tubules with calcification; negative for carcinoma

(All confirmed on paraffin sections)

MICROSCOPIC: The microscopic findings support the diagnosis given below.

FINAL DIAGNOSIS: Right testicle: Excisional biopsy: Atrophic tubules with focal microcalcification and increased fibrovascular soft tissue (See note.)

NOTE: PAS and PLAP immunostain were performed to rule out the possibility of a burned-out seminoma. However, these stains were negative for any residual intratubular germ cell neoplasia or seminoma.

This case was reviewed by several staff pathologists who agree with the diagnosis

Questions for Further Review: Case Study 8.8

1. What type of orchiectomy was performed?
   a. Simple orchiectomy with testicular prosthesis
   b. Simple orchiectomy without testicular prosthesis
   c. Partial orchiectomy
   d. Radical orchiectomy, inguinal approach
   e. Radical orchiectomy, abdominal approach

2. Was the procedure unilateral or bilateral?
   a. Unilateral
   b. Bilateral

3. CPT surgery code(s) and modifier(s):

Case Study 8.9

Read the following clinical document and answer the questions for further review.

OPERATIVE NOTE

AGE/SEX: 41/M

PREOPERATIVE DIAGNOSIS: Desire for permanent sterilization

OPERATION: Bilateral vasectomy

POSTOPERATIVE DIAGNOSIS: Desire for permanent sterilization

ANESTHESIA: Monitored anesthetic care

INDICATIONS: This is a 41-year-old gentleman who was seen in clinic as a potential vasectomy candidate. On examination his scrotum was felt to be relatively tight. It was very difficult to define his vas adequately. After discussion of the risks, benefits, and possible complications, it was decided to proceed to the operating room to perform this under intravenous sedation.

PROCEDURE: The patient was taken to the operative suite and placed in the supine position. After appropriate monitoring equipment was attached, he underwent adequate sedation. His genitalia were prepped and draped in the usual sterile manner. Attention was turned to the left vas deferens, which was isolated from surrounding cord structures. Local anesthetic consisting of 0.25% lidocaine plain was instilled in the skin and surrounding tissue. A puncture wound was made and the vas deferens was encircled, dissected free from surrounding structures, and doubly clamped and ligated. The lumen was cauterized using electrocautery. The distal end was tied using a Vicryl tie. The proximal end was oversewn using a chromic suture. There was no active bleeding. Attention was then turned to the right side, and in a similar fashion the vas deferens was identified. The skin was anesthetized and a puncture wound made. The vas deferens was encircled, dissected free from surrounding structures, and doubly clamped and divided. The lumen again was electrocauterized. The distal end was tied with a Vicryl tie and the proximal end was oversewn with a chromic suture. Again, no active bleeding was identified. At the conclusion of the case there was meticulous hemostasis. The vas deferens was retracted back into the scrotum, and postoperative bandages were placed. The patient was awakened from anesthesia and taken to the recovery room in stable condition. There were no complications.

Dr. B. was scrubbed and present throughout the entire case and available for postprocedural care.

Questions for Further Review: Case Study 8.9

1. What type of procedure was performed on the vas deferens?
   a. Vasotomy
   b. Vasovasostomy
   c. Percutaneous suture ligation
   d. Vasectomy

2. Was the procedure unilateral or bilateral?
   a. Unilateral
   b. Bilateral

3. The correct CPT code and modifier is 55250–50. Explain your answer.
   a. True
   b. False

   Explanation:

Case Study 8.10

Read the following clinical document and answer the questions for further review.

OPERATIVE NOTE

AGE/SEX: 55/M

PREOPERATIVE DIAGNOSIS: Adenocarcinoma of the prostate, Gleason 3 + 3, PSA 3.4

OPERATION: Ultrasound and template-guided iodine-125 transperineal implantation of the prostate

POSTOPERATIVE DIAGNOSIS: Adenocarcinoma of the prostate, Gleason 3 + 3, PSA 3.4

ANESTHESIA: Spinal

INDICATIONS: Patient is a 55-year-old gentleman recently diagnosed with adenocarcinoma of the prostate. After considering his various treatment options, he elected to undergo a radioactive seed implant of the prostate. This was carried out as described below.

PROCEDURE: The patient was brought to the operating room. Spinal anesthesia was induced, and the patient was placed in a lithotomy position on the operating table. The perineum was prepped and draped in the usual sterile fashion. A 12-French Foley catheter was inserted into the bladder, and 6 cc of sterile saline was injected into the balloon, as well as 60 cc of saline into the bladder. The scrotum was elevated onto the abdominal wall, and Venodyne stockings were placed over the patient's legs. Then 500 mg of ciprofloxacin was injected IV. Transrectal scanning was carried out at a frequency of 6 megahertz. When the image on the monitor correlated with the ultrasound volume study images, the transducer was anchored to the operating room table using a stabilizing device.

Beginning with the superior-most part of the prostate, implant needles were passed through predetermined apertures in the template and advanced toward the preselected ultrasound image planes, according to the planning worksheet. When the needle tips reached their correct coordinates and planes, the stylets were held stationary while the needle hubs were withdrawn. This left seeds and spacers in the prostate in the predetermined locations. A total of 18 needles were initially used.

Simulation was carried out using ultrasound scanning, and this indicated several potential gaps in coverage. A total of 6 additional needles containing 10 additional seeds were used. The total number of seeds in the implant was 91; each had an activity of 0.43 millicuries, for a total implant activity of 39.13 millicuries. The planned prescription dose was 150 gray.

Dr. B. fully participated in the procedure, including the transperineal placement of the seeds into the prostate. The patient tolerated the procedure well and was transferred directly to a hospital room for temporary admission. The Foley catheter was removed, and he was able to freely urinate and was discharged several hours later.

DISCHARGE MEDICATIONS:

1. Ciprofloxacin 250 mg b.i.d. x 10 days
2. Flomax 0.4 mg per day
3. Pyridium 200 mg t.i.d. p.r.n.

   The patient will return for follow-up in one month, at which time a post implant CT scan will be carried out for dosimetry verification purposes.

Questions for Further Review: Case Study 8.10

1. Was a cystoscopy performed?
   a. Yes
   b. No

2. Which of the following procedures was performed on the prostate?
   a. Prostatectomy
   b. Prostate biopsy
   c. Exposure of prostate for insertion of radioactive substance
   d. Transperineal placement of needles or catheters into prostate for interstitial radioelement application

3. How many needles were used in total?
   a. 18
   b. 24
   c. 6

4. How many seeds were implanted in total?
   a. 18
   b. 24
   c. 91
   d. 10

5. Which of the following codes classify this case?
   a. 55875
   b. 55875 and 76965

6. Which of the following pass-through device codes are needed for the seeds and needles?
   a. C1715 (brachytherapy needle)
   b. C1728 (catheter, brachytherapy seed administration)
   c. Both of the above

Case Study 8.11

Read the following clinical document and answer the questions for further review.

OPERATIVE REPORT

PREOPERATIVE DIAGNOSIS: Impotence

OPERATION: Malleable prosthesis placement

POSTOPERATIVE DIAGNOSIS: Same

ANESTHESIA: General endotracheal

ESTIMATED BLOOD LOSS: Less than 100 cc

IMPLANT: AMS 13 mm x 19 cm prosthesis with extenders

INDICATIONS: The patient is a 58-year-old man status post a radical prostatectomy. He has had problems with impotence. He is not satisfied with intracavernosal injections and is requesting placement of a malleable penile prosthesis.

PROCEDURE: After obtaining informed consent, the patient was brought to the operating room and placed on the operating table in the supine position. He underwent induction of general endotracheal anesthesia without complication. He had already been started on preoperative oral antibiotics and received IV antibiotics prior to the incision. The patient was prepped and draped in the usual fashion. A 16 French Foley catheter was placed, with 5 cc placed in the balloon and the catheter clamped.

A scrotal mid-raphe incision was made. This was carried down through dartos fascia and subcutaneous tissues in a hemostatic fashion. Both right and left corpora were dissected out. Stay sutures with 2-0 Prolene were placed, and an approximately 2- to 3-cm corporotomy was made bilaterally. These were dilated to 39 French or 13 mm distally and proximally. The right was measured to be 6 distally and 13 proximally; the left was measured to be 7 distally and 12 proximally.

Copious amounts of antibiotic solution were used to irrigate the corporal incisions. An AMS malleable prosthesis was used, 13 mm by 19 cm, and 3-cm extenders were placed. The prosthesis was then placed. This appeared to be slightly too short and 2-cm extenders were placed at the end of the 3-cm extenders and this proved to be the appropriate length, with a nice result.

The corporotomies were closed with running 2-0 Prolene suture. Dartos and subcutaneous tissues were reapproximated with running 3-0 Vicryl suture and the skin closed with a running 4-0 Vicryl subcuticular suture. The wound was cleaned and dried. Antibiotic ointment was applied. A Tegaderm dressing was applied. The penis was wrapped with Coban. The Foley catheter was unclamped, the bladder was drained and the Foley catheter removed.

The patient was awakened, extubated, and taken to the recovery room in satisfactory condition. Estimated blood loss was less than 100 cc. There were no complications.

Questions for Further Review: Case Study 8.11

1. What type of penile prosthesis was inserted?
   a. Noninflatable (semirigid)
   b. Inflatable (self-contained)
   c. Multicomponent inflatable

2. CPT surgery code(s) and modifier(s):

Case Study 8.12

Read the following clinical document and answer the questions for further review.

OPERATIVE REPORT

AGE: 59

OPERATION: Penile prosthesis implantation

ANESTHESIA: General endotracheal anesthesia

OPERATIVE INDICATIONS: The patient is a 59-year-old male with a recently diagnosed organic impotence. The patient has been on testosterone with no improvement in symptoms. The patient presents for elective prosthesis insertion: AMS 700 implant.

OPERATIVE PROCEDURE: The patient was taken to the operative suite after informed consent was obtained and was given general endotracheal anesthesia per the anesthesiologist. The patient was then placed in the lithotomy position in stirrups and prepped and draped in the usual sterile fashion. A ten-minute scrub was initiated. The patient's genitalia were shaved clean of any hair or foreign debris. After a prep of ten minutes, the patient was draped in the usual sterile fashion.

A Foley catheter was inserted. Urine was drained from the bladder. The Foley catheter was then plugged. This was a size #18 French Foley catheter. Next, the penoscrotal junction was identified and a 4-cm incision was made longitudinally along the penile shaft. The subcutaneous tissues were then dissected and the dartos fascia was separated down to the level of Buck's fascia. Buck's fascia was then opened and the corpora cavernosa were identified. A corporotomy approximately 2 centimeters long was made into the left corpora with special attention not to make the incision close to the urethra. This incision was made parallel to the urethra. The Hegar dilators were used to dilate the patient's corpora cavernosa approximately to #14 French and distally to #12 French. Upon adequate dilation, measurement was obtained. This revealed a measurement of 8 centimeters distally and 7 centimeters proximally. This was recorded. Next, a corporotomy was made in the same fashion on the opposite corpora. This was dilated to #14 French proximally and #12 French distally. Measurements were obtained and revealed 9 centimeters distally and 8 centimeters proximally.

It was decided that a 15-cm prosthesis would be used. The prosthesis was removed from its package and flushed for any air bubbles. The prosthesis was kept in antibiotic solution. Next, the corpora were thoroughly irrigated. The right prosthesis was then inserted and tested. Upon achieving adequate tumescence, it was deflated and corporotomy was then closed using #2-0 PDS suture. The opposite corpus was irrigated once again and the prosthesis was placed to the left corpora. It was decided that a 1-cm extension would be used on the right corpora and a 2-cm extension on the left corpora. This achieved maximum tumescence without any curvature.

Once again, the left prosthesis was inflated and tested. This was then deflated and the corporotomy closed in the repeat fashion using #2-0 PDS. The wound was then irrigated. Once again, a pouch was made for the reservoir. The reservoir was inserted. Next, the pouch was made into the scrotum for the pump mechanism. The pump mechanism was designed to connect to the reservoir, which sits in the retropubic space. These then were connected to the corporal prostheses. The device was then connected using connectors in the standard fashion as described by the manufacturer.

The dartos fascia was then reapproximated using #3-0 Vicryl suture over the prosthesis tubing. Upon completely enclosing the prosthesis under the dartos fascia, the skin was reapproximated using #4-0 Vicryl suture in a subcuticular fashion. Collodion was then applied to the wound. A dry sterile dressing was applied. The Foley was kept in place and connected to a bag. The patient had a scrotal support in place and the penis was in the semierect position up on the abdomen. The patient was then awakened from anesthesia and taken to the recovery room where he will be subsequently be transferred to the floor. The Foley will be removed on postoperative day one and the patient may go home on antibiotics. The patient was in good condition at the time of completion of the surgery.

Questions for Further Review: Case Study 8.12

1. What type of penile prosthesis was inserted?
    a. Noninflatable (semirigid)
    b. Inflatable (self-contained)
    c. Multicomponent inflatable

2. CPT surgery code(s) and modifier(s):

Case Study 8.13

Read the following clinical document and answer the questions for further review.

OPERATIVE REPORT

PREOPERATIVE DIAGNOSIS: History of urethral perforation with placement of penile prosthesis, with subsequent abandonment of placement of left cylinder

OPERATION: Revision of inflatable penile prosthesis with placement of a left corporal cylinder and repositioning of inflatable penile prosthesis pump

POSTOPERATIVE DIAGNOSIS: History of urethral perforation with placement of penile prosthesis, with subsequent abandonment of placement of left cylinder

ANESTHESIA: General endotracheal

ESTIMATED BLOOD LOSS: Minimal

DRAINS: None

SPECIMENS: None

COMPLICATIONS: None

INDICATIONS: The patient is a 71-year-old white male, who was status post placement of an inflatable penile prosthesis three months ago at another facility. At that time, the procedure was complicated by a urethral perforation with attempted placement of the left cylinder. The patient was brought back to the operating room now for placement of the left penile cylinder, as well as repositioning of the pump lower in the scrotum. The patient received broad-spectrum intravenous antibiotics preoperatively.

PROCEDURE: The patient was brought to the operating room and adequate general endotracheal anesthesia was obtained. He was prepped and draped in the usual sterile fashion in the supine position. A transverse incision was made at the midpoint of the symphysis pubis and carried down through the subcutaneous tissue using cutting cautery. The tubing to both of the penile cylinders and to the scrotal pump was isolated and was dissected out using the cutting current on the cautery proximally and distally. We found the tubing, which was intended for the left cylinder and isolated it. Stay stitches were then placed laterally on the left corpora. The corpus was opened using a scalpel and Mayo scissors, and the corpora was dilated to 33 French using Hegar dilators. The corpus was calibrated to approximately 17–18 cm. In both calibration and dilation, care was taken throughout to stay lateral and dorsal on the penis to avoid injury to the urethra. After dilation and calibration, we selected a 15-cm cylinder with a 2-cm rear-tip extender. A Furlow passer was used to place the cylinder in the left corporal body. The corporotomy was closed using a running 2-0 Prolene suture. The tubing was reconnected using the right-angle connectors and 3-0 Prolene suture, after all air had been removed from the tubing with Hypaque contrast material. Prior to closure, the pump to the penile prosthesis, which was in the right hemiscrotum, was repositioned somewhat lower and secured in place with a 3-0 Prolene suture. The subcutaneous tissue was closed using a running 3-0 Vicryl suture and the skin was closed using a running 4-0 Vicryl subcuticular stitch. Antibiotic ointment and sterile dressings were applied. Ice packs were applied.

The patient was awakened, extubated, and transferred to the postanesthesia recovery room in good condition.

Questions for Further Review: Case Study 8.13

1. What type of penile prosthesis did the patient have?
    a.   Noninflatable (semirigid)
    b.   Inflatable (self-contained)
    c.   Multicomponent inflatable

2. What type of procedure was performed?
    a.   Removal of all components of a multicomponent inflatable penile prosthesis without replacement
    b.   Repair of component(s) of a multicomponent inflatable penile prosthesis
    c.   Removal and replacement of all components of a multicomponent inflatable penile prosthesis at the same operative session
    d.   Removal and replacement of noninflatable (semirigid) penile prosthesis at the same operative session
    e.   Removal and replacement of an inflatable (self-contained) penile prosthesis at the same operative session
    f.   Removal and replacement of all components of a multicomponent inflatable penile prosthesis, through an infected field, at the same operative session
    g.   Removal and replacement of all noninflatable (semirigid) penile prosthesis, through an infected field, at the same operative session
    h.   Removal and replacement of all components of an inflatable (self-contained) penile prosthesis, through an infected field, at the same operative session

3. CPT surgery code(s) and modifier(s):

Case Study 8.14

Read the following clinical document and answer the questions for further review.

OPERATIVE REPORT

PREOPERATIVE DIAGNOSIS: Penile prosthesis malfunction

OPERATION: Removal of three-piece inflatable penile prosthesis Insertion of three-piece inflatable penile prosthesis

POSTOPERATIVE DIAGNOSIS: Penile prosthesis malfunction

ANESTHESIA: General

ESTIMATED BLOOD LOSS: Minimal

COMPLICATIONS: None

FINDINGS: Tubing to the right corporal body implant was frayed.

INDICATIONS: The patient is a 50-year-old male with a history of erectile dysfunction secondary to diabetes mellitus. The patient is status post insertion of penile prosthesis, a three-piece inflatable, nine years ago. However, this first penile prosthesis broke in 1999 and was replaced. Recently, the penile prosthesis #2 has not been properly inflating. Procedure, alternatives, and risks were fully discussed involving repair and possible removal and replacement of the penile prosthesis.

TECHNICAL DESCRIPTION: The patient was brought to the operating room and placed supine on the operating table. General anesthesia was induced. The patient's lower abdomen, penis, and scrotum were all prepped and draped in a normal sterile fashion. The Pfannenstiel incision from the prior operation was incised with the cutting current. Dissection was continued down to the tubing. The pocket was exposed. The prosthesis was tested. Upon further observation, it was found that there was a fraying of the tubing to the right corporal body implant. At this point, it was decided that we would remove the penile prosthesis and replace it with a Mentor three-piece inflatable prosthesis. Electrocautery was used to enter the reservoir pocket. The old prosthesis was removed. Hemostasis was achieved with electrocautery. The new penile prosthesis was inserted with the use of a Keith needle in the prior tracks. A 16-cm with a 3 + 1 back end extension piece was used bilaterally. These were placed into their old operative sites. The reservoir filled with 60 cc of Omnipaque contrast and was repositioned into the old pocket. The pump was placed in the right hemiscrotum. All tubing was connected in a normal fashion in the correct order. Care was taken to remove all air bubbles from the contraption. Prolene suture was used to approximate the tunica albuginea of the corporal bodies. Prolene suture was used to pursestring the opening to the reservoir pocket. The area of operation was copiously irrigated with antibiotic solution. Hemostasis at the end of the case was excellent. The penile prosthesis was pumped up, and appropriate erection was obtained. The penile prosthesis was deflated approximately halfway. The incision was closed in three layers of absorbable suture. Subcuticular suture was used to approximate skin edges. The patient's incision was cleansed and dried. A sterile dressing was applied. The patient was awakened from general anesthesia and transferred to the PACU in good condition.

Dr. B. was present, participated, and was available for postoperative questioning.

Questions for Further Review: Case Study 8.14

1. What type of penile prosthesis did the patient have before the surgery started?
   a. Noninflatable (semirigid)
   b. Inflatable (self-contained)
   c. Multicomponent inflatable

2. What type of procedure was performed?
   a. Removal of all components of a multicomponent inflatable penile prosthesis without replacement
   b. Repair of component(s) of a multicomponent inflatable penile prosthesis
   c. Removal and replacement of all components of a multicomponent inflatable penile prosthesis at the same operative session
   d. Removal and replacement of noninflatable (semirigid) penile prosthesis at the same operative session
   e. Removal and replacement of an inflatable (self-contained) penile prosthesis at the same operative session
   f. Removal and replacement of all components of a multicomponent inflatable penile prosthesis, through an infected field, at the same operative session
   g. Removal and replacement of all noninflatable (semirigid) penile prosthesis, through an infected field, at the same operative session
   h. Removal and replacement of all components of an inflatable (self-contained) penile prosthesis, through an infected field, at the same operative session

3. CPT surgery code(s) and modifier(s):

Chapter 9

Female Genital System and Maternity Care and Delivery

CPT codes 56405 through 59899 are used to report surgical and related procedures performed on the female genital system, which includes the vagina, cervix, uterus, and fallopian tubes. Common outpatient procedures involving the female genital system include dilation and curettage, hysteroscopies, and laparoscopies.

Dilation and Curettage

Dilation and curettage (D&C) involves the stretching and enlarging of the cervix and scraping of the endometrium. This procedure is performed for the removal of new growth or other abnormal tissue, or to obtain material for tissue diagnosis.

Coding Guidelines for Dilation and Curettage

The descriptions of female genital system excision codes must be read carefully. Often they provide for the removal of one or more fallopian tubes or ovaries.

Codes 59000–59899 are used to classify obstetrical D&Cs, which are found in the Maternity Care and Delivery subsection.

Nonobstetric D&Cs, which are found in the Female Genital System subsection, are distinguished from obstetric-related D&Cs, with codes varying according to the circumstances. For example:

- Code 58558 is assigned for a D&C with surgical hysteroscopy.

- Codes 57520 and 57522 are used for a D&C with cervical circumferential, or cone, biopsy.

- Code 57558 is the correct code for a D&C of a cervical stump.

- Code 58120 is assigned for a nonobstetrical diagnostic and/or therapeutic D&C.

- Codes 59840 and 59851 are used for an induced abortion by D&C.

APC	HCPCS	HCPCS Description	SI	Rel. Wt.	Payment Rate	OPPS OCE
0190			T	21.6576	1379.46	
	58558	Hysteroscopy, biopsy				Significant Procedure, Multiple Reduction Applies; Separate APC payment

Hysteroscopies

A hysteroscope is a thin telescope that can be inserted through the cervix into the uterus. Diagnostic hysteroscopies involve the direct visual inspection of the cervical canal and uterine cavity through a hysteroscope to examine the endometrium. For surgical hysteroscopies, very thin instruments can be inserted through channels in the hysteroscope to perform simple procedures, such as removing polyps or adhesions. Surgical laparoscopy always includes the diagnostic laparoscopy. To report a diagnostic laparoscopy (peritoneoscopy) (separate procedure), use 49320 (AMA 2008).

Coding Guideline for Hysteroscopies

Code 58558 should be assigned for surgical hysteroscopy with sampling biopsy and/or polypectomy, with or without D&C. The D&C should not be coded separately. The term *biopsy* means the removal and examination, usually microscopic, of tissue from the living body, performed to establish a precise diagnosis. Biopsy includes either the scrapings obtained with the curette or tissue taken using biopsy forceps. Either method is included when code 58558 is assigned (AMA 1994a).

Laparoscopies

Laparoscopies are performed for various diagnostic and surgical purposes. A laparoscopy permits visualization of the peritoneal cavity via a laparoscope inserted through the anterior abdominal wall. An endoscope is used to examine the pelvic viscera, such as the ovaries, fallopian tubes, and uterus.

Lysis of adhesions is an outpatient procedure commonly performed to break up and/or remove the abnormal fibrous bands that can form in and around the organs throughout the pelvic cavity as a result of postsurgical scarring, infection, or other trauma. Treatment is directed toward the relief of chronic pain and correction of fertility problems.

Laparoscopies are commonly performed for hysterectomies with salpingectomy and oophorectomy:

- Hysterectomy is the surgical removal of the uterus. In a salpingectomy, the fallopian tubes are removed, and in an oophorectomy, the ovaries are excised. Through the use of laparoscopic techniques, these lower abdominal surgeries in most instances can be performed transvaginally, eliminating the need for an abdominal incision, or laparoscopically.

- Code 58548, defined as a surgical laparoscope, with a radical hysterectomy, with a bilateral total pelvic lymphadenectomy and para-aortic lymph node sampling (biopsy), with removal of tube (s) and ovary (s), should be coded if all three procedures are performed.

Fallopian tube surgeries include:

- Salpingectomy, or removal of the fallopian tube
- Salpingostomy, or incision into the fallopian tube, such as to remove an ectopic pregnancy
- Fulguration or excision of unwanted tissue, such as with endometriosis
- Fimbrioplasty, which is performed to unblock the fimbria at the ends of the fallopian tube

Myomectomy is a procedure in which uterine fibroids are surgically removed from the uterus. Several different types of uterine fibromas, also known as uterine myomas, can be described as follows:

Intracavitary myomas are fibroids that are inside the uterus (for example, cornual).

Submucous myomas are fibroids found partially in the uterine cavity and partially in the wall of the uterus. Because these myomas are deep in the wall of the uterus, they are difficult to remove laparoscopically.

Intramural myomas are fibroids usually located in the wall of the uterus. Because the size can range from microscopic to larger than a grapefruit, these myomas take a lot more effort to remove than surface myomas.

- Pedunculated myomas are fibroids connected to the uterus by a stalk. These myomas are usually the easiest to remove laparoscopically.

Coding Guidelines for Laparoscopies

Code 49320 is assigned for a diagnostic laparoscopy.

Code 58541 should be assigned for surgical laparoscopy, supracervical hysterectomy, for uterus 250 g or less. Code 58542 should be used if the removal of tube (s) and/or ovary(ies) are also conducted.

Code 58543 should be assigned for surgical laparoscopy, supracervical hysterectomy, for uterus greater than 250 g. Code 58544 should be used if the removal of tube (s) and/or ovary (s) are also conducted.

Codes 58541–58544 should not be reported in conjunction with 49320, 57000, 57180, 57410, 58140–58146, 58545, 58546, 58561, 58661, 58670, 58671.

APC	HCPCS	HCPCS Description	SI	Rel. Wt.	Payment Rate	OPPS OCE
0131			T	45.5317	2900.10	
	58541	Laparoscopy, surgical, supracervical hysterectomy, for uterus 250 g or less				Significant Procedure, Multiple Reduction Applies; Separate APC payment

Following are codes that are assigned for lysis of adhesions, fallopian tube surgery, and myomectomies.

Lysis of Adhesions

Codes 44180 and 58660 should be assigned, as appropriate, for laparoscopic lysis of adhesions. Lysis of adhesions should be reported when documentation in the medical record states that adhesions:

- Are multiple or dense
- Cover the primary operative site
- Add considerable time to the operative procedure and increase the risk to the patient (AMA 1996b).

Fallopian Tube Surgery

The following codes apply to fallopian tube surgery:

- Code 58661 is used for surgical lysis of adhesions, partial or total oophorectomy and/or salpingectomy (includes removal of adnexal structures).
- Code 58662 is used for fulguration or excision of a fallopian tube lesion.
- Code 58670 is assigned for fulguration of fallopian tube(s) (with or without transection).

- Code 58671 is used for occlusion of fallopian tube(s) by devices such as band, clip, and Falope ring.
- Code 58672 is assigned for fimbrioplasty.
- Code 58673 is the correct code for salpingostomy (salpingoneostomy).

Fibroid Excision/Myomectomy

The codes for fibroid excision vary according to whether they are performed laparoscopically or hysteroscopically:

- Codes 58545 and 58546 are used for laparoscopic myomectomy.
- Code 58561 is assigned for hysteroscopic myomectomy (AMA 2003f).
- Codes 0071T and 0072T are used for focused ultrasound ablation of uterine leiomyomata (myoma).

Documentation Requirements for Female Genital System Procedures

The following clinical information must be documented in the medical record when a myomectomy is performed:

1. The total number of myomas/fibroid tumors present

2. The anatomical location of the myoma(s)/fibroid tumor(s):

   - Intramural
   - Surface

3. The total weight of the myoma/fibroid tumor:

   - 250 g or less
   - Greater than 250 g

4. The total volume of the myoma/fibroid tumor:

   - Less than 200 cc of tissue
   - 200 cc or more of tissue

5. The surgical approach used:

   - Open—abdominal
   - Open—vaginal
   - Laparoscopic
   - Hysteroscopic

Case Studies

This section contains actual operative reports from real-life cases. All identifiers have been removed or changed for confidentiality and privacy.

Carefully read the clinical documentation for each case study, which may include a procedure report as well as radiology and/or pathology reports, as applicable.

Answer all the questions for further review at the end of each case study. Use a current CPT codebook or HCPCS Level II code listing, as needed.

When appropriate, assign one or more of the following modifiers:

–50	Bilateral Procedure
–59	Distinct Procedural Service
–FA	Left hand, thumb
–F1	Left hand, second digit
–F2	Left hand, third digit
–F3	Left hand, fourth digit
–F4	Left hand, fifth digit
–F5	Right hand, thumb
–F6	Right hand, second digit
–F7	Right hand, third digit
–F8	Right hand, fourth digit
–F9	Right hand, fifth digit
–LT	Left side
–RT	Right side
–TA	Left foot, great toe
–T1	Left foot, second digit
–T2	Left foot, third digit
–T3	Left foot, fourth digit
–T4	Left foot, fifth digit
–T5	Right foot, great toe
–T6	Right foot, second digit
–T7	Right foot, third digit
–T8	Right foot, fourth digit
–T9	Right foot, fifth digit

Do not apply the current version of the Medicare CCI edits to any of these exercises; the focus is on the application of the coding guidelines and not on the application of edits that change on a quarterly basis. When coding in real life, of course, you will need to apply the CCI edits as appropriate for Medicare outpatient cases.

Case Study 9.1

Read the following clinical document and answer the questions for further review.

OPERATIVE REPORT

PREOPERATIVE DIAGNOSIS: Elective sterilization

POSTOPERATIVE DIAGNOSIS: Elective sterilization

PROCEDURE: Minilaparotomy, bilateral partial salpingectomy

ANESTHESIA: General endotracheal intubation

PROCEDURE: Under satisfactory general endotracheal intubation, the 26-year-old patient was placed in the lithotomy position. She was prepped and draped in the usual manner. A Merritt clamp was attached to the cervix and a straight catheter placed in the bladder.

A 3½-mm incision was made and fascia was incised. The incision was widened with Mayo scissors. The rectus muscles were identified. They were separated in the midline. The peritoneum was identified and opened without complication. The right tube was identified, grasped with Babcock clamps. A straight clamp was placed through an avascular space of the mesosalpinx, and two ligatures of #2-0 chromic were placed approximately 1 cm apart on this tube. The portion of tube between the two ligatures was then excised. The left tube was identified and treated in the same manner. Approximately a 2-cm portion of the tube was excised from the left tube. There was good hemostasis. The pelvic organs were allowed to fall back into the pelvis. The fascia was closed with a continuous suture of #2-0 Vicryl. Subcutaneous tissue was infiltrated with approximately 8 cc of 0.5% Marcaine. The skin was closed in a subcuticular fashion using a #3-0 Vicryl.

Sponge and needle counts were correct. All the instruments were removed from the cervix. The patient went to the Recovery Room in good condition.

SURGICAL PATHOLOGY RESULTS REPORT

CLINICAL HISTORY: Elective sterilization

OPERATION: Bilateral partial salpingectomy

GROSS DESCRIPTION: Received in two parts

Specimen #1: In formalin labeled "right tube" is a segment of tubular structure, representing a portion of excised fallopian tube, 2.0 cm in length and 0.4 cm in diameter. Representative section labeled 1A.

Specimen #2: In formalin labeled "left tube" is a segment of tubular structure, representing a portion of excised fallopian tube, 2.2 cm in length and 0.5 cm in diameter.
Representative section labeled 2A.

FINAL DIAGNOSIS:

Right (#1) and left (#2) fallopian tubes: Complete cross sections of bilateral fallopian tubes showing no significant histologic abnormalities.

Questions for Further Review: Case Study 9.1

1. What technique was used to perform the sterilization?
    a. Fulguration
    b. Excision
    c. Occlusion

2. Was the procedure unilateral or bilateral?
    a. Unilateral
    b. Bilateral

3. What approach was used for the procedure?
    a. Open
    b. Laparoscopic

4. CPT surgery code(s) and modifier(s):

Case Study 9.2

Read the following clinical document and answer the questions for further review.

OPERATIVE REPORT

PREOPERATIVE DIAGNOSIS: Incomplete spontaneous miscarriage

POSTOPERATIVE DIAGNOSIS: Incomplete spontaneous miscarriage

OPERATION: Suction dilation and curettage

ANESTHESIA: IV sedation and 10 cc of paracervical block with 1% Xylocaine plain

SPECIMENS: Products of conception

FINDINGS OF THE PROCEDURE: Moderate amounts of products of conception and eight-week-size uterus

ESTIMATED BLOOD LOSS: Minimal

URINE OUTPUT: Adequate prior to the procedure

IV FLUID REPLACEMENT: Crystalloid

DESCRIPTION OF PROCEDURE: The patient was prepped and draped in the usual sterile fashion. The surgeons were gowned and gloved. The patient was in the dorsal lithotomy position. A weighted speculum was placed against the posterior wall of the vagina; a Sims retractor was placed anteriorly. The cervix was grasped with a tenaculum. Products of conception were already coming through the os and were set aside for surgical pathology. When this was accomplished, a paracervical block was applied. It was 10 cc of 1% Xylocaine plain. This having been accomplished, the cervix was dilated using the Pratt dilators. When this was accomplished, the suction curettage was carried out using a size 8, curved suction curet. Suction curettage was carried out until clear. Both sharp and suction curettage were repeated over two passes to make sure that all the tissue had been removed. The suction curettage was done very gently to avoid scarring the endometrial lining. After the specimen had been collected and the procedure was accomplished, the tenaculum was removed. There was no bleeding from the tenaculum site. Then the patient was cleaned off and taken to the recovery room in stable condition. All instrument and sponge counts were correct at the end of the procedure.

COMPLICATIONS: There were no complications to the procedure.

SURGICAL PATHOLOGY REPORT

AGE/SEX: 27/F

SPECIMEN(S) RECEIVED: Uterine contents

GROSS: Specimen is received in formalin and consists of a 2 x 1 x 1 cm strip of dark brown soft tissue. Also received in a gauze sack are multiple separate fragments of dark brown and red soft tissue measuring 4 cm in aggregate. RSS—1 cassette

DIAGNOSIS: Uterus, curettage: Degenerating immature chorionic villi and decidualized secretory endometrium (See comment.)

COMMENT: Focal villar changes suggestive of partial mole are present. Follow-up Beta Hcg levels are recommended.

Questions for Further Review: Case Study 9.2

1. What type of abortion did this patient have?
   a. Elective
   b. Missed
   c. Incomplete

2. CPT surgery code(s) and modifier(s):

Case Study 9.3

Read the following clinical document and answer the questions for further review.

OPERATIVE RECORD

PREOPERATIVE DIAGNOSIS: Missed abortion

POSTOPERATIVE DIAGNOSIS: Missed abortion

OPERATION: Suction dilation and curettage

ANESTHESIA: General

INDICATIONS: This patient is a 25-year-old female who is para-2-0-0-2. The patient was seen in the office recently with chief complaint of bleeding during her first trimester of pregnancy. A sonogram was performed, which revealed a gestational sac with no fetal contents. The patient was informed of the diagnosis of missed abortion and of the potential need for D&C. She was allowed to wait for spontaneous abortion to occur over 48 hours, which did not occur. The patient then was advised to have suction D&C to remove the contents of the uterus.

Risks, complications, and benefits of the procedure were explained to the patient. She indicated she understood her counseling and asked that the procedure be performed.

PROCEDURE: The patient was brought to the operating room with an IV infusing well into her arm. Following administration of general anesthesia, she was prepped and draped in the usual sterile fashion.

The cervix was grasped with the single-toothed tenaculum and the uterus sounded to approximately 8 to 9 cm. A #7 French curved suction-tip catheter was placed inside the cervix, and the products of conception were removed. A sharp curette was then introduced to palpate any leftover products of conception, and none was noted.

The instrument nurse informed us that all sponge, needle, and instrument counts were correct.

The patient was taken to the recovery room in stable condition.

PATHOLOGY REPORT

AGE/SEX: 25/F

CLINICAL DIAGNOSIS: Missed abortion

TISSUE SUBMITTED: Products of conception

IMPORTANT CLINICAL DATA:

GROSS: PRODUCTS OF CONCEPTION: The specimen is received in formalin in a suction bag and consists of multiple fragments of hemorrhagic, brown tan and dark red soft friable tissue, in the aggregate measuring 10.0 x 8.0 x 2.0 cm, grossly consistent with products of conception without identified fetal tissue. Representative sections are submitted in a single cassette.

DIAGNOSIS: PRODUCTS OF CONCEPTION: Inflamed decidual tissue and hypersecretory endometrium with occasional chorionic villi

---

Questions for Further Review: Case Study 9.3

1. What type of abortion did this patient have?
   a. Elective
   b. Missed
   c. Incomplete

2. CPT surgery code(s) and modifier(s):

Case Study 9.4

Read the following clinical document and answer the questions for further review.

OPERATIVE REPORT

PREOPERATIVE DIAGNOSES: Multiparity and desires permanent sterilization

POSTOPERATIVE DIAGNOSES: Multiparity and desires permanent sterilization

OPERATION: Laparoscopic bilateral tubal ligation with bipolar cautery

PROCEDURE FINDINGS: Normal uterus, tubes, and ovaries. The rest of the abdominal contents were grossly within normal limits.

PROCEDURE: The patient was taken to the operating room where she was given general anesthesia. She was then prepped and draped in the normal dorsal lithotomy position. A bivalved speculum was then placed in the patient's vagina. Her cervix was grasped with a single-toothed tenaculum. A HUMI uterine manipulator was then placed in the patient's uterus for uterine manipulation, and a catheter was placed in the patient's bladder. Attention was then turned to the patient's abdomen where 5cc of 0.25% Marcaine were injected in her umbilicus. Then a 10-mm infraumbilical skin incision was made with a scalpel. Through this incision, a Veress needle was inserted into the abdomen after lifting up the anterior abdominal wall. Intra-abdominal placement was confirmed with a drop water test as well as demonstrating negative pressure when lifting up the anterior abdominal wall. A pneumoperitoneum was then obtained using 3 liters of CO_2 gas. The Veress needle was removed. A trocar was inserted in this infraumbilical skin incision under direct visualization using the Ethicon Visiport. Intra-abdominal placement was confirmed with the laparoscope. The abdomen was examined with the above-noted findings. Using a Kleppinger, the patient's right tube was then grasped and carried out to the fimbriated end. Then approximately 3 to 4 cm of the tube was completely cauterized. This was done ensuring that no adjacent sutures were injured during this cautery. Attention was then turned to the patient's left tube, which was also grasped and carried out to the fimbriated end. Approximately 3 to 4 cm of tube was completely cauterized again, making sure that no adjacent sutures were injured in this cautery. Pictures were taken demonstrating that the tube was completely cauterized for a 3 to 4 cm segment and that no additional structures were injured and demonstrating also that the tube was carried out to the fimbriated end. The ovaries were examined and found to be normal in anatomic appearance, as was the uterus. The liver edge was examined and also found to be normal in anatomic appearance. The trocar was then removed under direct visualization. The fascia at the trocar site was then closed with a figure-of-eight suture of a 0 Vicryl. Then the skin was closed with 3–0 Monocryl. There were no complications with this procedure. The estimated blood loss for this procedure was less than 20 cc. The instrument count was correct x 2. The HUMI and Foley were taken out. The patient was awakened, extubated, and taken to the postanesthetic care unit in good condition. Pictures were taken throughout procedure demonstrating the above-noted findings.

Questions for Further Review: Case Study 9.4

1. What operative approach was used for the procedure?
   a. Open
   b. Laparoscopic

2. What was the laterality of the procedure?
   a. Unilateral
   b. Bilateral

3. What type of procedure was performed?
   a. Lysis of fallopian tube adhesions
   b. Partial salpingectomy
   c. Total salpingectomy
   d. Fulguration of fallopian tubes
   e. Occlusion of fallopian tubes
   f. Salpingostomy
   g. Salpingoneostomy

4. CPT surgery code(s) and modifier(s):

Case Study 9.5

Read the following clinical document and answer the questions for further review.

OPERATIVE NOTE

PREOPERATIVE DIAGNOSES: Septate uterus, rule out didelphic uterus, and vaginal septum

POSTOPERATIVE DIAGNOSIS: Septate uterus and vaginal septum

OPERATIVE PROCEDURE: Diagnostic laparoscopy, diagnostic hysteroscopy, and excision of vaginal septum

ANESTHESIA: General

ESTIMATE BLOOD LOSS: 50 cc

FINDINGS: Examination under anesthesia revealed a complete vaginal septum from the introitus to the cervix. The cervix was duplicated, and inspection of the endometrial cavity with a hysteroscope revealed two separate cavities with one ostium coming into each side. The cavities were separated by a septum. The uterine cavity showed no evidence of polyps or submucous fibroids. At laparoscopy, the uterus was broad but otherwise had a normal shape. There was no evidence of indentation or separation of the two sides of the uterus. The tubes and ovaries were normal. There was no endometriosis or other pathology in the pelvis.

PROCEDURE: Under adequate general anesthesia, the patient was prepped and draped in the usual sterile fashion in the dorsal lithotomy position for vaginal and lower abdominal surgery. Examination under anesthesia was performed. A weighted speculum was placed in the vagina, and the tenaculum was placed on the left cervix. A Rubin's cannula was placed in the cervix, and attention was then turned to the abdomen. The subumbilical region was injected with 0.25% Marcaine, and a small incision was made in the inferior aspect of the umbilicus. A Veress needle was placed down in the peritoneal cavity; and the peritoneal cavity was insufflated with 3 L of CO_2 and the Veress needle was removed. The incision of the umbilicus was extended to 1 cm. The trocar and trocar sheath were placed down into the peritoneal cavity. The trocar was removed and the laparoscope placed. The pelvis was inspected with the findings as noted above. The findings were documented with a video printer. When the laparoscopy was complete, the laparoscope was removed, and the CO_2 was expelled. The trocar sheaths were removed. The incision in the umbilicus was closed with two subcuticular stitches of 3-0 Vicryl. Attention was then turned to the vagina, and the Rubin's cannula was removed from the left cervix. The uterus was sounded and the cervix was then dilated to #25 Pratt dilator. The diagnostic hysteroscope was sounded, and the cervix dilated to #25 Pratt dilator. The diagnostic hysteroscope was inserted into the endometrial cavity with the findings as noted above. Saline delivered with a hysteroscope pump was used for endometrial distention. The findings were documented with a video printer, and the hysteroscope was removed. After the vaginal septum had been removed, the hysteroscope was then placed up into the right cervix, and similar findings were identified and documented with a video printer. The vaginal septum was excised by grasping with Allis clamps for traction and excising the septum using the Bowie set at 25 cut. Bleeders were controlled with the Bowie coag also set at 25. The septum was gradually excised from the introitus all the way up to the cervix. The separations of the vaginal mucosa were closed anteriorly, with a running locking stitch of 2-0 Vicryl, and another small area was approximated with 2-0 chromic anteriorly and the posterior mucosa was approximated with a running locking stitch of 2-0 chromic catgut. The hemostasis was complete. The patient was given a dose of Ampicillin and Gentamicin in the operation room for prophylaxis and a prescription for Augmentin to take home. She is to return to my office in two days for follow-up. The estimated blood loss was 50 cc.

Questions for Further Review: Case Study 9.5

1. What type(s) of endoscopy was performed?
   a. Laparoscopy
   b. Hysteroscopy

2. What surgical procedure was performed?
   a. Hysteroscopic excision of intrauterine septum
   b. Open excision of vaginal septum
   c. Open partial vaginectomy
   d. Laparoscopic excision of vaginal septum

3. CPT surgery code(s) and modifier(s):

Case Study 9.6

Read the following clinical document and answer the questions for further review.

OPERATIVE NOTE

PREOPERATIVE DIAGNOSIS: Uterine synechia and endometrorrhagia

POSTOPERATIVE DIAGNOSIS: Uterine synechia and nometrorrhagia, with endometrial polyp

OPERATION: Hysteroscopy, lysis of synechia, removal of endometrial polyp, and dilation and curettage

ANESTHESIA: General anesthesia

PROCEDURE: With the patient under general anesthesia and in the lithotomy position, the abdomen and the peritoneum were adequately scrubbed and draped. The anterior lip of the cervix was caught with a single-toothed tenaculum. The cavity sounded 8.5 cm. Dilation was carried out with difficulty as probably synechia was being encountered, and dilation was done to a #10 Hegar dilator. Hysteroscopy was done; multiple uterine synechia could be seen joining the anterior and posterior walls of the uterine cavity. These were lysed with blunt dissection. Tubal ostium on the right was visualized. It was patent. The tubal ostia on the left were visualized and hardly patent. An endometrial polyp was on the right aspect of the uterine cavity. This was removed and sent to the lab for analysis. The endocervical canal was normal. All the synechia were lysed with blunt dissection. The cavity ended up being normal.

At this stage, hysteroscope was concluded. Then curettage was done with the retention of a moderate amount of tissue that was sent to the lab for analysis. The procedure was concluded. The estimated blood loss was minimal. The operative time was 30 minutes. The patient left the operating room for the recovery room in good condition.

SURGICAL PATHOLOGY REPORT

AGE: 35

GENDER: F

SPECIMEN(S) RECEIVED: Endometrial curretings/curettage

ENDOMETRIUM, CURETTAGE: Endometrial polyp(s), functional type

CLINICAL HISTORY: Synechial polyps

GROSS DESCRIPTION: The specimen is labeled "endometrial uterine curettings."

The specimen is submitted in formalin and consists of a Telfa pad on which are multiple irregular gray-tan soft tissue fragments measuring 1.5 x 1.2 x 0.3 cm in aggregate.

Multiple sections/one cassette

Entire specimen submitted.

Questions for Further Review: Case Study 9.6

1. What type(s) of endoscopy was performed?
    a. Colposcopy
    b. Laparoscopy
    c. Hysteroscopy

2. Which of the following procedures was performed?
    a. Lysis of intrauterine adhesions
    b. Polypectomy
    c. D&C
    d. All of the above

3. CPT surgery code(s) and modifier(s):

Case Study 9.7

Read the following clinical document and answer the questions for further review.

OPERATIVE REPORT

PREOPERATIVE DIAGNOSIS: Intrauterine fibroids

POSTOPERATIVE DIAGNOSES: Intrauterine fibroids and endometriosis

OPERATION: Laparoscopic myomectomy and excision of endometriosis

MEDICATION: General

OUTPATIENT CLASSIFICATION: Class2

ESTIMATED BLOOD LOSS: Minimal

PROCEDURE: The patient was placed supine on the operating room table and, following adequate general anesthesia and endotracheal intubation, she was placed in the modified lithotomy position in Allen stirrups. Her right arm was tucked by her side, and her left arm was extended to approximately 90 degrees. Her legs were comfortably raised in padded Allen stirrups. She had sequential compression stockings during the procedure.

The abdomen, vulva, and vagina were then prepped and draped in the usual sterile fashion. Examination under anesthesia revealed the uterus to be approximately the gestational size. A weighted vaginal speculum was then placed in the posterior vagina. A single-toothed tenaculum was placed on the anterior lip of the cervix. The uterus was sounded to 11 cm. A Pratt dilator was then placed in the endometrial cavity and tied to the tenaculum for manipulation of the uterus during laparoscopy. A Foley catheter was placed in the urinary bladder and the bulb inflated. The laparoscopy was then performed in the following fashion.

A 10-mm, 0-degree laparoscope was placed in transparent bladeless 12-mm Ethicon trocar. Direct entry into the peritoneal cavity was achieved. CO_2 was then insufflated. The abdomen was first inspected and it was normal. It should be mentioned that at initial entry, inspection of the abdomen did not reveal any evidence of traumatic entry. Inspection of the pelvis revealed endometrial implants on the left anterior aspect of the uterine serosa as well as on the left posterolateral pelvic sidewall. There was a dominant enlargement in the anterior aspect of the uterine serosa as well as on the left posterolateral pelvic sidewall. There was a dominant enlargement in the anterior inferior aspect of the uterus, approximately 5 cm, which was felt to be the previously identified intramural fibroid with submucous extension. Using Allis forceps and Endoshears, both areas of endometriosis were excised. Pitressin, prepared by mixing 20 units and 250 cc, was then injected into the myometrium. Following this, the uterus was incised with scissors and the incision carried down to the level of the fibroid. It should be mentioned that, following initial entry, we placed 3 additional 5-mm trocars, one suprapubic and the other two lateral, clear of the inferior epigastric vessels. Through these operating instruments, we utilized a combination of monopolar and bipolar electrosurgery and the fibroid was dissected with insignificant bleeding. The endometrial cavity was entered during this aspect of the procedure. The dilator could be identified and no other fibroids were evident.

After achieving homeostasis, with bipolar electrosurgery, I used a #1 Vicryl suture to close the uterine defect in two layers, using a running stitch. The pelvis was then copiously irrigated. The myoma was removed with the aid of the GYN care morcellator. The 12-mm paraumbilical trocar site was closed with #1 Vicryl, using the exit closure device. All trocars and instruments were then removed. Gas was expelled, and all skin incisions were then closed using #4-0 Vicryl cuticular stitches. It should be mentioned that in removing all the trocars from the abdomen, the final 5-mm trocar was withdrawn while the laparoscope was still in the peritoneal cavity. The laparoscope was withdrawn, inspecting the tract with the camera. There was no evidence of any bleeding or any withdrawal of any tissue into the tract. Then 0.5% Marcaine was injected into all surgical sites. Steri-Strips and Band-Aids were left on the abdomen. The patient was awakened and taken from the operating room to the recovery room in a very satisfactory condition.

SURGICAL PATHOLOGY REPORT

AGE/SEX: 24/F

SPECIMEN(S):
   A. Endometriosis
   B. Leiomyoma(s), myomectomy without uterus

FINAL DIAGNOSIS:
   A. Pelvic peritoneum, biopsy: endometriosis.
   B. Uterus, myomectomy (morcellated): Leiomyomas with focal infarction. Pressure atrophy of overlying endometrium.

CLINICAL HISTORY: Uterine fibroids; abnormal uterine bleeding

GROSS DESCRIPTION:

A. The specimen is labeled "endometriosis."

The specimen is received in formalin and consists of two fragments of pinkish-tan, soft tissue, ranging in size from 0.3 to 0.5 cm in greatest dimension each. The external surface is vaguely nodular. The entire specimen is submitted in a single cassette.

Multiple sections/1 cassette

Entire specimen submitted

B. The specimen is labeled "fibroid."

The specimen is received in formalin and consists of multiple cordlike white, firm tissues in aggregate 8.0 x 6.0 x 1.5 cm and weighing 35.0 grams. The cut surface demonstrates whorled-like pattern.

Multiple sections/5 cassettes

Representative sections submitted.

Questions for Further Review: Case Study 9.7

1. How many myomas/fibroid tumors were present?
   a. Two
   b. One

2. Where was the anatomical location of the myoma(s)/fibroid tumor(s)?
   a. Intramural
   b. Surface

3. What was the total weight of the myoma(s)/fibroid tumor(s)?
   a. 250 g or less
   b. Greater than 250 g

4. What surgical approach was used?
   a. Open, abdominal
   b. Open, vaginal
   c. Laparoscopic
   d. Hysteroscopic

5. Endometrial implants were also present and removed.
   a. True
   b. False

6. CPT surgery code(s) and modifier(s):

Case Study 9.8

Read the following clinical document and answer the questions for further review.

HISTORY AND PHYSICAL

HISTORY OF PRESENT ILLNESS: This is a 32-year-old female gravida 0 who presents to the office with complaints of worsening dysmenorrhea, low back pain, abnormal uterine bleeding that has been progressively worsening and refractory to medical therapy. She desires definitive diagnosis with treatment.

PAST MEDICAL HISTORY: Is negative for diabetes or hypertension

FAMILY HISTORY: Unremarkable

PAST SURGICAL HISTORY: Unremarkable

SOCIAL HISTORY: She denies tobacco or alcohol.

ALLERGIES: She has no known drug allergies.

PHYSICAL EXAMINATION:
Vital signs: She is afebrile; vital signs are within normal limits.

GENERAL: She is a well-developed, well-nourished female in no acute distress.
  HEENT: Pupils are equal and reactive to light and accommodation. Extraocular muscles are intact.
  Neck: No thyromegally or lymphadenopathy
  Chest: Clear
  Heart: Regular rate and rhythm without murmur
  Breasts: Without masses or discharge bilaterally
  Abdomen: Within normal limits
  Pelvic: External genitalia is normal, cervix without lesions. Uterus is tender. Adnexa is tender bilaterally.

ASSESSMENT: Worsening dysmenorrheal, abnormal uterine bleeding, rule out endometriosis.

PLAN: The patient will undergo dilation and curettage, hysteroscopy, diagnostic laparoscopy, and rule out uterine or pelvic pathology.

OPERATION REPORT

PREOPERATIVE DIAGNOSIS: Worsening pelvic pain, abnormal uterine bleeding

POSTOPERATIVE DIAGNOSIS: Sigmoid colon adhesions to left adnexa involving the round ligament, tube, ovary, and left pelvic sidewall, right ovarian cyst

OPERATIVE PROCEDURES:
D&C
Diagnostic hysteroscopy
Operative laparoscopy
Lysis of adhesions
Right ovarian cystotomy

ANESTHESIA: General endotracheal anesthesia

EBL: Minimal

INDICATIONS: The patient is a 32-year-old female with the above-mentioned presentation.

DESCRIPTION OF PROCEDURE: The patient was taken to the operating room, placed in the dorsal lithotomy position, prepped and draped in the usual fashion for laparoscopic surgery. After satisfactory induction of general endotracheal anesthesia, examination under anesthesia revealed an anteverted uterus, no adnexal masses. The cervix was grasped with the single-toothed tenaculum and dilated to allow a 5 French hysteroscope. Hysteroscopy of the endocervical canal was normal. The endometrial cavity showed lush endometrium; no submucous fibroids or polyps were noted. The tubal ostia were visualized bilaterally. The scope was removed and D&C performed with endometrial curetting sent to pathology. The HUMI catheter was placed and attention turned to the abdominal wall. A subumbilical incision was made, and the Veress needle was placed. Pneumoperitoneum with 2 liters of carbon dioxide gas was achieved. A 5-mm trocar was placed, and the video laparoscope was introduced through the trocar sleeve. Inspection of the insertion site showed no active bleeding or adhesions. On moving the scope in the pelvis, a suprapubic incision was made, and the 5-mm trocar was placed under direct visualization. At this time, systematic inspection of the pelvis was undertaken. The bladder flap was clean. The uterus was normal in size. The sigmoid colon was adhered to the left tube and ovary, round ligament, and left pelvic sidewall. Lysis of adhesions was performed with scissors with cautery, paying close attention to the course of the bowel. When this was complete, the left ovary appeared normal. The cul-de-sac was clean. The right ovary was adhered to the right pelvic sidewall, and this was freed up with blunt dissection. Also, a 3-cm cyst was present on the right ovary, which was opened and drained with good hemostasis noted. At this time, the pelvis was irrigated clean. Good hemostasis was noted throughout. No endometriosis was noted. The adhesions were lysed completely and the instruments were removed. The pneumoperitoneum was relieved and the incisions closed with subcuticular 4-0 Vicryl. The patient was taken to the recovery room in stable condition.

PATHOLOGY REPORT

SPECIMEN GROSS DIAGNOSIS: In formalin, labeled with the patient's name and endometrial curretings, is a 0.2 g aggregate of dark tan–tinged mucoid material. Totally submitted in one.

ENDOMETRIAL CURETTINGS:
Proliferative endometrium
Benign endocervical fragments with focal reserve cell hyperplasia

---

Questions for Further Review: Case Study 9.8

1. What type(s) of endoscopy was performed?
   a. Laparoscopy
   b. Hysteroscopy

2. A dilation and curettage was performed.
   a. True
   b. False

3. Where were the adhesions located?
   a. Sigmoid colon
   b. Left fallopian tube
   c. Left ovary
   d. Round ligament
   e. Left pelvic sidewall
   f. Right ovary
   g. Right pelvic sidewall
   h. All of the above

4. How was the right ovarian cyst treated?
   a. Open drainage, vaginal approach
   b. Open drainage, abdominal approach
   c. Laparoscopic drainage

5. CPT surgery code(s) and modifier(s):

Chapter 10

Nervous System

CPT Codes 61000 through 64999 are used to report surgical and related procedures performed on the nervous system, which includes the skull, meninges, and brain. Common outpatient procedures involving the nervous system include spinal injections and blocks, sacroiliac joint injections, and implantation of neurostimulators, catheters, reservoirs, and pumps.

Spinal Injections and Blocks

Spinal injections are performed to administer anesthesia or radiopaque substances. Spinal blocks are used to anesthetize specific areas of the body.

Common types of spinal injections and blocks are:

- Single injection: A one-time injection that is given either intrathecally or epidurally via lumbar puncture

- Differential injection: The injection of local anesthetics of varying strengths and a placebo to assist in the identification of a source of pain

- Continuous injection: An injection of drug therapy during a period of days to a week via a catheter placed either intrathecally or epidurally and connected to an external infusion pump, which mimics an implantable system and is used for assessment during the patient's normal daily activities

- Single-level block: Interrupts nerve function at a single dermatomal level (that is, the skin area that a single nerve supplies)

- Multiple-level block: Involves the interruption of nerve function of more than one dermatomal level

- Regional block: Involves the interruption of nerve function from a limb or area of the body, achieved by placement of local anesthetic along the course of the nerve or into the spinal space

Coding Guidelines for Spinal Injections and Blocks

The injection procedure codes are considered "unilateral" procedures and are reported *once* per level, per side (right or left), regardless of the number or types of injections performed on the right or left side at a specific spinal level. Thus, injection codes 62280–62282, 62310–62319, 64470–64484, and

64622–64627 are not reported for *each* substance injected on one side at a particular spinal level.

When both sides are injected at a specific spinal level, the appropriate injection codes should be reported with modifier –50 appended (AMA 1999c). For example, codes 64470–64476 are considered *unilateral* procedures. When injections are performed at both right *and* left paravertebral facet joints or paravertebral facet joint nerves, the bilateral procedure modifier –50 is appended to the appropriate code.

The paravertebral facet joint injection codes 64470–64476 should be reported per spinal level. Each vertebra in the spine is joined to the one above and the one below it by articular facet joints. There are four facet joints associated with each single vertebra in the spine below the level of C2 and above the level of S1. For example, at the L4 vertebral level, there is an L3-L4 facet joint at the upper end and also an L4-L5 facet joint at the inferior end.

Generally, each facet joint has dual innervation; one from the dorsal rami at the same level and one from the level above. For example, the L4-L5 lumbar facet joint is innervated by the medial branches of the dorsal rami from L3 and L4. The facet joint injection codes refer to the injection of a facet joint either by injection into the joint with one needle puncture or by anesthetizing the two medial branch nerves that supply each joint (two needle punctures).

The facet injection codes are reported once when the injection procedure is performed, irrespective of whether a single or multiple puncture is required to anesthetize the target joint at a given level and side. Commonly, physicians use a technique that involves insertion of the needle once, with attachment of a short piece of extension tubing through which the first drug is injected. The syringe is then changed, and the next drug is injected through the same tubing/needle. Should the physician choose to perform separate needle punctures, this multiple needle technique does not alter reporting.

To clarify, only one facet injection code should be reported at a specified level and side injected (for example, right L4-5 facet joint), regardless of the number of needle(s) inserted or number of drug(s) injected at that specific level. For example, a left-sided L4-L5 intra-articular injection performed with a single needle puncture would be coded as 64475. Injection of the L3 and L4 medial branch nerves supplying the L4–L5 facet joint would also be coded as 64475, even though two separate injections are performed to effect the same result.

Codes 64479–64484 are considered *unilateral* procedures. When both a right and a left transforaminal epidural injection is performed, the bilateral procedure modifier –50 is appended to the appropriate code.

For codes 62318 and 62319, a catheter is threaded through the needle and placed in the subarachnoid or epidural space. A continuous infusion is started through the catheter, which continues for several hours or days. Occasionally, as part of a detailed diagnostic or treatment regimen, multiple (3 or more) injections might be given through this catheter over a period of hours or 1–2 days. These multiple injections often involve different substances, such as placebo injection or varying amounts of narcotic (AMA 2000c, 4).

Codes 62290 and 72295 can be reported more than once when a discography is performed at multiple levels (such as at L2–3, L3–4, L4–5, and L5–S1) (AMA 2003c).

Injection Blood/Clot Patch

This procedure is performed following a spinal puncture to prevent spinal fluid leakage. The patient remains in a spinal tap position. The patient's blood is injected outside the dura to clot and plug the wound, preventing spinal fluid leakage.

Coding Guidelines for Injection, Epidural Blood or Clot Patch

Code 62273 is used for injection, epidural blood or clot patch. To report injection of diagnostic or therapeutic substance(s), code 62310, 62311, 62318, or 62319 is used (AMA 2008).

APC	HCPCS	HCPCS Description	SI	Rel. Wt.	Payment Rate	OPPS OCE
0206			T	4.0964	260.92	
	62273	Injection epidural patch				Significant Procedure, Multiple Reduction Applies; Separate APC payment

Sacroiliac Joint Injection

Arthrography is the radiographic examination of a joint after the injection of a dyelike contrast material and/or air to outline the soft tissue and joint structures on the images. Sometimes an anesthetic or steroid is also injected into the joint for pain relief or treatment.

Coding Guidelines for Sacroiliac Joint Injection

Under the official coding guidelines for CPT, a single code, 27096, is reported for injection procedure for sacroiliac joint, arthrography, and/or anesthetic/steroid. When bilateral sacroiliac joint arthrograms are performed, code 27096 should be reported using modifier –50 (AMA 1999c).

Under CMS reimbursement rules, two HCPCS codes are required to report injection procedures for sacroiliac joint with arthrography, depending on whether anesthetic/steroid is also provided, as follows:

- For Medicare hospital outpatients, HCPCS Level II code G0259 is reported for injection procedure for sacroiliac joint; arthrography.

- For Medicare hospital outpatients, HCPCS Level II code G0260 is reported for injection procedure for sacroiliac joint; provision of anesthetic, steroid, and/or other therapeutic agent and arthrography.

Coding Guidelines for Destruction by Neurolytic Agent

Codes 64622–64627 are considered *unilateral* procedures. When these procedures are performed on both the right and left sides, append the bilateral procedure modifier '–50' to the appropriate code (AMA 2003d).

Unlike facet joint nerve (medial branch) codes used to describe facet joint injection (64470–64484), facet nerve destruction codes 64622–64627 refer to individual nerve level destruction. Thus, although injection of the left L3 and L4 medial (facet joint) nerve would be coded as 64475, destruction of the L3 and L4 medial branch nerves would be coded as 64622 and 64623 (AMA 2004c).

The injection of contrast material is an inclusive component of codes 64622–64627 (AMA 2000e).

Neurostimulator Generators and Electrodes

A neurostimulator is a device used for chronic electrical excitation of the central or peripheral nervous systems.

Coding Guidelines for Neurostimulator Generators and Electrodes

The choice of neurostimulator CPT code(s) is based on:

- The anatomic site (intracranial, spinal nerve, peripheral nerve)
- The surgical approach (open incisional, percutaneous, subcutaneous)
- Initial system placement or subsequent revision or replacement of one or more components (for example, the entire device, or the pulse generator [transmitter] or electrode array only)

For spinal electrodes, codes 63650 and 63655 are used for insertion, and code 63660 is used for revision or removal.

For spinal pulse generator or receivers, code 63685 is assigned for insertion, and code 63688 is used for revision or removal.

APC	HCPCS	HCPCS Description	SI	Rel. Wt.	Payment Rate	OPPS OCE
0222			S	240.7990	15337.45	
	63685	Insertion or replacement of spinal neurostimulator pulse generator or receiver, direct or inductive coupling				Significant Procedure, Not Discounted when Multiple; Separate APC payment

Spinal Reservoir and Pump Implantation

Subcutaneous reservoirs or access ports consist of subcutaneously implanted rigid reservoirs with injection ports. The reservoirs are connected internally to catheters, terminating in a compartment such as the subarachnoid space or hepatic artery. They are manufactured from relatively biocompatible materials such as titanium, stainless steel polysulfone, or reinforced silicone, in a variety of sizes and volume capacities.

The reservoir controls the rate of drug delivery by passive diffusion, because drug concentration in the reservoir is greater than in the target compartment. There is no battery or other power source. Because the reservoir volume is small, it needs to be filled manually at frequent intervals (hours or days). Subcutaneous reservoirs have been used as permanent delivery systems and as temporary reservoirs for patients undergoing evaluation for permanent epidural or intrathecal drug delivery systems.

Implantable infusion pumps (IIPs) include an infusion pump and reservoir, bacteriostatic filters, fluid administration sets, and delivery catheters. The pumps are implanted in a subcutaneous pocket and connected to a dedicated catheter placed in the appropriate compartment. Constant or variable-rate infusions are possible over long periods of time (several weeks to years) with minimal human intervention (refilling or reprogramming), while the capability for external control of rate and volume of primary and supplemental drug delivery is retained.

IIPs are labeled for specific drugs and routes of administration, such as epidural morphine sulfate, intrathecal morphine sulfate, or intrathecal baclofen. Nonprogrammable pumps include pulsatile pumps and vapor pressure–powered pumps. Peristaltic pumps are programmable. (Although the brand name does not indicate whether a pump is programmable, the manufacturer's marketing literature and Web site may specify the pump's capabilities.)

Coding Guidelines for Spinal Reservoir and Pump Implantation

Two codes must be reported when a spinal reservoir or pump is implanted or replaced, one for the catheter implantation and another for the reservoir or pump, as follows:

- Code 62350 or 62351 is assigned for the implantation of the delivery catheter.
- Code 62360 is the correct code for a subcutaneous reservoir.
- Code 62361 or 62362 is used for an IIP.

To report implantable pump or reservoir refill, code 96522 is used. This code includes access of pump port.

Sympathetic Nerve Injections

Injection Anesthetic Agent, 64505–64530

APC	HCPCS	HCPCS Description	SI	Rel. Wt.	Payment Rate	OPPS OCE
0204			T	2.3213	147.85	
	64505	Nerve block, spenopalatine ganglion				Significant Procedure, Multiple Reduction Applies; Separate APC payment

Coding Guidelines for Injection, Anesthetic Agent

Code 64505 is used for injection, anesthetic agent into sphenopalatine ganglion. The physician injects the sphenopalatine ganglion nerve with an anesthetic agent to provide anesthesia to the nasal mucosa. The anesthesia is applied by entering through the nares and injecting cocaine posterior to the middle turbinate.

Code 64508 is assigned for injection, anesthetic agent into carotid sinus (separate procedure). The physician injects the carotid sinus nerve with an anesthetic agent to block sympathetically mediated pain or cardiovascular responses.

Code 64510 is used for injection, anesthetic agent into stellate ganglion (cervical sympathetic). The physician performs a nerve block on the stellate ganglion—also known as the cervicothoracic ganglion—by injecting an anesthetic agent to block sympathetically mediated pain. The stellate ganglion is located at the C7/T1 level vertebrae; its fibers distribute to the head, neck, heart, and upper limb. This block is used to provide anesthetic relief for pain in the face, neck, and upper extremity. Using separately reportable fluoroscopic imaging, the physician guides the needle into correct placement in the ganglion and injects the nerve block agent.

Code 64517 is assigned for injection, anesthetic agent into a superior hypogastric plexus. The physician performs a nerve block on the superior hypogastric plexus by injecting an anesthetic agent through a needle inserted in the L5/S1 interspace. The superior hypogastric plexus, also called the presacral nerve, is located in front of the upper part of the sacrum and is formed by lower lumbar nerves responsible for pain sensation in the pelvic area. This nerve block is done in such cases as severe, intractable menstrual pain and pain due to pelvic area metastases from cancer, such as prostatic malignancy. The patient is placed in the prone position and prepped. A 6-inch needle is guided under radiological imaging, such as fluoroscopy (reported separately), into the ventral lateral spine and through the L5/S1 interspace. Needle position is checked by injecting contrast material and aspirating for the return of any blood, urine, or cerebral spinal fluid. With negative aspiration results and imaging verifying that the needle position is in the prevertebral space and not within a blood vessel, a ureter, or spinal nerves, local anesthetic is injected on both sides.

Code 64520 is assigned for injection, anesthetic agent into the lumbar or thoracic (paravertrebral sympathetic) nerves. The physician performs a nerve block on lumbar or thoracic paravertebral sympathetic nerves by injecting an anesthetic agent to block sympathetically mediated pain. The lumbar or thoracic block provides anesthetic relief for pain in the torso, pelvis, and lower extremities. Using separately reportable fluoroscopic imaging, the physician guides the needle into correct placement into the paravertebral sympathetic nerve fibers and injects the nerve block agent.

Code 64530 is used for injection, anesthetic agent into the celiac plexus, with or without radiologic monitoring. The physician injects the celiac plexus with an anesthetic to block sympathetically mediated or visceral pain. Anesthesia is provided with or without radiologic monitoring (Merck Manual, 2008).

To report intracranial surgery on cranial nerves, use CPT codes 61450, 61460, and 61790. (AMA 2008).

Documentation Requirements for Nervous System Procedures

Each procedure is followed by clinical information that must be documented in the medical record when the procedure is performed.

Spinal Injections

Spinal injections are reported with CPT codes 62263, 62264, 62280–62282, 62310–62319, 64400 64530, and 64600–64681.

1. Substances injected into the spine:

    -   Lysis solution (for example, hypertonic saline, enzyme)
    -   Anesthetic
    -   Antispasmodic
    -   Opioid
    -   Steroid
    -   Neurolytic substance (for example, alcohol, phenol, iced saline solution, chemical, thermal, electrical, radiofrequency)
    -   Other solution—specify (for example, narcotic)

2. Whether the injection (continuous infusion or intermittent bolus) was performed via an indwelling catheter

- Type of injection:
- Single injection
- Differential injection
- Continuous injection
- Single-level block
- Multiple-level block
- Regional block
- Intermittent bolus

3. Site(s) of injection(s):

- Lumbar subarachnoid
- Cervical subarachnoid
- Thoracic subarachnoid
- Sacral subarachnoid
- Lumbar epidural
- Cervical epidural
- Thoracic epidural
- Sacral epidural
- Lumbar paravertebral facet joint or facet joint nerve
- Cervical paravertebral facet joint or facet joint nerve
- Thoracic paravertebral facet joint or facet joint nerve
- Sacral paravertebral facet joint or facet joint nerve
- Lumbar transforaminal
- Cervical transforaminal
- Thoracic transforaminal
- Sacral transforaminal
- Somatic nerve, specify:
  - Trigeminal, facial, greater occipital, vagus, phrenic, spinal accessory, cervical plexus, brachial plexus, axillary, suprascapular, intercostal, ilioinguinal, iliohypogastric, pudendal, paracervical (uterine), thoracic paravertebral, lumbar paravertebral, sacral paravertebral, coccygeal paravertebral, lumbar paravertebral facet joint, sciatic, lumbar plexus
- Sympathetic nerve, specify:
  - Sphenopalatine ganglion, carotid sinus, stellate ganglion/cervical sympathetic, lumbar paravertebral sympathetic, thoracic paravertebral sympathetic, celiac plexus, superior hypogastric plexus

4. Each vertebral level of the spine that is injected:

- Lumbar paravertebral facet joint or facet joint nerve
- Cervical paravertebral facet joint or facet joint nerve
- Thoracic paravertebral facet joint or facet joint nerve
- Sacral paravertebral facet joint or facet joint nerve
- Lumbar transforaminal
- Cervical transforaminal
- Thoracic transforaminal
- Sacral transforaminal

Spinal Catheter Implantation

Spinal catheter procedures are reported with CPT codes 62350–62355.

1. Type of catheter implanted:

- Intrathecal
- Epidural

2. Intrathecal or epidural catheterization procedure(s):

- Implantation for reservoir/pump with laminectomy
- Implantation for reservoir/pump without laminectomy
- Revision for reservoir/pump with laminectomy
- Revision for reservoir/pump without laminectomy
- Repositioning for reservoir/pump with laminectomy
- Repositioning for reservoir/pump without laminectomy
- Removal of previously implanted catheter

Spinal Reservoir/Pump Implantation

Spinal reservoir/pump procedures are reported with CPT codes 62360–62368.

1. Intrathecal or epidural subcutaneous reservoir procedure(s):

- Implantation of subcutaneous reservoir
- Replacement of subcutaneous reservoir
- Removal of subcutaneous reservoir
- Refilling and maintenance of subcutaneous reservoir

2. Intrathecal or epidural pump procedure(s):

- Implantation of nonprogrammable pump
- Implantation of programmable pump

- Replacement of nonprogrammable pump
- Replacement of programmable pump
- Removal of pump (nonprogrammable or programmable)
- Electronic analysis of programmable pump with reprogramming
- Electronic analysis of programmable pump without reprogramming
- Refilling and maintenance of implantable pump

Case Studies

This section contains actual operative reports from real-life cases. All identifiers have been removed or changed for confidentiality and privacy.

Carefully read the clinical documentation for each case study, which may include a procedure report as well as radiology and/or pathology reports, as applicable.

Answer all the questions for further review at the end of each case study. Use a current CPT codebook or HCPCS Level II code listing, as needed.

When appropriate, assign one or more of the following modifiers:

−50	Bilateral Procedure
−59	Distinct Procedural Service
−FA	Left hand, thumb
−F1	Left hand, second digit
−F2	Left hand, third digit
−F3	Left hand, fourth digit
−F4	Left hand, fifth digit
−F5	Right hand, thumb
−F6	Right hand, second digit
−F7	Right hand, third digit
−F8	Right hand, fourth digit
−F9	Right hand, fifth digit
−LT	Left side
−RT	Right side
−TA	Left foot, great toe
−T1	Left foot, second digit
−T2	Left foot, third digit
−T3	Left foot, fourth digit
−T4	Left foot, fifth digit
−T5	Right foot, great toe
−T6	Right foot, second digit
−T7	Right foot, third digit
−T8	Right foot, fourth digit
−T9	Right foot, fifth digit

Do not apply the current version of the Medicare CCI edits to any of these exercises; the focus is on the application of the coding guidelines and not on the application of edits that change on a quarterly basis. When coding in real life, of course, you will need to apply the CCI edits as appropriate for Medicare outpatient cases.

Case Study 10.1

Read the following clinical document and answer the questions for further review.

OPERATIVE REPORT

PREOPERATIVE DIAGNOSIS: L3–4, L4–5, and L5–S1 facet degenerative joint disease

PROCEDURE: Left L3–4 facet injection. Right L3–4 facet injection. Left L4–5 facet injection. Right L4–5 facet injection. Left L5–S1 facet injection. Right L5–S1 facet injection.

ANESTHESIA: 1% plain Lidocaine local

ESTIMATED BLOOD LOSS: Minimal

DRAINS: None

COMPLICATIONS: None

PATH SPECIMEN: None

INDICATIONS: This 56-year-old female is status post previous lumbar decompression and has had back pain that has improved with intermittent facet injections. She presents for repeat facet injections. Because of degenerative changes of the levels noted above, she will undergo bilateral facet injections.

PROCEDURE: In the prone position, sterile Betadine prep and draping, 1% lidocaine was used to infiltrate the skin and subcutaneous tissue over the projected needle insertion sites. This was determined using C-arm fluoroscopy. Then, 22-gauge spinal needles were placed down to the L3–4, L4–5, and L5–S1 facets bilaterally. Each level on each side was then injected with an equal mixture from a total of 80 mg of Depo-Medrol, 10 cc of 1% plain lidocaine, and 20 cc of 0.5% Marcaine without difficulty.

The patient tolerated the procedure well and was discharged home.

Questions for Further Review: Case Study 10.1

1. What substances were injected into the spine?
   a. Lysis solution
   b. Anesthetic
   c. Antispasmodic
   d. Opioid
   e. Steroid
   f. Neurolytic substance(s) (for example, alcohol, phenol, iced saline solution, chemical, thermal, electrical, radiofrequency)
   g. Other solution—specify (for example, narcotic)

2. Were the substances administered via an indwelling catheter?
   a. Yes
   b. No

3. What type of injection was performed?
   a. Single
   b. Multiple/regional block
   c. Differential
   d. Continuous infusion
   e. Intermittent bolus

4. Identify the anatomical site(s) of the injection(s).
   a. Lumbar subarachnoid
   b. Cervical subarachnoid

    c.   Thoracic subarachnoid
    d.   Sacral subarachnoid
    e.   Lumbar epidural
    f.   Cervical epidural
    g.   Thoracic epidural
    h.   Sacral epidural
    i.   Lumbar paravertebral facet joint or facet joint nerve
    j.   Cervical paravertebral facet joint or facet joint nerve
    k.   Thoracic paravertebral facet joint or facet joint nerve
    l.   Sacral paravertebral facet joint or facet joint nerve
    m.   Lumbar transforaminal
    n.   Cervical transforaminal
    o.   Thoracic transforaminal
    p.   Sacral transforaminal
    q.   Somatic nerve: Trigeminal facial greater occipital, vagus, phrenic, spinal accessory, cervical plexus, brachial plexus, axillary, suprascapular, intercostal, ilioinguinal, iliohypogastric, pudendal, paracervical (uterine), thoracic paravertebral, lumbar paravertebral, sacral paravertebral, coccygeal paravertebral, lumbar paravertebral facet joint, sciatic, lumbar plexus
    r.   Sympathetic nerve: Sphenopalatine ganglion, carotid sinus, stellate ganglion/cervical sympathetic, lumbar paravertebral sympathetic, thoracic paravertebral sympathetic, celiac plexus, superior hypogastric plexus

5.   List each vertebral level of the spine that was injected.

6.   CPT surgery code(s) and modifier(s):

Case Study 10.2

Read the following clinical document and answer the questions for further review.

OPERATIVE REPORT

OPERATION: Thoracic epidural catheter placement and thoracic sympathectomy

INTERIM HISTORY: This patient has done very well since his intralesional injections about a week ago for shingles. One area under his right axilla is ecchymotic and tender, and some areas around his right scapula are pruritic. Otherwise, his pain has significantly improved since last week. He presents today, since stopping his Coumadin on Friday, for epidural catheter placement for thoracic sympathectomy.

PROCEDURE: After obtaining an informed consent, the patient was placed in a sitting position. His back was prepped and draped in the usual sterile fashion using a Betadine solution. The area of shingles was located, and the corresponding interspace in the upper thoracic region was injected with a 1% lidocaine solution through the anesthetized area. An 18-gauge Tuohy needle was inserted using a loss-of-resistance technique. Good loss of resistance was obtained, and no blood or CSF was noted via the epidural needle. With the epidural needle in place, a solution of 0.5% lidocaine was obtained and injected through the needle with a volume of 3 cc. Following this, an epidural catheter was placed 3 cm and secured in place after withdrawing the needle. Through the catheter, an additional 3 cc of 0.5% lidocaine was injected. The patient was observed, and frequent blood pressures revealed good hemodynamic stability. After approximately 5 to 10 minutes, the patient reported that he had significant improvement in his symptomatology. One remaining section of area of itching was injected subcutaneously with 0.5% lidocaine with rapid resolution. The patient stated that he had significant improvement, and no further injections were performed. The catheter was secured in place, and he was scheduled for a repeat injection tomorrow.

ASSESSMENT: Good response to thoracic epidural catheter placement and dosing with 0.5% lidocaine

PLAN: The patient was instructed to come at 1:30 tomorrow for follow-up evaluation and possible repeat injection via the epidural catheter. If good relief is still obtained after repeat injection, the catheter will be removed. If he has a shorter duration of relief, however, the catheter can remain an additional day for reinjection.

Questions for Further Review: Case Study 10.2

1.   What type of catheter was inserted?
    a.   Intrathecal
    b.   Epidural

2.   How was the catheter inserted?
    a.   Surgically implanted
    b.   Percutaneous placement

3. What anatomical site was injected?
   a. Cervical
   b. Subarachnoid
   c. Thoracic
   d. Subdural
   e. Lumbar
   f. Caudal

4. What type of injection was performed?
   a. Single
   b. Differential
   c. Continuous

5. CPT surgery code(s) and modifier(s):

Case Study 10.3

Read the following clinical document and answer the questions for further review.

OPERATIVE REPORT

AGE: 42

DISCH: 08/11/200X

PREOPERATIVE DIAGNOSIS: Right C6 radiculitis

PROCEDURE: Right C6 transforaminal epidural steroid injection

CLINICAL NOTE: This patient previously underwent a right C6 injection. Her symptoms have now returned, and are, in fact, more severe, and she desires a repeat injection.

PROCEDURE: The patient was brought to the treatment room area. Informed consent was obtained. She was placed in the supine position on the fluoroscopy table, and her right neck was prepped with Betadine and draped with sterile drapes. The C5–6 neural foramen was identified using slightly oblique from the lateral fluoroscopic veins. The overlying skin was infiltrated with 1.5% lidocaine using a 30-gauge needle. A 22-gauge 3½-inch spinal needle was passed into the posterior portion of the neural foramen at C5–6, and advancement was stopped when the needle was found to lie just in the column of the facet joints on AP view.

After negative aspiration, 2 cc of a mixture containing 80 mg Depo-Medrol and 1 cc of 1.5% plain lidocaine was injected incrementally without problems.

Ten minutes after the procedure, the patient noted that she was numb in what appeared to be a C6 sensory distribution. She noted that even though she had numbness, she still had deep muscle aching.

Questions for Further Review: Case Study 10.3.

1. Identify the medical substance(s) injected into the spine.
   a. Lysis solution
   b. Anesthetic(s)
   c. Antispasmodic
   d. Opioid
   e. Steroid(s)
   f. Neurolytic substance(s) (for example, alcohol, phenol, iced saline solution, chemical, thermal, electrical, radiofrequency)
   g. Other solution—specify (for example, narcotic)

2. Were the substances administered via an indwelling catheter?
   a. Yes
   b. No

3. What type of injection was performed?
   a. Single

     b.   Multiple/regional block
     c.   Differential
     d.   Continuous infusion
     e.   Intermittent bolus

4.   Identify the anatomical site(s) of the injection(s).
    a.   Lumbar subarachnoid
    b.   Cervical subarachnoid
    c.   Thoracic subarachnoid
    d.   Sacral subarachnoid
    e.   Lumbar epidural
    f.   Cervical epidural
    g.   Thoracic epidural
    h.   Sacral epidural
    i.   Lumbar paravertebral facet joint or facet joint nerve
    j.   Cervical paravertebral facet joint or facet joint nerve
    k.   Thoracic paravertebral facet joint or facet joint nerve
    l.   Sacral paravertebral facet joint or facet joint nerve
    m.   Lumbar transforaminal
    n.   Cervical transforaminal
    o.   Thoracic transforaminal
    p.   Sacral transforaminal
    q.   Somatic nerve (circle one): Trigeminal facial greater occipital, vagus, phrenic, spinal accessory, cervical plexus, brachial plexus, axillary, suprascapular, intercostal, ilioinguinal, iliohypogastric, pudendal, paracervical (uterine), thoracic paravertebral, lumbar paravertebral, sacral paravertebral, coccygeal paravertebral, lumbar paravertebral facet joint, sciatic, lumbar plexus
    r.   Sympathetic nerve (circle one): Sphenopalatine ganglion, carotid sinus, stellate ganglion/cervical sympathetic, lumbar paravertebral sympathetic, thoracic paravertebral sympathetic, celiac plexus, superior hypogastric plexus

5.   List each vertebral level of the spine that was injected.

6.   CPT surgery code(s) and modifier(s):

Case Study 10.4

Read the following clinical document and answer the questions for further review.

OPERATIVE REPORT

PREOPERATIVE DIAGNOSIS: Lumbar facet arthropathy

POSTOPERATIVE DIAGNOSIS: Lumbar facet arthropathy

PROCEDURE: Medial branch neurolysis at L2, L3, L4, and L5, bilaterally, with radiographic guidance

INDICATIONS FOR PROCEDURE: Mr. Miller has undergone diagnostic facet joint injections at the L3–4, L4–5, and L5–S1 levels with significant relief of his low back pain. These diagnostic and therapeutic procedures were performed twice. The patient had significant relief after both sets of injections. His pain has returned somewhat at this time, and given his favorable response to facet joint injections, we have decided to proceed with facet joint nerve radiofrequency neurolysis. The patient understands the risks, benefits, and alternatives to the procedure, and he gave his informed consent.

OPERATIVE REPORT: Intravenous cannula was started preoperatively. The patient was placed in the prone position. His back was prepped with a Betadine solution and draped in a sterile fashion. Under fluoroscopy, his lumbar facets were identified bilaterally. The skin and subcutaneous tissues along the lines to the nerves which innervate these joints (medial branch nerves) were anesthetized with 1% lidocaine using a 25-gauge needle. Then 10-cm radiofrequency needles with 10-mm active tips were advanced to the medial branch nerve sites on both the right and left sides. This was accomplished at L2, L3, L4, and L5 on both the right and left sides. At each nerve site, sensory stimulation occurred at each site at 50 Hz with less than 1 mV. Motor testing at each site was negative at 2 Hz and 2 mV. Radiofrequency lesioning was then performed at each site after an injection of 1 cc of lidocaine by each needle. Radiofrequency lesioning was performed at 80°C for 90 seconds at each site. All needles were removed intact. There were no complications to the procedure. The patient tolerated the procedure well and remained conversant throughout the procedure. The patient was discharged with stable vital signs. He was given instructions to follow up with me in approximately 2½ weeks.

Questions for Further Review: Case Study 10.4

1. Identify the medical substance(s) injected into the spine.
   a. Lysis solution (for example, hypertonic saline, enzyme)
   b. Anesthetic(s)
   c. Antispasmodic(s)
   d. Opioid(s)
   e. Steroid(s)
   f. Neurolytic substance(s) (for example, alcohol, phenol, iced saline solution, chemical, thermal, electrical, radiofrequency)
   g. Other solution—specify (for example, narcotic)

2. Which of the following medial branches was/were treated?
   a. L2
   b. L3
   c. L4
   d. L5
   e. all of the above

3. How was the medial branch treatment performed?
   a. unilaterally
   b. bilaterally

4. CPT surgery code(s) and modifier(s):

Case Study 10.5

Read the following clinical document and answer the questions for further review.

OPERATIVE REPORT

PREOPERATIVE DIAGNOSIS: Dorsal injury of the lumbar area

POSTOPERATIVE DIAGNOSIS: Same

OPERATION PERFORMED: Trial spinal cord stimulator lead placement under fluoroscopic guidance

ANESTHESIA: Local/monitor

COMPLICATIONS: None

FINDINGS: Electrode position is T9/T10

PROCEDURE: The patient was brought to the OR and placed on the table in a prone position. The lumbar spine was prepped and draped in the usual sterile fashion. The patient was given 1 gram of Ancef through the intravenous. The patient was given 1 cc of Fentanyl intravenously and then 4 cc of Diprivan was given as a bolus dose. When this was done, the subcutaneous tissue was injected with 0.25% Marcaine with epinephrine at L2/L3 interspace. A 14-gauge modified Tuohy needle was inserted into the epidural canal without any complications, passed without resistance, and heme negative CSF was noted. When this was done, the Octrode ANS was placed through the needle into the spinal canal, the electrode positioned in the midline in the epidural canal at T10/T9, and patient was checked for concordant paresthesias. Good concordant paresthesias were obtained bilaterally in the both lower extremities down to his foot, as well as in his toes and into his lower back area, as well as the buttocks. When this was confirmed, AP lateral views were taken, the needle was removed from the epidural canal, the insertion site was applied with Bacitracin ointment, and dressings were applied. The patient tolerated the procedure well and was sent to the recovery room for recovery.

Questions for Further Review: Case Study 10.5

1. What was the surgical approach for this procedure?
   a. Incision and subcutaneous placement
   b. Percutaneous
   c. Laminectomy for implantation

2. What type of procedure was performed?
   a. Initial placement of electrode
   b. Initial placement of pulse generator or receiver

    c. Replacement of electrode
    d. Replacement of pulse generator or receiver
    e. Removal of electrode
    f. Removal of pulse generator or receiver
    g. Revision of electrode
    h. Revision of pulse generator or receiver

3. On what anatomic site was the procedure performed?
    a. Cranial nerve
    b. Epidural
    c. Peripheral nerve
    d. Autonomic nerve
    e. Sacral nerve
    f. Neuromuscular
    g. Transcutaneous
    h. Spinal cord

4. CPT surgery code(s) and modifier(s):

Case Study 10.6

Read the following clinical document and answer the questions for further review.

OPERATIVE REPORT

PREOPERATIVE DIAGNOSIS: Malfunction spinal cord stimulator

POSTOPERATIVE DIAGNOSIS: Same

OPERATION PERFORMED: Exploration of the connection of the spinal cord stimulator lead, as well as extension. Exploration of the IPG generator battery under fluoroscopy and replacement of the extension wire.

ANESTHESIA: Local/monitor

COMPLICATIONS: None

FINDINGS: In the distal end of extension was noted to be fractured electrode.

PROCEDURE: The patient was brought to the OR and placed on the table in the prone position. Lumbar spine, as well as the flank and right buttock area, was prepped and draped in the usual sterile fashion. Skin was injected with 0.25% Marcaine at midthoracic spine incision, where the connection of the spinal cord stimulator extension was, and the right buttock incision was also injected with local anesthetic. A #15 blade was utilized to open both incisions. The incisions were further dissected down to the subcutaneous pocket. The extension connection was removed from the pocket, and the spinal cord stimulator lead was released via hex wrench. At that point, the integrity of the spinal cord stimulator lead was checked with the outside connecting cable, and programming was done intraoperatively, where the patient reported good paresthesias in her left upper extremities. When this was confirmed, the generator was removed from the subcutaneous pocket and the extension wire was removed from the generator using a hex wrench. At removal of the extension wire, it was noted that there was a fracture of the distal electrode from the extension wire. The extension wire was removed from the subcutaneous pocket and the tunnel, and a new tunnel was passed from the midthoracic incision down to the right buttock area. New 30 cm-long extension was tunneled and connected to the spinal cord stimulator lead. Boot was placed over the connection and secured with 0-silk tie, which was utilized to secure the connection. The extension wire was connected to the IPG generator using hex wrench, as well as the boot was placed over the connection. The IPG generator was placed back in the subcutaneous pocket, and both incisions were irrigated with the antibiotic solution. Both incisions were closed with 3-0 Vicryl sutures. The skin was closed with Dermabond. Dressings were applied. The patient tolerated the procedure well and was sent back to the recovery room for a recovery period. We did utilize fluoroscopy for tracing of the connection, as well as checking the integrity of the system.

Questions for Further Review: Case Study 10.6

1. What was the surgical approach for this procedure?
    a. Open via incision
    b. Percutaneous
    c. Laminectomy

2. What type of procedure was performed?
   a. Initial placement of electrode
   b. Initial placement of pulse generator or receiver
   c. Replacement of electrode
   d. Replacement of pulse generator or receiver
   e. Removal of electrode
   f. Removal of pulse generator or receiver
   g. Revision of electrode
   h. Revision of pulse generator or receiver

3. On what anatomic site was the procedure performed?
   a. Cranial nerve
   b. Epidural
   c. Peripheral nerve
   d. Autonomic nerve
   e. Sacral nerve
   f. Neuromuscular
   g. Transcutaneous
   h. Spinal cord

4. CPT surgery code(s) and modifier(s):

Case Study 10.7

Read the following clinical document and answer the questions for further review.

OPERATIVE REPORT

PREOPERATIVE DIAGNOSIS: Dorsal injury, malfunction spinal cord stimulator

POSTOPERATIVE DIAGNOSIS: Same

OPERATION PERFORMED: Removal of spinal cord stimulator, as well as the receiver from the right buttock area

ANESTHESIA: Local/monitor

COMPLICATIONS: None

PROCEDURE: The patient is brought to the OR and positioned in the prone position. The spine, as well as thoracic spine, is prepped and draped in the usual sterile fashion. Under fluoroscopic guidance, the electrode implant levels are identified. The lead has been approximately entered at L1–2. There are 2 leads in the interspinal space. Under fluoroscopic guidance, they were identified. When this was done, the skin was injected with 0.25% Marcaine at the site of the lead, as well as the implant site of the IP receiver. A #15 blade was utilized for incision. The incisions were further dissected down to the supraspinous ligament at the lumber spine area. While we were dissecting down to the supraspinous ligament, there was an intrathecal jugular catheter at lower pole of the incision. This was carefully retracted, and, at that point, the spinal cord stimulator leads were dissected from the supraspinous ligaments. The anchor sites were dissected from the supraspinous ligaments with electrocautery. When the anchors were removed from the supraspinous ligaments, the leads were pulled from the epidural space without any difficulty. When this was done, attention was diverted to the right buttock area, where the receiver was implanted. Further dissection, down to the subcutaneous pocket was done with electrocautery, and the receiver was removed from the subcutaneous pocket without any difficulty. At that point, both leads were pulled from the buttock incisions without any difficulty. When this was achieved, both incisions were irrigated with antibiotic solution. Hemostasis was obtained. Both incisions were closed with 3-0 Vicryl sutures in an interrupted fashion. The skin was closed with Dermabond. Dressings were applied. The patient tolerated the procedure well and was sent to recovery room for a recovery period.

Questions for Further Review: Case Study 10.7

1. What was the surgical approach for this procedure?
   a. Open via incision
   b. Percutaneous
   c. Laminectomy

2. What types of procedures were performed?
   a. Initial placement of electrode
   b. Initial placement of pulse generator or receiver
   c. Replacement of electrode

    d.   Replacement of pulse generator or receiver
    e.   Removal of electrode
    f.   Removal of pulse generator or receiver
    g.   Revision of electrode
    h.   Revision of pulse generator or receiver

3.   On what anatomic site was the procedure performed?
    a.   Cranial nerve
    b.   Epidural
    c.   Peripheral nerve
    d.   Autonomic nerve
    e.   Sacral nerve
    f.   Neuromuscular
    g.   Transcutaneous
    h.   Spinal cord

4.   CPT surgery code(s) and modifier(s):

Case Study 10.8

Read the following clinical document and answer the questions for further review.

OPERATIVE REPORT

AGE: 75

OPERATION: Implantation of spinal cord stimulator

ANESTHESIA: MAC with sedation

PREOPERATIVE DIAGNOSIS: Bilateral polyneuropathy, peripheral vascular disease, arachnoiditis, and bilateral leg pain

POSTOPERATIVE DIAGNOSIS: Bilateral polyneuropathy, peripheral vascular disease, arachnoiditis, and bilateral leg pain

PATHOLOGICAL DIAGNOSIS: None

OPERATIVE FINDINGS: None

OPERATIVE PROCEDURE: The patient was brought to the operating room and placed in the prone position. He was prepared and draped in the usual sterile fashion. With fluoroscopic guidance, the location of the desired site for placement of the Integral Intrel II lead was identified, and a local anesthetic consisting of 0.75% bupivacaine and 1% lidocaine with epinephrine was injected subcutaneously over the area. An approximately 7-cm longitudinal incision was made from L1 to L2. The incision was dissected down to the supraspinous ligament. Hemostasis was established, and a self-retaining retractor was used to allow adequate visualization. A #15-gauge Tuohy needle was then introduced with a paraspinous approach under fluoroscopic guidance up to the L1–L2 interlaminar space. The entry of the Tuohy into the epidural space was verified by using the loss-of-resistance technique with a glass 20-cc syringe and air. A guide wire was then introduced through the needle to create a path for the lead. The lead was passed through the needle and up to the disc space between T9 and T10 with fluoroscopic guidance. The screen cable connector was then joined to the lead stylet handle, and the cable was connected to the screener. A test stimulation was performed, and the screen cable was removed from the lead. The stylet was then removed from the lead, and the Tuohy needle was displaced, leaving the lead in position. The lead was anchored to the supraspinous ligament with #3-0 nylon suture in a clove hitch fashion. The lead was then reconnected to the screen cable and retested for position and placement.

A pocket site was identified just below the right iliac crest. A local anesthetic was administered into the region, and a 3-cm incision was made. A subcutaneous pocket was then created with blunt dissection technique for placement of the Intrel II implantable pulse generator. Tunneling was done between the lead and the pocket site after the administration of additional local anesthetic subcutaneously. The tunneling tool with a wedge-tip attachment was introduced subcutaneously from the lead incision and guided to the pocket. The wedge tip was then removed, and the extension cable tip was attached to the tunneling tool. The carrier tip was attached to the tunnel and extension connector lead from the tunnel tool. An insulating boot was then slipped over the lead body and the lead connector inserted into the extension connection. Screws were tightened with a hex wrench. The silicone boot was slipped over the extension connector and sutured in place. The Intrel II extension connector pins were then inserted into the receptacles of the generator, and each was screwed tightly with the hex wrench. The generator was introduced into the pocket. Both surgical wounds were then irrigated with antibiotic solution and closed with #2-0 Vicryl sutures.

DRAINS: None were put in place.

COMPLICATIONS: None

ESTIMATED BLOOD LOSS: Minimal

Questions for Further Review: Case Study 10.8

1. What was the surgical approach for the electrode procedure?
   a. Incision and subcutaneous placement
   b. Percutaneous
   c. Laminectomy for implantation

2. What was the surgical approach for the generator procedure?
   a. Incision and subcutaneous placement
   b. Percutaneous
   c. Laminectomy for implantation

3. What types of procedures were performed?
   a. Initial placement of electrode
   b. Initial placement of pulse generator or receiver
   c. Replacement of electrode
   d. Replacement of pulse generator or receiver
   e. Removal of electrode
   f. Removal of pulse generator or receiver
   g. Revision of electrode
   h. Revision of pulse generator or receiver

4. On what anatomic site was the procedure performed?
   a. Cranial nerve
   b. Epidural
   c. Peripheral nerve
   d. Autonomic nerve
   e. Sacral nerve
   f. Neuromuscular
   g. Transcutaneous
   h. Spinal cord

5. CPT surgery code(s) and modifier(s):

Case Study 10.9

Read the following clinical document and answer the questions for further review.

OPERATIVE REPORT

PREOPERATIVE DIAGNOSIS: Dorsal injury, lumbar radiculopathy

POSTOPERATIVE DIAGNOSIS: Removal of SynchroMed programmable pump, as well as catheter, as well as the anchor

ANESTHESIA: Local/monitor

COMPLICATIONS: None

PROCEDURE: The patient was brought to the OR and placed on the table in the lateral decubitus position. The spine and the abdominal wall were prepped and draped in the usual sterile fashion. The left flank was prepped and draped in the usual sterile fashion. The skin was injected with 0.25% Marcaine at the previous implant site, as well as the lumbar spine incision area. A #15 blade was utilized for incision, followed by further dissecting down to the supraspinous ligament on the lumbar spine area, as well as incisions further dissecting down to the subcutaneous pocket and the abdominal wall area. Blunt dissection of the abdominal wall area was done, where the pouch and the pump were removed from the subcutaneous pocket without any difficulty. When this was done, good hemostasis was obtained with electrocautery. The pump was disconnected from the catheter. The anchor was removed from the supraspinous ligament from the spine site, and the catheter was removed from the intrathecal spine. The track was electrocauterized to close it and no leakage of CSF was noted. When this was confirmed, the catheter was removed from the spine incision. The connector was removed from the spine incision, and the rest of the catheter was pulled from the abdominal wall area. Both incisions were irrigated copiously with the antibiotic solution. Hemostasis was checked, and both incisions were closed with 3-0 Vicryl sutures in an interrupted fashion. The skin was closed with Dermabond. Dressings were applied. The patient tolerated the procedure well and was sent to the recovery room for a recovery period.

Questions for Further Review: Case Study 10.9

1. Which of the following procedures was performed?
   a. Removal of previously implanted catheter
   b. Implantation of nonprogrammable pump
   c. Implantation of programmable pump
   d. Replacement of nonprogrammable pump
   e. Replacement of programmable pump
   f. Removal of pump (nonprogrammable or programmable)
   g. Electronic analysis of programmable pump with reprogramming
   h. Electronic analysis of programmable pump without reprogramming
   i. Refilling and maintenance of implantable pump

2. CPT surgery code(s) and modifier(s):

Chapter 11

Eye and Auditory System

CPT codes 65091 through 69979 are used to report surgical and related procedures performed on the eye and auditory system, which includes all parts of the eyeball; the eyelid; and the external, middle, and inner ear. Common outpatient procedures involving the eye and auditory system involve aqueous shunts, trabeculectomy, vitrectomy, eyelid surgery, ventilating tubes, tympanoplasties, and stapedectomies.

The final code in the Surgical section of the CPT manual is the code used to report the use of an operating microscope, code 69900.

Aqueous Shunts

Aqueous shunts are used for reducing and controlling abnormally high intraocular pressure in glaucoma. A shunt consists of a plastic tube that is connected to a reservoir or drainage plate. One end of the tube is implanted into the anterior chamber, and the other end is attached to the reservoir positioned between the sclera and the conjunctiva (AMA 2003e).

The shunt drains some of the aqueous fluid from the anterior chamber into a reservoir beneath the conjunctiva, lowering the pressure in the eye. The fluid is eventually absorbed into nearby tissues.

To prevent the drainage tube from eroding through the conjunctiva, the surgeon may place a piece of processed, dehydrated human pericardial allograft over the drainage tube before closing the conjunctival flap. The allograft is cut to size and secured in place with nylon sutures, anchoring its edges to the sclera. Code 67255 describes scleral reinforcement with graft, such as a Tutoplast patch graft. According to the Web site of the manufacturer (IOP, Inc.), a Tutoplast patch graft is a preformed, processed human scleral shell. For aqueous shunt procedures, the application of the allograft is not coded separately.

Coding Guidelines for Aqueous Shunts

The following guidelines apply to the coding of aqueous shunts:

- Code 66180 describes the implantation of a shunt to an external reservoir that is sutured to the eye wall at the equator of the eye. A graft is placed over the shunt, and the conjunctiva is carefully closed over the entire apparatus to prevent leakage of fluid into the tear film. This procedure allows vision to be preserved; earlier modes of therapy saved the eyeball but often lost vision. The devices listed in code 66180 (Molteno, Schocket, and Denver-Krupin) are examples only. If a different glaucoma drainage device is implanted, code 66180 may be used to report it. Examples of other commonly used drainage devices are the Ahmed Glaucoma Valve and the Baerveldt Implant (AMA 2003e).

- Code 66185 describes revision of the shunt, which involves taking down the overlying conjunctiva, removing the tube from its present position, and either relocating it under another graft or cutting it so that it fits differently through the same hole. This procedure also may include removal of scar tissue that sometimes forms around the reservoir.

APC	HCPCS	HCPCS Description	SI	Rel. Wt.	Payment Rate	OPPS OCE
0673			T	39.7101	2529.30	
	66180	Implant eye shunt				Significant Procedure, Multiple Reduction Applies; Separate APC payment
	66185	Revise eye shunt				Significant Procedure, Multiple Reduction Applies; Separate APC payment

Trabeculectomy

Trabeculectomy is performed to treat glaucoma by reducing intraocular pressure from the normally present fluid in the anterior segment of the eye. Trabeculectomy involves surgical creation of a new opening between the eye's anterior chamber and the external eye. The opening serves as a conduit to drain fluid from the anterior chamber into an area between the sclera and conjunctiva, where it can be reabsorbed by the body (AMA 2003h).

Coding Guidelines for Trabuculectomy

The following guidelines apply to the coding of trabuculectomy:

Code 66170 is reported when an antifibrotic agent or other wound-healing retardant is used on an eye without previous surgery, scarring, or trauma. For patients in certain ethnic groups that are prone to scarring, wound-healing retardants may be used to prevent premature closure of the conduit created by the trabeculectomy, and subsequent failure of the procedure (AMA 2003g).

- The use or nonuse of an antifibrotic agent, such as Mitomycin C, does not affect code selection for trabeculectomy procedures, as it may be used in patients with or without scarring from previous ocular surgery or trauma.

- A peripheral iridectomy is not coded separately. Peripheral iridectomies are performed as a routine component of trabeculectomy to promote flow of aqueous from the posterior chamber to the anterior chamber by preventing the iris from blocking the drainage pathway (AMA 2003h).

- Code 66170 is also used for trabeculectomy performed in the absence of previous surgery or when trabeculectomy ab externo is performed after a failed laser procedure on the iris for treating glaucoma.

- Code 66172 is used only to report a trabeculectomy performed on an eye that has conjunctival scarring from previous ocular surgery or injury. Examples include history of cataract surgery, history of strabismus surgery, history of failed trabeculectomy ab externo, history of penetrating trauma to eyeball, or conjunctival lacerations. This code includes the injection of antifibrotic agents, such as 5-Fluorouracil (5-FU). The technique of injecting 5-FU is recognized as effective in reducing the number of failed procedures caused by the formation of scar tissue and fistula closure.

- Operative wound revision code 66250 is used for a repeat trabeculectomy performed in the absence of scarring. This code should not be used unless procedure records specifically state that no scarring is present.

Cataract Removal

Cataract removal is a procedure to remove a clouded lens from the eye. Cataracts are removed to improve vision. An artificial intraocular lens (IOL) is usually inserted to help the eye focus in the absence of the removed lens.

The normal lens of the eye is transparent (has no color or shade). It focuses light onto the inner surface of the eye (the retina) to create an image. As a cataract develops, the lens becomes cloudy and blocks the normal path of light entering the eye. Vision becomes obscured.

- Intracapsular cataract extraction (ICCE): The surgeon removes the entire lens and its capsule.

- Extracapsular cataract extraction (ECCE): The surgeon removes the front portion and nucleus of the lens, leaving the posterior capsule in place.

- Anterior chamber intraocular lens (Anterior IOL): The surgeon inserts the intraocular lens after the intracapsular cataract extraction.

- Posterior chamber intraocular lens (Posterior IOL): The surgeon inserts the intraocular lens after the extracapsular cataract extraction.

APC	HCPCS	HCPCS Description	SI	Rel. Wt.	Payment Rate	OPPS OCE
0246			T	23.8649	1520.05	
	66982	Cataract surgery, complex				Significant Procedure, Multiple Reduction Applies; Separate APC payment
	66983	Cataract surgery w/ IOL, 1 stage				Significant Procedure, Multiple Reduction Applies; Separate APC payment

Coding Guidelines for Cataracts

The following guidelines apply to the coding of cataracts:

- The two types of cataract extraction are extracapsular and intracapsular. Extracapsular extraction, which includes the removal of the lens material without removing the posterior capsule, is reported with codes 66840–66852, 66940, 66982 and 66984. Intracapsular extraction, which involves removal of the entire lens including the capsule, is reported using 66920, 66930 and 66983.

- Lateral canthotomy, iridectomy, iridotomy, anterior and posterior capsulotomy, the use of viscoelastic agents, enzymatic zonulysis, use of other pharmacologic agents, and subconjunctival or subtenon injections are included as part of the code for the extraction of lens. Do not code 66830–66999 separately.

- Use code 66986 for the exchange of an IOL. Use code 65920 for anterior chamber removal of implanted material, and use code 67121 for posterior chamber removal of implanted material; extraocular, and 67121 for intraocular (AMA 2008).

- Do not code injections of medications used in conjunction with cataract surgery. Code 66030, injection of medication into the anterior chamber, is considered part of the cataract procedure and should not be coded separately.

Vitrectomy

A vitrectomy is an ocular surgical procedure involving the removal of the vitreous humor from the vitreous chamber. The CPT manual lists ten vitrectomy procedure codes, each of which describes a different method or approach. The variety of choices often confuses coders faced with an operative report for a vitrectomy procedure. Four common procedures are:

- Anterior vitrectomy: The surgeon approaches from the front of the iris, for example, incision at the limbus.

- Pars plana vitrectomy: The surgeon approaches the vitreous from behind the iris and in front of the retina.

- Mechanical vitrectomy: The surgeon uses an instrument or probe.

- Nonmechanical vitrectomy: The vitreous is removed using handheld sponges and scissors.

Coding Guidelines for Vitrectomy

The following guidelines apply to the coding of vitrectomies:

- Code 67005 is assigned for a nonmechanical anterior vitrectomy, in which handheld Weck-Cel sponges and scissors are used to cut the vitreous.

- Code 67010 is used for a mechanical anterior vitrectomy, in which an instrument or probe is used in front of the iris to perform an anterior vitrectomy. The instrument is used to cut and suction the vitreous mechanically. Common instruments for mechanical anterior vitrectomy include an ocutome, Microvit, guillotine retractor, Haslin gravity cannula, Shimadzu dry technique, or Daisy vitrectomy cutter. For removal of vitreous by paracentesis of anterior chamber, use 65810.

- Code 67025 is reported for the injection of vitreous substitute, pars plana or limbal approach, (fluid-gas exchange), with or without aspiration (separate procedure). Two CPT codes describe these injections: CPT 67025, as stated above, and CPT 67028, Intravitreal injection of a pharmacologic agent, separate procedure. They are distinguished by the injected substance: vitreous substitute or pharmacologic agent; 67025 is a major surgery with a 90-day postop period; 67028 is a minor procedure with zero postop days.

- An intravitreal injection may be an incidental component of another procedure, such as CPT 67108, Repair of retinal detachment. As an integral component, it is not separately reimbursed. If the injection is a stand-alone procedure, a separate claim can be filed.

- Code 67027 is reported for the implantation of an intravitreal drug delivery system. A tiny pellet of a drug implant is placed inside the eye during a short surgical procedure. The pellet is wrapped so that the drug is released into the eye consistently for a long period of time, eliminating the need for daily or weekly treatment. This procedure is most often performed for the treatment of Cytomegalovirus (CMV) retinitis in AIDS patients. Although no drug kills the CMV virus, drugs such as ganciclovir greatly slow down its multiplication. This makes it possible for the patient to maintain vision in the parts of the retina that are unaffected by the virus. The implant remains active for approximately five to eight months. When the implant becomes inactive, the doctor will likely insert another implant. Clinical studies show that a second implant has been as effective as the first.

- Code 67039 is used for a pars plana vitrectomy with focal endolaser photocoagulation. After the vitreous is removed, a laser is used to treat the retinal disorder(s) with one or two small focal areas.

- Code 67040 also is used for a pars plana vitrectomy with panretinal endolaser photocoagulation. After the vitreous is removed, a laser is used to treat all four quadrants of the retina by scattering the laser treatment through each panretinal area. Note: For use of ophthalmic endoscope with 67036, 67039, 67040–67043, use code 66990 (use separately in addition to primary procedure; for an associated lensectomy, use 66850) (AMA 2008).

- Codes 67041–67043 are assigned for a pars plana vitrectomy with removal of the retinal membrane.

APC	HCPCS	HCPCS Description	SI	Rel. Wt.	Payment Rate	OPPS OCE
0237			T	27.8450	1773.56	
	67025	Replace eye fluid				Significant Procedure, Multiple Reduction Applies; Separate APC payment

Strabismus Surgery

Strabismus surgery involves making a small incision in the tissue covering the eye, which allows the ophthalmologist access to the underlying eye muscles. Which eye muscles are repositioned depends on the direction the eye is turning. It may be necessary to perform surgery on both eyes.

Strabismus is a visual defect in which the eyes are misaligned and point in different directions. Strabismus can occur early in childhood or later in adulthood, although the causes of the eye misalignment are different. Strabismus can be the first sign of a serious vision problem

The two most common types of strabismus are esotropia and exotropia.

Esotropia describes an inward turning eye and is the most common type of strabismus in infants. Young children with esotropia do not use their eyes together, and the risk of amblyopia or poor vision development is the major concern.

Exotropia, or an outward turning eye, is another common type. This occurs most often when a child is focusing on distant objects. Typically, exotropia has less severe consequences upon visual development. Both forms can typically be corrected medically or surgically.

Coding Guidelines for Strabismus Surgery

The following guidelines apply to the coding of strabismus surgery (strabismus surgery refers to each eye individually):

Horizontal muscles: Code 67311 is used for one horizontal muscle, and code 67312 is used for two muscles of the same eye.

Vertical muscles: Code 67314 is used for one vertical muscle, and code 67316 for two muscles for the same eye.

Codes 67320, 67331, 67332, 67334, 67335, and 67340 are considered add-on procedures codes to be used in addition to the strabismus procedure codes (67311–67318).

Code 67320 describes a transposition procedure where the extraocular muscles are transposed.

Code 67334 describes a posterior fixation suture technique in which the extraocular muscle is sutured to the eye posterior to its insertion.

Code 67335 describes an adjustable suture insertion in which the sutures are tied in such a way that will allow for adjustment when the anesthetic wears off.

APC	HCPCS	HCPCS Description	SI	Rel. Wt.	Payment Rate	OPPS OCE
0243			T	24.1291	1536.88	
	67311	Strabismus surgery, recession or resection procedure; one horizontal muscle				Significant Procedure, Multiple Reduction Applies; Separate APC payment
	67314	Strabismus surgery, recession or resection procedure; one vertical muscle (excluding superior oblique)				Significant Procedure, Multiple Reduction Applies; Separate APC payment

Eyelid Surgery

Outpatient eyelid surgeries typically involve one or more of the following four components:

The conjunctiva is the mucous membrane that lines the underside of each eyelid and continues to form a protective covering over the exposed surface of the eyeball.

The tarsus is a platelike framework within upper and lower eyelids that provides stiffness and shape.

The canthus is an angle formed by the inner or outer junction of the upper and lower eyelids.

The orbicularis muscle is the elliptical muscle sheet that surrounds the eye. This muscle is responsible for closing eyelids and is innervated by the seventh cranial nerve.

Coding Guidelines for Eyelid Surgery

The following guidelines apply to the coding of eyelid surgery:

Codes 67916, 67917, 67923, and 67924 reflect surgical repair of ectropion and entropion of the eyelids, and not blepharoplasty, which is synonymous with reduction of orbital fat prolapse and redundant skin around the orbit. Blepharoplasty procedures are included in codes 15820, 15821, 15822, and 15823. Note: Blepharoplasty previously included any plastic surgical procedure performed on the eyelids; however, a distinction has evolved over the years in the usage of the terminology applied to various types of eyelid surgeries. This distinction was made to facilitate correct coding and interpretation of eyelid surgeries included in the integumentary and ophthalmology sections of the CPT book. Integumentary repair of eyelids (orbital fat prolapse, redundant skin) and the ophthalmological repair of eyelids (ectropion, entropion) are not related (AMA 2003d).

Codes 67961, 67966, 67971, 67973, 67974, and 67975 are used for excision and repair of eyelid involving lid margin, tarsus, conjunctiva, canthus, or full thickness. Note: For canthoplasty, use 67950; for free skin grafts use 15120, 15121, 15260, 15261; for tubed pedicle flap preparation, use 15576; for delay, use 15630; for attachment, use 15650.

Ventilating Tubes

Ventilating or pressure equalization tubes are used in ocular procedures to relieve pressure and encourage drainage. Two outpatient procedures that involve piercing the eardrum are myringotomy and tympanostomy. For a bilateral myringotomy or tympanostomy, report the procedure twice by using the same five-digit code or by using the code once with modifier –50, as used for Medicare cases.

Coding Guidelines for Ventilating Tubes

The following guidelines apply to the coding of ventilating tubes:

- Myringotomy codes 69420 and 69421 involve the surgical incision of the tympanic membrane to relieve pressure and release pus from an infection. In this procedure, also known as tympanotomy, fluid is gently suctioned out of the middle ear.

- Codes 69433 and 69436 are used for myringotomy with insertion of ventilating tube and are not used in conjunction with codes 69420 or 69421. To confirm insertion of a ventilating tube, review the anesthesia sheet or operating room nursing sheet for a manufacturer's label identifying the ventilating tube.

- Code 69433 or 69436 is assigned for tympanostomy requiring insertion of ventilating tubes. Also, check the anesthesia record for the type of anesthesia used.

- Code 69424 is used for ventilating tube removal. Verify whether the ventilating tube removal was performed under general anesthesia and whether it was unilateral or bilateral.

- Code 69424 should not be used in conjunction with the following codes: 69205, 69210, 69420, 69421, 69433–69676, 69710–69745, and 69801–69930.

APC	HCPCS	HCPCS Description	SI	Rel. Wt.	Payment Rate	OPPS OCE
0251			T	2.5002	159.25	
	69420	Myringotomy including aspiration and/or eustachian tube inflation				Significant Procedure, Multiple Reduction Applies; Separate APC payment

Tympanoplasties

Tympanoplasty involves repairing or reconstructing the eardrum. The words *eardrum* and *tympanic membrane* may be used interchangeably. Mastoidectomies and ossicular chain reconstructions are common types of tympanoplasties. These procedures may or may not involve the canal wall.

In a mastoidectomy, mastoid cells are removed and the surgeon defines two or more boundaries. The tympanic membrane is repaired by inserting graft material into the hole, usually fascia, periosteum, or perichondrium. The affected boundaries may include facial nerve, labyrinth or lateral and/or posterior semicircular canal, digastric ridge, the mastoid tip, sigmoid plate, posterior phositdura, tegmen, and mastoid air cells.

Ossicles are the three small bones in the ear: malleus, incus, and stapes. In an ossicular chain reconstruction, these bones may be replaced with prosthetic bones. Examples of partial ossicular replacement prostheses (PORPs) are incus-stapes and malleus-incus. An example of total ossicular replacement prosthesis (TORP) is a malleus-incus-stapes.

The partition between the exterior ear canal and the mastoid space is the canal wall. If the procedure records list "intact canal wall" or there is no reference to the canal wall, the patient has not had a modified radical mastoidectomy. Nonintact canal wall is seen when the canal wall is down. Reconstructed canal wall, though uncommon, is usually rebuilt with cartilage from the knee. Cancer or cholesteatoma sometimes obliterates the canal wall altogether. The tympanic membrane is repaired by inserting graft material into the hole, usually fascia, periosteum, or perichondrium. Although there are a variety of ways to stabilize graft material, the most commonly performed stabilization technique in the United States is gel foam packing.

Coding Guidelines for Tympanoplasties

The following guidelines apply to the coding of tympanoplasties:

- Code 69610 is intended to describe tympanic membrane repair procedures in which the physician freshens the edges of the perforated area of the tympanic membrane. The physician may or may not apply a paper patch to the site (AMA 2001h).
- Codes 69641–69646 are used for tympanoplasty with mastoidectomy.
- Codes 69601–69676 refer to repairs and are listed by anatomy. Because temporalis fascia grafts, other tissue grafts, or fat plugs may not be needed, these procedures are not inclusive of the codes, and each is reported separately using the appropriate codes. For example, a temporalis fascia graft is reported with code 15732 (AMA 2003i).

APC	HCPCS	HCPCS Description	SI	Rel. Wt.	Payment Rate	OPPS OCE
0254			T	23.9765	1527.16	
	69610	Tympanic membrane repair, with or without site preparation of perforation for closure, with or without patch				Significant Procedure, Multiple Reduction Applies; Separate APC payment
	69620	Myringoplasty (surgery confined to drumhead and donor area)				Significant Procedure, Multiple Reduction Applies; Separate APC payment

Stapedectomies

A stapedectomy is the surgical removal of the stapes of the middle ear. Stapedectomies involve only the stapes and are coded separately from ossicular chain reconstructions.

Coding Guidelines for Stapedectomies

The following guidelines apply to the coding of stapedectomies:

- Codes 69660 and 69661 are used for stapedectomies. Code 69661 specifically refers to stapedectomy with footplate drillout. In otosclerotic patients, the footplate can be thickened many times its normal width. In such cases, a drill is used to remove bone so the disease process can be identified.
- Code 69662 is reported for stapedectomy revision.

Documentation Requirements for Eye and Auditory System Procedures

Each procedure is followed by clinical information that must be documented in the medical record when the procedure is performed.

Vitrectomy

Vitrectomies are reported with CPT codes 66852, 67005–67043, 67108, and 67112.

1. The type of vitrectomy performed:

   - Anterior approach
   - Posterior/pars plana approach.

2. The instrument(s) used to perform the vitrectomy:

   - Nonmechanical (for example, the use of Weck-cel sponges and scissors)
   - Mechanical (for example, the use of vitrector, Microvit, ocutome, retractor)

3. The type of procedure(s) performed:

   - Injection of vitreous substitute
   - Aspiration or release of vitreous
   - Discission of vitreous strands
   - Severing of vitreous strands
   - Intravitreal injection of pharmacologic agent
   - Implantation of intravitreal drug delivery system
   - Aspiration or release of vitreous
   - Epiretinal membrane stripping
   - Focal endolaser photocoagulation
   - Endolaser panretinal photocoagulation
   - Vitrectomy with pars plana lensectomy/removal of lens material
   - Vitrectomy for retinal detachment

Eyelid Repair/Reconstruction

Eyelid repair/reconstruction is reported with CPT codes 15820–15823, 67912, 67916, 67917, 67923, and 67924.

1. The diagnosis for each eyelid being operated on (for example, blepharochalasia, ectropion, entropion, lagophthalmos).

2. Each eyelid that is surgically treated:

- Left upper eyelid
- Right upper eyelid
- Left lower eyelid
- Right lower eyelid

3. The fraction of eyelid margin that is surgically treated (for example, one-fourth of lid margin)

4. The surgical technique used to repair each eyelid:

    - Implantation of upper eyelid load (for example, gold weight)
    - Blepharoplasty
    - Blepharoplasty with extensive lower eyelid herniated fat pad
    - Blepharoplasty with excessive skin weighting down upper eyelid
    - Tarsal wedge excision
    - Extensive repair
    - Tarsal strip operation
    - Capsulopalpebral fascia repair

Middle Ear Surgery

Middle ear surgery is reported with CPT codes 69502–69511 and 69601–69676.

1. Type of mastoidectomy:

    - Complete
    - Modified radical
    - Radical
    - Revision resulting in complete mastoidectomy
    - Revision resulting in modified radical mastoidectomy
    - Revision resulting in radical mastoidectomy
    - Revision resulting in tympanoplasty
    - Revision with apicectomy

2. Type of tympanic membrane surgery:

    - Tympanic membrane repair (with or without site preparation, perforation, or patch)
    - Tympanoplasty without mastoidectomy
    - Tympanoplasty with antrotomy
    - Tympanoplasty with mastoidotomy
    - Tympanoplasty with mastoidectomy
    - Ossicular chain reconstruction
    - Ossicular chain reconstruction and synthetic prosthesis (partial or total replacement)

3. External auditory canal wall status:

   • Intact

   • Reconstructed

4. Stapes surgery:

   • Stapedectomy

   • Stapedotomy

   • Footplate drillout

Case Studies

This section contains actual operative reports from real-life cases. All identifiers have been removed or changed for confidentiality and privacy.

Carefully read the clinical documentation for each case study, which may include a procedure report as well as radiology and/or pathology reports, as applicable.

Answer all the questions for further review at the end of each case study. Use a current CPT codebook or HCPCS Level II code listing, as needed.

When appropriate, assign one or more of the following modifiers:

−50	Bilateral Procedure
−59	Distinct Procedural Service
−FA	Left hand, thumb
−F1	Left hand, second digit
−F2	Left hand, third digit
−F3	Left hand, fourth digit
−F4	Left hand, fifth digit
−F5	Right hand, thumb
−F6	Right hand, second digit
−F7	Right hand, third digit
−F8	Right hand, fourth digit
−F9	Right hand, fifth digit
−LT	Left side
−RT	Right side
−TA	Left foot, great toe
−T1	Left foot, second digit
−T2	Left foot, third digit
−T3	Left foot, fourth digit
−T4	Left foot, fifth digit
−T5	Right foot, great toe
−T6	Right foot, second digit
−T7	Right foot, third digit
−T8	Right foot, fourth digit
−T9	Right foot, fifth digit

Do not apply the current version of the Medicare CCI edits to any of these exercises; the focus is on the application of the coding guidelines and not on the application of edits that change on a quarterly basis. When coding in real life, of course, you will need to apply the CCI edits as appropriate for Medicare outpatient cases.

Case Study 11.1

Read the following clinical document and answer the questions for further review.

OPERATIVE REPORT

PREOPERATIVE DIAGNOSIS: Exposure of tube from Krupin valve, left eye

POSTOPERATIVE DIAGNOSIS: Exposure of tube from Krupin valve, left eye

OPERATION: Revision of tube with placement of new scleral patch graft, left eye

ANESTHESIA: Peribulbar local anesthesia and IV sedation

COMPLICATIONS: None

PROCEDURE: The patient was anesthetized with peribulbar local anesthesia after receiving IV sedation. The patient was prepped and draped in the usual sterile fashion. A wire-lid speculum was used to keep the eye in the open position, and a conjunctival peritomy was performed over the location of the Krupin tube. The conjunctiva was dissected posteriorly to free attachments until the tube was exposed, and a scleral patch graft, trans-Z-graft tissue was then cut to the appropriate size to completely cover the tube and was sutured in place with two 9-0 nylon sutures at the anterior extent of the tube. The conjunctival peritomy was then closed using 8-0 Vicryl suture at the superior and inferior margins of the limbus such that the patch graft was completely covered.

An inferior injection of 0.5 cc Ancef and 0.5 cc dexamethasone was administered subconjunctivally. The eye was patched with TobraDex ointment, an eye patch, and a Fox shield. The patient will be seen tomorrow for follow-up.

Questions for Further Review: Case Study 11.1

1. What type of procedure was performed?
   a. Insertion of the Krupin valve aqueous shunt to extraocular reservoir
   b. Revision of the Krupin valve aqueous shunt to extraocular reservoir

2. CPT surgery code(s) and modifier(s):

Case Study 11.2

Read the following clinical document and answer the questions for further review.

OPERATIVE REPORT

PREOPERATIVE DIAGNOSIS: Uncontrolled open-angle glaucoma, left eye

POSTOPERATIVE DIAGNOSIS: Uncontrolled open-angle glaucoma, left eye

OPERATION: Trabeculectomy with mitomycin C, left eye

PROCEDURE: The patient was anesthetized with peribulbar local anesthesia. He was prepped and draped in the usual sterile fashion. A lid speculum was used to keep the eye in an open position, and a superior nasal peritomy was performed with the Westcott scissors. Local anesthesia was injected into the subconjunctival space, and hemostasis was obtained with wet field cautery. Mitomycin C 0.5 mg/ml was placed on two Weck-cel sponge fragments in the subconjunctival space for a total of three minutes. The subconjunctival space was then copiously irrigated with a full bottle of balanced salt solution. A triangular trabeculectomy flap 3 mm in length and height was then outlined with a #75 Superblade and dissected forward to clear cornea with a #57 beaver blade. A single 10-0 nylon suture was preplaced in the bed of the trabeculectomy flap at the apex. The paracentesis tract was made with the Superblade, and preservative free lidocaine was irrigated through the anterior chamber. A trabeculectomy window was then cut with the Superblade and the Kelly punch. Miochol solution was irrigated through the anterior chamber, and a peripheral iridectomy was performed. The trabeculectomy flap was sutured in place with preplaced nylon at the apex, and it was noted that the anterior chamber remained formed with leakage at the edges of the trabeculectomy flap with light pressure. The conjunctival peritomy was then closed in a watertight fashion using a 9-0 nylon on a Vas-100 vascular needle. Balanced salt solution was irrigated through the anterior chamber, and a large bleb formed in the supranasal quadrant without evidence of leakage. A single drop of atropine was placed on the eye. An inferior injection of Ancef with Dexamethasone 0.5 cc was administered sub-conjunctivally. The eye was then patched with TobraDex ointment, an eye patch, and a Fox shield. The patient will be seen tomorrow for follow-up.

Questions for Further Review: Case Study 11.2

1. What type of procedure was performed?
   a. Trabeculotomy
   b. Trabeculectomy in absence of previous surgery
   c. Trabeculectomy with scarring from previous ocular surgery or trauma
   d. Trabeculectomy with previous ocular surgery or trauma with no documentation of scarring

2. CPT surgery code(s) and modifier(s):

Case Study 11.3

Read the following clinical document and answer the questions for further review.

OPERATIVE REPORT

PREOPERATIVE DIAGNOSIS: Vitreous hemorrhage secondary to central retinal vein occlusion, left eye

POSTOPERATIVE DIAGNOSIS: Vitreous hemorrhage secondary to central retinal vein occlusion, left eye

OPERATION: Vitrectomy with panretinal photocoagulation, left eye

ANESTHESIA: Local with sedation

DESCRIPTION OF PROCEDURE: The patient was brought to the operating room and given sedation by vein before being given a retrobulbar block consisting of 7 cc of the standard mixture. The left eye was prepped and draped in the usual sterile fashion and prepared for a three-port pars plana vitrectomy with a 4-mm infusion cannula and all three sclerotomies 4.0 posterior to the limbus. A dense vitreous hemorrhage was encountered with fresh-greater-than-old blood. It was removed systematically. There was, fortunately, full posterior vitreous detachment, so the vitreous was trimmed as anteriorly as possible in this phakic patient. A significant amount of blood was layered on the macula, which was removed with passive extrusion. Following removal of the blood, panretinophotic coagulation was performed in a heavy pattern throughout the periphery. A total of 973 spots at 0.3 seconds duration of power were delivered. Scleral depression was then performed to assess for any pulls, tears, or breaks in the peripheral retina; there were none. The sclerotomies were then closed with #6-0 Vicryl, and the conjunctiva were closed with #6-0 plain gut. The patient was given subconjunctival Ancef and Decadron and topical scopolamine and TobraDex drops. The drapes were removed, and two sterile eye pads and an eye shield were taped over the eye. The patient was taken to the recovery area in good condition.

The estimated blood loss for this procedure was 5 cc. There were no complications.

Questions for Further Review: Case Study 11.3

1. What type of vitrectomy was performed?
   a. Anterior approach
   b. Posterior/pars plana approach

2. What type of procedure was performed?
   a. Nonmechanical (for example, use of Weck-cel sponges and scissors)
   b. Mechanical (for example, use of vitrector, Microvit, ocutome, retractor)
   c. Injection of vitreous substitute
   d. Intravitreal injection of pharmacologic agent
   e. Implantation of intravitreal drug delivery system (for example, Ganciclovir implant)
   f. Aspiration or release of vitreous
   g. Discission of vitreous strands
   h. Severing of vitreous strands
   i. Epiretinal membrane stripping
   j. Focal endolaser photocoagulation

      k.   Endolaser panretinal photocoagulation
      l.   Vitrectomy with pars plana lensectomy/removal of lens material
      m.   Vitrectomy for retinal detachment

3.   CPT surgery code(s) and modifier(s):

Case Study 11.4

Read the following clinical document and answer the questions for further review.

OPERATIVE REPORT

PREOPERATIVE DIAGNOSIS: Macular pucker, left eye

POSTOPERATIVE DIAGNOSIS: Macular pucker and small possible retinal hole, left eye

OPERATION: Vitrectomy with extensive membranectomy and focal laser, left eye

DESCRIPTION OF PROCEDURE: The patient was brought to the operating room and given sedation by vein before being given a retrobulbar block consisting of 7 cc of the standard mixture. The left eye was then prepped and draped in the usual sterile fashion and prepared for a three-port pars plana vitrectomy with a 4-mm infusion cannula and all three sclerotomies 3.5 mm posterior to the limbus.

A core vitrectomy was performed without incident. There was a significantly condensed opaque membrane causing a fold through the fovea and extending nearly horizontally through the macula from just temporal to the disc to one to two disc diameters temporal to the fovea. Using first a bent MVR blade as a pick and then a series of forceps and forceps/picks, this membrane was liberated in pieces. There was a mild amount of bleeding on the surface of the retina, but no holes were created. The residual membrane was removed without incident, and small amounts of blood were vacuumed off the surface of the macula with passive extrusion. The fundus was then examined, and there was a small break just below the macula with some blood. This was lasered, as was a small suspicious area with hemorrhage on the retina and in the retina just nasal to this. Both of these areas were outside the macula. Approximately 250 laser spots were used to completely surround these with photocoagulation. The remainder of the peripheral fundus was unremarkable. The sclerotomies were closed with #6-0 Vicryl and the conjunctiva with #6-0 plain gut. The patient was given subconjunctival Ancef and Decadron and topical scopolamine and TobraDex drops. The drapes were removed, and two sterile eye pads and an eye shield were taped over the eye. The patient was taken to the recovery area in good condition.

The estimated blood loss for this procedure was 10 cc. There were no complications.

Questions for Further Review: Case Study 11.4

1.   What type of vitrectomy was performed?
    a.   Anterior approach
    b.   Posterior/pars plana approach

2.   What types of procedures were performed?
    a.   Nonmechanical (for example, the use of Weck-cel sponges and scissors)
    b.   Mechanical (for example, the use of vitrector, Microvit, ocutome, retractor)
    c.   Injection of vitreous substitute
    d.   Intravitreal injection of pharmacologic agent
    e.   Implantation of intravitreal drug delivery system (for example, Ganciclovir implant)
    f.   Aspiration or release of vitreous
    g.   Discission of vitreous strands
    h.   Severing of vitreous strands
    i.   Epiretinal membrane stripping (for example, macular pucker)
    j.   Focal endolaser photocoagulation
    k.   Endolaser panretinal photocoagulation
    l.   Vitrectomy with pars plana lensectomy/removal of lens material
    m.   Vitrectomy for retinal detachment

3.   CPT surgery code(s) and modifier(s):

Case Study 11.5

Read the following clinical document and answer the questions for further review.

OPERATIVE REPORT

POSTOPERATIVE DIAGNOSIS: Macular pucker, left eye

OPERATIONS:

1. Pars plana vitrectomy, left eye
2. Removal of preretinal membranes, left eye

PROCEDURE/FINDINGS: The patient was taken to the operating room. The left eye had been dilated preoperatively. The left eye was prepped and draped in a sterile fashion.

Limited peritomies were performed of the conjunctiva. A standard pars plana vitrectomy setup was utilized 2.5 mm posterior to the surgical limbus. The end of the infusion cannula was visualized in the inferotemporal quadrant before infusion was begun. The end of the infusion cannula was visualized in the vitreous cavity before the infusion was begun.

Additional sclerotomies were made 3.5 mm posterior to the surgical limbus superiorly. A pars plana vitrectomy was performed. The posterior vitreous was detached. The pucker was identified. The pucker was peeled with a pick and end-grabbing forceps. There was a nice edge on the pucker on the superior margin. No retinal holes or tears were created. The peripheral retina was inspected. There were no retinal holes or tears. The retina was attached. There was good perfusion of the optic nerve.

The sclerotomies were cleaned and closed with 7-0 Vicryl suture. The conjunctiva was closed with 6-0 plain gut suture.

Dexamethasone 2 mg was injected subconjunctivally. Erythromycin, atropine, and a patch were applied to the left eye.

The patient left the operating room.

Questions for Further Review: Case Study 11.5

1. What type of vitrectomy was performed?
   a. Anterior approach
   b. Posterior/pars plana approach

2. What type of procedure was performed?
   a. Nonmechanical (for example, the use of Weck-cel sponges and scissors)
   b. Mechanical (for example, the use of vitrector, Microvit, ocutome, retractor)
   c. Injection of vitreous substitute
   d. Intravitreal injection of pharmacologic agent
   e. Implantation of intravitreal drug delivery system (for example, Ganciclovir implant)
   f. Aspiration or release of vitreous
   g. Discission of vitreous strands
   h. Severing of vitreous strands
   i. Removal of preretinal cellular membrane
   j. Focal endolaser photocoagulation
   k. Endolaser panretinal photocoagulation
   l. Vitrectomy with pars plana lensectomy/removal of lens material
   m. Vitrectomy for retinal detachment

3. CPT surgery code(s) and modifier(s):

Case Study 11.6

Read the following clinical document and answer the questions for further review.

OPERATIVE REPORT

PREOPERATIVE DIAGNOSIS:
1. Cataract, right eye
2. Preglaucoma

POSTOPERATIVE DIAGNOSIS: Cataract, right eye

ANESTHESIA: Monitored anesthesia care with retrobulbar

INDICATIONS FOR SURGERY: Patient with decreased vision in her right eye secondary to cataract. Patient's visual acuity is 20/100 with contrast sensitivity with 2+ nuclear cataract. The intraocular pressure is 23 in the right eye and 22 in the left eye, with 50–60% cupping OU. The patient is considered preglaucoma. The patient is here at this time for surgical correction.

OPERATION: Phacoemulsification with lens implantation, right eye.

PROCEDURE/FINDINGS: The patient was taken to the operating room and light general anesthesia was begun. A 2.5 cc modified Gills technique for akinesia and anesthesia. Light pressure was placed on for two minutes. The eye was then prepped and draped in the usual manner for eye surgery. The lid speculum was inserted and a fornix-based flap was made at the 12 o'clock position, 8 mm in length, and a groove was made 3.0 mm in length, 2 mm posterior to the blue line, dissected into clear cornea where entrance into the anterior chamber was made at the 12 o'clock position. Occucoat was injected.

A peritomy incision was made at the 2 o'clock position. The anterior capsulotomy was performed with continuous tear technique. Hydrodissection was done with balanced salt solution. Phacoemulsification was used for 1 minute 6 seconds to remove nuclear material. Irrigation and aspiration was used to remove cortical material and the cap-vac to polish the posterior capsule.

The incision was enlarged to 3.5 mm, internally and lens implant was inserted. It was a 22.5-diopter model LI61AO posterior chamber foldable Bausch and Lomb intraocular lens, serial number 4707924062. It was rotated to 180-degree position. The occucoat was removed. Balanced salt solution was used to refill the anterior chamber. Carbastat was used to inject in the anterior chamber. The incision was found to be watertight. Conjunctiva was pulled over the incision. Antibiotic and steroid drops were placed in the eye. A patch and shield were placed over the eye.

The patient was removed from the operating room without complications.

Questions for Further Review: Case Study 11.6

1. What type of cataract was removed?
   a. Nuclear cataract—Central part of the lens
   b. Cortical cataract—Peripheral part of the lens
   c. Idiopathic cataract—Posterior subcapsular part of the lens

2. What type of procedure was performed?
   a. Extracapsular cataract removal with insertion of IOL
   b. Intracapsular cataract removal with insertion of IOL
   c. Exchange of IOL only
   d. Use of ophthalmic endoscope

3. CPT surgery code(s) and modifier(s):

Case Study 11.7

Read the following clinical document and answer the questions for further review.

OPERATIVE REPORT

POSTOPERATIVE DIAGNOSIS:

1. Cytomegalovirus retinitis, both eyes
2. Cytomegalovirus optic neuritis, both eyes

OPERATION:

1. Pars plana vitrectomy, left eye
2. Vitrasert insert, left eye

PROCEDURE/FINDINGS: The patient was taken to the operating room. A retrobulbar block was administered to the left eye. The left eye was prepped and draped in a sterile fashion. The left eye was inspected with the indirect ophthalmoscope. The optic nerve was involved with cytomegalovirus. There was a retinitis extending along the arcade and in the superior nasal quadrant. The retina was attached. A limited peritomy was placed in the inferior temporal quadrant. A 5.5-mm sclerotomy was performed 4 mm posterior to the surgical limbus. The Vitrasert was trimmed approximately 3 mm and then was placed into the eye and attached to the sclerotomy lip with an #8-0 nylon suture. The wound was then closed with buried #8-0 nylon suture. The retina was inspected, and the retina was attached. The eye was of reasonable pressure. Vitreous was cleaned from the wound both at the time of incision and after implantation. The conjunctivae were closed with #6-0 plain gut suture. We injected 20 mg of dexamethasone and 20 mg of Nebcin subconjunctivally. The patient left the operating room without complications.

Questions for Further Review: Case Study 11.7

1. What type of vitrectomy was performed?
   a. Anterior approach
   b. Posterior/pars plana approach

2. What type of procedure was performed?
   a. Nonmechanical (for example, the use of Weck-cel sponges and scissors)
   b. Mechanical (for example, the use of vitrector, Microvit, oculome, retractor)
   c. Injection of vitreous substitute
   d. Intravitreal injection of pharmacologic agent
   e. Implantation of intravitreal drug delivery system (for example, Ganciclovir implant)
   f. Aspiration or release of vitreous
   g. Discission of vitreous strands
   h. Severing of vitreous strands
   i. Epiretinal membrane stripping
   j. Focal endolaser photocoagulation
   k. Endolaser panretinal photocoagulation
   l. Vitrectomy with pars plana lensectomy/removal of lens material
   m. Vitrectomy for retinal detachment

3. CPT surgery code(s) and modifier(s):

Case Study 11.8

Read the following clinical document and answer the questions for further review.

OPERATIVE REPORT

PREOPERATIVE DIAGNOSIS:

1. Bilateral upper lid dermatochalasis
2. Bilateral brow ptosis

POSTOPERATIVE DIAGNOSIS: Same

PROCEDURE:

1. Bilateral upper blepharoplasty
2. Bilateral direct brow pexy

ANESTHESIA: Mac

COMPLICATIONS: None

TISSUE TO PATHOLOGY: None

INDICATIONS FOR SURGERY: Patient with combined bilateral brow ptosis and dermatochalasis causing greater than a 20-degree superior visual field obstruction, here for surgical correction.

FINDINGS AND PROCEDURE: Appropriate preoperative consent was obtained on the 18th of June, 200X. The patient was taken to the holding area, where IV access was obtained. The patient was placed in a sitting position, and the upper lid creases were marked, and the redundant tissue above the creases was marked with a surgical marking pen. A proposed incision line was marked in the lateral two-thirds of the superior edge of the brow hair, and a 4–5 mm parallel marking was made above the brow. The patient was then transferred to the operating room and placed in supine position on the table. Routine vital sign monitoring equipment was placed. Brief IV sedating was given, during which 0.3 cc of 1% Xylocaine with epinephrine and .75% Marcaine were infiltrated in each of the upper eyelids and four cc of the same above-mentioned solution into the super brow region. Gentle pressure was maintained for several minutes, and the patient was then prepped and draped in the usual fashion.

Attention was first directed to the upper lids, where the previously made marking was incised with a scalpel. A full-thickness excision was performed removing the redundant skin, and a strip of pretarsal orbicularis was then directly excised. Herniated orbital fat was identified, cross-clamped, and excised and the pedicle cauterized. The wound was then closed with continuous running 6-0 fast absorbing gut.

Attention was then directed to the contralateral side where the same above-mentioned procedure was performed.

Attention was then directed to the right brow where an incision was made at the previously made marking with a beveling of the blade away from the hair follicles. An identical beveled incision in the superior limb of the marking and a 4–5-mm thick swath of the super brow skin was then excised. Discretion was continued to the periosteum, which was then incised and elevated, freeing the brow pad from the superorbital rim. After adequate homeostasis was obtained with bipolar cautery, the periosteum was advanced superiorly with 4-0 Vicryl sutures for reapposition. The wound was then closed in a layered fashion with 5-0 Vicryl suture for deep closure and 5-0 silk for superficial closure with alternating simple interrupted and vertical mattress for slight wound eversion.

Attention was then directed to the contralateral side where the same above-mentioned direct brow pexy procedure was performed. At the conclusion of the procedure, the wound was noted to be hemostatic.

A light pressure dressing was placed over the brows, and Bacitracin ointment and Maxitrol ophthalmic ointment were placed on the eyelids. The patient tolerated the procedure well and returned to the outpatient surgical area.

Questions for Further Review: Case Study 11.8

1. What is the diagnosis for the eyelid(s) treated?

2. Which eyelids were treated surgically?
   a. Left upper eyelid
   b. Right upper eyelid
   c. Left lower eyelid
   d. Right lower eyelid

3. What surgical technique was used to repair each eyelid?
   a. Implantation of upper eyelid load (for example, gold weight)
   b. Blepharoplasty
   c. Blepharoplasty with extensive lower eyelid herniated fat pad
   d. Blepharoplasty with excessive skin weighting down upper eyelid
   e. Tarsal wedge excision
   f. Extensive repair
   g. Tarsal strip operation
   h. Capsulopalpebral fascia repair
   i. Excision and repair of eyelid
   j. Transfer of tarsoconjunctival flap from opposing eyelid

4. Brow ptosis was performed.
   a. True
   b. False

5. CPT surgery code(s) and modifier(s):

Case Study 11.9

Read the following clinical document and answer the questions for further review.

OPERATIVE REPORT

PREOPERATIVE DIAGNOSIS: Biopsy-proven basal cell carcinoma, left lower lid

POSTOPERATIVE DIAGNOSIS: Biopsy-proven basal cell carcinoma, left lower lid

OPERATION:

1. Excision of basal cell carcinoma, left lower lid, with frozen section control
2. Reconstruction of left lower lid with primary closure and a myocutaneous advancement flap from the lateral canthus
3. Lateral canthotomy with cantholysis, left eye

DESCRIPTION OF PROCEDURE: After the patient was brought to the operating room and IV sedation was administered, the patient was infiltrated with 2% lidocaine with epinephrine 1:100,000 solution injected across the entire aspect of the left lower lid and the left lateral canthal region. The patient was then prepped and draped in the usual sterile fashion and attention directed to the left eye, where a large chalazion clamp was placed to the lid margin and the central aspect of the lid outlined surrounding the area of the biopsy-proven basal cell carcinoma. Leaving approximately a 1 to 1.5-mm margin around the obvious edge of the tumor, the area was outlined with a surgical marking pen and resected as a block resection and sent as the main tumor to be examined at a later date. The edges were then trimmed with a nasal inferior and temporal margin, and these were all sent off for frozen section and all returned negative.

To close the defect that had been created by resecting more than a third of the lower eyelid, a lateral canthotomy and cantholysis were necessary to advance the skin and muscle across to close the defect. In the lateral canthal angle, the undermining was taken out temporally to release in the suborbicularis plane to allow skin and muscle to be advanced in a nasal direction. When the tension on the central lid was found to be released sufficiently to allow for closure without undue tension, the wound was closed with #6-0 silk suture vertical mattress on the lid margin and tarsus to tarsus was anchored together using #6-0 Vicryl suture with a spatula needle. Orbicularis was closed similarly, and the skin was closed with #6-0 nylon on both sides of the lash line. All the sutures near the lid margin were hung down to the skin with a hang-back stitch to keep the suture ends from irritating the ocular surface. Interrupted #6-0 nylon was used to complete the skin closure. The lateral canthal incision was closed with a single #6-0 nylon stitch to close the skin, but leaving the defect. It is understood that, later on, this lateral canthal angle could be reformed when the primary closure was well healed and at little risk of opening up. At the completion of the case, Bacitracin ophthalmic ointment was applied to the eye and a gentle pressure patch was applied over that, and the patient went to the recovery room in excellent condition.

PATHOLOGY REPORT

AGE/SEX: 89/F

LOCATION: Outpatient surgery

AP CASE TYPE: Surgical

AP RESULT STATUS: Final

AP SPECIMEN DESCRIPTION:

1. Lesion, nasal margin, left lower lid, F.S.
2. Lesion, temporal margin, left lower lid, F.S.
3. Lesion, inferior margin, left lower lid, F.S.
4. Main tumor, left lower lid

GROSS:

1. Received is a 0.4-cm fragment of tan skin. ESS frozen section
   Frozen Section Diagnosis: No tumor seen.
2. Received fresh is a 0.4-cm fragment of tan tissue. ESS frozen section
   Frozen Section Diagnosis: No tumor seen.
3. Received fresh are two 0.5-cm strips of tan-red tissue. ESS frozen section
   Frozen Section Diagnosis: No tumor seen. (EJS)
4. Specimen consists of a wedge biopsy of tan skin measuring 0.6 x 0.5 x 0.5 cm in greatest dimension. The skin is etched in purple dye. The deep margin is inked. The specimen is bisected and ESS—1 cassette.

DIAGNOSIS:

1. Left lower eyelid, nasal margin: Negative for tumor
   Patchy chronic inflammation

2. Left lower eyelid, temporal margin:
   Negative for tumor
   Patchy mild chronic inflammation

3. Left lower eyelid, inferior margin:
   Negative for tumor
   Patchy mild chronic inflammation

4. Left lower eyelid, main tumor:
   Negative for tumor
   Patchy chronic inflammation and reactive fibrosis

Questions for Further Review: Case Study 11.9

1. Which eyelid was treated surgically?
   a. Left upper eyelid
   b. Right upper eyelid
   c. Left lower eyelid
   d. Right lower eyelid

2. What percentage of the eyelid margin was resected?
   a. Up to one-fourth of lid margin
   b. Over one-fourth of lid margin

3. What surgical technique was used to repair each eyelid?
   a. Implantation of upper eyelid load (for example, gold weight)
   b. Blepharoplasty
   c. Blepharoplasty with extensive lower eyelid herniated fat pad
   d. Blepharoplasty with excessive skin weighting down upper eyelid
   e. Tarsal wedge excision
   f. Extensive repair
   g. Tarsal strip operation
   h. Capsulopalpebral fascia repair
   i. Excision and repair of eyelid
   j. Transfer or tarsoconjunctival flap from opposing eyelid

4. CPT surgery code(s) and modifier(s):

Case Study 11.10

Read the following clinical document and answer the questions for further review.

OPERATIVE REPORT

PREOPERATIVE DIAGNOSIS:

1. Basal cell carcinoma, left lower eyelid, measuring 0.6 x 0.4 cm
2. New ulcerated lesion, right upper eyelid, measuring 0.2 x 0.3 cm at eyelid margin

POSTOPERATIVE DIAGNOSIS:

1. Basal cell carcinoma, left lower eyelid, measuring 0.6 x 0.4 cm
2. New ulcerated lesion, right upper eyelid, measuring 0.2 x 0.3 cm eyelid margin

OPERATION:

1. Excisional biopsy basal cell carcinoma, left lower eyelid, with frozen section and control
2. Greater than 50% full-thickness eyelid reconstruction with Tenzel myocutaneous advancement flap
3. Shave biopsy of lesion, right upper eyelid margin

ANESTHESIA:
MAC, local
2% Xylocaine with epinephrine

DISCHARGE STATUS: Condition is stable.

COMPLICATIONS: None

ESTIMATED BLOOD LOSS: Minimal, less than 10 cc

FINDINGS:

1. Frozen section and control of basal cell carcinoma of the left lower eyelid, measuring 0.6 x 0.5 cm
2. Permanent section of right upper eyelid ulcerated lesion, incisional biopsy, rule out basal cell carcinoma

INDICATIONS: The patient has a biopsy-proven basal cell carcinoma of the left lower eyelid, which she has had for several months. She is admitted for corrective surgery by frozen section control excision of the lesion with full-thickness eyelid reconstruction. She recently had a new onset of her ulcerated right upper eyelid margin lesion for which she will undergo an incisional biopsy.

PROCEDURE: After informed consent was obtained, the patient was taken to the operating room and placed supine on the operating table. After induction of local MAC, monitored anesthesia care, a 2% lidocaine injection was given to the left lower eyelid and lateral canthal region in the right upper eyelid. The patient was then prepped and draped sterilely. Attention was turned to a big lesion on the left lower eyelid, 3-mm margins were marked, and a wedge resection of the lower eyelid was excised and submitted for tissue pathology, frozen section. Silk suture was used for a skin marker orientation for the lesion. Hemostasis was maintained with Bovie cautery. While we were waiting for the pathologist, attention was turned to the right upper eyelid. A shave excision was performed at the right upper eyelid margin and submitted for permanent tissue pathology. Attention was turned back to the left lower eyelid margin. When the margins were reported to be clear by the pathologist, the eyelid defect measured greater than 50% of the left lower eyelid margin. A Tenzel myocutaneous flap was then fashioned. The eyelid skin was marked from the lateral canthus extending posteriorly in a semicircular fashion toward the temple. An incision was made along this mark. Dissection was begun with a lateral canthotomy and inferior cantholysis. A myocutaneous fat flap was then elevated with care to stay superficial posteriorly to avoid any risk or damage to the branch of the 7th nerve. The Tenzel flap was then advanced medially. At the eyelid margin defect, the eyelid margins were reapproximated with 6-0 silk sutures placed at the gray line and the lash line. Before this was tightened, 6-0 Vicryl sutures were placed through the ptosis, which was then reapproximated to itself. These were placed in an interrupted fashion. Before these were tied, a lateral canthal angle was reformed using deep sutures of 5-0 Vicryl, reattaching the new lower eyelid lateral canthus to the lateral orbital rim periosteum. This was intentionally superplaced. Deep sutures of interrupted 5-0 Vicryl were then placed along the myocutaneous flap, attaching it to the lateral orbital periosteum and deep temporal fascia. When deeper sutures were placed, skin sutures were closed at the eyelid defect in an interrupted fashion with 6-0 silk sutures. The eyelid margin sutures were left long and tied away from the globe. The lateral canthal sutures were closed in an interrupted fashion as well. When this was completed, erythromycin ophthalmic ointment was placed in both eyes. The left eye was then patched and covered with tape. The patient tolerated the procedure well without complications during surgery.

PATHOLOGY REPORT

AGE/SEX: 64/F

PROCEDURE: Excisional Biopsy BCC LT lower eyelid

TISSUE REMOVED:

A. LT lower eyelid

B. Lateral border

C. Shaving of upper right eyelid

FROZEN SECTION DIAGNOSIS:

1. Basal cell carcinoma with probable involvement of lateral margin; all other margins free of tumor
2. No residual BCCA detected

GROSS DESCRIPTION: Part A received labeled left lower eyelid, suture medial margin, frozen as 1.0 x 0.5 x 0.2-cm portion of eyelid with a black stitch attached to the specimen indicating medial margin. The medial margin is inked green, the lateral margin yellow, and the inferior margin black. The specimen is serially sectioned along the superior to inferior axis from medial to lateral. All submitted for frozen section examination.

Part B received labeled excision of lateral border, ink on lateral margin, is a 0.3 x 0.2 x 0.2 cm, pink-to-white tissue fragment with black ink on one side. The specimen is trisected and all submitted for frozen section examination.

Part C received labeled shaving of upper right eyelid, rule out basal cell carcinoma. The specimen consists of a skin-shave biopsy specimen measuring 0.2 cm in diameter and 0.1 cm in thickness, with a centrally located round pigmented macule present measuring 0.1 cm in diameter. Inked and submitted in C1.

PATH PROCEDURES: Path DLG, path FS, path FRS ADD, CEX X3, frozen section A, frozen section B

FINAL DIAGNOSIS: Part A skin of left lower eyelid, excisional biopsy: basal cell carcinoma identified on frozen section. Cannot rule out lateral margin involvement. The medial and deep margins appear clear of tumor.

Part B skin of lateral lower eyelid reexcision: Benign skin with no residual basal cell carcinoma detected

Part C right upper eyelid, shave biopsy: Keratotic debris and inflammatory scale crust. No squamous epithelium is present. The specimen is too superficial for diagnosis.

Questions for Further Review: Case Study 11.10

1. Which eyelid was treated surgically?
   a. Left upper eyelid
   b. Right upper eyelid
   c. Left lower eyelid
   d. Right lower eyelid

2. What percentage of the eyelid margin was resected?
   a. Up to one-fourth of lid margin
   b. Over one-fourth of lid margin

3. What surgical technique(s) was performed on each eyelid?
   a. Implantation of upper eyelid load (for example, gold weight)
   b. Blepharoplasty
   c. Blepharoplasty with extensive lower eyelid herniated fat pad
   d. Blepharoplasty with excessive skin weighting down upper eyelid
   e. Tarsal wedge excision
   f. Extensive repair
   g. Tarsal strip operation
   h. Capsulopalpebral fascia repair
   i. Excision and repair of eyelid
   j. Transfer or tarsoconjunctival flap from opposing eyelid
   k. Shave biopsy
   l. Excision

4. CPT surgery code(s) and modifier(s):

Case Study 11.11

Read the following clinical document and answer the questions for further review.

HOSPITAL OPERATIVE REPORT

PREOPERATIVE DIAGNOSIS: Retained myringotomy tube

POSTOPERATIVE DIAGNOSIS: Retained myringotomy tube, tympanic membrane perforations (left)

ANESTHESIA: General

PRELIMINARY NOTE: This 6-year-old young man presents with a history of retained myringotomy tube. He was very reluctant to have this removed in the office.

DESCRIPTION OF PROCEDURE: The patient was induced under general mask anesthesia. Examination of the left tympanic membrane revealed two tympanic membrane perforations, one approximately 20% and the other about 5% in size. In addition, a silicone myringotomy tube was lying adjacent to the tympanic membrane imbedded in a small amount of granulation tissue. Utilizing microforceps, the tube was removed uneventfully. Cortisporin drops were instilled. The patient was then taken to the recovery room in good condition.

SURGICAL PATHOLOGY REPORT

AGE/SEX: 6/M

TISSUE: Myringotomy tube (foreign body, retained P.E. tube)

DIAGNOSIS: Foreign body (ear): Myringotomy tube, gross description only

CLINICAL SUMMARY:
1. Retained myringotomy tube
2. Removal of myringotomy tube

GROSS DESCRIPTION: Specimen is received in formalin, labeled left myringotomy tube, and consists of a minute tube, measuring 0.4 x 0.4 x 0.3 cm in dimensions. It is submitted for photo only.

Questions for Further Review: Case Study 11.11

1. What type of anesthesia was used?

2. What type of procedure was performed?
    a. Insertion of myringotomy/ventilating tube, unilateral
    b. Insertion of bilateral myringotomy/ventilating tubes
    c. Removal of unilateral myringotomy/ventilating tube
    d. Removal of bilateral myringotomy/ventilating tubes

3. CPT surgery code(s) and modifier(s):

Case Study 11.12

Read the following clinical document and answer the questions for further review.

OPERATIVE REPORT

PREOPERATIVE DIAGNOSIS: Left mixed hearing loss and serous otitis media and retained myringotomy tube

POSTOPERATIVE DIAGNOSIS: Same

OPERATION PERFORMED: Left exploratory tympanotomy; removal of myringotomy tube and placement of paper patch

ANESTHESIA: Local IV sedation

HISTORY: This 32-year-old female has had a complicated otologic history. She has had an operative procedure of the left ear, performed by another otolaryngologist, where a myringotomy tube was apparently placed with difficulty. The patient noticed that after that operative procedure, she had a significant hearing loss and presented to me for evaluation. She was noted, preoperatively, to have a retained myringotomy tube and possible perforation of the tympanic membrane, marked crusting of the tympanic membrane, and a significant mixed hearing loss with almost a 50 db air–bone gap in the left ear, as well as a drop in the sensory neural hearing in the higher frequencies.

PROCEDURE: The patient was placed on the operating room table in the supine position. General anesthesia was induced through inhalation. The patient was prepped and draped in a sterile fashion. At this point, the Reuter bobbin was visible and removed from what appeared to be crusted material in and around tympanic membrane remnant. There was a large tympanic membrane perforation occupying approximately 75% of the pars tensa portion of the drum. The ossicles were examined, and there appeared to be an alteration and a long process of the malleolus that seemed to be foreshortened with bony overgrowth in that region. The landmarks were not clearly visualized with respect to the ossicles. At this point, the perimeter of the perforation was freshened. A tympanic membrane patch was placed over the hole and perforation that was present, following removal of tympanic membrane remnant. At this point, the patient was revived and returned to the recovery room in satisfactory condition.

Questions for Further Review: Case Study 11.12

1. What type of tympanic membrane surgery was performed?
    a. Tympanic membrane repair (with or without site preparation, perforation, or patch)
    b. Tympanoplasty without mastoidectomy
    c. Tympanoplasty with antrotomy
    d. Tympanoplasty with mastoidotomy
    e. Tympanoplasty with mastoidectomy
    f. Ossicular chain reconstruction
    g. Ossicular chain reconstruction and synthetic prosthesis (partial or total replacement)

2.   Code 69424, ventilating tube removal requiring general anesthesia, should be used for this case.
    a.   True
    b.   False

    Explanation:

3.   CPT surgery code(s) and modifier(s):

Case Study 11.13

Read the following clinical document and answer the questions for further review.

OPERATIVE REPORT

AGE/SEX: 30/F

OPERATION: Left modified radical mastoidectomy (canal wall down) with ossicular reconstruction (TORP)

ANESTHESIA: General endotracheal

PREOPERATIVE DIAGNOSIS: Left chronic otitis media, external auditory canal polyp

POSTOPERATIVE DIAGNOSIS: Left chronic otitis media, external auditory canal polyp, and left attic cholesteatoma

OPERATIVE INDICATIONS: The patient is a 30-year-old female with a long history of left otitis media. The patient failed numerous medical treatments. During the examination in the office, she was found to have a large polyp filling up the external auditory canal. There was also sign of infection.

OPERATIVE FINDINGS: Left external canal was filled with polyp and pus. Left mastoid was sclerotic and small. Left facial nerve was dehiscent in the tympanic segment. There was incus erosion of the long process noted. Stapes superstructure was destroyed. The stapes footplate showed decreased mobility. Attic pus under pressure and cholesteatoma.

OPERATIVE PROCEDURE: The patient was brought to the operating room and placed in the supine position. After general endotracheal anesthesia was obtained, the patient was positioned for examination of the left ear. The facial monitor was applied, and the left ear area was prepped and draped in routine fashion. The postauricular canal, tragus, and the external auditory canal were injected with 1% Lidocaine with 1:100,000 epinephrine.

The postauricular incision was made with the Bovie and carried down to the level of the fascia. A large graft of areola tissue was harvested. Then, the periosteum was entered in a T-fashion down to the cortex. The periosteum was elevated to the level of the external canal.

Then, a simple mastoidectomy was performed. It was noted that the mastoid was very small and sclerotic. The tegmen was identified and followed anteriorly. Then the canal wall was taken down and the facial recess was entered. It was noted that the left cranial nerve was dehiscent in the tympanic segment close to the oval window. The incus (long process) was eroded plus the stapes superstructure. The stapes footplate was found to have decreased mobility.

Then the attic was entered. It was found that it was filled with pus under pressure and cholesteatoma, which was removed. Subsequently, the polyp, which was filling up the external auditory canal, was removed. Then, the middle ear mucosa was cleaned with diamond bur. Subsequently, Gelfoam soaked with epinephrine was packed into the middle ear.

Then attention was brought to the tragus. The tragal cartilage with surrounding perichondrium was removed. The incision was closed with several Dexon sutures. Then the perichondrium was dissected off the anterior surface of the cartilage. Subsequently, prosthesis (TORP) was placed on the stapes footplate. This was covered by the tragal cartilage. Subsequently, the graft (areolar tissue) was placed over the prosthesis. The cavity was filled up with gel.

Subsequently, a meatoplasty was performed in the usual fashion and the excess of cartilage and soft tissue was excised. The skin was closed in two layers in the usual fashion. Then a pressure dressing was applied.

The patient was awakened and extubated in the operating room. The patient was then taken to the recovery room in satisfactory condition.

PATHOLOGY DIAGNOSIS: Pending

COMPLICATIONS: None

DRAINS: None

ESTIMATED BLOOD LOSS: About 50 cc

Questions for Further Review: Case Study 11.13

1. What type of mastoidectomy was performed?
   a. Simple
   b. Complete
   c. Modified radical
   d. Radical

2. What type(s) of tympanic membrane surgery was performed?
   a. Tympanic membrane repair (with or without site preparation, perforation, or patch)
   b. Tympanoplasty without mastoidectomy
   c. Tympanoplasty with antrotomy
   d. Tympanoplasty with mastoidotomy
   e. Tympanoplasty with mastoidectomy
   f. Ossicular chain reconstruction

3. What was the external auditory canal wall status?
   a. Intact
   b. Reconstructed
   c. Down

4. What was the donor site for the graft placed over the prosthesis?
   a. Nasal septum
   b. Areolar tissue
   c. Fascia lata

5. CPT surgery code(s) and modifier(s):

Case Study 11.14

Read the following clinical document and answer the questions for further review.

OPERATIVE REPORT

AGE/SEX: 62/F

OPERATION: Right tympanoplasty with mastoidectomy intact canal wall with ossicular reconstruction

ANESTHESIA: General endotracheal

PREOPERATIVE DIAGNOSIS: Right central tympanic membrane perforation

POSTOPERATIVE DIAGNOSIS: Right central tympanic membrane perforation

OPERATIVE PROCEDURE: With the patient in the supine position, general endotracheal anesthesia was administered without difficulty. The head was turned to the left, and the right ear was sterilely prepped and draped. The postauricular and canal injections of 1% Xylocaine with 1:100,000 adrenaline were given. The vascular strip incision was made. Margins of the central drum perforation were freshened. A postauricular incision was made and temporalis areolar tissue harvested for later use. The periosteum was elevated and inferior and superior canal skin flaps were elevated to enter the middle ear. Aside from the perforation, there was no disease within the middle ear. However, there was a fibrous band connecting the incus long process with the stapes, so this was divided. The incus was removed. The malleus head was removed. The tensor tympani tendon was transected. The malleus handle mobility was normal. Stapes mobility was normal. The chorda tympani nerve was sacrificed. A simple mastoidectomy was performed, and the facial recess was opened. There was no further disease. Hemostasis was good. Gelfoam pledgets were used to support the areolar tissue graft in an underlay fashion. This was then held with the skin flap up against the anterior wall while a Polycel PORP was introduced onto the stapes head. This was covered by tragal cartilage with perichondrium suspended up the canal wall. The tragal incision was closed with multiple 5–0 Dexon sutures. The drum and graft were then returned to their normal anatomic position over the cartilage and perichondrium. Care was taken to ascertain that all of the graft was then returned to its normal anatomic position over the cartilage and perichondrium. Care was taken to ascertain that all of the graft was medial to the drum remnant again. Neosporin was used to fill the anterior canal, and the vascular strip was then returned to its normal position. Ointment was placed in the remainder of the canal, and the postauricular tissues were closed in two layers with multiple 3–0 Vicryl sutures. A sterile dressing was applied, and the patient was transferred to the recovery room in good condition.

PATHOLOGY REPORT

FINAL DIAGNOSIS: Portion of right malleus incus and eardrum, biopsy—mild chronic inflammation and fragments of bone

SPECIMEN(S) SUBMITTED: Right malleus, incus, and drum

CLINICAL DATA: Right chronic TM perforation

GROSS DESCRIPTION: Received fresh are multiple osseous and tan, soft tissue fragments aggregating to 2.0 x 0.5 x 0.2 cm. The specimen is totally submitted in Holland's in cassette A1.

Questions for Further Review: Case Study 11.14

1. What type of mastoidectomy was performed?
   a. Simple
   b. Complete
   c. Modified radical
   d. Radical

2. What type(s) of tympanic membrane surgery was performed?
   a. Tympanic membrane repair (with or without site preparation, perforation, or patch)
   b. Tympanoplasty without mastoidectomy
   c. Tympanoplasty with antrotomy
   d. Tympanoplasty with mastoidotomy
   e. Tympanoplasty with mastoidectomy
   f. Ossicular chain reconstruction

3. What was the external auditory canal wall status?
   a. Intact
   b. Reconstructed
   c. Down

4. What was the donor site for the graft placed over the prosthesis?
   a. Nasal septum
   b. Areolar tissue
   c. Fascia lata

5. CPT surgery code(s) and modifier(s):

Case Study 11.15

Read the following clinical document and answer the questions for further review.

OPERATIVE REPORT

PREOPERATIVE DIAGNOSIS: Right conductive hearing loss, otosclerosis

POSTOPERATIVE DIAGNOSIS: Same

PROCEDURE: Right stapedectomy and myringotomy

ANESTHESIA: General endotracheal supplemented with local injection of 2% Xylocaine with 1:00,00 epinephrine

FINDINGS: The footplate was found to be fixated and relatively thick. The incus and malleus were found to be normal and mobile.

PROCEDURE: After adequate general endotracheal anesthesia was given to the patient, the right ear was prepped and draped in the usual fashion for stapedectomy.

A skin incision was performed in the area just above the auricle. An adequate amount of areolar tissue was removed for grafting material. The incision was closed with interrupted sutures of 5-0 chromic. The four quadrants of the ear canal were injected with less than 1 cc of the local anesthetic solution.

A Shea speculum holder was used to hold the speculum. The tympanomeatal flap was elevated to the middle ear and the middle ear was entered. The corti-tympani was identified and preserved throughout the procedure. The superoposterior bony canal wall was minimally curetted to gain good exposure of the oval window area. The palpation of the malleus revealed good mobility of this ossicular as well as of the incus. The stapes, however, was very fixated. The incostapedial joint was separated and the stapedial tendon was sectioned, and then the superstructure of the stapes was fractured toward the promontory and removed. Good visualization of the oval window was achieved. The distance from the footplate medial ostic of the incus was found to be 4 mm.

Using the Skeeter drill, a hole was performed in the middle portion of the footplate. Then, using a small right-angle hook, all the posterior footplate as well as a portion of the anterior was removed. No injury was performed to the vestibule of the inner ear.

The previously obtained areolar tissue was immediately placed over the oval window to cover this area. A Robinson 4-mm large well, thin shaft prosthesis was placed between the graft and the lenticular process of the incus. The wire of the bucket was brought over the long process of the incus and secured in position. Palpation of the malleus revealed good mobility of the prosthesis.

The tympanomeatal flap was brought back into its original position and was kept in place using pledgets of Gelfoam. A small myringotomy was performed superiorly anteriorly to prevent any negative pressure in the middle ear. Cotton was left in the most lateral aspect of the external otoratory canal and a piece of Band-Aid placed over the skin incision. The patient was awakened from the anesthesia and returned to the recovery room in satisfactory condition.

Questions for Further Review: Case Study 11.15

1. What type of anesthesia was used?

2. What type of stapes surgery was performed?
    a. Stapedectomy
    b. Stapedotomy
    c. Stapedectomy with footplate drillout
    d. Stapedotomy with footplate drillout

3. What type of myringotomy procedure was performed?
    a. Myringotomy, unilateral
    b. Myringotomy, bilateral
    c. Insertion of myringotomy/ventilating tube, unilateral
    d. Insertion of bilateral myringotomy/ventilating tubes
    e. Removal of unilateral myringotomy/ventilating tube
    f. Removal of bilateral myringotomy/ventilating tubes

4. CPT surgery code(s) and modifier(s):

Chapter 12

Ancillary Services and Departments

Although a significant number of outpatient services, such as surgical procedures, gastrointestinal laboratory procedures (both diagnostic and therapeutic), and cardiac catheterization procedures (both diagnostic and therapeutic), are provided in the ambulatory surgery settings of hospitals, many services are rendered in ancillary departments, including:

- Emergency department services
- Hospital-based clinic services
- Chemotherapy/oncology services
- Radiation therapy services
- Pulmonary services
- Rehabilitation services, such as physical therapy, occupational therapy, and speech–language pathology services

Various reimbursement methodologies are applied to these services, including fee schedules, additional APC assignment, or transitional pass-through payment.

Under OPPS, only minimal packaging applies; that is, payment for a procedure or medical visit does not include payment for the related ancillary services, such as laboratory tests or x-rays.

Payment for clinical diagnostic laboratory tests is made under the clinical laboratory fee schedule. Additional APCs are assigned for diagnostic radiology and other diagnostic and therapeutic services, such as respiratory services, therapeutic radiology, and pathological laboratory under OPPS. These payments are made in addition to the OPPS payment for a surgical procedure or medical visit performed on the same day. Various discounting methodologies may be applied, so that 100 percent of the allowable reimbursement is not received for every procedure reported.

APC payments include certain packaged items, such as anesthesia, most medical/surgical supplies, certain drugs, and the use of operating, recovery, and observation rooms. Some supplies, for example, implantable devices, such as pacemakers and some sophisticated intraocular lenses, are assigned their own APC reimbursement. Those devices for which a current pass-through ("C") code exists may be reimbursed in addition to the procedure, although these additional reimbursements do not continue indefinitely.

Outpatient rehabilitation services, such as physical and occupational therapy, are paid under the Medicare Physicians' Fee Schedule. Ambulance services also are paid under a fee schedule, as are screening mammograms and durable medical equipment (DME), provided the facility applies for and receives a DME provider number.

Medical Visit Coding Guidelines

Medical visits are coded with the CPT evaluation and management (E/M) codes in the range 99201–99215. The CPT code book provides definitions of certain key words and phrases used throughout the E/M section, which are intended to "reduce the potential for differing interpretations and to increase the consistency of reporting by physicians in differing specialties" (AMA 2004). Coders should become very familiar with these standard terms and definitions to ensure appropriate coding of E/M services.

Although there are rather specific guidelines for assignment of E/M levels for physician services, there are no such guidelines for facility coding. Currently, the CMS allows each facility to devise its own mechanism to assign E/M codes. These are typically based on the intensity of nursing interventions. The provider community awaits more specific guidance from the CMS on E/M code assignment, including the possible reduction from five levels to three.

Interventional Radiology Procedures

Coding for interventional radiology procedures requires the use of two codes, one from the radiology section (70000–79999) to reflect the radiological supervision and interpretation performed by the radiologist and one from the interventional (surgical) section (10000–69999) to reflect the injection portion or other invasive portion of the procedure.

The code for a specific study or intervention procedure is divided by the following sections: Head, neck and chest, abdominal, gastrointestinal, genitourinary, upper extremities, lower extremities, percutaneous drainage, venous, pulmonary, pain management, miscellaneous interventional radiology, and cardiac catheterization exams. With the exception of cardiac catheterization, each section has two parts: angiographic exams and interventional radiology procedures.

Medicare assigns a relative value unit (RVU) to all CPT/HCPCS codes for reimbursement purposes. The national figure is adjusted by a geographic index (GPCI) and then multiplied by a conversion factor (CF) to determine the actual payment for services. Medicare pays 100 percent for codes in the 7XXXX series, which are typically assigned a modifier –26 professional component. For CPT codes in the 10xxx to 69xxx range, Medicare pays 100 percent for the highest weighted RVU and 50 percent for codes 2–5. Medicare is moving toward a resource-based RVU, which applies to services and procedures that the provider has not performed in the past. CMS has also expanded RVUs for facility and nonfacility settings.

Modifiers and bundled codes directly impact reimbursement for interventional radiology. Procedures should be reported with the HCPCS/CPT codes that most comprehensively describe the services performed. Modifiers indicate when a service or exam was performed and is altered in some way, but do not change the overall definition of the code. Hospitals must assign modifiers to all the technical components for outpatient claims. Coders should check with their hospital FIs for an updated list of modifiers. As of January, 2008, the hospital OPPS CCI edits utilized by Medicare carriers are available on the Internet at www.cms.hhs.gov/NationalCorrectCodInitEd/NCCIE-HOPPS/list.asp#TopOfPage.

The Correct Coding Initiative (CCI) lists code groups and pairs that Medicare will not allow to be billed together on the same claim and same date. The CCI edits are used for both physician and hospital outpatient services. The edits are similar for both physician and hospitals. Hospital claims are processed with the Outpatient Code Editor (OCE) version of the CCI. See www.cms.hhs.gov/OutpatientCodeEdit for specific guidance.

For example, a transluminal angioplasty of the renal artery requires use of code 35471 to report the angioplasty, code 36245 for placement of the catheter and code 75966 for radiological supervision and interpretation.

This type of component coding also applies to nonvascular procedures such as imaging-guided biopsies and other invasive procedures. An ultrasound-guided biopsy of deep muscle is coded 20225 for the biopsy and 76942 for the radiological supervision and interpretation. Change of a biliary drainage tube is reported with two codes: 47525 or 47530 for the tube change; and the radiological supervision and interpretation code 75984 for the imaging portion of the procedure.

The CPT manual is the primary source for guidance on those procedures that require both an interventional and a radiological supervision and interpretation code. Careful reading of the instructional notes in both the surgical and imaging portions of the manual will assist the coding professional in assigning the appropriate combination of codes. See Exhibit 12.1 at the end of this chapter for an example of key CPT manual instructional notes.

Injection, Infusion, and Chemotherapy Coding

The reporting of drug administration for hospital outpatient services rendered under the OPPS has changed from HCPCS Level II codes in 2004, CPT codes in 2005, and then to a combination of HCPCS Level II codes and CPT codes in 2006. CMS has adopted the full set of CPT codes for reporting drug administration in CY 2007 for use under the OPPS. According to CMS' OPPS final rule published November 24, 2006, the list of C-codes then used to report drug administration services under the OPPS was discontinued effective December 31, 2006.

Coding for injections of immune globulins, vaccines, and toxoids also involves a combination of CPT codes. Codes in the range 90281–90399 identify only the immune globulin products and are reported along with codes for the product administration, codes from the range 90760–90761. Codes in the range 90471–90472 report only the administration of a vaccine, and codes in the range 90476–90749 are reported in addition to 90471–90472 codes to identify the specific vaccine given.

Prolonged intravenous infusions; hydration, are reported with codes 90760 (initial, 31 minutes to one hour) and 90761 (each additional hour). These codes are intended to report a hydration IV infusion to consist of a prepackaged fluid and electrolytes (for example, normal saline, D5-1/2 normal saline +30mEq KCl/liter), but are not used to report infusion of drugs or other substances. Hydration IV infusions typically require direct physician supervision for purposes of consent, safety oversight, or intraservice supervision of staff. Typically such infusions require little special handling to prepare or dispose of, and staff that administer these do not typically require advanced practice training. After initial set-up, infusion typically entails little patient risk and, thus, little monitoring.

Use 90761 in conjunction with 90760. Report 90761 for hydration infusion intervals of greater than 30 minutes beyond 1 hour increments. Report 90761 to identify hydration if provided as a secondary or subsequent service after a different initial service (90760, 90765, 90774, 96409, 96413) is administered through the same IV access (AMA 2008).

Do not report intravenous infusion for hydration of 30 minutes or less (AMA 2008).

APC	HCPCS	HCPCS Description	SI	Rel. Wt.	Payment Rate	OPPS OCE
0440			S	1.7998	114.64	
	90760	Intravenous infusion, hydration; initial, 31 minutes to 1 hour				Significant Procedure, Not Discounted when Multiple; Separate APC payment.

Subcutaneous tissue and intramuscular injections are reported with code 90772, intra-arterial injections with 90773, and intravenous infusions with 90774. Use code 90775 in conjunction with initial IV infusion (90765), IV push (90774) (96409), or chemotherapy administration (96413) to identify each additional push of a new substance/drug if provided as a secondary or subsequent service after a different initial service is administered through the same IV access.

Chemotherapy administration codes 96401–96549 apply to parenteral administration of non-radionuclide antineoplastic drugs; and also to antineoplastic agents provided for treatment of non-cancer diagnoses; or to substances such as monoclonal antibody agents and other biologic response modifiers. These services can be provided by any physician.

Chemotherapy services are typically highly complex and require direct physician supervision for any or all purposes of patient assessment, provision of consent, safety oversight and intraservice supervision of staff. Typically, such chemotherapy services require advanced practice training and competency for staff who provide these services; special considerations for preparation, dosage or disposal; and commonly, these services entail significant patient risk and frequent monitoring.

If performed to facilitate the infusion or injection, the following services are included and not reported separately:

- Use of local anesthesia
- IV start
- Access to indwelling IV, subcutaneous catheter or port
- Flush at conclusion of infusion
- Standard tubing, syringes and supplies
- Preparation of chemotherapy agent(s)

Report separate codes for each parenteral method of administration employed when chemotherapy is administered by different techniques. The administration of medications (for example, antibiotics, steroidal agents, antiemetics, narcotics, analgesics) administered independently or sequentially as supportive management of chemotherapy administration, should be separately reporting using 90760–90761, 90765, or 90779 as appropriate.

Report both the specific service as well as code(s) for the specific substances(s) or drug(s) provided. The fluid used to administer the drug(s) is considered incidental hydration and is not separately billable.

When administering multiple infusions, injections or combinations, only one "initial" service code should be reported, unless protocol requires that two separate IV sites must be used. The "initial" code that best describes the key or primary reason for the encounter should always be reported irrespective of the order in which the infusions or injections occur. If an injection or infusion is of a subsequent or concurrent nature, even if it is the first such service within that group of services, then a subsequent or concurrent code from the appropriate section should be reported (for example, the first IV push given subsequent to an initial one-hour infusion is reported using a subsequent IV push code).

When reporting codes for which infusion time is a factor, use the actual time over which the infusion is administered.

If a significant, separately identifiable E/M service is performed, the appropriate E/M service code should be reported using modifier 25 in addition to 96401–96549. For a same-day E/M service, a different diagnosis is not required. (AMA 2008.)

Effective January 1, 2007, hospitals report the following codes for Medicare outpatient chemotherapy and infusion therapy services:

96401	Chemotherapy administration, subcutaneous or intramuscular, nonhormonal antineoplastic
96402	Chemotherapy administration, subcutaneous or intramuscular, hormonal anti-neoplastic
96405	Chemotherapy administration, intralesional; up to and including 7 lesions
96406	Chemotherapy administration, intralesional; more than 7 lesions
96409	Chemotherapy administration, intravenous; push technique, single or initial substance/drug
+96411	Chemotherapy administration, intravenous; each additional substance/drug Add on code (List separately in addition to code for primary procedure.)
96413	Chemotherapy administration, intravenous; infusion technique, up to 1 hour, single or initial substance/drug
+96415	Chemotherapy administration, intravenous; infusion technique, each additional hour Add on code (List separately in addition to code for primary procedure.)
96416	Chemotherapy administration, intravenous; infusion technique, more than 8 hours, requiring the use of a portable or implantable pump
+96417	Chemotherapy administration, intravenous; infusion technique, each additional sequential infusion (different substance/drug), up to 1 hour Add on code (List separately in addition to code for primary procedure.)
96420	Chemotherapy administration, intra-arterial; push technique
96422	Chemotherapy administration, intra-arterial; infusion technique, up to one hour
+96423	Chemotherapy administration, intra-arterial; infusion technique, each additional hour Add on code (List separately in addition to code for primary procedure.)
96425	Chemotherapy administration, intra-arterial; infusion technique, initiation of prolonged infusion (more than 8 hours), requiring the use of a portable or implantable pump
96440	Chemotherapy administration into pleural cavity, requiring and including tho-racentesis
96445	Chemotherapy administration into peritoneal cavity, requiring and including peritoneocentesis
96450	Chemotherapy administration, into CNS (for example, intrathecal), requiring and including spinal puncture
96542	Chemotherapy injection, subarachnoid or intraventricular via subcutaneous reservoir, single or multiple agents
96549	Unlisted chemotherapy procedure
90760	Intravenous infusion, hydration; initial, 31 minutes to 1 hour

+90761   Intravenous infusion, hydration; each additional hour
Add on code (List separately in addition to code for primary procedure.)

90765   Intravenous infusion, for therapy, prophylaxis, or diagnosis (specify substance or drug); initial, up to 1 hour

+90766   Intravenous infusion, for therapy, prophylaxis, or diagnosis (specify substance or drug); each additional hour
Add on code (List separately in addition to code for primary procedure.)

+90767   Intravenous infusion, for therapy, prophylaxis, or diagnosis (specify substance or drug); additional sequential infusion, up to 1 hour
Add on code (List separately in addition to code for primary procedure.)

+90768   Intravenous infusion, for therapy, prophylaxis, or diagnosis (specify substance or drug); concurrent infusion
Add on code (List separately in addition to code for primary procedure.)

90769   Subcutaneous infusion for therapy or prophylaxis (specify substance or drug); initial, up to one hour, including pump set-up and establishment of subcutaneous infusion site(s)

90770   Subcutaneous infusion for therapy or prophylaxis (specify substance or drug); each additional hour (List separately in addition to code for primary procedure)

90771   Subcutaneous infusion for therapy or prophylaxis (specify substance or drug); additional pump set-up with establishment of new subcutaneous infusion site(s) (List separately in addition to code for primary procedure)

90772   Therapeutic, prophylactic, or diagnostic injection (specify substance or drug); subcutaneous or intramuscular

90773   Therapeutic, prophylactic, or diagnostic injection (specify substance or drug); intra-arterial

90774   Therapeutic, prophylactic, or diagnostic injection (specify substance or drug); intravenous push, single or initial substance/drug

+90775   Therapeutic, prophylactic, or diagnostic injection (specify substance or drug); each additional sequential intravenous push or a new substance/drug
Add on code (List separately in addition to code for primary procedure.)

90776   Therapeutic, prophylactic, or diagnostic injection (specify substance or drug); each additional sequential intravenous push of the same substance/drug provided in a facility (List separately in addition to code for primary procedure)

90779   Unlisted therapeutic, prophylactic, or diagnostic intravenous or intra-arterial injection or infusion

Infusion Therapy and Physician Supervision

CMS has affirmed that hospitals may report CPT codes 90760 (intravenous infusion, hydration, initial, 31 minutes to 1 hour) and 90761 (each additional hour)

CMS views their general requirements regarding physician supervision (with respect to payment for services that are incident to a physician's service in the outpatient hospital setting) as meeting the physician supervision aspect of the codes 90760 and 90761, and thus, do not believe that use of the codes in the hospital outpatient setting would be prevented by the inclusion of the language in the code definition.

Physician work related to hydration, injection and infusion service, predominantly involves affirmation of treatment plan and direct supervision of staff.

If a significant separately identifiable Evaluation and Management (E/M) service is performed, the appropriate E/M service code should be reported using modifier 25 in addition to 90760–90779. For same day E/M service, a different diagnosis is not required.

CPT 2008 includes a parenthetical remark immediately following CPT code 90772 (Therapeutic, prophylactic, or diagnostic injection; [specify substance or drug]; subcutaneous or intramuscular.) It states, "Physicians do not report 90772 for injections given without direct physician supervision. To report, use 99211. Hospitals may report 90772 when the physician is not present."

This coding guideline does not apply to Medicare patients. If the RN, LPN or other auxiliary personnel furnishes the injection in the office, and the physician is not present in the office to meet the supervision requirement, which is one of the requirements for coverage of an incident to service, then the injection is not covered. The physician would also not report 99211, as this would not be covered as an incident to service, according to the National Correct Coding Policy Manual, Physician Version 14.0, Effective January 1, 2008.

Infusion Therapy and Other Services During Same Encounter

CPT codes 90760 and 90761 are assigned to status indicator S, which is not discounted when multiple.

Because the costs of space, utilities, and staff attendance are duplicated when the beneficiary is receiving another service at the same time as infusion therapy, in particular when the patient is in observation, CMS believes that it is appropriate to apply a multiple procedure reduction to infusion therapy, particularly when the patient is in observation status.

Multiple visits per day for antibiotic infusion are common, and the drug administration policies should permit such visits to be paid separately.

The reporting and payment for these multiple visits and services will not be an issue once payment for drug administration under the OPPS is made based on CPT code-specific data. However, until such time, hospitals will need to use modifier 59 (distinct procedure) when billing charges for services furnished during multiple visits that follow the initial visit.

When multiple occurrences of any APC that represents drug administration are assigned in a single day, modifier –59 is required on the code(s) to permit payment for multiple units of that APC, up to a specified maximum; additional units above the maximum are packaged. If modifier –59 is not used, only one occurrence of any drug administration APC is allowed, and any additional units are packaged.

Payments for Drug Administration Services

For CY 2007, OPPS drug administration APCs have been restructured, resulting in a six-level hierarchy where active HCPCS codes have been assigned according to their clinical coherence and resource use. Contrary to the CY 2006 payment structure that bundled payment for several instances of a type of service (nonchemotherapy, chemotherapy by infusion, noninfusion chemotherapy) into a per-encounter APC payment, the CY 2007 structure provides a separate APC payment for each reported unit of a separately payable HCPCS code.

Hospitals should note that the transition to the full set of CPT drug administration codes provides for conceptual differences when reporting, such as those noted here.

- In CY 2006, hospitals were instructed to bill for the first hour (and any additional hours) by each type of infusion service (nonchemotherapy, chemotherapy by infusion, noninfusion chemotherapy). In CY 2007, the first hour concept no longer exists. CY 2007 CPT codes allow for only one initial service per encounter, for each vascular access site, no matter how many types of infusion services are provided; however, hospitals will receive an APC payment for the initial service and separate APC payment(s) for additional hours of infusion or other drug administration services provided that are separately payable.

- In CY 2006, hospitals providing infusion services of different types (nonchemotherapy, chemotherapy by infusion, noninfusion chemotherapy) received payment for the associated per-encounter infusion APC even if these infusions occurred during the same time period. In CY 2007, CPT instructions allow reporting of only one initial drug administration service, including infusion services, per encounter, for each distinct vascular access site, with other services through the same vascular access site being reported via the sequential, concurrent or additional hour codes.

For CY 2008 APC payment rates, refer to Addendum B on the CMS Web site: www.cms.hhs.gov/HospitalOutpatientPPS.

Infusions Started Outside the Hospital

Hospitals may receive Medicare beneficiaries for outpatient services who are in the process of receiving an infusion at their time of arrival at the hospital (for example, a patient who arrives via ambulance with an ongoing intravenous infusion initiated by paramedics during transport). Hospitals are reminded to bill for all services provided using the HCPCS code(s) that most accurately describe the service(s) they provided. This includes hospitals reporting an initial hour of infusion, even if the hospital did not initiate the infusion, and additional HCPCS codes for additional or sequential infusion services if needed (CMS, 2006).

Emergency Department Screening

Every patient who presents to an emergency department (ED) and requests a screening or has requested a screening on his or her behalf must be screened in accordance with the Emergency Medical Treatment and Active Labor Act (EMTALA). This 1986 federal antidumping law prohibits hospitals from transferring or discharging patients known to have emergency conditions, regardless of ability to pay. If the physician or other hospital staff who performs the screening determines that no medical emergency exists, the patient can be referred to one of the hospital's clinics or another provider (for example, a physician's office) for further treatment, or ED personnel can decide to treat the patient in the ED. If nonemergency treatment is furnished, the appropriate emergency room visit should be billed and not the screening.

Similarly, if the screening reveals that an emergency does exist and treatment is instituted immediately, the screening should not be billed; the screening is subsumed into the further treatment.

If no treatment is furnished, the CMS would expect screening to be billed with a low-level ED visit code.

If an emergency room physician feels the need to consult with another physician before deciding whether the patient needs emergency treatment, the consultation is part of the original screening and the hospital should bill for only one screening visit (if a bill for screening is appropriate) as described earlier.

Critical Care

Critical care is the direct delivery by a physician(s) of medical care for a critically ill or critically injured patient. Critical care differs from ED treatment reported with the E/M codes in the range 99201–99215 in that it is inclusive of a number of other, minor procedures, and because it represents the highest level of intervention and is based on time.

Guidelines do not require that a patient be in a critical care area for the critical care codes to be assigned; however, just because a patient is in a critical care area does not justify use of these codes. Guidelines for use of the critical care codes by facilities include the following: Under the outpatient PPS, the hospital can use CPT 99291 in place of, but not in addition to, a code for a medical visit or an ED service. Thus, it would be inappropriate for the hospital to code both an ED visit code (such as 99285) and critical care code 99291 for a single outpatient encounter.

Code 99291 is used to report the first 30–74 minutes of critical care on a given date. It should be used only once per date even if the time spent by the physician is not continuous on that date.

Code 99292 is used to report additional block(s) of time of up to 30 minutes beyond the first 74 minutes.

Example: Appropriate E/M Codes Less than 30 minutes

99291 X 1	30–74 minutes (30 minutes–1 hr 14 minutes)
99291 X 1 and 99292 X 2	75–104 minutes (1 hr 45 minutes–2 hr 14 minutes)
99291 X 1 and 99292 X 3	135–164 minutes (2 hr 15 minutes–2 hr 44 minutes)
99291 X 1 and 99292 X 4	165–194 minutes (2 hr 45 minutes–3 hr 14 minutes)

When other services, such as surgery, x-rays, or cardiopulmonary resuscitation, are furnished on the same day as the critical care services, the CMS allows the hospital to bill for them separately.

Radiation Oncology

Radiation therapy is reimbursed under OPPS in the form of additional APC payments. Radiation oncology services are typically "cycle billed" on a monthly basis. Included in the APC reimbursement are any drugs, anesthesia, and supplies provided during the treatment.

Coding for radiation oncology services is divided into technical and professional components, with different sets of CPT codes, as follows:

- Codes in the range 77261–77263 are physician services, used to report treatment-planning services.

- Codes 77280–77299, used to report simulation-aided field testing, are technical (facility) codes.

- Codes 77300–77399 (Medical Radiation Physics, Dosimetry, Treatment Devices, and Special Services) represent technical services as well. Radiation physicists are typically hospital employees.

- Codes 77401–77421 represent the actual delivery of the treatment and are technical codes. They cover the direct and indirect costs associated with the delivery equipment and are based on the types of devices used.

- Codes 77427–77432 are professional codes, but code 77470 represents a type of procedure and is thus a technical code.

- Codes 77520–77525 are used to report treatment via a proton beam delivery system and are technical codes, as are codes 77600–77620 for reporting hyperthermia. Codes 77750–77799 are technical codes used to report clinical brachytherapy.

The following excerpt provides additional coding guidelines for the coding of radiation therapy treatment for Medicare patients:

"CPT Codes 77401 through 77416 may be reported more than once per date of service only when radiation treatment is provided during completely different sessions. Only one of these codes may be reported for each treatment session no matter how many areas are treated or no matter how much radiation is delivered. CPT Codes 77402 through 77406 describe treatment delivery for a single treatment area. CPT Codes 77407 through 77411 describe treatment delivery to two treatment areas. CPT Codes 77412 through 77416 describe treatment delivery or three or more treatment areas. In the cases of CPT codes 77407 through 77416, the number of distinct treatment areas and complexity of the treatment determine which code series to report, which is then modified by the selection of energy (i.e., MeV). For example, if three treatment areas are each treated with 11 MV, then the proper code to bill is 77414. It is incorrect to report 77404–77414 (for "11–19 MeV") three times. However, if there is a distinct break and the same region or regions are treated again the same day then a second charge describing the energy and level of complexity is appropriate" (CMS 2003 [January 3]).

Steps in Radiation Therapy

A course of radiation therapy is composed of six steps that involve distinct activities of varying complexity. A clinical team, led by the radiation oncologist, provides the medical services associated with the steps in the process of care. Other team members in the patient's planning and treatment regimen include the medical physicist, the dosimetrist, the radiation therapist, and nursing staff. Many of the procedures in each step are completed before the patient's care is taken to the next step; other activities occur and recur during the course of treatment.

Each of these distinct steps involves medical evaluation, interpretation, management, and decision making by the radiation oncologist. Of necessity, certain steps are repeated during treatment due to patient tolerance, changes in tumor size, necessity for boost field or port size changes, and protection of normal tissue or as other clinical circumstances require.

Steps in the course of radiation therapy are as follows.

1. Consultation: The radiation oncologist has an initial encounter with the patient to evaluate the patient's history and clinical status and ascertain whether he or she is a candidate for radiation therapy. This initial consultation is reported using E/M codes from the 99241–99255 series of CPT.

2. Tumor mapping and clinical treatment planning: If the determination is made that the patient should receive radiation treatment, clinical treatment planning occurs. In this step, the disease-bearing area is determined and a treatment plan is devised, including the type of radiation to be utilized, areas to be treated, techniques for treatment, dose to be delivered, and duration of therapy. CPT codes corresponding to clinical treatment planning are 77261–77263.

3. Simulation: Following the completion of clinical treatment planning, including tumor mapping, the treatment portals must be established to deliver the radiation to the volume selected. Therapeutic radiology simulation is the process of establishing radiation treatment portals that most efficiently and precisely encompass the treatment volume. Simulation may be performed more than once during a course of therapy, but only once per day. (See codes 77280–77295 for simulation.)

4. Medical radiation physics services, dosimetry services, treatment devices, and special services: This phase of the process of care involves the radiation oncologist in collaboration with the medical physicist, the dosimetrist, and the radiation therapist staff. This team develops dosimetry, builds treatment devices to modify and refine treatment delivery, and performs other special services required for the measurement of precision dose delivery, including quality assurance and the identification and review of complicated situations requiring special medical physics consultation. The CPT codes used are in the 77300–77399 series.

5. Radiation treatment delivery and radiation treatment management: Radiation treatment delivery described by CPT codes 77401–77418 and 77520–77525 are technical codes only and describe the delivery of external-beam radiation therapy. Brachytherapy CPT codes for interstitial implants are described in the 77750–77799 series and include both professional work and technical reimbursement.

While the patient is undergoing radiation therapy, the radiation oncologist is responsible for the care of the patient and the overall management of the course of treatment. External-beam services are covered by codes 77427, 77431, 77432, and 77470, which are used depending on the complexity and modality of treatment. For external-beam radiation therapy, radiation therapy treatment management is reported in units of five fractions or treatment sessions.

The professional services furnished during the treatment management typically consist of:

- Review of port films
- Review and modification of dosimetry, dose delivery, and treatment parameters
- Review of treatment setup
- Examination of the patient for medical evaluation and management

Management of brachytherapy treatment is included in the brachytherapy code.

6. Patient follow-up: This final step in the course of radiation therapy is covered by CPT codes for follow-up evaluation of an established patient under the 99261–99263 series of E/M codes.

Additional resources for radiation oncology, which include a case study, a table of radiation oncology treatments, and a list of clinical terms, are contained in Exhibits 12.2, 12.3, and 12.4, respectively.

Case Studies

This section contains actual ancillary department reports from real-life cases. All identifiers have been removed or changed for confidentiality and privacy.

Carefully read each case study's clinical documentation, which may include a procedure report as well as radiology and/or pathology reports, as applicable.

Answer all the questions for further review at the end of each case study. Use a current CPT codebook or HCPCS Level II code listing, as needed.

Case Study 12.1

Read the following clinical document and answer the questions for further review.

EMERGENCY DEPARTMENT RECORD

ADDENDUM NOTE: On 2/16/200X at approximately 16:02—Mom returned with child today for the rest of the sutures to be removed. States the tape closures have been in place the entire time. Adhesive bandage removed, tape closures, and three middle sutures removed. The middle 1 cm of the wound has edges that are not approximated. The two ends have 1-cm areas that are well approximated and look good. Tape closures replaced with benzoin and covered with adhesive bandage. Mom instructed on how to reapply if they come off. Otherwise to see PMD in 5 days for tape closure removal and wound evaluation. After tape closures applied, the wound edges were well approximated and I expect the wound will heal without problems.

VITALS BP: 89/52 mm   Hg sitting 14:38
P: 109/min. 14:38   Resp: 14/min. 14:38
Wgt.: 11.8 kg 14:38   Temp: 97.8 F Axillary 14:38

CC:

1. Suture removal.
2. Wound check: Sutures under chin need to be removed.

SYMPTOM AND PROBLEM LIST: Suture removal; drug allergy; history of prior drug allergy; postop trauma repair check

ALLERGIES: Amoxicillin

MEDICATION: Zithromax

ACUITY: 14:36 Triage acuity level is 4, Single problem patient assigned to Minor Acute Care.

TRIAGE & NURSING HISTORY: Injury occurred (5) days ago.

PAST MEDICAL HISTORY: No significant past medical history available

PRE ARRIVAL TREATMENT: Child brought to facility by parents via personal transportation.

IMMUNIZATIONS: Tetanus status is N/A; up-to-date with childhood immunization schedule

LANGUAGE: Verbal with age-appropriate speech; English-speaking household

DEMEANOR: Domestic violence question N/A. Alert, interactive, and appears to have age-appropriate behavior. (DB) Age less than 15 (KI)

NURSING NOTE

NURSING ASSESSMENT:

DERMATOLOGIC EXAM: 14:45 Initial assessment: Child has sutures noted under chin covered with adhesive bandage. No redness or swelling noted on site. Child playing happily w/mom and dad next to him.

RN CONTINUATION NOTES: 14:42 Update: Child ambulated to room #2 in MACU from triage area. 14:52 NP/PA: Vicki Day NP with patient. 15:15 Update: Vicki Day NP removed some of the sutures, leaving some in. Vicki Day NP dressed wound after applying tape closures to wound. Child was immobilized w/pillow case and bath blanket w/ RN holding child's head. Parents remained in room w/child. (KI)

NURSING DISPOSITION: Condition: Stable. 15:29 Patient discharged from department to home. Left ambulatory. Accompanied by family members. Minor left with parents. Instructions given to parents who understand Rx and plan. No outstanding psychosocial needs. (KI)

CLINICIAN NOTE

HISTORY: 15:09 The onset of the presenting problem began (5) days ago. Was at the doctor's office, and they were unable to remove the sutures so they sent them here. History available from mother. Overall, the history seems quite reliable.

Problem #1 Wound check: Routine suture removal. Sutures have been in place for (5) days. No other specific complaints, doing well.

PHYSICAL EXAM:

GENERAL PRESENTATION: Well-developed, well-nourished nontoxic child in no acute distress

PSYCHIATRIC AND MENTAL STATUS: Age-appropriate behavior; interactive with examiner and environment

PROGRESS NOTES: There is an approximate 3-cm wound located over the lower part of face. Advised to cover with simple adhesive bandage. Tape closures were placed on wound. Attending physician in department. (ID)

PROCEDURE NOTES: 15:10 Wound looks good. The wound's edges looked well approximated. Sutures removed from each end, a thin scab had formed and as it pulled away, the wound started bleeding slightly at both ends. The wound's edges are approximated, and I feel it would be best to leave the center sutures in for two more days and reinforce the wound with sterile tape closures in the meantime. Exam reveals (after removing two sutures from each end) the edges began bleeding slightly and didn't seem to be strongly approximated. Three central sutures left in, benzoin and tape closures applied, then adhesive bandage. (ID)

PRIMARY DIAGNOSIS: Partial suture removal

PHYSICIAN DISPOSITION: Patient discharged. Told to return in three days. 15:13 Patient seen with physician support available in the department. (ID)

Question for Further Review: Case Study 12.1

1. Using Exhibit 1.2 on page 62, assign the E/M level for this case.
   a. Low level
   b. Mid level
   c. High level

Case Study 12.2

Read the following clinical document and answer the questions for further review.

INFUSION CLINIC NOTE

AGE: 60 **SEX**: M

TREATMENT NOTE:

Diagnosis: Lymphoma
Indication for transfusion/infusion: Relapse
Previous Reaction: Fever
Component to be infused: MTX/ARA-C

PT arrived on unit via 2/c escort with friend at 1050. PT is ambulatory with use of cane but requires w/c for long distances. PT's VSS, labs monitored, and PT afebrile. PT is ordered for MTX/ARA-C infusions every other week x 3 doses. PT with L CW GROSHONG with + blood return. PT was premedicated with Zofran 8 mg in 50 cc of NS via IV infusion over 20 minutes at 1120 and Decadron 10 mg via slow IVP at 1140. PT then received Methotrexate 40 mg via IVP through side of free-flowing NX over 2 minutes at 1155. PT then received ARA-C 500 mg in 100 cc of NS via IV infusion over 30 minutes at 1200. PT's GROSHONG was with + blood return pre/intra and post all chemotherapy treatments. PT tolerated all treatments received, and VSS throughout. PT's GROSHONG was flushed with NX post infusion. PT left unit ambulatory with use of cane and without complaint at 1250.

Question for Further Review: Case Study 12.2

1.   Which of the following codes correctly classify this case?
     a.   90760: Intravenous infusion, hydration; initial, 31 minutes to 1 hour
     b.   96409: Chemotherapy administration, intravenous; push technique single or initial substance/drug
     c.   +96411: Chemotherapy administration, intravenous; each additional substance/drug
     d.   All of the above
     e.   90760 and 96409 only

Case Study 12.3

Read the following clinical document and answer the questions for further review.

INFUSION AND CLINIC NOTE

AGE: 60 **SEX**: M

TREATMENT NOTE:
Diagnosis: Lymphoma
Previous reaction: Fevers
Component to be infused: MTX/ARA-C

PT arrived on unit via W/C escort and stable at 1015. PT ambulatory with use of cane for shorter distances. PT's VSS, labs monitored and PT afebrile. PT with L CW GROSHONG with + blood return. Today is dose 2 of 8 doses of MTX/ARA-C. PT received premedication of dexamethasone 10 mg via slow IVP over 1 minute at 1057, then received Zofran 30 mg in 100 cc of NS via IV infusion over 20 minutes at 1100. PT then received methotrexate 40 mg via IVP through free-flowing NS over three minutes. PT then received ARA-C 500 mg in 100 cc of NS via IV infusion over 30 minutes at 1130. PT tolerated all therapies received, and PT's GROSHONG was with + blood return pre/intra and post infusions. PT's GRO-SHONG was flushed with NS post-infusion. PT received 40,000U of Procrit via SQ injection in his LUE, and an adhesive bandage was applied to site for his trip home. PT left unit ambulatory and without complaint at 1240.

Question for Further Review: Case Study 12.3

1.   Which of the following codes correctly classify this case?
     a.   90760: Intravenous infusion, hydration; initial, 31 minutes to 1 hour
     b.   96409: Chemotherapy administration, intravenous; push technique single or initial substance/drug
     c.   +96411: Chemotherapy administration, intravenous; each additional substance/drug
     d.   90772–59: Injection, subcutaneous—Distinct procedural service
     e.   All of the above
     f.   90760 and 96409 only

Case Study 12.4

Read the following clinical document and answer the questions for further review.

RADIOLOGY REPORT

DOB: 8/14/1947
SEX: F

FINAL REPORT
Bilateral Screening Mammography
Indication: Screening

Mediolateral and craniocaudal view of both breasts was obtained. Previous outside mammograms unavailable for comparison. There is a mildly dense fibroglandular pattern.

There is a 1-cm ill-defined nodule within the right breast approximately 7 cm posterior from the nipple. Patient should return for spot compression views and sonography.

There are no suspicious pleomorphic microcalcifications. The skin and nipple contours are unremarkable.

Impression: 1-cm ill-defined nodule right breast
Overall assessment: Category 0. Incomplete additional imaging required
Patient should return for spot compression views and sonography of the right breast.

1. Which code correctly classifies this case?
   a. 77055
   b. 77056
   c. 77057
   d. 77057–50

Case Study 12.5

Read the following clinical document and answer the questions for further review.

RADIOLOGY REPORT

MRN:
AGE: 88
SEX: F

Procedure/Reason for Study: CT Scan/OP

FINAL REPORT

CT scan of the Brain

History: Status post fall

Technique: Noncontrast head CT was performed from vertex to skull base in 5-mm serial axial images.

Findings:
There is no evidence of epidural, subdural, subarachnoid, or intracerebral hemorrhage.
No masses are identified.
There is age-related parenchymal involutional change with associated ventricular and sulcal prominence. Periventricular white matter hypoattenuation changes are noted representing small vessel disease. There is no evidence of acute territorial infarct.
No fractures identified.

Impression: Cerebral atrophy
No acute infraction or hemorrhage

Question for Further Review: Case Study 12.5

1. Which code correctly classifies this case?
   a. 70450
   b. 70460
   c. 70470

Case Study 12.6

Read the following clinical document and answer the questions for further review.

RADIOLOGY REPORT

MRN:
AGE: 46
SEX: F

FINAL REPORT

Radionuclide Thyroid Scan

A history: Rule out cold nodule

24-hour images of the thyroid gland obtained following oral ingestion of 286 uCi of I-123.

Normal configuration of the thyroid gland seen with homogeneous uptake of the radio-tracer

The 24-hour radioiodine uptake is 66.6%.

Impression: Findings consistent with hyperthyroidism; no photon-deficient regions noted

---

Question for Further Review: Case Study 12.6

1. Which code correctly classifies this case?
   a. 78000
   b. 78006
   c. 78007

Case Study 12.7

Read the following clinical document and answer the questions for further review.

RADIOLOGIST REPORT

HYSTEROSALPINGOGRAM:

History: 37-year old female, status post tubal ligation and subsequent tuboplasty now with persistent infertility

Procedure: Following obtaining informed consent, with a risk explained, including but not limited to, contrast reaction, the patient was placed on the fluoroscopy table in the lithotomy position. After the usual sterile prep and drape, the speculum was placed within the vagina and the external os and cervix identified.

This was prepped, and a pediatric Foley catheter was advanced through the external os into the uterine cavity. The balloon was inflated. Contrast injection was performed under fluoroscopic visualization with spot film imaging. Following removal of the catheter, a delayed image of the pelvis was obtained, following patient ambulation for several minutes.

Impression: Unremarkable uterine cavity with persistent right fallopian tube complete occlusion. The left fallopian tube is patent with loculated intraperitoneal spill present. A rounded filling defect is identified with the pool of loculated contrast in the left adnexa consistent with the ovary.

Question for Further Review: Case Study 12.7

1. Which code pairs correctly classify both the injection and the imaging components of this case?
   a. 58340 and 74742
   b. 74740 and 58340
   c. 58340 and 58340–59

Case Study 12.8

Read the following clinical document and answer the questions for further review.

RADIOLOGIST REPORT

ABDOMINAL ULTRASOUND: Visualized portions of the liver were normal in echogenicity without evidence of space occupying lesion. Gallbladder was not visualized secondary to previous cholecystectomy. Surgical clip is noted in the gallbladder fossa. No evidence of intra- or extrahepatic biliary dilatation. Common duct measures 4 mm. The head and body of the pancreas were normal. Both kidneys were normal in echogenicity without evidence of hydronephrosis. Spleen was normal in size and echogenicity.

CONCLUSIONS: The patient is status post previous cholecystectomy. The examination otherwise is unremarkable.

Question for Further Review: Case Study 12.8

1. Which code correctly classifies this case?
   a. 76775
   b. 76770
   c. 76705
   d. 76700

Case Study 12.9

Read the following clinical document and answer the questions for further review.

CLINICAL NOTE

A 15-month-old female presented with bilateral retinoblastoma. The right eye had a large dome-shaped tumor, extending from the nasal margin of the optic disc to almost the ora serrata with total retinal detachment. Additional small tumors were seen inferiorly and temporally. The left eye also had a large nasal tumor similar in configuration to the right one. Again, there was total retinal detachment and subretinal seeding. No vitreous cells were seen. CT scans were negative for evidence of CNS or optic nerve involvement. A multidiscipline team decided that a curative goal with the desirable preservation of vision would best be met by bilateral irradiation with proton beams. A central line was placed for the purpose of daily anesthesia.

An immobilization device was fitted to the baby for use during CT scanning and proton treatment. CT scans were obtained in the treatment position with suction cups holding the eyes in the neutral position. The CT scans were transferred to the proton treatment planning system, and the physician drew the tumor contours on each of the CT cross sections. The dosimetrist calculated a three-dimensional treatment plan on the reconstructed tumor volumes using the physician's prescription for the tumor doses and the doses to the normal ocular structures and temporal bones. The treatment plan included one beam for each of the eyes and the designs of two treatment apertures and two tissue compensators that corrected for the nonuniform surfaces, tissue inhomogeneities, and the shapes of the distal surface of the target volumes. Reconstructed digital radiographs for both treatment beams and dose-volume histograms for the two tumors were calculated. The treatment plans were presented to the multidisciplinary tumor conference for review and were approved.

The child was given 22 treatment fractions at 2 Gy/fraction for a total dose of 44 Gy to the tumor in each eye. For the left eye, a very satisfactory regression of the tumor was noted after 24 Gy, and the treatment aperture was reduced anteriorly in order to minimize the dose to the lens. No field change was made for the right eye. Each treatment was given with the child under general anesthesia, with the eye suction cup in place to stabilize the eyes. Both eyes were sequentially treated each day. For each treatment fraction, the treatment setup coordinates were obtained through the use of stereotactic x-rays of the bony orbit. After the correct treatment position was obtained, a beam's-eye-view verification film was obtained and approved by the physician each day. The child tolerated treatment very well and had no problems with the daily anesthesia. She developed the expected skin reaction in the region of the treatment beam entrance near the lateral orbit but experienced no desquamation. After completion of treatment, the baby had a complete evaluation and a course of follow-up was determined.

Question for Further Review: Case Study 12.9

1. What type of proton beam treatment delivery was performed?
   a. 77520—Simple. Proton treatment delivery to a single treatment area utilizing a single nontangential/oblique port, custom block without compensation
   b. 77522—Simple. Proton treatment delivery to a single treatment area utilizing a single nontangential/oblique port, custom block with compensation
   c. 77523—Intermediate. Proton treatment delivery to one or more treatment areas utilizing two or more ports or one or more tangential/oblique ports, with custom blocks and compensators
   d. 77525—Complex. Proton treatment delivery to one or more treatment areas utilizing two or more ports per treatment area with matching or patching fields and/or multiple isocenters, with custom blocks and compensators

   Explanation:

Exhibit 12.1. Instructional notes for coding angiography and venography performed with transcatheter procedures

Diagnostic angiography and venography (radiological supervision and interpretation) codes 75600–75893 should not be used with transcatheter interventional procedures (codes 75894–75989) when associated with the following services, because this work is captured in the interventional procedure code(s):

    1.   Contrast injections, angiography, roadmapping, and/or fluoroscopic guidance for the intervention
    2.   Vessel measurement
    3.   Post-angioplasty/stent angiography

Diagnostic angiography performed at the time of an interventional procedure is separately reportable if:

    1.   No prior catheter-based angiographic study is available and a full diagnostic study is performed, and the decision to intervene is based on the diagnostic study, OR
    2.   Prior study is available, but as documented in the medical record:
        a.   The patient's condition with respect to the clinical indication has changed since the prior study, OR
        b.   There is inadequate visualization of the anatomy and/or pathology, OR
        c.   There is a clinical change during the procedure that requires new evaluation outside the target area of intervention.

Diagnostic angiography performed at a separate setting from an interventional procedure is separately reported. Diagnostic angiography performed at the time of an interventional procedure is not separately reportable if it is specifically included in the interventional code descriptor.

Source: *2008 CPT* codebook.

Exhibit 12.2. Case study for radiation treatment management code 77427*

A 61-year-old was found to have a 4-cm near-circumferential, moderately differentiated adenocarcinoma of the rectum (8–12 cm above the anal verge) on evaluation of three months rectal bleeding, four weeks of dyspareunia, and two weeks of dull lower pelvic pain.

Workup findings included anemia (Hct 33%, Hgb 10.9 g/dL), CEA 7.3, and no evidence of adenopathy or distant metastasis on CTs of pelvis and abdomen and chest x-ray. KPS was 80 percent. She did well after low anterior resection, with pathologic findings of tumor into perirectal fat, three of eight nodes involved (TNM stage III). Recommendations for adjuvant chemotherapy and radiotherapy were accepted.

Four weeks after Mediport placement and simulation, treatment began with continuous 24-hour infusion (for four weeks) 5-FU and concurrent three-field pelvic radiotherapy to an intended total dose of 4,500 cGy in 25 daily treatments over five weeks, with a planned boost thereafter to the posterior pelvis of 540 cGy in three daily treatments, all with 10-mV photons.

Treatment in the prone position ("belly board" technique) in the first week was awkward and uncomfortable for the patient because of the infusion pump, incisional pain, and hip osteoarthritis. Analgesic drugs and dosing were modified.

Mild nausea in the second week was controlled with a phenothiazine antiemetic prn. Nutrition was appropriate.

Nausea increased during the third week, and intermittent semiwatery diarrhea developed. Mild neutropenia appeared. Weight dropped by two pounds. Postoperative oral iron therapy was stopped. Strict adherence to a low-residue diet, frequent smaller feedings, and nutritional supplements was advised. Atropine sulfate and diphenoxylate hydrochloride (Lomotil) was prescribed in the fourth week. The patient's symptoms were stable. Mild neutropenia persisted. Radiodermatitis in the gluteal cleft was topically managed.

In week five, watery diarrhea, urinary frequency, dysuria, and mild stomatitis developed. WBC was 2500/nl, platelets 100,00/nl. Stool culture for *Clostridium difficile* was negative, urinalysis/culture confirmed urinary tract infection, antibiotic was prescribed, and inflamed hemorrhoids were topically treated. Treatment was not given Thursday and Friday to give irradiated bowel a four day rest from therapy. Chemotherapy infusion was completed.

The patient's GI status was improved in the fifth week; stools were semiformed, one to three times per day with some tenesmus. Moist desquamation in the gluteal cleft was treated with mupirocin. WBC was 2800/nl. Stomatitis/uL and cystitis resolved.

Posterior pelvic boost completed the patient's treatment in week six. GI function was unchanged from week five. At end of radiotherapy, net weight loss was five pounds and KPS was 80%. She was seen two and four weeks after radiotherapy, with progressive recovery.

Chemotherapy resumed four weeks after radiotherapy. When the patient was seen again two months after radiotherapy, skin was healed. GI symptoms were mild and controlled by minor diet adjustment. Sexual counseling was given. Return visit in six months was scheduled.

* Other nonradiation oncology CPT codes could be assigned for the case study above if detailed documentation is available elsewhere in the medical record.

Exhibit 12.3. Radiation oncology treatments

Type of Treatment	Simple	Intermediate	Complex
Therapeutic Radiology Treatment Planning	77261—Simple planning requires a single treatment area of interest encompassed in a single port or simple parallel opposed ports with simple or no blocking.	77262—Intermediate planning requires three or more converging ports, two separate treatment areas, multiple blocks, or special time dose constraints.	77263—Complex planning requires highly complex blocking, custom shielding blocks, tangential ports, special wedges or compensators, three or more separate treatment areas, rotational or special beam considerations, combination of therapeutic modalities.
Therapeutic Radiology Simulation-Aided Field Setting	77280—Simple simulation of a single treatment area with either a single port or parallel opposed ports. Simple or no blocking.	77285—Intermediate simulation of three or more converging ports, two separate treatment areas, multiple blocks.	77290—Complex simulation of tangential portals, three or more treatment areas, rotation or arc therapy, complex blocking, custom shielding blocks, brachytherapy source verification, hyperthermia probe verification, any use of contrast materials. 77295—Computer-generated three-dimensional reconstruction of tumor volume and surrounding critical normal tissue structures from direct CT scans and/or MRI data in preparation for non-coplanar or coplanar therapy. The simulation utilizes documented three-dimensional beam's eye view volume-dose displays of multiple or moving beams. Documentation with three-dimensional volume reconstruction and dose distribution is required.
Teletherapy Isodose Plan	77305—Simple—one or two parallel opposed unmodified ports directed to a single area of interest.	77310—Intermediate—three or more treatment ports directed to a single area of interest.	77315—Complex—mantle or inverted Y, tangential ports, the use of wedges, compensators, complex blocking, rotational beam, or special beam considerations.
Brachytherapy Isodose Plan	77326—Simple—calculation made from single plane, one to four sources/ribbon application, remote afterloading brachytherapy, 1 to 8 sources.	77327—Intermediate—multiplane dosage calculations, application involving 5 to 10 sources/ribbons, remote afterloading brachytherapy, 9 to 12 sources.	77328—Complex—multiplane isodose plan, volume implant calculations, over 10 sources/ribbons used, special spatial reconstruction, remote afterloading brachytherapy, over 12 sources.
Treatment Devices, Design and Construction	77332—Simple block, simple bolus.	77333—Intermediate—multiple blocks, stents, bite blocks, special bolus.	77334—Complex—irregular blocks, special shields, compensators, wedges, molds, or casts.
Proton Beam Treatment Delivery	77520/77522—Simple—Proton treatment delivery to a single treatment area utilizing a single non-tangential/oblique port, custom block with compensation (77522) and without compensation (77520).	77523—Intermediate—Proton treatment delivery to one or more treatment areas utilizing two or more ports or one or more tangential/oblique ports, with custom blocks and compensators.	77525—Complex—Proton treatment delivery to one or more treatment areas utilizing two or more ports per treatment area with matching or patching fields and/or multiple isocenters, with custom blocks and compensators.
Intracavitary Radiation Source Application	77761—Simple—application has one to four sources/ribbons.	77762—Intermediate—application has five to ten sources/ribbons.	77763—Complex—application has greater than ten sources/ribbons.
Interstitial Radiation Source Application	77776—Simple—application has one to four sources/ribbons.	77777—Intermediate—application has five to ten sources/ribbons.	77778—Complex—application has greater than ten sources/ribbons.

Source: AMA 2008.

Exhibit 12.4. Clinical terminology for radiation oncology

Applicator: A mechanical contrivance that has one or more internal compartment(s) into which small sources of radioactive material may be loaded. The geometry of the applicator can usually be varied.

Beam: A beam of photons or electrons emitted from a radiation treatment machine such as a linear accelerator. The beam is made up of the radiation being emitted from the machine.

Block: A device, usually made of lead or other heavy metal, that is interposed between the radiation beam and a portion of the patient's body, which requires protection from the radiation beam. These blocks are known as shielding blocks because they shield the normal structures from the radiation beam. A custom shielding block is one that has been designed specifically in its shape to follow natural and normal anatomic boundaries rather than simple square or circular geometric lines.

Brachytherapy: The use of radioactive sources placed directly into a tumor-bearing area to generate local regions of high-intensity radiation.

Compensators: Blocks specifically designed in shape to follow natural and normal anatomic boundaries requiring direct input from the physician for design, selection, and ultimate placement, which shape the lateral dimensions of the treatment beam.

Dose calculation points: Specific areas within the body requiring an exact dose of radiation to be calculated from each treatment or an accumulative dose from many treatments.

Electron: A small negatively charged particle that is accelerated by a high electrical potential to either bombard a target and produce x-rays or be released directly from the machine and used as the treatment beam.

Field: The area of interest that is being treated. A field usually consists of a specific area of the body that is involved with the malignancy and often encompasses the surrounding areas of potential spread of the malignancy.

Fraction: A single session of radiation treatment delivered to a specific area of interest at one setting.

Fractionation: The schedule of fractions of treatment as it is delivered. It is usually expressed as the number of fractions or treatment sessions delivered over a specific period of time.

Hyperfractionation: Any technique of radiation treatment that delivers more than one treatment session per day. Hyperfractionation is usually twice—and occasionally three times—per day treatment separated by a period of at least four to six hours.

Hyperthermia: The use of heat, generated by either microwave, ultrasound, or other heat-developing means to raise the temperature of a specific area of the body in an attempt to increase cell metabolism, thereby increasing the potential cell killing in a malignancy. Hyperthermia is generally used in conjunction with conventional radiation therapy treatments.

Interstitial: The placement of needles through the skin directly into tissues.

Intracavitary: The placement of a probe or other source directly into a body cavity.

Isodose plan: A plotting of lines of the same dosage within a given treatment field. An isodose plan is usually derived from a combination of treatment beams impinging upon a particular field of interest. The levels of doses to be delivered are expressed in percentages within this area of interest.

Linear accelerator: A type of high-energy x-ray machine, usually ranging from 4 to as high as 25 million volts of x-ray energy.

Per oral cone: A shielded tubelike structure that is placed directly in the mouth to irradiate cancers located in the oral cavity.

Photon: A bundle of electromagnetic energy, such as x-ray or light.

(Continued on next page)

Exhibit 12.4. (Continued)

Portal: A point of entry on the skin where the radiation treatment beam enters the body and converges on the field of interest.

Portal films: X-rays taken during the delivery of radiation treatment, utilizing the treatment beam of the machine. Portal films demonstrate the exact shape, size, and area covered by the treatment beam during an actual treatment.

Rad: A unit of radiation-absorbed dose. The newer radiation literature also includes the term *Gray,* abbreviated Gy. One Gray equals 100 rads of absorbed dose.

Radiation sensitizer: A drug, such as cis-Platinum, used in small quantities to sensitize the cancer to the radiation and thereby enhance the effect.

Ribbons: Small plastic tubes that have radioactive sources, generally Iridium-192, spaced at regular lengths along the ribbon. The ribbon may be cut into specific lengths to tailor the size of the area of radiation treatment.

Seeds: Tiny (usually 1 millimeter or smaller) sources of radioactive material used for permanent implantation into tumors.

Simulation: The act of determining the configuration of the radiation treatment portals. Simulation is performed without actually delivering a treatment, but utilizing all of the parameters of the treatment to be delivered.

Source: A radioactive element packaged in a small configuration used as a source of radiation in the treatment of malignancy.

Treatment delivery: The act of utilizing a radiation treatment machine to deliver an actual treatment to a patient.

Treatment management: The ongoing medical management of a patient receiving a course of radiation treatment, usually expressed in sets of five during a week.

Treatment planning: The cognitive process carried out by the physician to determine all of the parameters of a given course of radiation therapy.

Part III

Ensuring Coding and Billing Integrity under OPPS

Chapter 13

APCs and Data Quality

Under OPPS, for outpatient ambulatory payment classifications (APCs), in *most* hospitals, the individuals with formal coding training assign the ICD-9-CM diagnosis codes and CPT/HCPCS procedure codes that determine the APC groups for the *surgical* procedures only (revenue code 360, 450). Clinical or nonclinical staff members who have no formal coding training—physicians, physician assistants, nurses, technicians—assign the CPT/HCPCS procedure codes that determine the APC groups for the *nonsurgical* services (revenue code 250, 510), such as:

- Separately reimbursable supplies and implantables
- Drugs, pharmaceuticals, and biologicals
- Radiology and radiation therapy
- Clinic visits or emergency visits
- Diagnostic services and tests
- Surgical pathology
- Chemotherapy
- Partial hospitalization

In some outpatient settings, such as a cardiology department, all codes assigned may be generated by the chargemaster. The HIM coding department might not need to assign any additional codes if the cardiology department charged for all services provided.

Chargemaster Overview

The chargemaster drives the process for assigning CPT codes for outpatient services typically not coded by HIM coders. The process of assigning CPT codes from the chargemaster is known as hard coding, whereas HIM-assigned coding is soft coded. In some outpatient departments, the facility may create a policy and procedure that outlines which department is responsible for assigning codes. This process can assist with preventing duplicate charging. Also referred to as a charge description master or a service description master, the chargemaster is an electronic file that lists the following information for every chargeable item or service in the hospital:

- Service code or charge code, which is a specific internal code assigned by the hospital
- Charge code description, which is an abbreviated description assigned by the hospital

- Revenue code, which is reported on the UB-04 claim form
- CPT/HCPCS code, which is listed when a code exists but is not reported by a coding specialist
- The hospital's charge for the item or service

Most hospitals use either a manual or automated process to ensure that codes for nonsurgical services are reported through the chargemaster process.

Manual Chargemaster Process

The manual chargemaster process comprises the following steps:

1. Patient XYZ receives outpatient care during a visit.

2. The designated staff members report the items and services provided to patient XYZ by manually completing a charge ticket.

3. The charge ticket for patient XYZ is batched with all other charge tickets for patients seen. At the end of the day, a designated staff member picks up all of the charge tickets.

4. Designated staff members enter the data on all of the charge tickets into a computer terminal containing the hospital's billing software.

5. Patient XYZ's charge ticket data eventually appears on his or her UB-04 claim form.

> **Example:** Patient is seen in the USA Medical Center's Echocardiography (ECHO) Lab. She has a color flow study and a two-dimensional echocardiogram performed. The ECHO technician completes the ECHO charge ticket by writing in the date of service and the patient's name and medical record number and by indicating that the patient had quantity 1 color flow study and quantity 1 2D ECHO performed. (See Figure 13.1 for a sample charge ticket.)

Designated staff members enter the following data from patient's ECHO charge ticket into a computer terminal containing the hospital's billing software:

- Date of service   03/26/08
- Medical record number   123456
- Each service code and quantity   03320017   1
                                     03396496   1

The service codes entered by the staff trigger the hospital's information system to pull the following data from the chargemaster for this patient's bill:

- For service code 03320017   483   93325 $430.00
- For service code 03396496   483   93307 $600.00

An excerpt from a sample hospital chargemaster is shown in Figure 13.2.

Figure 13.1. Sample hospital echocardiography (ECHO) lab charge ticket

USA MEDICAL CENTER
ECHO LAB

DATE 03/26/X   PATIENT NAME XXXXXXX   MED REC# 123456

FREQUENTLY USED ITEMS

SRV CDE	DESCRIPTION	CPT CODE	REV CODE	QTY
03320017	COLOR FLOW	93325	480	1
03320009	CONTRAST ECHO	93307	480	
03320033	DOBUTAMINE STRESS ECHO	93350	480	
03396496	ECHOCARDIOGRAM 2D	93307	480	1
03396306	EKG	93005	730	
03396553	EKG RHYTHM STRIP	93005	730	
03396314	EKG TRACING ONLY	93005	730	
03396504	HOLTER MONITOR 26M RECORDING	93225	731	
03396512	HOLTER MONITOR 26M SCANNING	93226	731	
03395704	INTRAOPERATIVE ECHO	93312	480	
03320025	PULSED/CONTINOUS WAVE DOPPLER	93320	480	
03396603	SIGNAL AVERAGED EKG	93278	730	
03396462	STRESS ECHO	93350	480	
03396322	TRANSESOPHAGEAL ECHO	93312	480	

SPECIAL-USE ITEMS

SRV CDE	DESCRIPTION	CPT CODE	REV CODE	QTY
03396611	DOPPLER, F/U OR LTD	93321	480	
03396629	TEE, CONGENITAL ANOMAL	93315	480	

Figure 13.2. Sample hospital chargemaster excerpt: ECHO lab

SERVICE CODE	DESCRIPTION CODE	REV CODE	HCPCS	CHARGE
3320017	**COLOR FLOW**	**480**	**93325**	**$430.00**
3320009	CONTRAST ECHO	480	93307	$440.25
3320033	DOBUTAMINE STRESS ECHO	480	93350	$750.00
3396496	**ECHOCARDIOGRAM 2D**	**480**	**93307**	**$600.00**
3396306	EKG	730	93005	$80.00
3396553	EKG RHYTHM STRIP	730	93005	$110.75
3396314	EKG TRACING ONLY	730	93005	$74.00
3396504	HOLTER MONITOR 26M RECORDING	731	93225	$170.00
3396512	HOLTER MONITOR 26M SCANNING	731	93226	$294.00
3395704	INTRAOPERATIVE ECHO	480	93312	$550.00
3320025	PULSED/CONTINOUS WAVE DOPPLER	480	93320	$430.00
3396603	SIGNAL AVERAGED EKG	730	93278	$319.00
3396462	STRESS ECHO	480	93350	$700.00
3396322	TRANSESOPHAGEAL ECHO	480	93312	$900.00
3396611	DOPPLER, F/U OR LTD	480	93321	$430.00
3396629	TEE, CONGENITAL ANOMAL	480	93315	$540.00

The chargemaster data for this patient eventually appears on her UB-04 claim form. (See Figure 13.3.)

Figure 13.3. UB-04 claim form excerpt: ECHO lab charge ticket data billed

42 REV.CD.	43 DESCRIPTION	44 HCPCS/RATES	45 SERV.DATE	46 SERV.UNITS	47 TOTAL CHARGES
483	CARDIOGRAPHY	93325	032620XX	1	430.00
483	CARDIOGRAPHY	93307	032620XX	1	600.00

Automated Chargemaster Process

Some hospitals use electronic processes to ensure that codes for nonsurgical services are reported through the chargemaster process. The electronic chargemaster process comprises the following steps:

1. The patient receives the outpatient care during a visit.

2. Designated staff members enter charge-specific data about the items and services rendered during online order-entry into a computer terminal containing the hospital's charge-entry software.

3. The charge-entry software accesses the hospital's chargemaster database.

4. The charge-specific data eventually appears on the UB-04 claim form for the patient.

Note: An online order-entry system contains a menu of charges by department within the hospital's software.

Sample automated charge-entry screens are shown in Figures 13.4 and 13.5. The italicized text in the figures reflects the data entered by the designated staff.

Role of HIM in Chargemaster Maintenance

To ensure that the chargemaster contains accurate CPT/HCPCS codes and revenue codes, hospitals must constantly review and update their chargemasters to adhere to changes to the OPPS. HIM professionals can be invaluable in the chargemaster maintenance process because of their knowledge and expertise in the areas of coding and reimbursement.

Following are key steps to the successful maintenance of the chargemaster:

1. Each line item on the chargemaster should be reviewed for the CPT/HCPCS code description, revenue code, and charging accuracy using these resources:

   - Current CPT codebook
   - Current HCPCS Level II code listing
   - Current Medicare fee schedules (for example, clinical diagnostic laboratory services, outpatient rehabilitation)
   - Regulatory notices, bulletins, newsletters, advisories, and Internet postings from the Medicare fiscal intermediary (FI) and the CMS

Figure 13.4. Radiology charge-entry sample screen #1

```
Phy #1:      Age: 21        Type: E/R       Sex: M          Adm Date: 03/26/XX
Phy #2:      Age: 21        Room:           Wgt:            Dis Date:
Allergies:
                          Order Entry Maintenance: RADIOLOGY
Film No.: 122776
Order#: 23497 <=X-RAY ORDER=> .......      3099994         By:     Date:    Time:
1.    STAT (Y/N ...................... N    Ordered: JD      0528XX1843
2.    Physician....................XXXXX    10.  Collect:
3.    Schedule Date: .......... 0326XX1843  11.  Received:
                                            12.  Complete: TW 0326XX 1854
                                                 Results: GC 0327XX 1038
6.    Isolation:........................N
7.    Batch Code: ......................     Signed: _____
8.    Assoc. Items

Comments Below:
31.   Procedure(s): LEFT WRIST X-RAY   _____
32.   Reason for Procedure(s): POST REDUCTION _____
33.   Transportation: Stretcher _____ IV? N_____ 02?_____ N_____
34.   E/R Room#: ER ROOM ORTHO RIGHT _____
                          Status = COMPLETED
Enter: (0—More "H"elp "C"an "DC" "R"esult "S"end
```

Figure 13.5. Radiology charge-entry sample screen #2

```
Enter Extremity Orders        Enter Info        03/26/XX          0953
PATIENT   F   33    /         RAD     Pt#: 13445093
Atn Dr.: XXXXXXXX             IMAG
Adm Dt.: 03/26/XX    OA       Isol.                          Mr: 1140444

Svc. Desc/Code: ELBOW< THREE VIEWS X-RAYS       RAD2350
Priority: TODAY        Dly Freq: ONCE           Wkly Freq: ONCE
?TODAY                 ?DOWNTIME     ?ONCE
?ROUTINE
?STAT
?PREOP
?URGENT
Start Dt/Tm: 03/26/XX      09 : 53 Duration: O H
Left/Right Ind: ____ Body Site: _____ Transport Meth: _____
                      Ordering Dr. 005777  XXXXXX
                                         Modifiers: ____ ____ ____
Reason:        _____
Comments:      _____
               _____
               _____

Indicators: IV? O2? Monitor? Dye Allergy? Stand? Pregnant?
! F1 Master Menu        ! F6 Skip Order                 ! F 11 Signoff
! F2 Order Menu         ! F5 Enter W/O Printing Requisite   & Enter
```

Coding and reimbursement managers, revenue cycle managers, and HIM staff can assist with the interpretation of guidelines published in these resources.

2. The chargemaster should be reviewed for missing information. For example, a procedure is performed in a department but is not listed, a procedure is listed without its CPT/HCPCS code, or a procedure is listed without its revenue code.

3. All procedure line items must be coded with valid CPT/HCPCS codes. Charges submitted without codes or with codes that do not accurately reflect the procedures performed may be deemed medically unnecessary and thus denied. Also, most CPT/HCPCS codes must be accompanied by compatible UB-04 revenue codes to ensure appropriate payment and to avoid claim rejections or denials.

4. Technical staff, such as radiology and lab technicians, should participate in the review to ensure that the assigned codes reflect the test or procedure. Moreover, there should be interaction and cooperation among responsible staff of various departments to ensure successful implementation of the changes.

When the chargemaster review has been completed, the following should take place:

1. The department managers approve the revisions.

2. The chief financial officer or some other appropriate executive reviews the charges and authorizes the appropriate staff to make the necessary changes in the hospital information system.

3. Designated staff members input the chargemaster changes.

4. The revised chargemaster is distributed to department directors to verify its accuracy.

5. The revised chargemaster is distributed to the HIM department to prevent the listing of codes on the chargemaster for items/services that are already coded by HIM coding specialists.

6. The charge-entry screens and/or charge tickets are revised.

7. The hospital tests and verifies that the codes are transferring appropriately from the chargemaster to the UB-04 claim forms.

8. The hospital trains the staff who will be responsible for either completing the charge tickets or entering the charge data into the charge-entry software.

9. Formal annual chargemaster reviews are performed to ensure that all CPT and HCPCS Level II additions, revisions, and deletions that affect outpatient services rendered in the hospital have been addressed. The review also ensures that any new procedures performed or items used in the departments have been included.

Chargemaster Data Quality

A current and well-maintained chargemaster greatly reduces—but does not eliminate—UB-04 claims data quality issues. Below are some recommendations for troubleshooting billing data reported via the chargemaster.

Supplies

Supply charges are reported with their affiliated supply revenue codes and are not bundled into the charges for the outpatient procedure or service. The following bill excerpt is in error because it does not reflect a separate revenue code and charge for a splint, even though CPT code 29515 classifies the application of a splint. The appropriate supply code for a splint also should appear on this bill.

42 REV.CD.	43 DESCRIPTION	44 HCPCS/RATES
450	EMERG RM	9928325
450	EMERG RM	29515

Implantable Items

Implantables are classified as packaged (when payment for the device is included in the APC payment for the service to which the item relates) or separately reimbursable.

Packaged Implantables

Bills with HCPCS Level II C codes for packaged implantables should carry the correct C code to classify the implantable used during the outpatient visit. The following bill excerpt inappropriately reflects packaged code C1784 (ocular device) instead of packaged code C1781 (implantable mesh). The CPT code 49568 that was billed classifies the application of mesh performed during the patient's incisional/ventral hernia repair.

42 REV.CD.	43 DESCRIPTION	44 HCPCS/RATES
278	SUPPLY/IMPLANTS	C1784
360	OPERATING RM	49561
360	OPERATING RM	49568

Separately Reimbursable Implantables

Bills containing HCPCS Level II C codes for separately reimbursable implantables should correctly classify the implantable used during the outpatient visit. The following bill excerpt inappropriately reflects nonexistent code C1873 instead of separately reimbursable code C1783 (ocular implant, aqueous drainage assist device). The CPT code 66180 that was billed classifies the placement of an aqueous shunt to the extraocular reservoir.

42 REV.CD.	43 DESCRIPTION	44 HCPCS/RATES
278	SUPPLY/IMPLANTS	C1873
360	OPERATING RM	66180

Drugs, Pharmaceuticals, and Biologicals

Revenue codes listed next to the HCPCS Level II drug codes are reimbursed under the OPPS and reported next to revenue code 636 as required by Medicare. The following bill excerpt inappropriately lists an OPPS reimbursable drug code J9280 next to revenue code 250. Code J9280 has a K status indicator; therefore, it should be reported next to revenue code 636.

42 REV.CD.	43 DESCRIPTION	44 HCPCS/RATES
250	PHARMACY	J9280

Surgical Procedures

Bills should not contain duplicate codes reported by the chargemaster and HIM-based coding specialists. This duplication may lead to the hospital being overpaid under the OPPS. The following bill excerpt inappropriately lists upper gastrointestinal endoscopy code 43235 twice. The coding specialist reported the code 43235 that appears next to revenue code 360, but the GI endoscopy suite nurse reported the charge that triggered the code 43235 which appears next to revenue code 750. The procedure was performed only once, so the code should appear only once.

42 REV.CD.	43 DESCRIPTION	44 HCPCS/RATES
360	OPERATING RM	43235
750	GI SERVICES	43235

Radiology and Radiation Therapy

Bilateral procedure modifier –50 is used when there is no bilateral CPT code to classify the bilateral radiology service. The following bill excerpt inappropriately lists shoulder x-ray code 73020–LT and 73020–RT to classify the bilateral shoulder x-rays that were performed on the outpatient. The bill should reflect 73020–50 to classify the bilateral shoulder x-rays.

42 REV.CD.	43 DESCRIPTION	44 HCPCS/RATES	45 SERV.DATE	46 SERV.UNITS
320	DX X-RAY	73020LT	032620XX	1
320	DX X-RAY	73020RT	032620XX	1

Clinic Visits

It is appropriate to report a procedure in addition to an evaluation and management (E/M) code if both services are supported by the medical record documentation. The following bill excerpt inappropriately omits a CPT code 31505 for the indirect laryngosocopy that was performed and documented in the Clinic Note.

42 REV.CD.	43 DESCRIPTION	44 HCPCS/RATES	45 SERV.DATE	46 SERV.UNITS
510	CLINIC	99213	032620XX	1

Emergency Department Visits

A separate charge is listed for the visit code and for the procedure(s) performed. The following bill excerpt inappropriately bundles the charge for the wound repair (code 12004) into the charge for the visit (code 99283–25). The bill should reflect a charge of $175.00 next to code 99283–25 and a charge of $240.00 next to code 12004.

42 REV.CD.	43 DESCRIPTION	44 HCPCS/RATES	45 SERV.DATE	46 SERV.UNITS	47 TOTAL CHARGES
450	EMERG RM	9928325\	032620XX	1	**415.00**
450	EMERG RM	12004	032620XX	1	0

Critical Care

A visit code is not reported along with a critical care code when a patient received critical care services. Medicare guidelines do not allow the reporting of another visit code when the critical code is billed. The following bill excerpt inappropriately lists visit code 99285 in addition to the critical care code 99291. Only code 99291 should appear because this patient received critical care during the emergency department visit before being stabilized and transferred to another hospital.

42 REV.CD.	43 DESCRIPTION	44 HCPCS/RATES	45 SERV.DATE
450	EMERG RM	**99285**	032620XX
450	EMERG RM	99291	032620XX

Diagnostic Services and Other Diagnostic Tests

The repeat procedure modifier –76 (Repeat Procedure by Same Physician) or –77 (Repeat Procedure by Another Physician) is used when an outpatient has multiple diagnostic services or tests (except clinical laboratory tests) ordered and performed during a single visit. When multiple clinical laboratory tests are ordered and performed in the same calendar day, modifier –91 is reported on the second and all subsequent occurrences of the code.

The following bill excerpt inappropriately lists two units of service for spirometry (code 94010). This outpatient had two spirometry tests ordered by the same physician and performed by respiratory technicians on the same date of service, so this case should be billed as 94010 with one unit of service on one line item and 94010–76 with one unit of service on the next line item.

42 REV.CD.	43 DESCRIPTION	44 HCPCS/RATES	45 SERV.DATE	46 SERV.UNITS
460	RESP SVC	94010	032620XX	2

Surgical Pathology

A surgical pathology code and charge should be listed when a tissue specimen was biopsied during the outpatient surgical visit. The following bill excerpt inappropriately omits a surgical pathology code from the 88300–88309 range. The CPT code that was billed, 11100, classifies a biopsy of skin, subcutaneous tissue, or mucous membrane; however, the actual pathological examination of the biopsy specimen was not coded or charged.

42 REV.CD.	43 DESCRIPTION	44 HCPCS/RATES	45 SERV.DATE	46 SERV.UNITS
750	GI SERVICES	**11100**	032620XX	1

Chemotherapy

A chemotherapy drug is coded and charged when a charge and a code are listed for chemotherapy administration. The following bill excerpt reflects chemotherapy infusion code 96413; however, no code is listed for the chemotherapy drug that was infused. Code J9060 (Cisplatin, 10 mg injection) with five units of service is missing for the 50 mg of Cisplatin infused on 03/26/20XX.

42 REV.CD.	43 DESCRIPTION	44 HCPCS/RATES	45 SERV.DATE	46 SERV.UNITS
335	CHEMO IV	96413	032620XX	1

Preventive Services Furnished to Healthy Persons

A preventive code is not billed with a therapeutic code for the same service. The following bill inappropriately reflects the colorectal cancer screening colonoscopy code G0105 in addition to the colonoscopy with biopsy code 45380. Medicare guidelines require the omission of the preventive code when a therapeutic procedure is performed during the session. Only code 45380 should be reported on this bill.

42 REV.CD.	43 DESCRIPTION	44 HCPCS/RATES	45 SERV.DATE	46 SERV.UNITS
750	GI SERVICES	G0105	032620XX	1
750	GI SERVICES	45380	032620XX	1

Partial Hospitalization for the Mentally Ill

Partial hospitalization program (PHP) bills should contain a mental health ICD-9-CM diagnosis code and at least three partial hospitalization HCPCS codes for each day of service, one of which must be a psychotherapy HCPCS code other than brief psychotherapy codes that group to APC 0322. Below are the CMS-approved partial hospitalization codes (including those that group to APC 0322*):

Description	HCPCS Code
Occupational therapy (partial hospitalization)	G0129
Activity therapy (partial hospitalization)	G0176
Education training (partial hospitalization)	G0177
Psychiatric general services	90801, 90802, 90875, 90876, 90899*
Individual psychotherapy	90816*, 90817*, 90818, 90819, 90821, 90822, 90823*, 90824,* 90826, 90827, 90828, 90829
Group psychotherapy	90849, 90853, 90857
Family psychotherapy	90846, 90847, 90849
Psychiatric testing	96101, 96116, or 96118

*Brief psychotherapy codes that group to APC 0322

The following bill excerpt contains three PHP codes for the same date of service; however, Medicare requires that at least one of the PHP codes be a psychotherapy HCPCS code other than brief psychotherapy for each PHP day of service. None of the codes on this bill reflects psychotherapy: G0129 classifies occupational therapy, G0176 classifies activity therapy, and G0177 classifies educational training.

42 REV.CD.	43 DESCRIPTION	44 HCPCS/RATES	45 SERV.DATE
913	PARTIAL HOSP	G0129	032620XX
913	PARTIAL HOSP	G0176	032620XX
913	PARTIAL HOSP	G0177	032620XX

Inpatient Procedures for Patients Who Expire

Outpatient bills that contain inpatient procedures for patients who die prior to inpatient admission should be reviewed carefully to verify that the modifier –CA (Procedure Payable Only in the Inpatient Setting When Performed Emergently on an Outpatient Who Dies Before Admission) is appended to the inpatient procedure CPT code being billed.

The following bill excerpt is in error because it omits the appendage of modifier –CA to the open-chest heart massage code 32160. For the Medicare FI to pay this claim, the code must be billed as 32160–CA.

42 REV.CD.	43 DESCRIPTION	44 HCPCS/RATES	45 SERV.DATE
450	EMERG RM	32160	032620XX

Coding Specialist Data Quality

For the outpatient APCs, in *most* hospitals, the coding specialists assign the ICD-9-CM diagnosis codes and CPT/HCPCS procedure codes that determine the APC groups for the surgical procedures only. The data quality for codes reported by coding specialists is just as important as the chargemaster-driven data. Recommendations for troubleshooting billing data reported by the coding specialists are listed here:

- **Chargemaster–HIM duplication:** Codes should not be duplicated by the chargemaster and HIM-based coding specialists.

- **Ongoing bill reviews:** Ongoing monitors and review processes should be in place to ensure that modifiers, ICD-9-CM diagnosis, CPT, and/or HCPCS Level II procedure codes are not omitted, transposed, or duplicated inappropriately on the outpatient UB-04s, and that the originally reported codes appear appropriately on the outpatient UB-04s.

- **Unlisted procedure codes:** When unlisted procedure codes are assigned, another coding team member should review the procedure/service report and the current edition of the CPT codebook and HCPCS Level II code listing to verify that no code is available to describe the procedures performed.

- **Invalid modifiers:** Modifiers that are nonexistent and/or not permitted for hospital reporting to Medicare should not be listed. For example, modifier –E5 does not exist, only modifiers –E1 through –E4 exist for the four eyelids.

- **Inherently bilateral codes:** Modifier –50 should not be reported with CPT codes that contain "bilateral" in the code description.

- **Incompatible anatomic-site CPT modifier:** Anatomic site-specific modifiers should be listed only with compatible CPT codes. For example, a toe modifier should not be appended to a metatarsal repair CPT code.

- **Coronary artery modifiers:** Coronary artery modifiers –LC, –LD, and –RC should be reported only with CPT codes 92980, 92981, 92982, 92995, and 92996.

- **Modifier –52 with anesthesia:** Modifier –52 (Reduced Services) should be avoided with procedures that require anesthesia (*Federal Register*, April 7, 2000). It is used to indicate a procedure that did not require anesthesia or a procedure that was terminated after the patient was prepared for the procedure, including sedation and transport to the room where the procedure was to be performed.

- **Multiple HCPCS level II modifiers:** Only one anatomic-site modifier can be reported next to a CPT code on a single line item. FIs cannot process more than one HCPCS Level II modifier appended to a CPT code. For example, 26055-FA-F1 should be reported as two separate codes: 26055–FA and 26055–F1.

- **Multiple procedures with discontinuation:** If multiple procedures are planned but one or more of them is not attempted, the canceled procedure(s) should be neither coded nor billed. It would be incorrect to list the canceled procedure code and either modifier –73 (Discontinued Outpatient Procedure Prior to the Administration of Anesthesia) or –74 (Discontinued Outpatient Procedure After Administration of Anesthesia).

- **Canceled diagnosis code with modifiers:** Discontinued procedure modifiers –73 and/or –74 should not be reported without ICD-9-CM diagnosis code V61, V64.2, or V64.3 (procedure not carried out) being reported as a secondary diagnosis on the same claim.

- **Multiple-occurrence CPT codes:** Modifiers –50 (Bilateral Procedure), –LT (Left side), and –RT (Right side) next to CPT codes should be avoided with codes including multiple occurrences in the description. For example, the code for needle electromyography of three extremities, 95863, would not carry these modifiers.

Information Technology Used for APC Data Quality

Many hospitals use information technology and software to identify, correct, and prevent APC data quality issues.

Overview of Hospital Information Systems

Hospitals must use, and sometimes interface with, numerous information systems, many of which facilitate the successful management of APC data:

- **Admission/discharge/transfer (ADT):** ADT data assist the hospital in identifying Medicare outpatients who have multiple medical visits on the same date of service. In order for both visits to be paid, both visits must be reported on the UB-04 claim form with separate E/M codes.

- **Patient care system:** Patient care information is the cornerstone for documentation, coding, and billing of Medicare outpatient services.

- **Automated order/charge-entry system:** This system allows the hospital to build logic or artificial intelligence into the reporting of modifiers for services that are charged via the automated order/charge-entry system. For example, the order-entry system may be programmed to flag visits where duplicate codes appear because one or more of the codes may require a modifier such as: –50 (Bilateral Procedure), –59 (Distinct Procedural Service), –76 (Repeat Procedure by Same Physician), –77 (Repeat Procedure by Another Physician), –91 (Repeat Clinical Diagnostic Laboratory Test), –E1 through –E4 (eyelid repair), –FA through –F9 (finger repair), or –TA through –T9 (toe repair).

- **Electronic patient data/record:** The availability of on-line clinical results, such as pathology and radiology, and/or dictated reports, facilitates the accurate and expedient coding and billing of outpatient services.

- **Clinical data abstracting:** Outpatient data abstracting facilitates the hospital's analysis of Medicare outpatient data for case mix, outcomes, and other elements.

- **Billing system:** The UB-04 claim is used to assign the data that generate the APC groups and reimbursement for the hospital.

- **APC grouper:** Some hospitals use an APC grouper to determine the expected APC groups and payment prior to submission of the claim to the Medicare fiscal intermediary.

- **Cost accounting:** Cost-accounting software allows hospital management to plan, monitor, and control outpatient operations under Medicare's multiple outpatient payment methodologies.

- **Contract management:** Contract management software facilitates the hospital's projection of expected payments from Medicare under APCs and the other Medicare reimbursement systems (for example, clinical diagnostic laboratory fee schedule).

- **Decision support system:** Decision support software facilitates the hospital's management of the Medicare outpatient data under the APC system.

- **Report writer:** Report writer software facilitates the hospital's management of the Medicare outpatient data under the APC system.

- **Clinical data repository:** For each Medicare outpatient encounter, the modifier and APC-related data elements should be transferred to the clinical data repository.

APC Management Reports

More advanced software packages enable the automated generation of case-mix and error reports.

APC Case-Mix Report

Some APC grouper software packages allow hospitals to generate APC case-mix reports for Medicare. APC case-mix data are paramount to the hospital's outpatient care: performance measurement, outcomes analysis, marketing, and strategic planning initiatives.

Following are sample data elements that may be included in the report, depending on the needs of the hospital:

- Medical record/patient account number

- Admission and discharge dates

- Site of service

- Primary ICD-9-CM diagnosis code, with or without secondary diagnosis codes

- CPT and HCPCS Level II codes, all or only those impacting APC payment, per the hospital's discretion

- APC payment group for each code

- APC Medicare program payment amount for each APC group

- APC beneficiary copayment amount for each APC group

- APC outlier payment for case, if applicable

- Total outpatient charges for each case
- APC case-mix index for the encounter
- Other data elements as specified by the hospital.

Figure 13.6. Sample APC case-mix report excerpt

Mrec: 55585 Pat: 9998623 Admit Date: 10/02/XX Dschg Date: 10/03/XX Tot Chrgs Amt: 3,142.87 Pat Type Desc: AMBULATORY SURGERY Dx 01: 72768 Dx Desc: RUPTURE TENDON FOOT NEC **Cpt Code: 27691** Serv Ind: T **Apc Code: 51** **28300** T **56** P550 Payment 11/10/XX 1,395.70
Mrec: 555230 Pat: 9998550 Admit Date: 10/02/XX Dschg Date: 10/02/XX Tot Chrgs Amt: 1,357.58 Pat Type Desc: AMBULATORY SURGERY Dx 01: 6210 Dx Desc: POLYP OF CORPUS UTERI **Cpt Code: 58558** Serv Ind: T **Apc Code: 190** P550 Payment 11/10/XX 536.68
Mrec: 555904 Pat: 9997961 Admit Date: 10/06/XX Dschg Date: 10/06/XX Tot Chrgs Amt: 1,671.77 Pat Type Desc: AMBULATORY SURGERY Dx 01: 72402 Dx Desc: SPINAL STENOSIS-LUMBAR **Cpt Code: 62311** Serv Ind: T **Apc Code: 212** P550 Payment 11/10/XX 144.17
Mrec: 555805 Pat: 9998688 Admit Date: 10/02/XX Dschg Date: 10/02/XX Tot Chrgs Amt: 1,054.55 Pat Type Desc: AMBULATORY SURGERY Dx 01: 53510 Dx Desc: ATROPHIC GASTR WO HEMORRH **Cpt Code: 43239** Serv Ind: T **Apc Code: 141** P550 Payment 11/13/XX 236.37
Mrec: 555383 Pat: 9993761 Admit Date: 10/01/XX Dschg Date: 10/01/XX Tot Chrgs Amt: 99.00 Pat Type Desc: EMERGENCY ROOM PT. Dx 01: 88100 Dx Desc: OPEN WOUND OF FOREARM **Cpt Code: 12001** Serv Ind: T **Apc Code: 24** **99281** V **610** P550 Payment 11/02/XX 146.39
Mrec: 555575 Pat: 9998039 Admit Date: 10/11/XX Dschg Date: 10/11/XX Tot Chrgs Amt: 2,060.42 Pat Type Desc: AMBULATORY SURGERY Dx 01: 36610 Dx Desc: SENILE CATARACT NOS **Cpt Code: 66984** Serv Ind: T **Apc Code: 246** P550 Payment 11/13/XX 826.00

APC Error Report

Some billing software packages allow hospitals to:

- Load comprehensive, front-end coding and billing edits for such elements as coding validity, revenue code validity, and type of bill validation. Such software assists the hospitals in decreasing the number of claims that are rejected by the Medicare FI and increase the number of error-free claims that are paid within fourteen days by the Medicare FI.

- Generate error reports for those outpatient claims that do not pass internal coding and billing edits. Such software is used to identify patterns or trends in the invalid or incorrect coding and billing data reported throughout the facility. These patterns and trends may identify the need for chargemaster revisions, coder training, or physician education. (See Figure 13.7 and Table 13.1.)

Figure 13.7. APC error summary report

Error	1/16/XX Number of Claims	3/2/XX Number of Claims	1/16/XX Claim Amount	3/2/XX Claim Amount	Comments
01 – Invalid Dx	190	10	$79,285	$1,020	Programming is complete to prevent this from occurring. Remaining claims are "reference visits." Neither HIM nor PFS can correct. Will recommend for write-off.
06 – Invalid procedure code	27	22	$56,722	$24,228	HIM continues to resolve these as they occur to determine correct code, update chargemaster, and so on.
12 – Questionable service	12	25	$29,590	$70,062	These will continue to occur, and HIM will forward to PFS to push through after review and approval. These are most commonly plastic surgery procedures, where confirmation of medical necessity is required.
15 – Service units out of range	37	36	$135,140	$104,113	High-dollar ones since 1/01 are radiation oncology dosimetry for stereotactic radiosurgery. HIM and radiation oncology believe ranges are correct. Working with radiation oncology and outside resources to confirm this. When research is complete, this may require a clinical appeal through the FI and CMS to relax edit and facilitate billing beyond 10 units. Remaining claims also appear to be correct. Continue to research and work with our APC software vendor on logic behind this edit.
16 – Multiple bilateral procs w/out modifier 50	21	21	$23,206	$39,549	Ongoing education to departments to correct

Table 13.1.   APC error report distribution

Edit	Edit Type	Disposition	Responsible Party
1. Invalid diagnosis	Diagnosis edit	Claim returned to provider	HIM
2. Diagnosis and age conflict	Diagnosis edit	Claim returned to provider	HIM
3. Diagnosis and sex conflict	Diagnosis edit	Claim returned to provider	HIM
4. Medicare secondary payer alert	———	Claim suspension	PFS
5. E-code as reason for visit	Diagnosis edit	Claim returned to provider	HIM
6. Invalid procedure code	Procedure edit	Claim returned to provider	HIM
7. Procedure and age conflict[a]	Procedure edit	Claim returned to provider	HIM
8. Procedure and sex conflict	Procedure edit	Claim returned to provider	HIM
9. Noncovered service	Procedure edit	Line item denial	Edit overridden
10. Service submitted for verification of denial (condition code 21)	Procedure edit	Claim denial	PFS
11. Service submitted for review (condition code 20)	Procedure edit	Claim suspension	PFS
12. Questionable covered service	Procedure edit	Claim suspension	Edit overridden
13. Separate payment for services not provided by Medicare	Procedure edit	Claim returned to provider	Edit overridden
14. Code indicates a site of service not included in OPPS	Procedure edit	Claim returned to provider	NA
15. Service unit out of range for procedure[b]	Procedure edit	Claim returned to provider	HIM
16. Report code once with modifier –50 when performed bilaterally during the same session	Procedure edit	Claim returned to provider	HIM
17. Inappropriate specification of bilateral procedure	Procedure edit	Claim returned to provider	HIM
18. Inpatient procedure	Procedure edit	Line item denial	HIM
19. Mutually exclusive procedure that is not allowed even when appropriate modifier is present	Procedure edit	Line item rejection	HIM
20. Component of a comprehensive procedure that is not allowed even when appropriate modifier is present	Procedure edit	Line item rejection	HIM
21. Medical visit on same day as a type T or S procedure without modifier –25	Procedure edit	Line item rejection	Clinical departments
22. Invalid modifier	Modifier edit	Claim returned to provider	HIM
23. Invalid date	Date edit	Claim returned to provider	PFS
24. Date out of OCE range	Date edit	Claim suspension	PFS
25. Invalid age	Age edit	Claim returned to provider	HIM/PFS
26. Invalid sex	Sex edit	Claim returned to provider	HIM
27. Only incidental services reported	———	Claim returned to provider	PFS
28. Code not recognized by Medicare; alternate code for same service available	Procedure edit	Claim returned to provider	HIM
29. Partial hospitalization service for non–mental health diagnosis	Partial hospitalization edit	Claim returned to provider	HIM
30. Insufficient services on day of partial hospitalization	Partial hospitalization edit	Claim suspension	HIM/Psychiatry
31. Partial hospitalization on same day as ECT or type T procedure	Partial hospitalization edit	Claim suspension	HIM/Psychiatry

Table 13.1. (Continued)

Edit	Edit Type	Disposition	Responsible Party
32. Partial hospitalization claim spans 3 or fewer days with insufficient services, or ECT or significant procedure on at least one of the days	Partial hospitalization edit	Claim suspension	HIM/Psychiatry
33. Partial hospitalization claim spans more than 3 days with insufficient number of days having mental health services	Partial hospitalization edit	Claim suspension	HIM/Psychiatry
34. Partial hospitalization claim spans more than 3 days with insufficient number of days meeting partial hospitalization criteria	Partial hospitalization edit	Claim suspension	HIM/Psychiatry
35. Only activity therapy and/or occupational therapy services provided	Mental health edit	Claim returned to provider	HIM/Rehab therapies
36. Extensive mental health services provided on day of ECT or significant procedure	Mental health edit	Claim suspension	HIM/Psychiatry
37. Terminated bilateral procedure or terminated procedure with units greater than one	Procedure edit	Claim returned to provider	HIM
38. Implanted device without implantation procedure	Procedure edit	Claim returned to provider	HIM
39. Mutually exclusive procedure that would be allowed if appropriate modifier were present	Procedure edit	Claim returned to provider	HIM
40. Component of a comprehensive procedure that would be allowed if appropriate modifier were present	Procedure edit	Line item rejection	HIM
41. Invalid revenue code	Revenue code edit	Claim returned to provider	PFS/HIM
42. Multiple medical visits on same day with same revenue code without condition code G0	Procedure edit	Line item rejection	PFS
43. Transfusion or blood product exchange without specification of blood product	Procedure edit	Claim returned to provider	PFS
44. Observation revenue code on line item with non-observation HCPCS code	Procedure edit	Claim returned to provider	PFS
45. Service not appropriate for type of bill	Not activated	Line item rejection	————
46. Partial hospitalization condition code 41 not approved for type of bill	Partial hospitalization edit	Claim returned to provider	PFS
47. Service is not separately payable	Procedure edit	Line item rejection	PFS
48. -Revenue center requires HCPCS	Revenue code edit	Claim returned to provider	PFS

HIM = Health information management; PFS = Patient financial services

[a] Currently not used.
[b] Units for all line items with the same HCPCS code are added together when applying this edit.

Chapter 14

Coding and Incomplete Clinical Data

An AHIMA practice brief on data quality states that coding professionals should maintain a positive working relationship with physicians through ongoing communication and open dialogue. It also states that coding professionals should not misrepresent the patient's clinical picture through incorrect coding or add diagnoses or procedures unsupported by the documentation in order to optimize reimbursement or meet insurance policy coverage requirement (AHIMA 2003).

Each entity is somewhat different in what documentation is required prior to coding and releasing the bill to the payer. Coders should have, at a minimum, a history and physical, operative report (if applicable), short stay summary (should include a final impression), and culture and pathology reports. Some entities do not hold billing for final impression. If a coder determines the information in the existing record has sufficient documentation to accurately code, the hospital may choose to release the bill. This is opposite to best practices when an operative report is not available during coding. Many procedures vary, and the coder cannot ensure accuracy by only coding from a diagnostic or procedural statement. It is recommended to hold the billing until a pathology report is final, however, many entities will bill without the documentation as oftentimes the coding does not impact reimbursement in the outpatient setting. However, the coding specificity of the ICD-9-CM code may attribute to a denial due to a procedure being performed that lacks medical necessity, based on the diagnosis.

To accurately code outpatient services when the physician's documentation is unclear or incomplete, coding specialists must find a way to communicate with physicians. Many hospitals use query forms or written correspondence to ask the physician to clarify missing or unclear clinical documentation. Figures 14.1 through 14.4 offer examples of different types of query forms.

Query Form Process

Following are recommended steps for implementing a query form process:

1. Use feedback from the coding specialists to identify patterns of outpatient conditions or procedures that are not thoroughly documented by physicians.

2. Create query forms based on the documentation needed to assign appropriate codes and to adhere to any coding guidelines that apply. Use codebooks and official guidelines as references.

Figure 14.1. Sample Emergency Department Query form

EMERGENCY DEPARTMENT QUERY

Dear Dr._____   Date: _____

Patient Name: _____

Acct.#: _____

D.O.S.: _____

Please see the attached record for the above patient to whom you provided emergency care. Additional information is needed to complete the coding of this record. Please complete the following portion of the attached record:

[ ] History: _____

[ ] Physical: _____

[ ] Diagnosis: _____

[ ] Procedure note: _____

[ ] Laceration length: _____

[ ] Laceration complexity: _____

[ ] Other: _____

_____

_____

This form will be maintained as part of the permanent medical record.

Record Completion Review: _____
                          (Initials/Date)

Coder Review:_____
                          (Initials/Date)

Figure 14.2. Sample Bladder Lesion Query form

Pt. Name:_____

MR#: _____

Acct#: _____

D/C Date: _____

PHYSICIAN QUERY:
SIZE OF BLADDER LESION/TUMOR?

Dear Dr._____

Please provide documentation to support the **selection of the correct CPT code.**

Please document below the **size of the bladder lesion/tumor.**

In the future, when dictating the operating report, please document this description within the **statement of the operation** to be performed. Thank you.

Date Submitted:_____

Physician Response:

_____

_____

_____

_____

_____

Physician Signature/Title

Source: Peterson (unpublished data)

Figure 14.3.   Sample Skin Lesion/Wound Query form

Pt. Name:_____

MR#: _____

Acct#: _____

D/C Date: _____

PHYSICIAN QUERY:
SIZE OF LESION/MASS/TUMOR/WOUND REPAIR SITE?

Dear Dr._____

Please provide complete the "Physician Response" section below to support the selection of the correct CPT code.

In the future, when dictating the operating report, please document this information within the statement of the operation to be performed. Thank you.

Date Submitted:_____

Physician Response:

[ ] Please document the size of: _____

[ ] Lesion/mass/tumor of the: _____

_____

[ ] Wound repair site

[ ] Is the lesion/mass/tumor

    [ ] subcutaneous? or of the [ ] soft tissue?

_____

Physician Signature/Title

Source: Peterson (unpublished data)

Figure 14.4.   Sample query sticker that is affixed to a chart document

Case Number: _____

Name: _____

Dear Doctor:_____

At the time of dictation the following was omitted:

[ ] **History**

[ ] Chief complaint	[ ] Family history
[ ] Present illness	[ ] Social history
[ ] Past history	[ ] Review systems

[ ] **Physical examination**

Operative Record

[ ] Preoperative diagnosis	[ ] Name of operation
[ ] Postoperative diagnosis	[ ] Findings and technique
[ ] Please fill in blanks	

Remarks:_____

_____

_____

3. Develop a policy regarding whether to file the query forms in the medical record as permanent documents in the chart.

4. Develop a policy that defines the deadline for physician response to the query form (for example, the physician must respond within 48 hours of the form being completed) and seek feedback from hospital executives to determine how to handle a physician nonresponse (for example, suspension of admitting privileges).

5. House query forms in a location where physicians will see them immediately.

6. Log queries to track cases that are pending because the coding specialist is awaiting a response. Such a log can be automated in clinical data abstracting software packages. Report tracking to monthly medical staff meetings and make available to administration and the chief of staff.

There are alternative ways to reach physicians who do not respond to query forms. Examples include:

- Arranging medical staff meetings for a nonresponding physician's specialty to present a brief documentation training session

- Writing an article for the medical staff newsletter that addresses documentation requirements for conditions or procedures that are repeatedly incomplete

- Meeting with the nonresponding physician in his or her office to discuss documentation deficiencies

Coding Issues Not Officially Addressed

First and foremost, coders are instructed to use the official coding resources supported by the Cooperating Parties:

- Coding conventions and alphabetic index of the ICD-9-CM codebook
- ICD-9-CM Official Guidelines for Coding and Reporting
- AHA *Coding Clinic for ICD-9-CM*
- AHA *Coding Clinic for HCPCS*

When the documentation is clear and complete, coding specialists still may find it difficult to code a case for which there is no official coding guideline. The following suggestions may be helpful in addressing coding issues that have no formal coding guidelines:

- The Internet is a good place to search for clinical information about the condition or procedure, especially CMS, OIG, and AMA Web sites for coding, billing, or reimbursement guidelines.

- The hospital's medical library sometimes has additional clinical details about the condition or procedure.

- Physicians may be willing to discuss the issue to help a coding specialist learn more about the clinical nature of the condition or procedure.

- Medical societies and associations that have expertise in the diagnosis and/or treatment of the condition or procedure may provide general information.

Any information found should be documented and shared with the entire coding team during the coding meetings. If the facility develops a policy of its own to address the issue, the policy should be added to the department's coding manual.

However, coders should be aware that many payers do not follow the official coding guidelines, making coding challenging. Typically in the outpatient setting, coders must review the record based on payer coding and billing guidelines or the claim will be denied. For example, coding guidelines state to use "V57.1: encounter for physical therapy" as the primary diagnosis; however, most commercial payers require the diagnosis that is most relevant to warrant the treatment for the therapy. The CPT code reveals which therapy is provided to the patient, and with only the V code as a listed diagnosis, the payer cannot determine if the reason for the visit is medically necessary.

Coding managers should try to communicate to payers via a formal letter explaining their policy is against coding guidelines; however, if the payer does not change or continues to require conflicting guidelines, coders should submit the requested codes.

The coding department should keep a file on all payer-specific policies that differ from the official coding guidelines. In the event of an external audit, the coding department should provide the information to the auditor.

Coding queries should be nonleading and ask a specific question that relates to the case. The query should always state the relevant clinical indicators of the case and utilize terminology that is clear, concise, and open-ended. Verbal discussions are beneficial to educating a physician, however, avoid verbal queries unless the physician can document the information in the record at the time of discussion.

Exhibits 14.1 and 14.2 offer additional readings on ethics in coding and the physician query process.

Exhibit 14.1. Ethics in Coding

Ethical Coding in the Physician Office

Peg Austin, RHIA, CPC, and Mary H. Stanfill, RHIA

Data quality has never been more scrutinized than it is today. Health Care Financing Administration [now CMS] rules and contractual obligations from various insurance companies complicate the notion of correct coding. At the same time, numerous trade associations publish coding guidelines that occasionally differ from the HCFA [CMS], American Medical Association, or American Hospital Association (AHA) interpretation. However well meaning, the intent of some guidelines is to get a claim paid. There have been numerous discussions recently in coding and compliance circles regarding the contradictions that exist between the Health Information Management (HIM) coding perspective and the Balanced Budget Act (BBA) billing perspective.

The medical code of ethics directs the physicians to "first do no harm," so he or she will act in the best interest of the patient and think about documentation secondarily. Physicians may feel pressured by coding staff who continually ask for more complete documentation or appear to be questioning the physician's medical judgment. Meanwhile, the coder's intent may be simply to instruct or notify the physician of proper coding practices. Thus, the development of an honest, supportive relationship with physicians will help them understand the importance of proper documentation and its trickle-down effect on coding and resulting reimbursement. Threats about the consequences of false claims and improper coding make the most negative impression on physicians. Instead, they need someone to guide them through the labyrinth of coding guidelines and government regulations regarding reimbursement.

In some cases, however, all efforts at physician education are met with resistance or threats along with explicit instructions to "code it anyway." Or the inquisitive nature of coders may reveal a coding practice that had previously been regarded as insignificant until someone researched it further and discovered an inappropriate monetary result.

So, what should the coding professional do when faced with ethical dilemmas? Consider the following scenarios, which are followed by an analysis and ethical response based on the AHIMA Standards of Ethical Coding.

Scenario 1

Dr. Miller codes an office visit 99215 with a long list of diagnoses that are minor or "history of" conditions. The only diagnosis that Jill, the coder, can find that was actually treated was vaginitis (616.10). Because this is a Medicare patient, she is concerned about billing for a level V office visit. After discussion with Dr. Miller, it appears that the patient was actually in for an annual physical, and Jill suggests a preventive medicine code. Dr. Miller is adamant that this patient not have to pay and says, "Just tell me what I need to dictate to be able to bill the 99215 without getting into trouble."

Several of AHIMA's Standards of Ethical Coding can be applied in this situation. Jill correctly applied standard #4: Only codes that are clearly and consistently supported by physician documentation in the medical record should be coded. Standard #5 indicates that the coder should consult physicians for clarification and additional documentation prior to code assignment when there is ambiguous data in the health record. What should she tell Dr. Miller to dictate and how far does her responsibility extend in this case? Jill also needs to keep in mind standard #6, which directs the coders not to change codes or the narrative of codes so that meanings are misrepresented; #7, which calls on coders to advocate proper documentation practices; and #10, which cautions the coders to remember that it is unethical and illegal to maximize payment by means that contradict regulatory guidelines. Above all, Dr. Miller should be advised to document the service he provided to this patient and not embellish the details in order to justify the claim.

The ethical response to this scenario:

- Advise Dr. Miller to document the service he provided, point out specific areas in his dictation where his services are unclear, and obtain a dictated addendum
- Obtain coding advice on this visit from an appropriate source, such as a coding supervisor, peer coder, or coding consultant on retainer
- Follow up with Dr. Miller regarding what codes are appropriate for the documented service, provided it is consistent with official coding guidelines and Medicare requirements. A possible solution might be use of HCPCS level II codes for a pap, pelvic, and breast exam along with the appropriate-level office visit and modifier –25 to treat the vaginitis.

Exhibit 14.1. (Continued)

Ethical Coding Best Practices

- Educate coders on the ethical standards and annually review them at the time of performance evaluations.
- Follow official coding guidelines and advice published in resources such as *CPT Assistant and Coding Clinic*.
- Develop tools to provide solutions to ethical dilemmas, such as a compliance plan, facility-specific coding guidelines, facility-specific procedures for responding to coding errors, or potential false claim submissions.
- Establish a good working relationship with the compliance officer and compliance committee.
- Physicians are best influenced by peers: find an advocate in the medical staff and work to keep this individual informed of ethical coding practices.
- Avoid focusing on penalties, such as fines and imprisonment, as a way to motivate physicians.
- Focus on consistent and accurate reporting of coded information for the purpose of quality healthcare data.
- Limit presentations to physician groups to 30–45 minutes, and avoid sandwiching presentations on ethics and compliance into larger meeting agendas.
- Tailor presentations to "real" practice-specific problems, rather than broad or general issues, with specific recommendations and tools for data quality improvement.

Scenario 2

Coders at XYZ clinic are responsible for coding from the dictated office notes and assigning CPT codes for ancillary services. Dr. Smith always circles the CPT code for his office visit appropriately, but does not circle anything else. When the coders review his dictation, they correctly circle other services provided and assign ICD-9 codes as dictated. Dr. Smith becomes very angry with the coding staff, saying that he told his patients that he would only charge them for the office visit, and the coders are creating additional charges for which patients will subsequently complain to him.

Analysis of this scenario shows that coding standards #1 and #3 have been appropriately applied. As coding professionals, they are expected to support the importance of accurate, complete, and consistent coding practices for the production of quality healthcare data. Also, coding professionals should use their skills and knowledge of currently mandated coding and classification systems and official resources to select the appropriate diagnostic and procedural codes. Standard #6 states that coders should not change codes or the narratives of codes on the billing abstract so that meanings are misrepresented. Diagnoses or procedures should not be inappropriately included or excluded because payment or insurance policy coverage requirements will be affected. Standard #10 states that coding professionals should strive for optimal payment for which the facility is legally entitled, remembering that it is unethical and illegal to maximize payment by means that contradict regulatory guidelines.

The ethical response to this scenario:

- Reassure Dr. Smith that coding guidelines for the clinic are being followed to report codes accurately, regardless of payment source, and he is being treated the same as all of the clinic's physicians.
- Caution Dr. Smith that the coding system cannot be used to manage accounting issues, and that acts of benevolence can be handled appropriately on the accounting side, in accordance with insurance plan requirements.
- Discuss the issue with the appropriate compliance plan representative of the practice or the practice administrator for resolution by the medical staff.

These types of scenarios can be very difficult for any coding professional, yet turning a blind eye to questionable claims and coding practices can lead to serious consequences for the physicians.

Cases to Consider

Court cases involving the Office of the Inspector General (OIG) can take years to resolve. Following are two current cases:

A urologist in Arkansas was charged with Medicare overpayment by unbundling lab codes and performing medically unnecessary tests. Review of claims paid over a period of six years showed overpayment of $708,812. Medicare argued that the physician had reason to be aware of the coding changes during that time frame, but submitted erroneous claims regardless and was paid for tests he did not perform. In addition, some tests were done for screening purposes, and occasionally tests were repeated at close intervals without justification. The physician appealed, stating that the sampling methodology was flawed, but the original decision was upheld. This particular case has been ongoing since the mid-1990s.

A physician in La Mesa, CA, pled guilty in December 2000 to charges of fraudulently billing Medicare for medically unnecessary cardiac rehabilitation, billing for office visits plus other procedures when only the rehabilitation procedure was done, and billing for monitored cardiac rehabilitation when only unmonitored rehabilitation was performed. The physician agreed to reimburse Medicare $50,000 and [was] sentenced/fined in April 2001.

(Continued on next page)

Exhibit 14.1. (Continued)

Circumstances like the above would certainly present an ethical challenge to an alert coding staff employed by these physicians. Regardless of whether or not your facility has an active compliance plan and committee, the following are general steps the coding professional should take when approaching a tough situation:

- Gather the facts regarding the situation and the standards that may apply. Get copies of the standards from their source.
- Follow the chain of authority specific to your organization. Do not surprise your immediate supervisor by going over his or her head, but use hotlines or other anonymous reporting mechanisms, if necessary, to get the issues addressed.
- At each level, explain the problem and the risk to the organization. Offer a solution, rather than just reporting the problem.
- Document each meeting or conversation including date, time, issues discussed, who was involved with the discussion, and whether the problem was resolved.
- If the practice continues, a formal letter is recommended to those in the chain of authority summarizing all of the previous steps.
- If there is no hope of resolution, it is suggested that the coder should terminate his or her position, rather than condone the practice by continued employment.
- The worst-case scenario would obligate the coder to report the problem to the OIG or to the US Attorney's office.

Coding professionals will inevitably be faced with ethical gray areas in their career. Diligence is necessary to apply guidelines in a consistent manner and to remain alert for questionable practices, even when no fraudulent intent exists. By using the resources available and establishing a positive working relationship with physicians, most coders will succeed in their efforts to code ethically and preserve data quality.

Additional Resources for Ethical Coding

The following are additional resources for ethical coding:

- AHIMA's Standards of Ethical Coding
- "Ethics in the Age of Compliance" Program in a Box by Linda Kloss, MA, RHIA, available at www.ahima.org
- *Ethical Challenges in the Management of Health Information* by Laurinda Harman, PhD, RHIA, available from Aspen Publishers
- Health Care Compliance Association Web site at http://www.hcca-info.org
- "Health Information Management Compliance: A Model Program for Healthcare Organizations" by Sue Prophet, RHIA, CCS, available at www.ahima.org
- Fighting Fraud and Abuse: Medicare Integrity Program available at http://www.hcfa.gov/medicare/fraud
- Office of the Inspector General. Available at http://www.oig.hhs.gov/index.htm. Contains the OIG Work Plan, fraud and abuse guidelines, and other reference materials

Notes

1. CCH Research Network. Available at http://health. cch.com/network.
2. Health Care Compliance Association. This Week in Corporate Compliance 2, no. 50 (December 22, 2000).

Source: Austin, Peg, and Mary H. Stanfill. "Ethical Coding in the Physician Office." *Journal of AHIMA* 72, no.3 (2001): 65–67.

Exhibit 14.1. (Continued)

Standards of Ethical Coding

In this era of payment based on diagnostic and procedural coding, the professional ethics of health information coding professionals continue to be challenged. A conscientious goal for coding and maintaining a quality database is accurate clinical and statistical data. The following standards of ethical coding, developed by AHIMA's Coding Policy and Strategy Committee and approved by AHIMA's Board of Directors, are offered to guide coding professionals in this process.

1. Coding professionals are expected to support the importance of accurate, complete, and consistent coding practices for the production of quality healthcare data.

2. Coding professionals in all healthcare settings should adhere to the ICD-9-CM (International Classification of Diseases, 9th revision, Clinical Modification) coding conventions, official coding guidelines approved by the Cooperating Parties,* the CPT (Current Procedural Terminology) rules established by the American Medical Association, and any other official coding rules and guidelines established for use with mandated standard code sets. Selection and sequencing of diagnoses and procedures must meet the definitions of required data sets for applicable healthcare settings.

3. Coding professionals should use their skills, their knowledge of currently mandated coding and classification systems, and official resources to select the appropriate diagnostic and procedural codes.

4. Coding professionals should only assign and report codes that are clearly and consistently supported by physician documentation in the health record.

5. Coding professionals should consult physicians for clarification and additional documentation prior to code assignment when there is conflicting or ambiguous data in the health record.

6. Coding professionals should not change codes or the narratives of codes on the billing abstract so that meanings are misrepresented. Diagnoses or procedures should not be inappropriately included or excluded because payment or insurance policy coverage requirements will be affected. When individual payer policies conflict with official coding rules and guidelines, these policies should be obtained in writing whenever possible. Reasonable efforts should be made to educate the payer on proper coding practices in order to influence a change in the payer's policy.

7. Coding professionals, as members of the healthcare team, should assist and educate physicians and other clinicians by advocating proper documentation practices, greater specificity, and resequencing or inclusion of diagnoses or procedures when needed to more accurately reflect the acuity, severity, and the occurrence of events.

8. Coding professionals should participate in the development of institutional coding policies and should ensure that coding policies complement, not conflict with, official coding rules and guidelines.

9. Coding professionals should maintain and continually enhance their coding skills, as they have a professional responsibility to stay abreast of changes in codes, coding guidelines, and regulations.

10. Coding professionals should strive for optimal payment to which the facility is legally entitled, remembering that it is unethical and illegal to maximize payment by means that contradict regulatory guidelines.

Revised 12/99

* The Cooperating Parties are the American Health Information Management Association, American Hospital Association, Health Care Financing Administration, and National Center for Health Statistics. All rights reserved. Reprint and quote only with proper reference to AHIMA's authorship.

Source: American Health Information Management Association. "Standards of Ethical Coding." *Journal of AHIMA* 71, no.3 (2000): insert after p.8.

Exhibit 14.2. Developing a physician query process

Principles of Medical Record Documentation

Medical record documentation is used for a multitude of purposes, including:

- Serving as a means of communication between the physician and the other members of the healthcare team providing care to the patient
- Serving as a basis for evaluating the adequacy and appropriateness of patient care
- Providing data to support insurance claims
- Assisting in protecting the legal interests of patients, healthcare professionals, and healthcare facilities
- Providing clinical data for research and education

To support these various uses, it is imperative that medical record documentation be complete, accurate, and timely. Facilities are expected to comply with a number of standards regarding medical record completion and content promulgated by multiple regulatory agencies.

The Joint Commission

The Joint Commission's 2000 Hospital Accreditation Standards state, "the medical record contains sufficient information to identify the patient, support the diagnosis, justify the treatment, document the course and results, and promote continuity among health care providers" (IM.7.2). The Joint Commission Standards also state, "medical record data and information are managed in a timely manner" (IM.7.6).

Timely entries are essential if a medical record is to be useful in a patient's care. A complete medical record is also important when a patient is discharged, because information in the record may be needed for clinical, legal, or performance improvement purposes. The Joint Commission requires hospitals to have policy and procedures on the timely entry of all significant clinical information into the patient's medical record, and they do not consider a medical record complete until all final diagnoses and complications are recorded without the use of symbols or abbreviations.

Joint commission standards also require medical records to be reviewed on an ongoing basis for completeness and timeliness of information, and action is taken to improve the quality and timeliness of documentation that affects patient care (IM.7.10). This review must address the presence, timeliness, legibility, and authentication of the final diagnoses and conclusions at termination of hospitalization.

Medicare

The Medicare *Conditions of Participation* require medical records to be accurately written, promptly completed, properly filed and retained, and accessible.

Records must document, as appropriate, complications, hospital-acquired infections, and unfavorable reactions to drugs and anesthesia. The conditions also stipulate that all records must document the final diagnosis with completion of medical records within 30 days following discharge.

Relationship between Coding and Documentation

Complete and accurate diagnostic and procedural coded data must be available, in a timely manner, in order to:

- Improve the quality and effectiveness of patient care
- Ensure equitable healthcare reimbursement
- Expand the body of medical knowledge
- Make appropriate decisions regarding healthcare policies, delivery systems, funding, expansion, and education
- Monitor resource utilization
- Permit identification and resolution of medical errors
- Improve clinical decision making
- Facilitate tracking of fraud and abuse
- Permit valid clinical research, epidemiological studies, outcomes and statistical analyses, and provider profiling
- Provide comparative data to consumers regarding costs and outcomes, average charges, and outcomes by procedure

Physician documentation is the cornerstone of accurate coding. Therefore, assuring the accuracy of coded data is a shared responsibility between coding professionals and physicians. Accurate diagnostic and procedural coded data originate from collaboration between physicians, who have a clinical background, and coding professionals, who have an understanding of classification systems.

Exhibit 14.2. (Continued)

Expectations of Physicians

Physicians are expected to provide complete, accurate, timely, and legible documentation of pertinent facts and observations about an individual's health history, including past and present illnesses, tests, treatments, and outcomes. Medical record entries should be documented at the time service is provided. Medical record entries should be authenticated. If subsequent additions to documentation are needed, they should be identified as such and dated. (Often these expectations are included in the medical staff or house staff rules and regulations.) Medical record documentation should:

- Address the clinical significance of abnormal test results.
- Support the intensity of patient evaluation and treatment and describe the thought processes and complexity of decision making.
- Include all diagnostic and therapeutic procedures, treatments, and tests performed, in addition to their results.
- Include any changes in the patient's condition, including psychosocial and physical symptoms.
- Include all conditions that coexist at the time of admission, that subsequently develop, or that affect the treatment received and the length of stay. This encompasses all conditions that affect patient care in terms of requiring clinical evaluation, therapeutic treatment, diagnostic procedures, extended length of hospital stay, or increased nursing care and monitoring.
- Be updated as necessary to reflect all diagnoses relevant to the care or services provided.
- Be consistent and discuss and reconcile any discrepancies (this reconciliation should be documented in the medical record).
- Be legible and written in ink, typewritten, or electronically signed, stored, and printed.

Expectations of Coding Professionals

The AHIMA Code of Ethics sets forth ethical principles for the HIM profession. HIM professionals are responsible for maintaining and promoting ethical practices. This Code of Ethics states, in part: "Health information management professionals promote high standards for health information management practice, education, and research." Another standard in this code states, "Health information management professionals strive to provide accurate and timely information." Data accuracy and integrity are fundamental values of HIM that are advanced by:

- Employing practices that produce complete, accurate, and timely information to meet the health and related needs of individuals
- Following the guidelines set forth in the organization's compliance plan for reporting improper preparation, alteration, or suppression of information or data by others
- Not participating in any improper preparation, alteration, or suppression of health record information or other organization data

A conscientious goal for coding and maintaining a quality database is accurate clinical and statistical data. AHIMA's Standards of Ethical Coding were developed to guide coding professionals in this process. As stated in the standards, coding professionals are expected to support the importance of accurate, complete, and consistent coding practices for the production of quality healthcare data. These standards also indicate that coding professionals should only assign and report codes that are clearly and consistently supported by physician documentation in the medical record. It is the responsibility of coding professionals to assess physician documentation to assure that it supports the diagnosis and procedure codes reported on claims.

Dialogue between coding professionals and clinicians is encouraged, because it improves coding professionals' clinical knowledge and educates the physicians on documentation practice issues. AHIMA's Standards of Ethical Coding state that coding professionals are expected to consult physicians for clarification and additional documentation prior to code assignment when there is conflicting or ambiguous data in the health record.

Coding professionals should also assist and educate physicians by advocating proper documentation practices, further specificity, and resequencing or inclusion of diagnoses or procedures when needed to more accurately reflect the acuity, severity, and the occurrence of events. It is recommended that coding be performed by credentialed HIM professionals. It is inappropriate for coding professionals to misrepresent the patient's clinical picture through incorrect coding or add diagnoses or procedures unsupported by the documentation to maximize reimbursement or meet insurance policy coverage requirements. Coding professionals should not change codes or the narratives of codes on the billing abstract so that meanings are misrepresented. Diagnoses or procedures should not be inappropriately included or excluded, because payment or insurance policy coverage requirements will be affected. When individual payer policies conflict with official coding rules and guidelines, these policies should be obtained in writing whenever possible. Reasonable efforts should be made to educate the payer on proper coding practices in order to influence a change in the payer's policy.

(Continued on next page)

Exhibit 14.2. (Continued)

Proper Use of Physician Queries

The process of querying physicians is an effective and, in today's healthcare environment, necessary mechanism for improving the quality of coding and medical record documentation and capturing complete clinical data. Query forms have become an accepted tool for communicating with physicians on documentation issues influencing proper code assignment. Query forms should be used in a judicious and appropriate manner. They must be used as a communication tool to improve the accuracy of code assignment and the quality of physician documentation, not to inappropriately maximize reimbursement. The query process should be guided by AHIMA's Standards of Ethical Coding and the official coding guidelines. An inappropriate query—such as a form that is poorly constructed or asks leading questions—or overuse of the query process can result in quality-of-care, legal, and ethical concerns.

Query Process

The goal of the query process should be to improve physician documentation and coding professionals' understanding of the unique clinical situation, not to improve reimbursement. Each facility should establish a policy and procedure for obtaining physician clarification of documentation that affects code assignment. The process of querying physicians must be a patient-specific process, not a general process. Asking "blanket" questions is not appropriate. Policies regarding the circumstances when physicians will be queried should be designed to promote timely, complete, and accurate coding and documentation.

Physicians should not be asked to provide clarification of their medical record documentation without the opportunity to access the patient's medical record. Each facility also needs to determine if physicians will be queried concurrently (during the patient's hospitalization) or after discharge. Both methods are acceptable. Querying physicians concurrently allows the documentation deficiency to be corrected while the patient is still in-house and can positively influence patient care.

The policy and procedure should stipulate who is authorized to contact the physician for clarifications regarding a coding issue. Coding professionals should be allowed to contact physicians directly for clarification, rather than limiting this responsibility to supervisory personnel or a designated individual.

The facility may wish to use a designated physician liaison to resolve conflicts between physicians and coding professionals. The appropriate use of the physician liaison should be described in the facility's policy and procedures.

Query Format

Each facility should develop a standard format for the query form. No "sticky notes" or scratch paper should be allowed. Each facility should develop a standard design and format for physician queries to ensure clear, consistent, appropriate queries. The query form should:

- Be clearly and concisely written.
- Contain precise language.
- Present the facts from the medical record and identify why clarification is needed.
- Present the scenario and state a question that asks the physician to make a clinical interpretation of a given diagnosis or condition based on treatment, evaluation, monitoring, and/or services provided. "Open-ended" questions that allow the physician to document the specific diagnosis are preferable to multiple-choice questions or questions requiring only a "yes" or "no" response. Queries that appear to lead the physician to provide a particular response could lead to allegations of inappropriate upcoding.
- Be phrased such that the physician is allowed to specify the correct diagnosis. It should not indicate the financial impact of the response to the query. The form should not be designed so that all that is required is a physician signature.

Exhibit 14.2. (Continued)

Include:

- Patient name
- Admission date
- Medical record number
- Name and contact information (phone number and e-mail address) of the coding professional
- Specific question and rationale (that is, relevant documentation or clinical findings)
- Place for physician to document his or her response
- Place for the physician to sign and date his or her response

The query forms should not:

- "Lead" the physician
- Sound presumptive, directing, prodding, probing, or as though the physician is being led to make an assumption
- Ask questions that can be responded to in a "yes" or "no" fashion
- Indicate the financial impact of the response to the query
- Be designed so that all that is required is a physician signature

When Is a Query Appropriate?

Physicians should be queried whenever there is conflicting, ambiguous, or incomplete information in the medical record regarding any significant reportable condition or procedure. Querying the physician only when reimbursement is affected will skew national healthcare data and might lead to allegations of upcoding.

Every discrepancy or issue not addressed in the physician documentation should not necessarily result in the physician being queried. Each facility needs to develop policies and procedures regarding the clinical conditions and documentation situations warranting a request for physician clarification. For example, insignificant or irrelevant findings may not warrant querying the physician regarding the assignment of an additional diagnosis code. Also, if the maximum number of codes that can be entered in the hospital information system has already been assigned, the facility may decide that it is not necessary to query the physician regarding an additional code. Facilities need to balance the value of marginal data being collected against the administrative burden of obtaining the additional documentation.

Members of the medical staff in consultation with coding professionals should develop the specific clinical criteria for a valid query. The specific clinical documentation that must be present in the patient's record to generate a query should be described. For example, anemia, septicemia, and respiratory failure are conditions that often require physician clarification. The medical staff can assist the coding staff in determining when it would be appropriate to query a physician regarding the reporting of these conditions by describing the specific clinical indications in the medical record documentation that raise the possibility that the condition in question may be present.

When Is a Query Not Necessary?

Queries are not necessary if a physician involved in the care and treatment of the patient, including consulting physicians, has documented a diagnosis and there is no conflicting documentation from another physician. Medical record documentation from any physician involved in the care and treatment of the patient, including documentation by consulting physicians, is appropriate for the basis of code assignment. If documentation from different physicians conflicts, seek clarification from the attending physician, as he or she is ultimately responsible for the final diagnosis.

Queries are also not necessary when a physician has documented a final diagnosis and clinical indicator such as test results that do not appear to support this diagnosis. While coding professionals are expected to advocate complete and accurate physician documentation and to collaborate with physicians to realize this goal, they are not expected to challenge the physician's medical judgment in establishing the patient's diagnosis. However, because a discrepancy between clinical findings and a final diagnosis is a clinical issue, a facility may choose to establish a policy that the physician will be queried in these instances.

(Continued on next page)

Exhibit 14.2. (Continued)

Documentation of Query Response

The physician's response to the query must be documented in the patient's medical record. Each facility must develop a policy regarding the specific process for incorporating this additional documentation in the medical record. For example, this policy might stipulate that the physician is required to add the additional information to the body of the medical record. As an alternative, a form, such as a medical record "progress note" form, might be attached to the query form and the attachment is then filed in the medical record. However, another alternative is to file the query form itself in the permanent medical record. Any documentation obtained post-discharge must be included in the discharge summary or identified as a late entry or addendum.

Any decision to file this form in the medical record should involve the advice of the facility's corporate compliance officer and legal counsel, due to potential compliance and legal risks related to incorporating the actual query form into the permanent medical record (such as its potential use as evidence of poor documentation in an audit, investigation, or malpractice suit, risks related to naming a nonclinician in the medical record, or quality-of-care concerns if the physician response on a query form is not clearly supported by the rest of the medical record documentation).

If the query form will serve as the only documentation of the physician's clarification, the use of "open-ended" questions (that require the physician to specifically document the additional information) are preferable to multiple- choice questions or the use of questions requiring only a "yes" or "no" answer. The query form would need to be approved by the medical staff/medical records committee before implementation of a policy allowing this form to be maintained in the medical record. Also keep in mind that the Joint Commission hospital accreditation standards stipulate that only authorized individuals may make entries in medical records (IM.7.1.1). Therefore, the facility needs to consider modifying the medical staff bylaws to specify coding professionals as individuals authorized to make medical record entries prior to allowing query forms to become a permanent part of the medical record.

Auditing, Monitoring, and Corrective Action

Ideally, complete and accurate physician documentation should occur at the time care is rendered. The need for a query form results from incomplete, conflicting, or ambiguous documentation, which is an indication of poor documentation. Therefore, query form usage should be the exception rather than the norm. If physicians are being queried frequently, facility management or an appropriate medical staff committee should investigate the reasons why.

A periodic review of the query practice should include a determination of what percentage of the query forms are eliciting negative and positive responses from the physicians. A high negative response rate may be an indication that the coding staff are not using the query process judiciously and are being overzealous.

A high positive response rate may indicate that there are widespread poor documentation habits that need to be addressed. It may also indicate that the absence of certain reports (for example, discharge summary, operative report) at the time of coding is forcing the coding staff to query the physicians to obtain the information they need for proper coding. If this is the case, the facility may wish to reconsider its policy regarding the availability of certain reports prior to coding. Waiting for these reports may make more sense in terms of turnaround time and productivity rather than finding it necessary to frequently query the physicians. The question of why final diagnoses are not available at the time of discharge may arise at the time of an audit, review by the peer review organization, or investigation.

The use of query forms should also be monitored for patterns, and any identified patterns should be used to educate physicians on improving their documentation at the point of care. If a pattern is identified, such as a particular physician or diagnosis, appropriate steps should be taken to correct the problem so the necessary documentation is present prior to coding in the future and the need to query this physician, or to query physicians regarding a particular diagnosis, is reduced. Corrective action might include targeted education for one physician or education for the entire medical staff on the proper documentation necessary for accurate code assignment.

Patterns of poor documentation that have not been addressed through education or other corrective action are signs of an ineffective compliance program. The Department of Health and Human Services Office of Inspector General has noted in its *Compliance Program Guidance for Hospitals* that "accurate coding depends upon the quality of completeness of the physician's documentation" and "active staff physician participation in educational programs focusing on coding and documentation should be emphasized by the hospital."

Exhibit 14.2. (Continued)

The format of the queries should also be monitored on a regular basis to ensure that they are not inappropriately leading the physician to provide a particular response. Inappropriately written queries should be used to educate the coding staff on a properly written query. Patterns of inappropriately written queries should be referred to the corporate compliance officer.

Prepared by Sue Prophet, RHIA, CCS

Acknowledgments

AHIMA Advocacy and Policy Task Force
AHIMA's Coding Practice Team
AHIMA Coding Policy and Strategy Committee
AHIMA Society for Clinical Coding
Dan Rode, MBA, FHFMA

Notes

1. Joint Commission on Accreditation of Healthcare Organizations. *Comprehensive Accreditation Manual for Hospitals: The Official Handbook.* Oakbrook Terrace, IL: Joint Commission, 2000.

2. Health Care Financing Administration, Department of Health and Human Services. "Conditions of Participation for Hospitals." *Code of Federal Regulations*, 2000. 42 CFR, Chapter IV, Part 482.

3. Official ICD-9-CM Guidelines for Coding and Reporting developed and approved by the American Hospital Association, American Health Information Management Association, Health Care Financing Administration, and the National Center for Health Statistics.

4. AHIMA is the professional organization responsible for issuing several credentials in health information management: Registered Health Information Administrator (RHIA), Registered Health Information Technician (RHIT), Certified Coding Specialist (CCS), and Certified Coding Specialist—Physician-based (CCS-P).

5. Office of Inspector General, Department of Health and Human Services. *Compliance Program Guidance for Hospitals.* Washington, DC: Office of Inspector General, 1998.

References

AHIMA Code of Ethics, 1998.
AHIMA Standards of Ethical Coding, 1999.
AHIMA Coding Policy and Strategy Committee. "Practice Brief: Data Quality." *Journal of AHIMA* 67, no. 2 (1996).

Source: Prophet, Sue. "Developing a Physician Query Process (AHIMA Practice Brief)." *Journal of AHIMA* 72, no.9 (2001): 88I–M.

Chapter 15

APC Compliance Strategies

The Office of Inspector General (OIG) provides hospitals with guidance on an effective and working compliance plan to ensure accuracy of coding and documentation requirements. Given the diversity of the hospital industry, there is no single "best" hospital compliance program. The OIG recognizes the complexities of the hospital industry and the differences among hospitals and hospital systems. Some hospital entities are small and may have limited resources to devote to compliance measures; others are affiliated with well-established, large, multifacility organizations with a widely dispersed workforce and significant resources to devote to compliance. The OIG strongly encourages hospitals to identify and focus their compliance efforts on those areas of potential concern or risk that are most relevant to their individual organizations. Compliance measures adopted by a hospital to address identified risk areas should be tailored to fit the unique environment of the organization (including its structure, operations, resources, and prior enforcement experience). In short, the OIG recommends that each hospital adapt the objectives and principles underlying this guidance to its own particular circumstances. For additional information, go to (http://oig.hhs.gov/fraud/docs/complianceguidance/012705HospSupplementalGuidance.pdf)

Compliance programs are especially critical in reimbursement and payment areas, where claims and billing operations are often the object of government scrutiny. This chapter outlines issues and strategies to assist specific hospital departments in the development of effective internal ambulatory payment classification (APC) coding and billing policy and procedure for more timely, accurate, and comprehensive coding and billing data. Included are pointers for patient access (admissions/registration), medical staff, patient financial services, chargemaster team, ancillary departments, the laboratory department, and the health information management (HIM) department.

Patient Access (Admissions/Registration)

Assignment of an APC payment to a service or procedure does not mean that Medicare automatically covers the service or procedure or that it may only be payable when furnished in an outpatient setting. An effective registration process is key to ensuring final payment for services provided to the patient. The registration clerical staff should have access to coverage guidelines during pre-scheduling of outpatient surgeries or tests. Physicians may order a test or surgery with a diagnosis that is not considered medically necessary and can be a denial for payment to the facility. (See the Medicare Coverage Database at www.cms.hhs.gov/mcd/search.asp? for more information.)

Advance Beneficiary Notice (ABN)

The facility should issue an Advance Beneficiary Notice (ABN) to any patient whose services may not covered by Medicare. The patient should be educated about the circumstances, informed that the service that was ordered by the physician may not be covered by Medicare, and given the available options for payment. The CMS Web site states: "The ABN is a notice given to beneficiaries in Original Medicare to convey that Medicare is not likely to provide coverage in a specific case. "Notifiers" include physicians, providers (including institutional providers like outpatient hospitals), practitioners, and suppliers paid under Part B. They must complete the ABN as described below, and deliver the notice to affected beneficiaries or their representative before providing the items or services that are the subject of the notice." (Available online at www.cms.hhs.gov/BNI/02_ABNGABNL.asp.)

The ABN must be verbally reviewed with the beneficiary or his/her representative and any questions that arise during that review must be answered before it is signed. The ABN must be delivered far enough in advance that the beneficiary or representative has time to consider the options and make an informed choice. ABNs are never required in emergency or urgent care situations. Once all blanks are completed and the form is signed, a copy is given to the beneficiary or representative. In all cases, the hospital must retain the original notice on file. (See Figure 15.1 for a CMS sample ABN form.)

Coverage Determinations

Medicare coverage is limited to items and services that are reasonable and necessary for the diagnosis or treatment of an illness or injury (and within the scope of a Medicare benefit category). National coverage determinations (NCDs) are made through an evidence-based process, with opportunities for public participation. In some cases, CMS' own research is supplemented by an outside technology assessment and/or consultation with the Medicare Coverage Advisory Committee (MCAC). In the absence of a national coverage policy, an item or service may be covered at the discretion of the Medicare contractors based on a local coverage determination (LCD).

CMS defers final coverage for most outpatient services to Medicare fiscal intermediaries (FIs), who in turn communicate their coverage requirements to hospitals via local medical review policies (LMRPs) and local coverage determinations (LCDs).

LMRPs are the coverage policies that are developed by the Medicare Insurance Carriers and apply directly to claims made to the Insurance Carrier for Coverage under Medicare. LMRPs outline how local carriers will review claims to ensure that they meet Medicare coverage and coding requirements. They specify under what clinical circumstances a service is covered and correctly coded. An LMRP includes a description of the service, specific procedure codes, and for each of these procedures, a list of covered and noncovered diagnostic codes.

LMRPs are issued separately for types of medical services, including psychiatry and psychological services, so hundreds of LMRPs are in existence for each local carrier. In general, carriers have wide freedom to determine coverage; the only restriction is that their policies not directly conflict with a National Coverage Decision issued by CMS on the same issue. For more information visit www.cms.hhs.gov/DeterminationProcess.

Many hospitals are experiencing numerous denials for medically unnecessary ancillary tests. (See Figure15.2 for a sample LMRP.)

Figure 15.1. CMS sample ABN form

(A) **Notifier(s):**
(B) **Patient Name:** _____   *(C)* **Identification Number:** _____

ADVANCE BENEFICIARY NOTICE OF NONCOVERAGE (ABN)

<u>*NOTE:*</u> If Medicare doesn't pay for *(D)*_____ below, you may have to pay.

Medicare does not pay for everything, even some care that you or your health care provider have good reason to think you need. We expect Medicare may not pay for the *(D)*_____ below.

*(D)*_____	*(E)* **Reason Medicare May Not Pay:**	*(F)* **Estimated Cost:**

WHAT YOU NEED TO DO NOW:

- Read this notice, so you can make an informed decision about your care.
- Ask us any questions that you may have after you finish reading.
- Choose an option below about whether to receive the *(D)*_____ listed above.
  Note: If you choose Option 1 or 2, we may help you to use any other insurance that you might have, but Medicare cannot require us to do this.

(G) OPTIONS: **Check only one box. We cannot choose a box for you.**

❑ **OPTION 1.** I want the *(D)*_____ listed above. You may ask to be paid now, but I also want Medicare billed for an official decision on payment, which is sent to me on a Medicare Summary Notice (MSN). I understand that if Medicare doesn't pay, I am responsible for payment, but **I can appeal to Medicare** by following the directions on the MSN. If Medicare does pay, you will refund any payments I made to you, less co-pays or deductibles.

❑ **OPTION 2.** I want the *(D)*_____ listed above, but do not bill Medicare. You may ask to be paid now as I am responsible for payment. **I cannot appeal if Medicare is not billed.**

❑ **OPTION 3.** I don't want the *(D)*_____ listed above. I understand with this choice I am **not** responsible for payment, and **I cannot appeal to see if Medicare would pay.**

(H) Additional Information:

This notice gives our opinion, not an official Medicare decision. If you have other questions on this notice or Medicare billing, call **1-800-MEDICARE** (1-800-633-4227/**TTY**: 1-877-486-2048).

Signing below means that you have received and understand this notice. You also receive a copy.

(I) **Signature:**	*(J)* **Date:**

According to the Paperwork Reduction Act of 1995, no persons are required to respond to a collection of information unless it displays a valid OMB control number. The valid OMB control number for this information collection is 0938-0566. The time required to complete this information collection is estimated to average 7 minutes per response, including the time to review instructions, search existing data resources, gather the data needed, and complete and review the information collection. If you have comments concerning the accuracy of the time estimate or suggestions for improving this form, please write to: CMS, 7500 Security Boulevard, Attn: PRA Reports Clearance Officer, Baltimore, Maryland 21244-1850.

Form CMS-R-131 (03/08)   Form Approved OMB No. 0938-0566

Figure 15.1.   Sample LMRP

Diagnostic mammography codes 76090 and 76091 are paid under APCs. Below are the criteria used by one Medicare fiscal intermediary in the Southeast for a diagnostic mammography.

CRITERIA: ICD-9-CM CODES FOR DIAGNOSTIC MAMMOGRAPHY

(76090, 76091) THAT SUPPORT MEDICAL NECESSITY

Code	Description
174.0	Cancer of breast, nipple and areola
174.1	Cancer of breast, central position
174.2	Cancer of breast, upper-inner quadrant
174.3	Cancer of breast, lower-inner quadrant
174.4	Cancer of breast, upper-outer quadrant
174.5	Cancer of breast, lower-outer quadrant
174.6	Cancer of breast, axillary tail
174.8	Cancer of breast, other specified sites of female breast
175.0	Cancer of male breast, nipple and areola
175.9	Cancer of male breast, other and unspecified sites
198.2	Secondary malignant neoplasm of skin of breast
198.81	Secondary malignant neoplasm of breast
217	Benign neoplasm of breast
233.0	Carcinoma in situ of breast
238.3	Neoplasm of uncertain behavior
610.0	Solitary cyst of breast
610.1	Diffuse cystic mastopathy
610.2	Fibroadenosis of breast
610.3	Fibrosclerosis of breast
610.4	Mammary duct ectasis
610.8	Other specific benign mammary dysplasias
611.0	Inflammatory disease of breast
611.1	Hypertrophy of breast
611.2	Fissure of nipple
611.3	Fat necrosis of breast
611.4	Atrophy of breast
611.5	Galactocele
611.6	Galactorrhea not associated w/ childbirth
611.71	Mastodynia
611.72	Lump or mass in breast
611.79	Other
611.8	Other specified disorders of breast
793.8	Nonspecific abnormal findings on radiological and other examination of breast
879.0	Open wound of breast, w/o mention of complication
879.1	Open wound of breast, complicated
996.54	Mechanical complicated due to breast prosthesis
V10.3	Personal history of malignant neoplasm, breast
V15.89	Personal history of benign breast disease
V 71.1	Observation for suspected malignant lesion

Manual Medical Necessity Validation

Medicare FI outpatient denial information should be kept in a database for monitoring. This database can allow the hospital's compliance team to track, monitor, and report denials. The database should identify:

- Reasons for denial
- Type of test
- Service type (emergency department, outpatient lab, radiology, rehabilitation, same-day surgery, and so on)

- ICD-9-CM diagnosis codes used
- Dollars denied

Analysis of why the denials have occurred can help prevent similar denials in the future. For example, the database may reveal that coders were not coding the reason the physicians ordered chest x-rays or EKGs and that the coders were not used to looking at the medical necessity for ordering tests on emergency department records.

Members of the compliance team should meet with the appropriate physicians to provide educational sessions on better documentation for supporting medical necessity.

Creation of a Medicare compliance criteria book can assist coding professionals in reviewing criteria on each ancillary test. The book also can be provided to HIM, physician offices, ancillary departments, and patient financial services as a reference.

Automated Medical Necessity Validation

Some hospitals have developed or purchased software that contains the medical necessity criteria for various ancillary tests based on the LMRPs and/or LCDs of the hospital's Medicare FI. When a patient is registered for an outpatient service, hospital staff members such as registrars enter the narrative description or code assignment for the reason for the visit and the ordered services or procedures. The software checks its database of medical necessity guidelines to determine coverage criteria for the procedure.

Medical Staff

Specific services or procedures may be reimbursable only in an inpatient setting, and the facility claim will be denied if incorrectly coded. Medicare does not deny payment for physicians' services when an inpatient-only procedure is performed in the hospital outpatient setting; however, it will deny the outpatient facility claim submitted by the hospital. The Medicare inpatient-only list is not binding on Medicare HMO/Medicare Plus Choice plans when within the network. For out-of-area payment, the inpatient-only list does apply. The inpatient-only list does not apply to Medicaid programs.

The medical staff should be provided a current electronic copy of the Medicare inpatient-only list. The list also should be distributed to the office managers of the medical staff for their reference prior to calling the hospital to schedule a Medicare patient for outpatient surgery. The inpatient-only list is usually addendum E to the OPPS Final Rule for each fiscal year and can be found on the CMS Web site at www.cms.hhs.gov/HospitalOutpatientPPS/HORD/itemdetail.asp?.

Medicare updates the inpatient-only list as frequently as every quarter. Providing updates to the medical staff will ensure that additions to, and deletions from, the list will be distributed to the office managers for their reference prior to calling the hospital to schedule a Medicare patient for outpatient surgery.

Patient Financial Services

Each Medicare FI applies more than sixty Medicare outpatient code editor (OCE) edits to all hospital outpatient claims subject to the APC system. Medicare outpatient claims can be verified for the OCE edits by using specialized software or by contracting with an electronic claims-processing clearinghouse prior to submission to the FI.

To validate the required units of service, a random sample of outpatient records should be audited on a regular basis to verify that the number of units reported on each UB-04 line item complies with Medicare's definitions and that the units are supported by the medical documentation.

The sample should include UB-04 claim forms and medical records for Medicare outpatients representing various outpatient types. The record sample should consistently represent all outpatient types, such as:

- Series/recurring patients
- Ambulatory/day surgery
- Emergency department
- Ancillary referrals
- Outpatient

Chargemaster Team

Under APCs, duplicate reporting of a procedure or service may generate additional APC payments that the hospital is not entitled to and/or expose the hospital to compliance violations. OCE software can identify cases that trigger OCE edits specifically designed to detect erroneous duplication of CPT/HCPCS codes and over reporting of units of service.

It may be helpful to form a chargemaster duplication workgroup. Such a group should:

- Consist of representatives from finance, patient accounts, and HIM, including at least one outpatient coder and outpatient biller
- Review a current printout of the chargemaster with a primary sort by CPT/HCPCS code numbers in ascending order
- Identify CPT/HCPCS codes that should be reported by HIM coding specialists due to the documentation review requirements and code assignment options that exist for specific outpatient procedures
- Formally document in an administrative policy the specific outpatient procedures that will be coded by HIM and not reported via the chargemaster
- Re-review a printout of the chargemaster on a quarterly basis after the designated staff member conducts the quarterly chargemaster update protocols

Ancillary Departments

Modifier –52 is used to indicate procedure order change or cancellation. Per the April 7, 2000, *Federal Register*, "Modifier –52 (Reduced Services) would be used to indicate a procedure that did not require anesthesia (local, regional, general), but was terminated after the patient has been prepared for the procedure, including sedation when provided and taken to the room where the procedure is to be performed."

Many radiology and other diagnostic services provided by hospitals do not require anesthesia. In addition, many of these services are reported via the chargemaster. Medicare guidelines require hospitals to assign a code that classifies the extent of the procedure that was performed before it was terminated, assuming that a codeable procedure was in fact completed. If no code exists for the completed procedure, hospitals are to report the originally intended procedure code with modifier –52.

It may be necessary to develop, and educate the appropriate staff on, the policy and procedure for reporting reduced-service procedures. The policy should indicate whether the original orders should be canceled and whether limited or reduced procedures should be reordered. "Orders" in this sense pertains to the charge submitted via the chargemaster.

Laboratory Department

Modifier –91, Repeat Clinical Diagnostic Laboratory Test, was established to indicate that a test was performed more than once on the same day for the same patient only when it is necessary to obtain multiple results in the course of treatment. Modifier –91 *may only be used* for laboratory tests paid under the clinical diagnostic laboratory fee schedule; it *may not be used when*:

- Tests are rerun to confirm initial results due to testing problems with specimens or equipment, or for any other reason when a normal, one-time, reportable result is all that is required.
- Standard HCPCS codes are available that describe the series of results (for example, glucose tolerance tests or evocative/suppression testing).

Modifier –59, Distinct Procedural Service, can be used when two procedures are reported that are not normally reported together. Microbiology CPT codes 87001–87999 require the use of modifier –59 for multiple specimens or sites. The CPT codebook also specifies: "If additional studies involve molecular probes, chromatography, or immunologic techniques, these should be separately coded in addition to definitive identification codes (87140–87158)."

Modifier –91 should be used to report repeat laboratory tests performed on the same day. Additional recommendations for laboratory coding accuracy are as follows:

- The current Medicare Clinical Diagnostic Laboratory Fee Schedule should be obtained.
- The appropriate laboratory staff members should review the fee schedule to identify clinical diagnostic lab tests that are likely to be repeated on the hospital's Medicare outpatients.

It is valuable to establish a charge code that will trigger a repeat clinical lab test CPT code with modifier –91 appended when a clinical diagnostic lab test is repeated on the same day for the same outpatient. For example, if a Medicare outpatient has two bacterial blood cultures performed on the same date of service, the UB-04 data would appear as follows:

42 REV.CD.	43 DESCRIPTION	44 HCPCS/RATES	45 SERV.DATE	46 SERV.UNITS	47 TOTAL CHARGES
306	LAB	87040	032620XX	1	75.00
306	LAB	8704091	032620XX	1	75.00

Only one unit should be reported for each clinical diagnostic lab test line item on the UB-04 claim form.

Carefully review the modifier –59 and–91 guidelines for reporting laboratory tests in the Medicare Program Memorandum Carriers/Intermediaries Transmittal No. AB-02-030 (March 2002).

HIM Department

The following subsections discuss compliance tips for the HIM department with regard to outpatient coding reviews and APC coding audits.

Outpatient Coding Reviews

The Office of Inspector General's *Compliance Program Guidance for Hospitals* recommends "performance of regular, periodic compliance audits by internal or external auditors who have expertise in federal and state health care studies, regulations and federal health care program requirements. ... These audits should be designed to address the hospital's compliance with laws governing kickback arrangements, the physicians self-referral prohibition, CPT/HCPCS, ICD-9-CM coding, claim development and submission, reimbursement, cost reporting and marketing" (HHS 1998).

Following are some suggestions to assist HIM staff in conducting internal audits:

- One or more staff members should perform regular quality reviews on a random sample of all outpatient case types in order to validate the ICD-9-CM, CPT, HCPCS Level II, and modifier coding accuracy.

- Results of the coding quality reviews should be documented: all results and findings, corrective action plans, and follow-up reviews scheduled to correct adverse coding quality.

The technical nature of the CPT coding system can be very challenging for coding specialists—and even more challenging for HIM professionals performing coding compliance and data quality reviews of outpatient medical records. However, based on official resources, HIM professionals can utilize several edits to target, analyze, and support their outpatient coding reviews. These categories are the foundation of an accurate and comprehensive outpatient procedure data quality review.

Specific Coding Guidelines

Many of the audit tips provided below are based on specific guidelines inherent in the code's description, the AMA's CPT coding conventions, or CPT coding guidelines listed in AMA's *CPT Assistant* newsletter.

- Source for code edits: The data quality reviewer should always document the source for each CPT code edit. Sources include specific CPT coding notes or guidelines and guidelines published in *CPT Assistant*.

- Coding analysis recommended action: For each code edit, a recommendation is provided on how the reviewer can analyze the chart or claims data to determine if the edit has in fact been violated.

- APC compliance issue: For each code edit, the risk or opportunity under the APC methodology is provided.

APC Coding Compliance Audit Tips

This section provides APC audit tips/CPT coding edits, analyses, and recommended actions based on official guidelines from the AMA, CMS, and/or physician advisors who have performed these procedures.

Adjacent Tissue Transfer or Rearrangement

The CPT code and description for adjacent tissue transfer or rearrangement is 14000, Adjacent tissue transfer or rearrangement, trunk; defect 10 sq cm or less.

Code Edits

Codes in the range 14000–14350 include the excision of a lesion at the site where the adjacent tissue transfer/rearrangement is created.

Recommended Action

Verify that there are no CPT codes for excision of lesion from trunk (code range 11400–11406, 11600–11606) reported with the 14000 code. Reporting the excision of lesion from trunk codes is only appropriate when the lesion is not at the same site where the adjacent tissue transfer/rearrangement is created.

Code Edits Source

The code edits source is the note in the second paragraph above code 14000 in the CPT codebook.

APC Compliance Issues

Adjacent tissue transfer or rearrangement codes in the range 14000–14350 group to a surgical service APC. Prevent the inappropriate generation of an additional APC payment from the surgical service APC groups for codes 11400–11406 and 11600–11606.

Free Skin Graft Site Preparation

The CPT code and description for free skin graft site preparation is in the range 15050–15400, such as 15100, Split graft, trunk, scalp, arms, legs, hands, and/or feet (except multiple digits); 100 sq cm or less, or each one percent of body area of infants and children (except 15050).

Code Edits

An additional code should be reported for the repair of a skin graft donor site that is closed with a skin graft or local flap(s).

Recommended Action

Verify the closure technique performed on the anatomical site that was used as the skin graft donor site.

Code Edits Source

The code edits source is the note in the third paragraph above code 15000 in the CPT codebook.

APC Compliance Issue

Appropriately capture an additional APC group from a surgical service APC group for application of a local flap or graft to the graft donor site.

Eyelid Blepharoplasty

The CPT codes and descriptions for eyelid blepharoplasty are 15820, Blepharoplasty, lower eyelid; 15821, Blepharoplasty, lower eyelid; with extensive herniated fat pad; 15822, Blepharoplasty, upper eyelid; and 15823, Blepharoplasty, upper eyelid; with excessive skin weighting down lid.

Code Edits

For blepharorhytidectomy correction of the disorder blepharochalasis, see codes 15820–15823. Do not assign CPT codes 67900–67924 from the eye and ocular adnexa section to report the repair of blepharochalasis.

Recommended Action

Verify that no CPT code from the 679XX series was reported on the abstract/claim for a diagnosis of blepharochalasis (ICD-9-CM diagnosis code 374.34, acquired, or 743.62, congenital).

Code Edits Source

The source of code edits is the fifth parenthetical note beneath code 67938 in the CPT codebook.

APC Compliance Issue

Appropriately generate a lower-paying surgical service APC for a 1582X code, instead of a higher-paying surgical service APC group, for a 679XX code.

Destruction of Benign or Premalignant Lesions

The codes and descriptions for the destruction of benign or premalignant lesions are 17000, Destruction by any method, including laser, with or without surgical curettement, all benign or premalignant lesions (for example, actinic keratoses) in any location, other than skin tags or cutaneous vascular proliferative lesions, including local anesthesia; first lesion; 17003, second through 14 lesions, each (list separately in addition to code for first lesion); and 17004, 15 or more lesions.

Code Edits

Code 17003 is an add-on code that can only be reported in addition to code 17000. It is not appropriate to report code 17004 in addition to either code 17000 and/or 17003, as 17004 is a stand-alone code reported for the destruction of 15 or more lesions.

Recommended Action

Verify that code 17004 does not appear with either code 17000 or 17003 on the abstract/claim for the same patient during the same encounter.

Code Edits Source

The code edits source is the parenthetical note above code 17004 in the CPT codebook.

APC Compliance Issue

Prevent the inappropriate generation of two surgical service APCs for CPT codes 17000 and 17004 when 15 or more lesions are destroyed. When 15 or more lesions are destroyed and only code 17004 is reported, one surgical service APC will be generated.

Excisional Breast Biopsy via Marker

The CPT code and description for excisional breast biopsy via marker is 19125, Excision of breast lesion identified by preoperative placement of radiological marker; single lesion.

Code Edits

The code edits for excisional breast biopsy via marker include:

- Code 19125 can only be reported if a radiological marker (such as a breast needle wire, intravenous dye, button) was present at the breast site where the lesion was excised.
- When a needle localization wire is the radiological marker placed on the breast, code 19290 also must appear on the abstract/claim to classify the actual placement of the wire. (This edit is applicable to facilities that perform both the surgery and radiology components.)
- When a needle localization wire is the radiological marker placed on the breast, code 77032 also must appear on the abstract/claim for the radiological imaging used during the placement of the wire. (This edit is applicable to facilities that perform both the surgery and radiology components.)

Recommended Action

The following actions are recommended with regard to excisional breast biopsy via marker:

- Verify that a radiological marker was in fact present at the breast excision site.
- When the radiological marker placed on the breast is a needle localization wire, verify that codes 19290 and 77032 are present in addition to code 19125. (This edit is applicable to facilities that perform both the surgery and radiology components.)

Code Edits Source

The source of code edits for excisional biopsy for breast via marker are the descriptions for CPT codes 19125 and 19290 and the parenthetical note beneath code 19291 in the CPT codebook.

APC Compliance Issue

Appropriately generate a surgical service APC for *each* code 19125 and 19290 reported for each lesion that is excised.

Breast Implant Capsulectomy

The CPT code and description for breast implant capsulectomy is 19371, Periprosthetic capsulectomy, breast.

Code Edit

A capsulectomy procedure involves removal of the capsule that has formed around the implant; it includes removal of the breast implant, but not reinsertion of the breast implant or insertion of a new breast implant.

Recommended Action

The following actions are recommended with regard to breast implant capsulectomy:

- Verify that a removal of breast implant code is not reported for a breast that has undergone capsulectomy during the same encounter.
- Verify that a separate code is reported for reinsertion of the breast implant or the insertion of a new breast implant (if performed).

Code Edits Source

The code edits source for breast implant capsulectomy is the August 1996 issue of *CPT Assistant*.

APC Compliance Issues

The following APC compliance issues apply to breast implant capsulectomy:

- Prevent the generation of an additional surgical service APC for removal of breast implant codes 19328 and 19330 because it is included in code 19371.
- Appropriately generate an additional surgical service APC for insertion of a new breast implant (if performed). This would most likely be coded as 19380, Revision of reconstructed breast.

Partial Palmar Fasciectomy

The CPT code and description for partial palmar fasciectomy is 26125, Fasciectomy, partial palmar with release of single digit including proximal interphalangeal joint, with or without Z-plasty, other local tissue rearrangement, or skin grafting (includes obtaining graft); each additional digit. (List separately in addition to code for primary procedure.)

Code Edits

Code 26125 is an add-on code that classifies the release of each additional digit after the first digit was released during fasciectomy. This code must appear on an abstract/claim along with code 26123, which classifies the release of the first digit.

Recommended Action

The following actions are recommended with regard to partial palmar fasciectomy:

- Verify that code 26125 appears along with 26123 on an abstract/claim.
- Verify that code 26125 is reported for each digit that was released (after the first digit). (For example, if three digits are released, codes 26123 and 26125 x 2 should appear.) Please note that "F" finger modifiers would be required to distinguish the fingers involved in this surgery.

Code Edits Source

The source of code edits for partial palmar fasciectomy is found in the parenthetical note beneath code 26123 in the CPT codebook.

APC Compliance Issue

Appropriately generate a surgical service APC for *each* digit released after the first digit.

Hernia Mesh Insertion

The CPT code and description for hernia mesh insertion is 49568, Implantation of mesh or other prosthesis for incisional hernia repair. (List separately in addition to code for the incisional hernia repair.)

Code Edits

Code 49568, which classifies the insertion of mesh or other prosthesis during incisional hernia repair, is an add-on code that can only be reported with incisional hernia repair code 49560 or 49561.

Recommended Action

Verify that code 49568 is reported with either 49560 or 49561 on an abstract/claim.

Code Edits Source

The code edits source for hernia mesh insertion are in the descriptions for CPT codes 49560, 49561, and 49568.

APC Compliance Issue

Appropriately generate an additional surgical service APC for the application of the mesh (code 49568).

Endoscopic Biopsy with Lesion Removal

The CPT codes and descriptions for endoscopic biopsy with lesion removal include, for example, 45380, Colonoscopy, flexible, proximal to splenic flexure; with biopsy, single or multiple; and 45385, Colonoscopy, flexible, proximal to splenic flexure; with removal of tumor(s), polyp(s), or other lesion(s) by snare technique.

Code Edits

When the same lesion is biopsied and subsequently removed during the same operative session, report only the code for removal of the lesion. When one lesion is biopsied and a separate lesion is removed during the same operative session, it would be appropriate to report a code for the biopsy of one lesion and an additional code for removal of the separate lesion. When one lesion is biopsied and a separate lesion is removed, it would be appropriate to append modifier –59 to the code reported for the biopsy procedure.

For example, if a patient has a colonoscopy with biopsy of a descending colon polyp and snare removal of a transverse colon polyp, the cases would be coded as follows: 45380–59 (colonoscopic biopsy, distinct procedural service) and 45385 (colonoscopic snare removal of polyp/lesion).

Recommended Action

The following actions are recommended with regard to endoscopic biopsy with lesion removal:

- Verify that two separate lesions were, in fact, biopsied and removed/destroyed.
- Verify that no existing single CPT code is available to classify both the biopsy and the removal procedures.

Code Edits Source

The source of code edits for endoscopic biopsy with lesion removal is the February 1999 issue of *CPT Assistant*.

APC Compliance Issue

Prevent inappropriate payment and ensure appropriate payment for an additional surgical service APC. The APC group and payment depend on the anatomical site of the biopsy and lesion removal procedures.

Urinary Catheterization

The CPT code and description for urinary catheterization is 52005, Cystourethroscopy, with ureteral catheterization, with or without irrigation, instillation, or ureteropyelography, exclusive of radiologic service.

Code Edits

Code 52005 classifies cystoscopic ureteral catheterization, which is also included in the descriptions for codes 52320–52330, 52352, and 52353. Code 52005 should not be reported in addition to codes 52320–52330, 52352, and 52353.

Recommended Action

Verify that code 52005 does not appear when any of the following codes appear on a claim for the same date of service: 52320–52330, 52352, and 52353. These codes have "including ureteral catheterization" or "ureteral catheterization is included" in their descriptions.

Code Edits Source

Sources of code edits for urinary catheterization include the descriptions for CPT codes 52005, 52320–52330, 52352, and 52353.

APC Compliance Issue

Prevent inappropriate generation of an additional surgical service APC for code 52005 when another code that includes ureteral catheterization is being reported.

Urinary Stent Placement

The CPT code and description for urinary stent placement is 52332, Cystourethroscopy, with insertion of indwelling ureteral stent (for example, Gibbons or double-J type).

Code Edits

Code 52332 can only be reported when a self-retaining ureteral stent is left inside the patient at the conclusion of the cystourethroscopic procedure. Further, it can only be reported for indwelling ureteral stents, not stents placed temporarily during the urology procedure and removed prior to completion.

Recommended Action

Verify that the ureteral stent was in a self-retaining stent that was left indwelling inside the patient at the conclusion of the urology procedure.

Code Edits Source

The source of code edits for urinary stent placement is the note in the second paragraph above code 52320 in the CPT codebook.

APC Compliance Issue

Prevent inappropriate generation of a surgical service APC when a stent is not left indwelling.

Hydrocelectomy

The CPT codes and descriptions for hydrocelectomy are 55040, Excision of hydrocele; unilateral; 55041, Excision of hydrocele; bilateral; and 55500, Excision of hydrocele of spermatic cord, unilateral (separate procedure).

Code Edits

Hydroceles excised from the tunica vaginalis (codes 55040 or 55041) group to a higher-paying surgical service APC. Hydroceles excised from the spermatic cord (code 55500) group to a lower-paying surgical service.

Recommended Action

Verify the anatomic site from which the hydrocele was excised (this is, tunica vaginalis versus spermatic cord).

Code Edits Source

APC payment rates are published annually by CMS in the *Federal Register*.

APC Compliance Issue

Prevent receipt of a higher-paying surgical service APC when the hydrocele was not excised from the tunica vaginalis. Hydroceles excised from the spermatic cord (code 55500) group to a lower-paying surgical service APC.

Laparoscopic Lysis of Adhesions

The CPT codes and descriptions are 58660, Laparoscopy, surgical; with lysis of adhesions (salpingolysis, ovariolysis) (separate procedure); and 44180, Laparoscopy, surgical; enterolysis (freeing of intestinal adhesion) (separate procedure).

Code Edits

Lysis of adhesions should be reported when the following elements are documented in the medical record: adhesions are multiple or dense, cover the primary operative site, add considerable time to the operative procedure, or increase the risk to the patient.

Recommended Action

The following actions are recommended with regard to laparoscopic lysis of adhesions:

- Verify that the operative report provides documentation of one of the above elements when laparoscopic lysis code(s) is/are reported on the abstract/claim.
- Verify that the adhesions involved the fallopian tube(s) and/or ovary(ies) when reporting code 58660.
- Verify that the adhesions involved the large (colon) or small intestine(s) (duodenum, jejunum, ileum) when reporting code 44180.

Code Edits Source

Sources of code edits for laparoscopic lysis of adhesions are the January 1996 issue of *CPT Assistant* and the descriptions for codes 44180 and 58660.

APC Compliance Issue

Prevent the inappropriate payment for "incidental" adhesiolysis procedures under a surgical service APC.

Endoscopic Surgery

Examples of the CPT codes and descriptions for endoscopic surgery include:

- 49491–49590: Various open repair hernia codes
- 49650: Laparoscopy, surgical; repair initial inguinal hernia
- 49651: Laparoscopy, surgical; repair recurrent inguinal hernia
- 49659: Unlisted laparoscopy procedure, hernioplasty, herniorrhaphy, herniotomy
- 30901–30906: Various open nasal hemorrhage control codes
- 31238: Nasal/sinus endoscopy, surgical; with control of epistaxis
- 64721: Neuroplasty and/or transposition; median nerve at carpal tunnel
- 29848: Endoscopy, wrist, surgical, with release of transverse carpal ligament

Code Edits

A number of procedures group to higher-paying APCs when the procedure is performed via an endoscopic as opposed to an open surgical approach.

Recommended Action

When an endoscopic code is assigned, verify that an endoscopic procedure was, in fact, documented.

Code Edits Source

APC payment rates are published annually by CMS in the *Federal Register*.

APC Compliance Issue

Prevent the generation of higher-paying surgical service APCs when a procedure is not performed through an endoscope. For example:

- Open hernia repair codes 49491–49590 group to higher-paying surgical service APCs than endoscopic hernia repair codes do.

- Open nasal hemorrhage control codes 30901–30906 group to higher-paying surgical service APCs than endoscopic nasal hemorrhage control code 31238 does.

- Open carpal tunnel repair code 64721 groups to a higher-paying surgical service APC than endoscopic carpal tunnel repair code 29848 does.

Coding Pass-Through Devices

The Social Security Act provides for temporary additional payments called transitional pass-through payments for medical devices that meet certain criteria established by CMS. Eligible categories for pass-through payments generally involve innovative, expensive technologies. The device payments are mandated by Congress to ensure that Medicare beneficiaries have access to costly new services and that hospitals are not grossly undercompensated when these services are rendered.

Hospitals receive OPPS payments for both the device and the surgical procedure when the pass-through devices are coded and billed. The payment amount is based on the cost of the device less the amount that is already included in the APC rate associated with the device.

Following is a list of implants that are eligible for pass-through payment under OPPS:

2008 Codes for Pass-Through Devices

CPT/HCPCS	SI	Description	APC
C1821	H	Interspinous implant	1821
C2616	H	Brachytx, non-str, Yttrium-90	2616
C2634	H	Brachytx, non-str, HA, I-125	2634
C2635	H	Brachytx, non-str, HA, P-103	2635
C2636	H	Brachy linear, non-str, P-103	2636
C2638	H	Brachytx, stranded, I-125	2638
C2639	H	Brachytx, non-stranded, I-125	2639
C2640	H	Brachytx, stranded, P-103	2640
C2698	H	Brachytx, stranded, NOS	2698
C1821	H	Interspinous implant	1821
C2616	H	Brachytx, non-str, Yttrium-90	2616
C2634	H	Brachytx, non-str, HA, I-125	2634

APC pass-through data are published annually by CMS in the Federal Register. Specific manufacturer brands and models of implants have been approved by CMS, and a manufacturer's label may be affixed in the medical record for some implants.

The coding professional should verify the correct coding and billing of implants based on documentation in the health record and the presence of the implant on the list of eligible devices for pass-through payment under APCs.

Exhibit 15. 1. NCD edits

Coding Guidelines for All NCD Edits

1. Any claim for a clinical diagnostic laboratory service must be submitted with an ICD-9-CM diagnosis code. Codes that describe symptoms and signs, as opposed to diagnosis, should be provided for reporting purposes when a diagnosis has not been established by the physician. (Based on Coding Clinic for ICD-9-CM, Fourth Quarter 1995, page 43).

2. Screening is the testing for disease or disease precursors so that early detection and treatment can be provided for those who test positive for the disease. Screening tests are performed when no specific sign, symptom, or diagnosis is present and the patient has not been exposed to a disease. The testing of a person to rule out or to confirm a suspected diagnosis because the patient has a sign and/or symptom is a diagnostic test, not a screening. In these cases, the sign or symptom should be used to explain the reason for the test. When the reason for performing a test is because the patient has had contact with, or exposure to, a communicable disease, the appropriate code from category V01, Contact with or exposure to communicable diseases, should be assigned, not a screening code, but the test may still be considered screening and not covered by Medicare. For screening tests, the appropriate ICD-9-CM screening code from categories V28 or V73-V82 (or comparable narrative) should be used. (From Coding Clinic for ICD-9-CM, Fourth Quarter 1996, pages 50 and 52).

3. A three-digit code is to be used only if it is not further subdivided. Where fourth-digit and/or fifth-digit sub-classifications are provided, they must be assigned. A code is invalid if it has not been coded to the full number of digits required for that code. (From Coding Clinic for ICD-9-CM. Fourth Quarter, 1995, page 44).

4. Diagnoses documented as "probable," "suspected," "questionable," "rule-out," or "working diagnosis" should not be coded as though they exist. Rather, code the condition(s) to the highest degree of certainty for that encounter/visit, such as signs, symptoms, abnormal test results, exposure to communicable disease or other reasons for the visit. (From Coding Clinic for ICD-9-CM, Fourth Quarter 1995, page 45).

5. When a non-specific ICD-9 code is submitted, the underlying sign, symptom, or condition must be related to the indications for the test.

Exhibit 15. 1.   (Continued)

Additional Coding Guidelines

190.12 – Urine Culture, Bacterial

1. Specific coding guidelines:

    a. Use CPT 87086 Culture, bacterial, urine; quantitative, colony count where a urine culture colony count is performed to determine the approximate number of bacteria present per milliliter of urine. The number of units of service is determined by the number of specimens.

    b. Use CPT 87088 where a commercial kit uses manufacturer defined media for isolation, presumptive identification, and quantitation of morphotypes present. The number of units of service is determined by the number of specimens.

    c. Use CPT 87088 where identification of morphotypes recovered by quantitative culture or commercial kits and deemed to represent significant bacteriuria requires the use of additional testing, for example, biochemical test procedures on colonies. Identification based solely on visual observation of the primary media is usually not adequate to justify use of this code. The number of units of service is determined by the number of isolates.

    d. Use CPT 87184 or 87186 where susceptibility testing of isolates deemed to be significant is performed concurrently with identification. The number of units of service is determined by the number of isolates. These codes are not exclusively used for urine cultures but are appropriate for isolates from other sources as well.

    e. Appropriate combinations are as follows: CPT 87086, 1 per specimen with 87088, 1 per isolate and 87184 or 87186 where appropriate.

    f. Culture for other specific organism groups not ordinarily recovered by media used for aerobic urine culture may require use of additional CPT codes (for example, anaerobes from suprapubic samples).

    g. Identification of isolates by non-routine, nonbiochemical methods may be coded appropriately (for example, immunologic identification of streptococci, nucleic acid techniques for identification of N. gonorrhoeae).

    h. While infrequently used, sensitivity studies by methods other than CPT 87184 or 87186 are appropriate. CPT 87181, agar dilution method, each antibiotic or CPT 87188, macrotube dilution method, each antibiotic may be used. The number of units of service is the number of antibiotics multiplied by the number of unique isolates.

2. ICD-9-CM code 780.02, 780.9 or 799.3 should be used only in the situation of an elderly patient, immunocompromised patient or patient with neurologic disorder who presents without typical manifestations of a urinary tract infection but who presents with one of the following signs or symptoms, not otherwise explained by another co-existing condition: increasing debility; declining functional status; acute mental changes; changes in awareness; or hypothermia.

3. In cases of post renal-transplant urine culture used to detect clinically significant occult infection in patients on long term immunosuppressive therapy, use code V58.69.

Exhibit 15. 1. (Continued)

190.13 – Human Immunodeficiency Virus (HIV) Testing (Prognosis Including Monitoring)

1. Specific coding guidelines:

    a. Temporary code G0100 has been superseded by code 87536 effective January 1, 1998.

    b. CPT codes for quantification should not be used simultaneously with other nucleic acid detection codes for HIV-1 (that is, 87534, 87535) or HIV-2 (that is, 87537, 87538).

2. Codes 647.60-647.64 should only be used for HIV infections complicating pregnancy.

190.14 - Human Immunodeficiency Virus (HIV) Testing (Diagnosis)

1. Specific coding guidelines:

    a. CPT 86701 or 86703 is performed initially. CPT 86702 is performed when 86701 is negative and clinical suspicion of HIV-2 exists.

    b. CPT 86689 is performed only on samples repeatedly positive by 86701, 86702, or 86703.

    c. CPT 87534 or 87535 is used to detect HIV-1 RNA where indicated. CPT 87537 or 87538 is used to detect HIV-2 RNA where indicated.

190.16 – Partial Thromboplastin Time (PTT)

1. When patients are being converted from heparin therapy to warfarin therapy, use code V58.61 to document the medical necessity of the PTT.

2. When coding for Disseminated Intravascular Coagulation (DIC), use 286.6 or code for the signs and symptoms clinically indicating DIC.

3. If a specific condition is known and is the reason for a pre-operative test, submit the clinical text description or ICD-9-CM code describing the condition with the order/referral. If a specific condition or disease is not known, and the pre-operative test is for pre-operative clearance only, assign code V72.84.

4. Assign codes 289.8 – other specified disease of blood and blood-forming organs only when a specific disease exists and is indexed to 289.8, (for example, myelofibrosis). Do not assign code 289.8 to report a patient on long term use of anticoagulant therapy (for example, to report a PTT value or re-check need for medication adjustment.) Assign code V58.61 to referrals for PTT checks or re-checks. (Reference AHA's Coding Clinic, March-April, pg 12 – 1987, 2nd quarter pg 8 – 1989)

190.17 – Prothrombin Time (PT)

1. If a specific condition is known and is the reason for a pre-operative test, submit the text description or ICD-9-CM code describing the condition with the order/referral. If a specific condition or disease is not known, and the pre-operative test is for pre-operative clearance only, assign code V72.84.

2. Assign codes 289.8 – other specified disease of blood and blood-forming organs only when a specific disease exists and is indexed to 289.8 (for example, myelofibrosis). Do not assign code 289.8 to report a patient on long term use of anticoagulant therapy

Exhibit 15. 1. (Continued)

(e.g. to report a PT value or re-check need for medication adjustment.) Assign code V58.61 to referrals for PT checks or re-checks. (Reference AHA's Coding Clinic, March-April, pg 12 – 1987, 2nd quarter pg 8 – 1989)

190.19 – Collagen Crosslinks, Any Method

1. When the indication for the test is long-term administration of glucocorticosteroids, use ICD-9-CM code V58.69.

190.20 – Blood Glucose Testing

1. A diagnostic statement of impaired glucose tolerance must be evaluated in the context of the documentation in the medical record in order to assign the most accurate ICD-9-CM code. An abnormally elevated fasting blood glucose level in the absence of the diagnosis of diabetes is classified to Code 790.6 - other abnormal blood chemistry. If the provider bases the diagnostic statement of impaired glucose tolerance" on an abnormal glucose tolerance test, the condition is classified to 790.2 -- normal glucose tolerance test. Both conditions are considered indications for ordering glycated hemoglobin or glycated protein testing in the absence of the diagnosis of diabetes mellitus.

2. When a patient is under treatment for a condition for which the tests in this policy are applicable, the ICD-9-CM code that best describes the condition is most frequently listed as the reason for the test.

3. When laboratory testing is done solely to monitor response to medication, the most accurate ICD-9-CM code to describe the reason for the test would be V58.69 -- long term use of medication.

4. Periodic follow-up for encounters for laboratory testing for a patient with a prior history of a disease, who is no longer under treatment for the condition, would be coded with an appropriate code from the V67 category -- follow-up examination.

5. According to ICD-9-CM coding conventions, codes that appear in italics in the Alphabetic and/or Tabular columns of ICD-9-CM are considered manifestation codes that require the underlying condition to be coded and sequenced ahead of the manifestation. For example, the diagnostic statement, "thyrotoxic exophthalmos (376.21)," which appears in italics in the tabular listing, requires that the thyroid disorder (242.0-242.9) is coded and sequenced ahead of thyrotoxic exophthalmos. Therefore, a diagnostic statement that is listed as a manifestation in ICD-9-CM must be expanded to include the underlying disease in order to accurately code the condition.

190.21 – Glycated Hemoglobin/Glycated Protein

1. A diagnostic statement of impaired glucose tolerance must be evaluated in the context of the documentation in the medical record in order to assign the most accurate ICD-9-CM code. An abnormally elevated fasting blood glucose level in the absence of the diagnosis of diabetes is classified to Code 790.6 - other abnormal blood chemistry. If the provider bases the diagnostic statement of impaired glucose tolerance" on an abnormal glucose tolerance test, the condition is classified to 790.2 -- normal glucose tolerance test. Both conditions are considered indications for ordering glycated hemoglobin or glycated protein testing in the absence of the diagnosis of diabetes mellitus.

Exhibit 15. 1. (Continued)

190.22 – Thyroid Testing

1. When a patient is under treatment for a condition for which the tests in this policy are applicable, the ICD-9-CM code that best describes the condition is most frequently listed as the reason for the test.

2. When laboratory testing is done solely to monitor response to medication, the most accurate ICD-9-CM code to describe the reason for the test would be V58.69 - long term use of medication.

3. Periodic follow-up for encounters for laboratory testing for a patient with a prior history of a disease, who is no longer under treatment for the condition, would be coded with an appropriate code from the V67 category -- follow-up examination.

4. According to ICD-9-CM coding conventions, codes that appear in italics in the Alphabetic and/or Tabular columns of ICD-9-CM are considered manifestation codes that require the underlying condition to be coded and sequenced ahead of the manifestation. For example, the diagnostic statement "thyrotoxic exophthalmos (376.21)," which appears in italics in the tabular listing, requires that the thyroid disorder (242.0-242.9) is coded and sequenced ahead of thyrotoxic exophthalmos. Therefore, a diagnostic statement that is listed as a manifestation in ICD-9-CM must be expanded to include the underlying disease in order to accurately code the condition.

5. Use code 728.9 to report muscle weakness as the indication for the test. Other diagnoses included in 728.9 do not support medical necessity.

6. Use code 194.8 (Malignant neoplasm of other endocrine glands and related structures, Other) to report multiple endocrine neoplasia syndromes (MEN-1 and MEN-2). Other diagnoses included in 194.8 do not support medical necessity.

190.26 – Carcinoembryonic Antigen

1. To show elevated CEA, use ICD-9-CM 790.99 (Other nonspecific findings on examination of blood) only if a more specific diagnosis has not been made. If a more specific diagnosis has been made, use the code for that diagnosis.

190.31 – Prostate Specific Antigen

1. To show elevated PSA, use ICD-9-CM code 790.93 (Elevated prostate specific antigen). If a more specific diagnosis code has been made, use the code for that diagnosis.

References and Bibliography

AHIMA. 2008. Analysis of Final Rule for 2008 Revisions to the Medicare Hospital Outpatient Prospective Payment System. Available online at www.ahima.org/dc/documents/MicrosoftWord-OP-PPSanalysis_CY08.pdf.

AHIMA. 2003 (July 2). Managing and improving data quality (updated). AHIMA Practice Brief. *Journal of American Health Information Management Association* 74(7): 64A-C.

American Academy of Head and Neck Surgery. 2007. *Middle Turbinate 2-Concha Bullosa.* Alexandra, VA.

American Medical Association. 1994a (fall). *CPT Assistant.* Chicago: American Medical Association.

American Medical Association. 1994b (spring). *CPT Assistant.* p. 3. Chicago: American Medical Association.

American Medical Association. 1995 (fall). *CPT Assistant.* Chicago: American Medical Association.

American Medical Association. 1996b (January). *CPT Assistant.* Chicago: American Medical Association.

American Medical Association. 1996a (March). *CPT Assistant.* Chicago: American Medical Association.

American Medical Association. 1996d (May). *CPT Assistant.* Chicago: American Medical Association.

American Medical Association. 1996c (August). *CPT Assistant.* Chicago: American Medical Association.

American Medical Association. 1997a (January). *CPT Assistant.* Chicago: American Medical Association.

American Medical Association. 1997c (November). *CPT Assistant.* Chicago: American Medical Association.

American Medical Association. 1997b (November 13–14). CPT 1998 Coding Symposium (handout). Chicago: American Medical Association.

American Medical Association. 1998a (February). *CPT Assistant.* Chicago: American Medical Association.

American Medical Association. 1998b (December). *CPT Assistant.* p. 10. Chicago: American Medical Association.

American Medical Association. 1999e (February). *CPT Assistant.* Chicago: American Medical Association.

American Medical Association. 1999b (June). *CPT Assistant.* Chicago: American Medical Association.

American Medical Association. 1999a (July). *CPT Assistant.* Chicago: American Medical Association.

American Medical Association. 1999d (November). *CPT Assistant.* Chicago: American Medical Association.

American Medical Association. 1999c. *CPT Changes 2000: An Insider's View.* Chicago: American Medical Association.

American Medical Association. 2000c (January). *CPT Assistant.* Chicago: American Medical Association.

American Medical Association. 2000e (March). *CPT Assistant.* p. 12. Chicago: American Medical Association..

American Medical Association. 2000b (April). *CPT Assistant.* p. 10. Chicago: American Medical Association.

American Medical Association. 2000d (November). *CPT Assistant.* p. 10. Chicago: American Medical Association.

American Medical Association. 2000a. *CPT Changes 2001: An Insider's View.* Chicago: American Medical Association.

American Medical Association. 2001g (January). *CPT Assistant.* Chicago: American Medical Association.

American Medical Association. 2001h (March). *CPT Assistant.* Chicago: American Medical Association.

American Medical Association. 2001i (April). *CPT Assistant.* Chicago: American Medical Association.

American Medical Association. 2001c (May). *CPT Assistant.* Chicago: American Medical Association.

American Medical Association. 2001d (July). *CPT Assistant.* Chicago: American Medical Association.

American Medical Association. 2001a (August). *CPT Assistant.* Chicago: American Medical Association.

American Medical Association. 2001e (September). *CPT Assistant.* Chicago: American Medical Association.

American Medical Association. 2001b (October). *CPT Assistant.* Chicago: American Medical Association.

American Medical Association. 2001f. *CPT Changes 2002: An Insider's View.* Chicago: American Medical Association.

American Medical Association. 2001j (November). CPT 2002 Coding Symposium (handout). Chicago: American Medical Association.

American Medical Association. 2002c (January). *CPT Assistant.* Chicago: American Medical Association.

American Medical Association. 2002a (February). *CPT Assistant.* Chicago: American Medical Association.

American Medical Association. 2002d (October). *CPT Assistant.* Chicago: American Medical Association.

American Medical Association. 2002b (December). *CPT Assistant.* Chicago: American Medical Association.

American Medical Association. 2002e. *CPT Changes 2003: An Insider's View.* Chicago: American Medical Association.

American Medical Association. 2002f (November 14-15). CPT 2003 Coding Symposium (handout). Chicago: American Medical Association.

American Medical Association. 2002g (November). *CPT Assistant.* Chicago: American Medical Association.

American Medical Association. 2003c (April). *CPT Assistant.* Chicago: American Medical Association.

American Medical Association. 2003a (May). *CPT Assistant.* Chicago: American Medical Association.

American Medical Association. 2003f (June). *CPT Assistant.* Chicago: American Medical Association.

American Medical Association. 2003g (July). *CPT Assistant.* Chicago: American Medical Association.

American Medical Association. 2003e (September). *CPT Assistant.* Chicago: American Medical Association.

American Medical Association. 2003b (October). *CPT Assistant.* Chicago: American Medical Association.

American Medical Association. 2003h (November). *CPT Assistant.* Chicago: American Medical Association.

American Medical Association. 2003d. *CPT Changes 2004: An Insider's View.* Chicago: American Medical Association.

American Medical Association. 2003j. *2004 Current Procedural Terminology.* Chicago: American Medical Association.

American Medical Association. 2003i (September 5). *CPT Information Services letter.* Chicago: American Medical Association.

American Medical Association. 2004. *CPT 2005*. Chicago: American Medical Association, p. 1.

American Medical Association. 2004a (January). *CPT Assistant*. Chicago: American Medical Association.

American Medical Association. 2004b (May). *CPT Assistant*. Chicago: American Medical Association.

American Medical Association. 2004c (September). *CPT Assistant*. Chicago: American Medical Association

American Medical Association 2007a. *CPT 2007*. Chicago: American Medical Association.

American Medical Association. 2007b. *CPT Changes 2007: An Insider's View*. Chicago: American Medical Association.

American Medical Association. 2007c. *CPT 2007 Professional Edition*. Chicago: American Medical Association.

American Medical Association. 2008. *CPT 2008*. Chicago: American Medical Association.

Centers for Medicare and Medicaid Services (n.d.). *Medicare Hospital Manual*. Section 442.7. Available online at (http://www.cms.hhs.gov/Manuals/PBM/itemdetail.asp?filterType=none&filterByDID=-99&sortByDID=1&sortOrder=ascending&itemID=CMS021912

Centers for Medicare and Medicaid Services, Regional Office VI. 1999. *CMS Regional PRO Letter No. 91-18*. Dallas, TX: Centers for Medicare and Medicaid Services.

Centers for Medicare and Medicaid Services, Department of Health and Human Services. 2000 (August 17). Medicare Program; Standards for Electronic Transactions and Code Sets. *Federal Register* 65 (50312).

Centers for Medicare and Medicaid Services, Department of Health and Human Services. 2002 (May 31). Medicare Program; Health Insurance Reform: Modifications to Electronic Data Transaction Standards and Code Sets. Proposed Rule. *Federal Register* 45 (173). Available online at: http://www.cms.hhs.gov/TransactionCodeSetsStands/Downloads/ModificationstoElectronicDataTransactionStandardsandCodeSets.pdf.

Centers for Medicare and Medicaid Services, Department of Health and Human Services. 2002 (November 1). Medicare Program; Changes to the Hospital Outpatient Prospective Payment System and Calendar Year 2003 Payment Rates; Final Rule. *Federal Register* 67:(148).

Centers for Medicare and Medicaid Services. 2003 (January 3). Medicare Program Memorandum Intermediaries, Transmittal A-02-129. Available on-line at http://www.cms.gov/manuals/pm_trans/A02129.pdf.

Centers for Medicare and Medicaid Services. 2003 (April 2). CMS Program Memorandum A-03-020.

Centers for Medicare and Medicaid Services. 2003 (August 1). Medicare Program Memorandum Carriers/Intermediaries, Transmittal AB-03-114.

Centers for Medicare and Medicaid Services. 2003 (August 8). Medicare Program Memorandum Intermediaries, Transmittal No. A-03-066, Hospital Outpatient Prospective Payment System (OOPS) Implementation Instructions.

Centers for Medicare and Medicaid Services, Department of Health and Human Services. 2003 (November 7). Medicare Program; Changes to the Hospital Outpatient Prospective Payment System and Calendar Year 2004 Payment Rates; Final Rule. *Federal Register* 68(216).

Centers for Medicare and Medicaid Services. 2003 (December 19). CMS Manual System, Pub. 100-20 One-Time Notification, Transmittal No. 32.

Centers for Medicare and Medicaid Services. 2003 (December 22). CMS Manual System, Pub. 100-04 Medicare Claims Processing, Transmittal No. 53.

Centers for Medicare and Medicaid Services, Department of Health and Human Services. 2004 (January 6). Medicare Program; Hospital Outpatient Prospective Payment Reform for Calendar Year 2004. *Federal Register* 69(3).

Centers for Medicare and Medicaid Services. 2004. *Hospital Manual* . Chapter 2, Section 210 and Section 230.1, Baltimore: Centers for Medicare and Medicaid Services.

Centers for Medicare and Medicaid Services. 2006 (December 22). Medicare Program Memorandum Intermediaries, Transmittal 1139. Available online at http://www.cms.gov/manuals/pm_trans/ R1139CP.pdf.

Centers for Medicare and Medicaid Services. 2007 (November 27). Final Changes to the Hospital Outpatient Prospective Payment System and CY 2008 Payment Rates. Available online at http://www.cms.hhs.gov/HospitalOutpatientPPS/HORD/list.asp#TopOfPage.

Centers for Medicare and Medicaid Services, Department of Health and Human Services. 2007 (November 27). Medicare Program; Final Rule Regarding Composite APCs, Year 2008. *Federal Register* 72 (227).

Centers for Medicare and Medicaid Services. 2008 (March). Beneficiary Notices Initiative (BNI). Available online at http://www.cms.hhs.gov/BNI/02_ABNGABNL.asp.

Health Care Financing Administration, Department of Health and Human Services. 1998 (September 8). Medicare Program; Prospective Payment System for Hospital Outpatient Services; Proposed Rules. *Federal Register* 63(173).

Health Care Financing Administration, Department of Health and Human Services. 2000 (April 7). Medicare Program Prospective Payment System for Hospital Outpatient Services; Final Rule. *Federal Register* 65(68).

Jones, Lolita M. 2002. *Modifier Clinic: A Guide to Hospital Outpatient Issues.* Marblehead, MA: HCPro.

Jones, Lolita M. 2004. *ASC Clinic: Multi-Specialty Procedures.* Fort Washington, MD: Lolita M. Jones Consulting Services.

Jones, Lolita M., and Deborah J. Thgoman. 2001 (August 9). Coding for APCs. AHIMA audioconference.

Merck Manual Medical Library: *The Merck Manual of Diagnosis,* Online version of *Merck Manual of Diagnosis and Therapy.* Available online at: www.merck.com/mmpe/index.html.

NCCI. 2007. National Correct Coding Policy Manual, Hospital APC Version 13.0, Effective April 1, 2007. *Chapter VI Surgery: Digestive System* CPT Codes 40000–49999 (NCCI 12.3), Washington, DC.

NCCI. 2007. National Correct Coding Policy Manual, Hospital APC Version 13.0, Effective April 1, 2007. *Chapter VII Surgery: Urinary, Male Genital, Female Genital, Maternity Care and Delivery Systems* CPT Codes 50000–59999 (NCCI 12.3), Washington, DC.

New York Eye and Ear Infirmary. 2008. Dept. of Otolaryngology. Caldwell-Lue Procedure. Available online at www.NYEE.edu.

Office of the *Federal Register.* 2004. *APC Payment Rates Published Annually by CMS.* Washington, DC: National Archives and Records Administration.

Office of Inspector General. 1998. *Compliance Program Guidance for Hospitals.* Washington, DC: Office of Inspector General.

Office of Inspector General. 2005. *OIG Supplemental Compliance Program Guidance for Hospitals.* Washington, DC: Office of Inspector General. Available online at http://oig.hhs.gov/fraud/docs/complianceguidance/012705HospSupplementalGuidance.pdf.

Schaefer, Steven D. 2007. *Caldwell-Luc Procedure-Definition.* New York, NY: The New York Eye and Ear Infirmary.

Appendix A

Glossary and Acronyms

Glossary

Ambulatory patient group (APG): A classification system used until 2000 to categorize ambulatory patients according to case types as a pricing mechanism for outpatient services provided to Medicare and Medicaid beneficiaries

Ambulatory payment classification (APC) system: The prospective payment system used since 2000 for reimbursement of hospitals for outpatient services provided to Medicare and Medicaid beneficiaries

Ambulatory surgical center (ASC): Under Medicare, an outpatient surgical facility that has its own national identifier; is a separate entity with respect to its licensure, accreditation, governance, professional supervision, administrative functions, clinical services, record keeping, and financial and accounting systems; has as its sole purpose the provision of services in connection with surgical procedures that do not require inpatient hospitalization; and meets the conditions and requirements set forth in the Medicare Conditions of Participation

Ancillary services: Tests and procedures ordered by a physician to provide information for use in patient diagnosis or treatment

APC relative weight: A number that reflects the expected resource consumption for cases associated with each APC, relative to the average of all APCs, that is used in determining payment

Balanced Budget Act (BBA) of 1997: Public Law 105-33, enacted by Congress on August 5, 1997, that mandated a number of additions, deletions, and revisions to the original Medicare and Medicaid legislation; the legislation that added penalties for healthcare fraud and abuse to the Medicare and Medicaid programs

Budget neutral/neutrality: Financial protections to ensure that overall reimbursement under the APC system is not greater than it would have been had the APC system not been in effect

Centers for Medicare and Medicaid Services (CMS): The division of the Department of Health and Human Services that is responsible for developing healthcare policy in the United States and for administering the Medicare program and the federal portion of the Medicaid program; called the Health Care Financing Administration (HCFA) prior to 2001

Compliance plan: A process that helps an organization, such as a hospital, to accomplish its goal of providing high-quality medical care and efficiently operating a business under various laws and regulations

Conversion factor: A monetary multiplier that converts relative value units into payments

Current Procedural Terminology (CPT): A comprehensive, descriptive list of terms and numeric codes used for reporting diagnostic and therapeutic procedures and other medical services performed by physicians; published and updated annually by the American Medical Association

Encounter: A direct personal contact between a patient and a physician or other person who is authorized by state licensure law and, if applicable, by medical staff bylaws to order or furnish healthcare services for diagnosis or treatment of the patient

Fiscal intermediary (FI): An organization that contracts with the Centers for Medicare and Medicaid Services to serve as the financial agent between providers and the federal government in the local administration of Medicare Part B claims

Freestanding facility: In Medicare terminology, an entity that furnishes healthcare services to beneficiaries and is not integrated with any other entity as a main provider, a department of a provider, or a provider-based entity

Healthcare Common Procedure Coding System (HCPCS): A classification system composed of three levels: I, Current Procedural Terminology codes; II, codes for equipment, supplies, and services not covered by CPT codes, as well as modifiers that can be used with all levels of codes; and III, local codes developed by regional Medicare Part B carriers and used to report physicians' services and supplies to Medicare for reimbursement

Hold harmless: A term used to refer to the financial protections that ensure that cancer hospitals recoup all losses due to the differences in their APC payments and the pre-APC payments for Medicare outpatient services

Information system (IS): An automated system that uses computer hardware and software to record, manipulate, store, recover, and disseminate data (that is, a system that receives and processes input and provides output); often used interchangeably with information technology (IT)

Inpatient: A patient who is provided with room, board, and continuous general nursing services in an area of an acute care facility where patients generally stay at least overnight

International Classification of Diseases, 9th Revision, Clinical Modification (ICD-9-CM): A classification system used in the United States to report morbidity and mortality information

Large urban area: An urban area with a population of more than one million

Local medical review policies (LMRPs): Documents that define Medicare coverage of outpatient services via lists of diagnoses defined as medically reasonable and necessary for the services provided

Low-volume hospital: A hospital with fewer than 5,000 outpatient visits per year

Main provider: A provider that either creates or owns another entity in order to deliver additional healthcare services under its name, ownership, and financial and administrative control

Major teaching hospital: A teaching hospital with 100 or more residents

National Correct Coding Initiative (CCI): A series of code edits on Medicare Part B claims

National Drug Codes (NDC): Codes that serve as product identifiers for human drugs, currently limited to prescription drugs and a few over-the-counter products

Office of the Inspector General (OIG): The office through which the federal government established compliance plans for the healthcare industry

Other urban area: An urban area with a population of one million or fewer

Outlier: A case for which the costs were unusually high for the diagnosis-related group to which the case was assigned; also, an extreme statistical value that falls outside the normal range

Outpatient: A patient who receives ambulatory care services in a hospital-based clinic or department

Outpatient code editor (OCE): A software program linked to the National Correct Coding Initiative that applies a set of logical rules to determine whether various combinations of codes are correct and appropriately represent the services provided

Outpatient prospective payment system (OPPS): The Medicare prospective payment system used for hospital-based outpatient services and procedures and predicated on the assignment of ambulatory payment classifications

Packaging: A payment under the Medicare outpatient prospective payment system that includes items such as anesthesia, supplies, certain drugs, and the use of recovery and observation rooms

Payment status indicator (PSI): An alphabetic code assigned to CPT/HCPCS codes to indicate whether a service or procedure is to be reimbursed under the Medicare OPPS

Provider-based entity: A provider of healthcare services, a rural health clinic, or a federally-qualified health clinic, as defined in section 405–2401 of the *Code of Federal Regulations*, that is either created or acquired by a main provider for the purpose of furnishing healthcare services under the name, ownership, and administrative and financial control of the main provider, in accordance with the provisions of the proposed rule

Provider-based status: The relationship between a main provider and a provider-based entity or a department of a provider that complies with the provisions of the final rule on ambulatory payment classifications

Quality improvement organization (QIO): The organization that performs medical peer review of Medicare and Medicaid claims, including review of validity of hospital diagnosis and procedure coding information; completeness, adequacy, and quality of care; and appropriateness of prospective payments for outlier cases and nonemergent use of the emergency room; formerly known as peer review organizations, or PROs

Rebasing: The redetermination of the APC weights to reflect changes in relative resource consumption

Recalibration: The adjustment of all APC weights to reflect changes in relative resource consumption

Risk corridor: Limits established to prevent immediate large financial gains or losses for hospitals because of implementation of a prospective payment system

Significant procedure APC: A procedure that constitutes the reason for the visit and dominates the time and resources rendered during the visit; and that is not subject to payment reduction/discounting

Small rural hospital: A hospital with fewer than 100 beds that is located outside a medical savings account plan

Social Security Act (SSA): The 1935 federal legislation that originally established the Social Security program, as well as unemployment compensation and support for mothers and children; amended in 1965 to create the Medicare and Medicaid programs

Trauma hospitals: Hospitals with level-one trauma centers

UB-04: A Medicare form for standardized uniform billing; also called CMS-1450 (like its predecessor UB-92)

Acronyms

APC:	Ambulatory payment classification
APG:	Ambulatory patient group
ASC:	Ambulatory surgical center
AWP:	Average wholesale price
BBA:	Balanced Budget Act of 1997
BBRA 1999:	Balanced Budget Refinement Act of 1999
CAH:	Critical access hospital
CAT:	Computerized axial tomography
CCI:	[CMS] Correct Coding Initiative
CCR:	Cost center–specific cost-to-charge ratio
CCU:	Coronary care unit
CDM:	Charge description master
CHAMPUS:	Civilian Health and Medical Program of the Uniformed Services
CMHC:	Community mental health center

CMP:	Civil money penalty
CMS:	Centers for Medicare & Medicaid Services
CORF:	Comprehensive outpatient rehabilitation facility
CPI:	Consumer Price Index
CPT:	[Physicians'] Current Procedural Terminology, copyrighted by the American Medical Association
DME:	Durable medical equipment
DMEPOS:	DME, prosthetics, prosthetic devices, prosthetic implants and supplies
DRG:	Diagnosis-related group
EACH:	Essential access community hospital
EBAA:	Eye Bank Association of America
ED:	Emergency department
EDI:	Electronic data interchange
EMS:	Emergency medical services
EMTALA:	Emergency Medical Treatment and Active Labor Act
ENT:	Ear/Nose/Throat
ESRD:	End-stage renal disease
FDO:	Formula-driven overpayment
FI:	Medicare Fiscal Intermediaries
FQHC:	Federally qualified health center
HCPCS:	Healthcare Common Procedure Coding System
HHA:	Home health agency
HHS:	Department of Health and Human Services
HIM:	Health information management
HIPAA:	Health Insurance Portability and Accountability Act of 1996
HOP QDRP:	Hospital Outpatient Quality Data Reporting Program
HQA:	Hospital Quality Alliance
ICD-9-CM:	International Classification of Diseases, Ninth Edition, Clinical Modification
ICU:	Intensive care unit
IHS:	Indian Health Service
IME:	Indirect medical education
IOL:	Interlobular lens
IPPS:	Inpatient prospective payment system
LTH:	Long-term hospital

LMRPs:	Local medical review policies
MAC:	Medicare Administrative Contractors
MDC:	Major diagnostic category
MDH:	Medicare-dependent hospital
MedPAC:	Medicare Payment Advisory Commission
MEDPAR:	Medicare Provider Analysis and Review
MRI:	Magnetic resonance imaging
MSA:	Metropolitan statistical area
NCDs:	National coverage decisions
NDC:	National drug codes
NECMA:	New England County Metropolitan Area
NPI:	National Provider Identifier
NQF:	National Quality Forum
NUBC:	National Uniform Billing Committee
OBRA:	Omnibus Budget Reconciliation Act
OIG:	Office of the Inspector General
OT:	Occupational therapy
PFS:	Patient financial services
PPO:	Preferred provider organization
PPS:	Prospective payment system
RFA:	Regulatory Flexibility Act
RHC:	Rural health clinic
RHQDAPU:	Reporting Hospital Quality Data for Annual Payment Update
RPCH:	Rural primary care hospital
RRC:	Rural referral center
SCH:	Sole community hospital
SGR:	Sustainable growth rate
SI:	Status indicator
SNF:	Skilled nursing facility
TEFRA:	Tax Equity and Fiscal Responsibility Act of 1982
TPA:	Tissue Plasminogen Activator

Appendix B

Answer Key

Case Study 3.1

1. What is the morphology of *each* lesion (for example, benign, premalignant, malignant)?
   All three lesions were benign; they were lipomas.

2. What are the dimensions of *each* lesion *plus* the margin (if known)?
   3.5 cm—right greater trochanter
   3 cm—right anterior thigh
   2.5 cm—left anterior thigh

3. What is the anatomical site of *each* lesion?
   Right greater trochanter
   Right anterior thigh
   Left anterior thigh

4. What surgical technique was used to remove *each* lesion?
   a. Excision
   b. Shaving
   c. Destruction (indicate the method of destruction)
   d. Mohs' micrographic surgery (chemosurgery)

5. What surgical technique was used to close *each* lesion defect site?
   a. Adhesive strip application
   b. Chemical or electrocauterization
   c. Simple repair
   d. Layer closure
   e. Complex repair
   f. Adjacent tissue transfer/rearrangement
   g. Split-thickness skin graft
   h. Full-thickness skin graft

6. CPT surgery code(s) and modifier(s): **11403, 11403–59, 11404**

Case Study 3.2

1. What is the morphology of *each* lesion (for example, benign, premalignant, malignant)?
   The lesion was benign; it was an epidermal inclusion cyst.

2. What are the dimensions of *each* lesion *plus* the margin (if known)?
   3 cm x 1.5 cm x 1.0 cm (We code based on the largest side, which is 3 cm.)

3. What is the anatomical site of *each* lesion?
   Posterior neck

4. What surgical technique was used to remove *each* lesion?
   a. Excision
   b. Shaving
   c. Destruction (indicate the method of destruction)
   d. Mohs' micrographic surgery (chemosurgery)

5. What surgical technique was used to close *each* lesion defect site?
   a. Adhesive strip application
   b. Chemical or electrocauterization
   c. Simple repair
   d. Layer closure
   e. Complex repair
   f. Adjacent tissue transfer/rearrangement
   g. Split-thickness skin graft
   h. Full-thickness skin graft

6. CPT surgery code(s) and modifier(s): **11423 and 12042**

Case Study 3.3

1. What is the morphology of *each* lesion (for example, benign, premalignant, malignant)?
   The lesion has benign components (solar elastosis) and malignant components (infiltrating well-differentiated keratinizing squamous cell carinoma).

2. What are the dimensions of *each* lesion *plus* the margin (if known)?
   2 cm

3. What is the anatomical site of *each* lesion?
   Tip of nose

4. What surgical technique was used to remove *each* lesion?
   a. Excision
   b. Shaving
   c. Destruction (indicate the method of destruction)
   d. Mohs' micrographic surgery (chemosurgery)

5. What surgical technique was used to close *each* lesion defect site?
   a. Adhesive strip application
   b. Chemical or electrocauterization
   c. Simple repair
   d. Layer closure
   e. Complex repair
   f. Adjacent tissue transfer/rearrangement
   g. Split-thickness skin graft
   h. Full-thickness skin graft

6. CPT surgery code(s) and modifier(s): **11442 and 12051**

Case Study 3.4

1. What are the dimensions of *each* wound?
   1.5 cm

2. What are the anatomical sites of *each* wound?
   Right thumb

3. What surgical method was used to repair *each* wound?
   a. Adhesive strip application in combination with other material or as a sole material
   b. Chemical or electrocauterization
   c. Debridement
   d. Simple repair
   e. Layer closure
   f. Complex repair
   g. **Secondary wound repair**
   h. Blood vessel, tendon, nerve repair
   i. Ligation and/or exploration of vessels
   j. Adjacent tissue transfer/rearrangement
   k. Split-thickness skin graft
   l. Full-thickness skin graft

4. CPT surgery code(s) and modifier(s): **13160**

Case Study 3.5

1. What type of skin graft was applied?
   Split-thickness

2. What was the anatomical site for the donor skin graft?
   Left upper thigh

3. What surgical technique was used to repair the donor site?
   The donor area was dressed.

4. What was the size (in square centimeters) of the defect site (recipient) on which the graft was applied?
   6 x 15 cm (90 sq cm)

5. On what anatomical site (recipient) was the graft applied?
   Left forearm

6. CPT surgery code(s) and modifier(s): **15002 and 15100**

Case Study 3.6

1. What type of skin graft was applied?
   Split-thickness skin graft

2. What was the anatomical site for the donor skin graft?
   Anterior and anterolateral left thigh

3. What surgical technique was used to repair the donor site?
   None. The donor site was covered with Xeroform gauze, 4 x 4s, and ABDs.

4. What was the size (in square centimeters) of the defect site (recipient) on which the graft was applied?
   15 cm x 15 cm = 225 sq cm

5. On what anatomical site (recipient) was the graft applied?
   Left axilla

6. CPT surgery code(s) and modifier(s): **15002, 15003 x 2, 15100, 15101 x 2**

Case Study 3.7

1. What type of skin graft was applied?
   Apligraf, which is a bilaminate skin substitute/neodermis.

2. What was the anatomical site for the donor skin graft?
   Because the graft was a skin substitute, there was no donor site.

3. What surgical technique was used to repair the donor site?
   Because the graft was a skin substitute, there was no donor site.

4. What was the size (in square centimeters) of the defect site (recipient) on which the graft was applied?
   Approximately 40 to 45 sq cm

5. On what anatomical site (recipient) was the graft applied?
   Left dorsal foot and left medial foot

6. CPT surgery code(s) and modifier(s): **15004 (for the dorsal foot wound debridement), 15004 (for the medial foot wound debridement), 15175 (for the Apligraf)**

Case Study 3.8

1. Was the biopsy unilateral or bilateral?
   a. Unilateral
   b. Bilateral

2. How many biopsies were performed on the breast(s)?
   One biopsy

3. Was imaging guidance used?
   Yes. Stereotactic imaging was used.

4. Was a radiological marker(s) used?
   a. Yes
   b. No

5. What type of biopsy(ies) was performed?
   a. Catheter lavage of mammary duct (specify number of ducts)
   b. Open
   c. Percutaneous needle core
   d. Percutaneous automated vacuum-assisted biopsy
   e. Percutaneous rotating biopsy device
   f. Excisional (specify number of lesions excised per breast)
   g. Microwave phased array thermotherapy

6. Was a surgical clip placed?
   a. Yes
   b. No

7. CPT surgery code(s) and modifier(s): **19103–RT and 19295–RT**

Case Study 3.9

1. Was the procedure unilateral or bilateral?
   a. Unilateral
   b. Bilateral

2. What type of breast excision was performed?
   a. Open excision of malignant breast tumor
   b. Partial mastectomy
   c. Subcutaneous mastectomy

3. What type of lymph node dissection was performed?
   a. Superficial needle biopsy of axillary lymph nodes
   b. Open biopsy of deep axillary lymph nodes

4. Which of the following correctly classifies this case?
   a. 19302–RT
   b. 38525
   c. 19301–RT
   d. 19301–RT and 38525

Explanation: Per the operative report, after the partial mastectomy site was closed, a new incision was made to biopsy the axillary lymph nodes.

Case Study 3.10

1. The patient had bilateral augmentation performed a number of years ago.
   a. True
   b. False

2. Which of the following procedures was performed?
   a. Removal of right intact mammary implant
   b. Removal of left intact mammary implant
   c. Removal of right mammary implant material
   d. Removal of left mammary implant material

3. Which of the following procedures was performed?
   a. Bilateral mammaplasty augmentation with prosthetic implants
   b. Bilateral immediate insertion of breast prostheses in reconstruction
   c. Bilateral delayed insertion of breast prostheses in reconstruction

4. CPT surgery code(s) and modifier(s): **19330–RT, 19328–LT, 19325–50**

Case Study 3.11

1. What was the anatomical site of any lesion(s) excised?
   Ear—helical dome

2. What were the dimensions in sq cm of the primary defect (the original defect to be closed)?
   2 cm x 2 cm

3. What was the donor site for the adjacent tissue transfer/rearrangement?
   Superior area from the helical dome

4. What were the dimensions in sq cm of the secondary defect (the defect created by the movement of tissue necessary to close the primary defect)?
   3 x 1.5 cm

5. What type of adjacent tissue transfer/rearrangement was performed?
   a. Advancement flap
   b. V-Y plasty
   c. Y-V plasty
   d. W-plasty
   e. Z-plasty
   f. Rotation flap
   g. Transpositional flap
   h. Sliding flap
   i. Interpolational
   j. Nasolabial flap
   k. Other (specify)

6. What technique was used to close the donor site for the adjacent tissue transfer/rearrangement?
   Advancement flaps

7. CPT surgery code(s) and modifier(s): **14060 and 14060–59**

Case Study 3.12

1. What was the anatomical site of any lesion(s) that is/are excised?
   Right ear

2. What were the dimensions in sq cm of the primary defect (the original defect to be closed)?
   Not documented

3. What was the donor site for the adjacent tissue transfer/rearrangement?
   Anterior-based position of the right ear

4. What were the dimensions in sq cm of the secondary defect (the defect created by the movement of tissue necessary to close the primary defect)?
   5 x 6 cm = 30 sq cm

5. What type of adjacent tissue transfer/rearrangement was performed?
   a.   Advancement flap
   b.   V-Y plasty
   c.   Y-V plasty
   d.   W-plasty
   e.   Z-plasty
   f.   Rotation flap
   g.   Transpositional flap
   h.   Sliding flap
   i.   Interpolational
   j.   Nasolabial flap
   k.   Other (specify)

6. What technique was used to close the donor site for the adjacent tissue transfer/rearrangement?
   This is not documented.

7. CPT surgery code(s) and modifier(s): **14061**

Case Study 3.13

1. What surgical technique was used to remove the basal cell carcinoma, left infra-auricular?
   a.   Excision
   b.   Shaving
   c.   Destruction (indicate the method of destruction)
   d.   Mohs' micrographic surgery (chemosurgery)

2. What surgical technique was used to close the basal cell carcinoma, left infra-auricular defect site?
   a.   Adhesive strip application
   b.   Chemical or electrocauterization
   c.   Simple repair
   d.   Layer closure
   e.   Complex repair
   f.   Adjacent tissue transfer/rearrangement
   g.   Split-thickness skin graft
   h.   Full-thickness skin graft

3. What surgical technique was used to remove the preauricular lesion?
   a.   Excision
   b.   Shaving
   c.   Destruction (indicate the method of destruction)
   d.   Moh's micrographic surgery (chemosurgery)

4. What surgical technique was used to close the preauricular lesion defect site?
   a.   Adhesive strip application
   b.   Chemical or electrocauterization
   c.   Simple repair
   d.   Layer closure
   e.   Complex repair
   f.   Adjacent tissue transfer/rearrangement
   g.   Split-thickness skin graft
   h.   Full-thickness skin graft
   i.   No closure

5. CPT surgery code(s) and modifier(s): **14060, 11311–59**

Case Study 4.1

1. What was the reason for the injection(s)?
   a. Therapeutic
   b. Prophylactic
   c. Diagnostic

2. What was the anatomical site of the injection?
   a. Single trigger point in one muscle
   b. Multiple trigger points in one muscle
   c. Multiple trigger points in multiple muscles

3. What substance(s) was/were injected?
   a. Anesthetic
   b. Chemotherapy
   c. Steroid

4. What dosage of medication/pharmaceutical substance was injected?
   1 cc of 2% Lidocaine

5. CPT surgery code(s) and modifier(s): **20553**

Case Study 4.2

1. What was the patient's diagnosis?
   Nondisplaced and minor impacted fracture of the distal radius

2. What was the anatomical site of the disorder?
   Distal radius

3. What type of treatment was provided?
   a. Application of cast and/or strapping for stabilization or comfort
   b. Restorative treatment: Application of cast and/or strapping
   c. Restorative treatment: Closed manipulation/reduction
   d. Restorative treatment: Open reduction
   e. Restorative treatment: Internal fixation
   f. Restorative treatment: Percutaneous skeletal fixation
   g. Restorative treatment: Skin or skeletal traction
   h. Restorative treatment: External fixation
   i. Restorative treatment: Soft tissue repair

4. What discharge instructions were provided to the patient?
   a. To follow up with this physician
   b. To follow up with another physician for removal of cast/strapping
   c. To follow up with another physician for orthopedic consultation
   d. To follow up with another physician for restorative treatment
   e. To follow up with another physician for other reason (specify)
   f. None of the above

5. CPT surgery code(s) and modifier(s): **25600–LT**

Case Study 4.3

1. What was the patient's diagnosis?
   Colles fracture of the left wrist

2. What was the anatomical site of the disorder?
   Left wrist

3. What type of treatment was provided?
   a. Application of cast and/or strapping for stabilization or comfort
   b. Restorative treatment: Application of cast and/or strapping
   c. Restorative treatment: Closed manipulation/reduction
   d. Restorative treatment: Open reduction
   e. Restorative treatment: Internal fixation
   f. Restorative treatment: Percutaneous skeletal fixation
   g. Restorative treatment: Skin or skeletal traction
   h. Restorative treatment: External fixation
   i. Restorative treatment: Soft tissue repair

4. What discharge instructions were provided to the patient?
   a. To follow up with this physician
   b. To follow up with another physician for removal of cast/strapping
   c. To follow up with another physician for orthopedic consultation
   d. To follow up with another physician for restorative treatment
   e. To follow up with another physician for other reason (specify)
   f. None of the above

5. CPT surgery code(s) and modifier(s): **29105–LT**

Case Study 4.4

1. What was the anatomic site of the fracture or dislocation?
   Left great toe proximal phalanx fracture, interarticular

2. Was the treatment open or closed?
   Closed

3. Was manipulation (reduction) involved?
   Yes

4. Was traction applied?
   No

5. Was percutaneous skeletal fixation applied?
   Yes

6. Was internal fixation applied?
   No

7. Was an external fixation system applied?
   No

8. Was soft-tissue closure performed?
   No

9. CPT surgery code(s) and modifier(s): **28496–LT**

Case Study 4.5

1. What was the anatomic site of the fracture or dislocation?
   Articular fracture, middle phalanx, right middle finger, with involvement of the proximal interphalangeal joint

2. Was the treatment open or closed?
   Open

3. Was manipulation (reduction) involved?
   Yes

4. Was traction applied?
   No

5. Was percutaneous skeletal fixation applied?
   No

6. Was internal fixation applied?
   No

7. Was an external fixation system applied?
   No

8. Was soft-tissue closure performed?
   No

9. CPT surgery code(s) and modifier(s): **26746–F7**

Case Study 4.6

1. What was the diagnosis for the right fourth and fifth toes?
   Hammertoe

2. Where was the patient's bunion located?
   a. Right great toe
   b. Left great toe
   c. Right fifth metatarsal
   d. Left fifth metatarsal

3. Which procedure was performed on the fifth metatarsal?
   a. Ostectomy, complete excision
   b. Ostectomy, partial excision
   c. Metatarsectomy

4. Which of the following techniques was used to repair the right fourth and right fifth digits?
   a. Partial phalangectomy
   b. Interphalangeal fusion
   c. Total phalangectomy

5. CPT surgery code(s) and modifier(s): **28285–T8, 28285–T9, 28110–RT**

Case Study 4.7

1. What procedure was performed on the toe?
   a. Amputation of metatarsal with toe
   b. Amputation toe, metatarsophalangeal joint
   c. Amputation toe, interphalangeal joint

2. On which toe was the procedure performed? **Left second toe**

3. CPT surgery code(s) and modifier(s): **28820–T1**

Case Study 4.8

1. Which of the following procedures was performed?
   a. Hallux valgus correction with resection of joint and insertion of implant
   b. Subtalar arthrodesis
   c. Arthrodesis great toe, interphalangeal joint
   d. Arthrodesis great toe, metatarsophalangeal joint

2. CPT surgery code(s) and modifier(s): **28750–RT**

Case Study 4.9

1. Was the hallux valgus/bunion deformity unilateral or bilateral?
   Bilateral

2. What bunion repair technique was used?
   Silver bunionectomy

3. CPT surgery code(s) and modifier(s): **28290–50**

Case Study 4.10

1. Was the hallux valgus/bunion deformity unilateral or bilateral?
   Unilateral

2. What bunion repair technique was used?
   Resection of joint with implant

3. CPT surgery code(s) and modifier(s): **28293–RT**

Case Study 4.11

1. Which of the following techniques was used to repair the right second hammertoe?
   a. Partial phalangectomy
   b. Interphalangeal fusion
   c. Total phalangectomy

2. Which of the following techniques was used to repair the right second metatarsophalangeal joint contracture?
   a. Capsulotomy
   b. Capsulotomy with tendon lengthening

3. What bunion repair technique was used?
   Chevron osteotomy

4. CPT surgery code(s) and modifier(s): **28285–T6, 28270–T6–59, 28296–RT**

Case Study 4.12

1. The patellar bone graft was harvested to repair which condition?
   a. Left anterior cruciate ligament disruption
   b. Lateral posterior horn meniscal tear

2. Which technique was used to repair the lateral compartment posterior horn tear?
   a. Open meniscectomy
   b. Arthroscopic meniscectomy
   c. Arthroscopic meniscal repair
   d. Open meniscal repair

3. Which of the following procedures were performed to correct the left anterior cruciate ligament disruption?
   a. Notchplasty
   b. Use of the drill to chamfer out the tibia hole
   c. Placement of the patellar bone plug graft
   d. All of the above

4. CPT surgery code(s) and modifier(s): **29888–LT, 29882–LT**

Case Study 4.13

1. Which technique was used to repair the meniscal tear?
   a. Arthroscopic medial meniscectomy
   b. Arthroscopic lateral meniscectomy
   c. Arthroscopic medial and lateral meniscectomy

2. In which of the following compartments of the knee was the chondromalacia debridement performed?
   a. Suprapatellar pouch
   b. Intercondylar pouch
   c. Medial compartment
   d. Lateral compartment

3. CPT surgery code(s) and modifier(s): **29881–RT, 29877–59–RT**

Case Study 4.14

1. What procedures were performed on the eburnated subchondral bone?
   a. Arthroscopic microfracture
   b. Arthroscopic abrasion arthroplasty
   c. Arthroscopic chondroplasty

2. From which compartments of the knee was synovium removed?
   a. Suprapatellar pouch
   b. Intercondylar pouch
   c. Medial compartment
   d. Lateral compartment

3. Which technique was used to repair the meniscal tear?
   a. Arthroscopic medial meniscectomy
   b. Arthroscopic lateral meniscectomy
   c. Arthroscopic medial and lateral meniscectomy

4. What procedure was performed for post-op pain control?
   a. Intra-articular/joint injection of medication
   b. Peripheral nerve injection of medication

5. CPT surgery code(s) and modifier(s): **29879, 29880, 29876, 20610**

Case Study 4.15

1. Which of the following techniques was used to repair the SLAP lesion?
   a. Arthroscopic distal clavicle excision
   b. Arthroscopic excision of subacromial bursa
   c. Arthroscopic placement of a suture anchor on the anterior superior glenoid rim

2. Arthroscopic subacromial decompression is supported by which of the following operative report excerpts?
   a. "...subacromial space was entered."
   b. "...excised enough of the subacromial bursa."
   c. "...removing inferior AC joint ligaments."
   d. "...removed the osteophyte. . . acromion."
   e. All of the above

3. Which of the following procedures was performed on the clavicle?
   a. Open total claviculectomy
   b. Open partial claviculectomy
   c. Arthroscopic distal claviculectomy

4. CPT surgery code(s) and modifier(s): **29807–RT, 29826–RT, 29824–RT**

Case Study 4.16

1. The removal of the distal clavicle is also called a:
   a. Mumford procedure
   b. SLAP repair
   c. Bankhart repair

2. The massive rotator cuff tear involved which of the following muscles and tendons?
   a. Supraspinatus
   b. Infraspinatus
   c. Teres minor
   d. All of the above

3. What procedure was performed on the biceps tendon?
   a. Tenodesis
   b. Resection
   c. Transplantation

4. Code 23420 includes an acromioplasty.
   a. True
   b. False

5. CPT surgery code(s) and modifier(s): **23120–RT, 23420–RT, 23430–59–RT**

Case Study 4.17

1. The patient had an anterior shoulder dislocation.
   a. True
   b. False

2. Which of the following codes classifies the procedure performed?
   a. 23450 Capsulorrhaphy, anterior; Putti-Platt procedure or Magnuson type operation
   b. 23455 Capsulorrhaphy, anterior; with labral repair (for example, Bankart procedure)

Case Study 4.18

1. Which of the following procedures was performed?
   a. Percutaneous palmar fasciotomy
   b. Open partial palmar fasciotomy
   c. Palm-only fasciectomy
   d. Partial palmar fasciectomy with release of single digit
   e. Partial palmar fasciectomy with release of multiple digits

2. Which digits were released?
   a. Right thumb
   b. Right middle finger
   c. Right ring finger

3. CPT surgery code(s) and modifier(s): **26123–F5, 26125–F7**

Case Study 4.19

1. The trapezium is a:
   a. Carpal bone
   b. Metacarpal bone
   c. Phalanx

2. The flexor carpi radialis tendon was harvested from which site?
   a. Wrist
   b. Hand
   c. Proximal forearm

3. The operative report states: "The tendon was then passed up through this hole and folded down on itself." What type of arthroplasty is this?
   a. Interposition
   b. Intermission

4. CPT surgery code(s) and modifier(s): **25447–RT, 25310–RT**

Case Study 4.20

1. Which joint was repaired in the little finger?
   a. Proximal interphalangeal (PIP) joint
   b. Distal interphalangeal (DIP) joint

2. Which of the following procedures was performed?
   a. Arthrodesis interphalangeal joint with autograft
   b. Arthrodesis interphalangeal joint with internal fixation
   c. Arthrodesis interphalangeal joint without internal fixation

3. CPT surgery code(s) and modifier(s): **26862–F4**

Case Study 5.1

1. What was the disease process for *each* turbinate?
   Hypertrophy of the bilateral inferior turbinates

2. What type of procedure was performed on *each* turbinate?
   a. Excision
   b. Submucous resection
   c. Superficial cauterization/ablation
   d. Intramural cauterization/ablation
   e. Therapeutic fracture
   f. Reduction

3. Was each turbinate procedure unilateral or bilateral?
   a. Unilateral
   b. Bilateral

4. What was the surgical approach used for the turbinate surgery?
   a. Open
   b. Endoscopic

5. CPT surgery code(s) and modifier(s): **30140–50**

Case Study 5.2

1. What type of bronchoscopy was performed?
   a. Diagnostic
   b. Therapeutic

2. What was the laterality of *each* therapeutic procedure performed?
   Unilateral: Endobronchial biopsy
   Bilateral: Bronchoalveolar lavage (BAL)

3. Identify *each* therapeutic procedure performed.
   a. Brushing
   b. Protected brushing
   c. Bronchial alveolar lavage (BAL)
   d. Biopsy
   e. Dilation, tracheal or bronchial
   f. Closed reduction of fracture
   g. Tracheal stent placement
   h. Foreign body removal
   i. Tumor excision
   j. Tumor destruction
   k. Stenosis relief using other than excision (for example, laser therapy, cryotherapy)
   l. Catheter(s) placement for intracavitary radioelement application
   m. Initial aspiration of tracehobronchial tree
   n. Subsequent aspiration of tracheobronchial tree
   o. Contrast injection for segmental bronchography

4. Identify each biopsy technique performed.
   a. Bronchial/endobronchial biopsy
   b. Transbronchial lung biopsy (specify *each* lobe)
   c. Transbronchial needle aspiration biopsy (specify *each* lobe)

5. CPT surgery code(s) and modifier(s): **31624–50, 31625**

Case Study 5.3

1. Was the laryngoscope rigid or flexible fiberoptic?
   Flexible (because an operating microscope was attached to it)

2. Was the laryngoscopy indirect or direct?
   Direct

3. What type of anesthesia was administered?
   General

4. Was an operating microscope used?
   Yes

5. CPT surgery code(s) and modifier(s): **31541 and 31571**

Case Study 5.4

1. What procedure was performed to correct the deviated septum?
   a. Primary rhinoplasty
   b. Septal dermatoplasty
   c. Septoplasty

2. What type of bilateral sphenoidotomy was performed?
   a. Endoscopic sphenoidotomy
   b. Endoscopic sphenoidotomy with removal of tissue from the sphenoid sinus

3. What type of bilateral ethmoidectomy was performed?
   a. Open partial (anterior only)
   b. Open total (anterior and posterior)
   c. Endoscopic partial (anterior only)
   d. Endoscopic total (anterior and posterior)

4. Endoscopic frontal sinus exploration with removal of tissue from frontal sinus was performed?
   a. Unilaterally
   b. Bilaterally

5. CPT surgery code(s) and modifier(s): **30520, 31288–50, 31255–80, 31276–50**

Case Study 5.5

1. What procedure was performed to correct the deviated septum?
   a. Primary rhinoplasty
   b. Septal dermatoplasty
   c. Septoplasty

2. What type of bilateral ethmoidectomy was performed?
   a. Open partial (anterior only)
   b. Open total (anterior and posterior)
   c. Endoscopic partial (anterior only)
   d. Endoscopic total (anterior and posterior)

3. What type of bilateral maxillary antrostomy was performed?
   a. Endoscopic maxillary antrostomy
   b. Endoscopic maxillary antrostomy with removal of tissue from the maxillary sinus
   c. Open maxillary antrostomy

4. CPT surgery code(s) and modifier(s): **30520, 31254–50, 31256–50**

Case Study 5.6

1. What type of ethmoidectomy was performed?
   a. Endoscopic unilateral partial (anterior only)
   b. Endoscopic unilateral total (anterior and posterior)
   c. Endoscopic bilateral partial (anterior only)
   d. Endoscopic bilateral total (anterior and posterior)

2. What type of maxillary antrostomy was performed?
   a. Endoscopic unilateral maxillary antrostomy
   b. Endoscopic unilateral maxillary antrostomy with removal of tissue from the maxillary sinus
   c. Endoscopic bilateral maxillary antrostomy
   d. Endoscopic bilateral maxillary antrostomy with removal of tissue from the maxillary sinus

3. How was the endoscopic frontal sinus surgery performed?
   a. Unilaterally
   b. Bilaterally

4. CPT surgery code(s) and modifier(s): **31276–50, 31255–50, 31256–50**

Case Study 5.7

1. The ENT Trak image-guided system is a stereotactic computer-assisted volumetric device.
   a. True
   b. False

2. What type of maxillary antrostomy was performed?
   a. Endoscopic unilateral maxillary antrostomy
   b. Endoscopic unilateral maxillary antrostomy with removal of tissue from the maxillary sinus
   c. Endoscopic bilateral maxillary antrostomy
   d. Endoscopic bilateral maxillary antrostomy with removal of tissue from the maxillary sinus

3. What type of ethmoidectomy was performed?
   a. Endoscopic unilateral partial (anterior only)
   b. Endoscopic unilateral total (anterior and posterior)
   c. Endoscopic bilateral partial (anterior only)
   d. Endoscopic bilateral total (anterior and posterior)

4. Endoscopic frontal sinus surgery was performed?
   a. Unilaterally
   b. Bilaterally

5. CPT surgery code(s) and modifier(s): **31267–RT, 31276–RT, 31254–RT, 61795**

Case Study 5.8

1. Which of the following correctly classifies the procedure performed?
   a. Code 30400, Rhinoplasty, primary; lateral and alar cartilages and/or elevation of nasal tip
   b. Code 30430, Rhinoplasty, secondary; minor revision (small amount of nasal tip work)
   c. Code 30460, Rhinoplasty for nasal deformity secondary to congenital cleft lip and/or palate, including columellar lengthening; tip only
   d. Code 30462, Rhinoplasty for nasal deformity secondary to congenital cleft lip and/or palate, including columellar lengthening; tip, septum, osteotomies
   e. Code 21235, Graft; ear cartilage, autogenous, to nose or ear (includes obtaining graft)

Case Study 5.9

1. Which of the following correctly classifies the procedure performed?
    a. Code 30400, Rhinoplasty, primary; lateral and alar cartilages and/or elevation of nasal tip
    b. Code 30430, Rhinoplasty, secondary; minor revision (small amount of nasal tip work)
    c. Code 30460, Rhinoplasty for nasal deformity secondary to congenital cleft lip and/or palate, including columellar lengthening; tip only
    d. Code 30462, Rhinoplasty for nasal deformity secondary to congenital cleft lip and/or palate, including columellar lengthening; tip, septum, osteotomies
    e. Code 21235, Graft; ear cartilage, autogenous, to nose or ear (includes obtaining graft)

Case Study 6.1

1. What is the age of the patient?
    69

2. Identify each device that was involved in this case.
    a. Single catheter
    b. Multicatheter device (Tesio)
    c. Subcutaneous port
    d. Subcutaneous pump

3. What type of procedure(s) was performed?
    a. Insertion
    b. Replacement (specify if same or different venous access site is being used)
    c. Repair
    d. Removal of device(s)
    e. Removal of obstructive material—pericatheter
    f. Removal of obstructive material—intraluminal
    g. Repositioning under fluoroscopic guidance

4. What was the catheter entry site?
    a. Jugular
    b. Subclavian
    c. Femoral vein
    d. Inferior vena cava
    e. Basilic vein
    f. Cephalic vein
    g. Other (specify)

5. Was the catheter tunneled?
    a. Yes
    b. No

6. CPT surgery code(s) and modifier(s): **36561**

Case Study 6.2

1. What is the age of the patient?
   42

2. Identify each device involved in this case.
   a. Single catheter
   b. Multicatheter device (Tesio)
   c. Subcutaneous port
   d. Subcutaneous pump

3. What type of procedure(s) was performed?
   a. Insertion
   b. Replacement—same access site is being used
   c. Replacement—different venous access site is being used
   d. Repair
   e. Removal of device(s)
   f. Removal of obstructive material—pericatheter
   g. Removal of obstructive material—intraluminal
   h. Repositioning under fluoroscopic guidance

4. What was the catheter entry site?
   a. Jugular
   b. Subclavian
   c. Femoral vein
   d. Inferior vena cava
   e. Basilic vein
   f. Cephalic vein
   g. Other (specify)
   h. Not applicable

5. Was the catheter tunneled?
   a. Yes
   b. No

6. CPT surgery code(s) and modifier(s): **36589, 36589–59, 36565**

Case Study 6.3

1. What is the age of the patient?
   49

2. Identify each device involved in this case.
   a. Single catheter
   b. Multicatheter device (Tesio)
   c. Subcutaneous port
   d. Subcutaneous pump

3. What type of procedure(s) was performed?
   a. Insertion
   b. Replacement—same access site is being used
   c. Replacement—different venous access site is being used
   d. Repair
   e. Removal of device(s)
   f. Removal of obstructive material—pericatheter
   g. Removal of obstructive material—intraluminal
   h. Repositioning under fluoroscopic guidance

4. What was the catheter entry site?
   a. Jugular
   b. Subclavian
   c. Femoral vein
   d. Inferior vena cava
   e. Basilic vein
   f. Cephalic vein
   g. Other (specify)
   h. Not applicable

5. Was the catheter tunneled?
   a. Yes
   b. No

6. CPT surgery code(s) and modifier(s): **36589**

Case Study 6.4

1. What is the age of the patient?
   73

2. Identify each device involved in this case.
   a. Single catheter
   b. Multicatheter device (Tesio)
   c. Subcutaneous port
   d. Subcutaneous pump

3. What type of procedure(s) was performed?
   a. Insertion
   b. Replacement—same access site is being used
   c. Replacement—different venous access site is being used
   d. Repair
   e. Removal of device(s)
   f. Removal of obstructive material—pericatheter
   g. Removal of obstructive material—intraluminal
   h. Repositioning under fluoroscopic guidance

4. What was the catheter entry site?
   a. Jugular
   b. Subclavian
   c. Femoral vein
   d. Inferior vena cava
   e. Basilic vein
   f. Cephalic vein
   g. Other (specify)
   h. Not applicable

5. Was the catheter tunneled?
   a. Yes
   b. No

6. CPT surgery code(s) and modifier(s): **36590, 36561**

Case Study 6.5

1. What is the age of the patient?
74

2. Identify each device involved in this case.
   a. Single catheter
   b. Multicatheter device (Tesio)
   c. Subcutaneous port
   d. Subcutaneous pump

3. What type of procedure(s) was performed?
   a. Insertion
   b. Replacement—same access site is being used
   c. Replacement—different venous access site is being used
   d. Repair
   e. Removal of device(s)
   f. Removal of obstructive material—pericatheter
   g. Removal of obstructive material—intraluminal
   h. Repositioning under fluoroscopic guidance

4. What was the catheter entry site?
   a. Jugular
   b. Subclavian
   c. Femoral vein
   d. Inferior vena cava
   e. Basilic vein
   f. Cephalic vein
   g. Other (specify)
   h. Not applicable (not documented)

5. Was the catheter tunneled?
   a. Yes
   b. No

6. CPT surgery code(s) and modifier(s): **36556**

Case Study 6.6

1. Does the patient have a congenital cardiac anomaly?
   a. Yes
   b. No

2. What side(s) of the heart was catheterized?
   a. Left side
   b. Right side
   c. Right and left sides

3. If left heart catheterization, what method was used to access the left side of the heart?
   a. Percutaneous retrograde from the brachial artery, axillary artery, or femoral artery
   b. Retrograde
   c. Transseptal through intact septum
   d. Left ventricular puncture (with or without retrograde left heart catheterization)
   e. Not applicable

4. Was angiography performed?
   a. Yes
   b. No

   If yes, on which site(s)?
   a. Pulmonary
   b. Right ventricular
   c. Right atrial
   d. Left ventricular
   e. Left atrial
   f. Selective coronary (injection of radiopaque material may be by hand)
   g. Aortic root
   h. All sites listed above

5. Was selective visualization/opacification of bypass graft(s) performed?
    a.   Yes
    b.   No

    If yes, on which site(s)?
    a.   Arterial conduits (for example, internal mammary)
    b.   Aortocoronary venous bypass grafts

6. Which additional code(s) should be assigned to classify the imaging supervision, interpretation, and report for the injection procedure(s) performed during the cardiac catheterization?
    a.   93555
    b.   93555, 93556

7. CPT surgery code(s) and modifier(s): **93526, 93543, 94544, 93545, 93555, 93556**

Case Study 6.7

1. Does the patient have a congenital cardiac anomaly?
    a.   Yes
    b.   No

2. What side(s) of the heart was catheterized?
    a.   Left side
    b.   Right side
    c.   Right and left sides

3. If left heart catheterization, what method was used to access the left side of the heart?
    a.   Percutaneous retrograde from the brachial artery, axillary artery, or femoral artery
    b.   Retrograde
    c.   Transseptal through intact septum
    d.   Left ventricular puncture (with or without retrograde left heart catheterization)

4. Was angiography performed?
    a.   Yes
    b.   No

    If yes, on which site(s)?
    a.   Pulmonary
    b.   Right ventricular
    c.   Right atrial
    d.   Left ventricular
    e.   Left atrial
    f.   Selective coronary (injection of radiopaque material may be by hand)
    g.   Aortic root
    h.   All sites listed above

5. Was selective visualization/opacification of bypass graft(s) performed?
    a.   Yes
    b.   No

6. Which additional code(s) should be assigned to classify the imaging supervision, interpretation, and report for the injection procedure(s) performed during the cardiac catheterization?
    a.   93555
    b.   93555, 93556

7. CPT surgery code(s) and modifier(s): **93510, 93543, 93545, 93555, 93556**

Case Study 6.8

1. Does the patient have a congenital cardiac anomaly?
   a. Yes
   b. No

2. What side(s) of the heart was catheterized?
   a. Left side
   b. Right side
   c. Right and left sides

3. If left heart catheterization, what method was used to access the left side of the heart?
   a. Percutaneous retrograde from the brachial artery, axillary artery, or femoral artery
   b. Retrograde
   c. Transseptal through intact septum
   d. Left ventricular puncture (with or without retrograde left heart catheterization)

4. Was angiography performed?
   a. Yes
   b. No

   If yes, on which site(s)?
   a. Pulmonary
   b. Right ventricular
   c. Right atrial
   d. Left ventricular
   e. Left atrial
   f. Selective coronary (injection of radiopaque material may be by hand)
   g. Aortic root
   h. All sites listed above

5. Was selective visualization/opacification of bypass graft(s) performed?
   a. Yes
   b. No

   If yes, on which site(s)?
   a. Arterial conduits (for example, internal mammary)
   b. Aortocoronary venous bypass grafts

6. Which additional code(s) should be assigned to classify the imaging supervision, interpretation, and report for the injection procedure(s) performed during the cardiac catheterization?
   a. 93555
   b. 93556
   c. 93555, 93556

7. What type of angioplasty was performed?
   a. Percutaneous transluminal pulmonary artery balloon angioplasty
   b. Open transluminal balloon angioplasty, aortic
   c. Open transluminal balloon angioplasty, venous
   d. Percutaneous transluminal coronary balloon angioplasty
   e. Percutaneous transluminal balloon angioplasty, aortic
   f. Percutaneous transluminal balloon angioplasty, venous

8. On how many vessels was the angioplasty performed?
   a. One vessel
   b. Two vessels

9. CPT surgery code(s) and modifier(s): **93510, 93539, 93540, 93545, 93556, 92982–LD**

Case Study 6.9

1. Does the patient have a congenital cardiac anomaly?
   a. Yes
   b. No

2. What side(s) of the heart was catheterized?
   a. Left side
   b. Right side
   c. Right and left sides
   d. Not done

3. Was angiography performed?
   a. Yes
   b. No

   If yes, on which site(s)?
   a. Pulmonary
   b. Right ventricular
   c. Right atrial
   d. Left ventricular
   e. Left atrial
   f. Selective coronary (injection of radiopaque material may be by hand)
   g. Aortic root
   h. All sites listed above

4. Was selective visualization/opacification of bypass graft(s) performed?
   a. Yes
   b. No

   If yes, on which site(s)?
   a. Arterial conduits (for example, internal mammary)
   b. Aortocoronary venous bypass grafts

5. Which additional code(s) should be assigned to classify the imaging supervision, interpretation, and report for the injection procedure(s) performed during the cardiac catheterization?
   a. 93555
   b. 93556
   c. 93555, 93556

6. What type of angioplasty was performed?
   a. Percutaneous transluminal pulmonary artery balloon angioplasty
   b. Open transluminal balloon angioplasty, aortic
   c. Open transluminal balloon angioplasty, venous
   d. Percutaneous transluminal coronary balloon angioplasty
   e. Percutaneous transluminal balloon angioplasty, aortic
   f. Percutaneous transluminal balloon angioplasty, venous

7. On how many vessels was the angioplasty performed?
   a. One vessel
   b. Two vessels

8. CPT surgery code(s) and modifier(s): **93544, 93545, 93556, 92982–RC**

Case Study 6.10

1. What procedure was performed?
   a. Needle biopsy
   b. Excisional biopsy—superficial
   c. Excisional biopsy—deep

2. On which lymph node(s) was the procedure performed?
   Supraclavicular cervical node

3. CPT surgery code(s) and modifier(s): **38510**

Case Study 6.11

1. What type of arteriovenous fistula was surgically created?
   a. Open arteriovenous anastomosis by upper basilic vein transposition
   b. Open arteriovenous anastomosis direct from an artery to a vein
   c. Creation of arteriovenous fistula by autogenous graft
   d. Creation of arteriovenous fistula by nonautogenous graft

2. CPT surgery code(s) and modifier(s): **36821**

Case Study 6.12

1. What type of arteriovenous fistula was surgically created?
   a. Open arteriovenous anastomosis by upper basilic vein transposition
   b. Open arteriovenous anastomosis direct from an artery to a vein
   c. Creation of arteriovenous fistula by autogenous graft
   d. Creation of arteriovenous fistula by nonautogenous graft

2. CPT surgery code(s) and modifier(s): **36830**

Case Study 6.13

1. What type of arteriovenous (AV) fistula did this patient have at the beginning of this procedure?
   a. Congenital fistula
   b. Traumatic fistula
   c. Surgically created fistula

2. What type of procedure was performed?
   a. Percutaneous thrombectomy
   b. Open thrombectomy
   c. Open revision of AV fistula with thrombectomy
   d. Open revision of AV fistula without thrombectomy

3. What devices were used to perform this procedure?
   a. Endarterectomy dissector
   b. Foley catheter
   c. Fogarty catheter
   d. Balloon catheter

4. CPT surgery code(s) and modifier(s): **36833**

Case Study 6.14

1. What type of arteriovenous (AV) fistula did this patient have at the beginning of this procedure?
    a. Congenital fistula
    b. Traumatic fistula
    c. Surgically created fistula

2. What types of procedures were performed?
    a. Percutaneous thrombectomy
    b. Open thrombectomy
    c. Open revision of AV fistula with thrombectomy
    d. Open revision of AV fistula without thrombectomy
    e. Percutaneous transluminal balloon venous angioplasty

3. How many times was an AV fistulogram performed?
    Twice

4. CPT surgery code(s) and modifier(s): **36870, 35476, 75978, 36145, 36145–59, 75790**

Case Study 7.1

1. Identify *each* anatomical site examined with the endoscope.
    a. Esophagus
    b. Stomach
    c. Duodenum
    d. Small intestine
    e. Anus
    f. Rectum
    g. Sigmoid colon
    h. Descending colon
    i. Transverse colon
    j. Ascending colon
    k. Cecum

2. Was an endoscopic ultrasound examination performed?
    a. Yes
    b. No

3. Was a transendoscopic device placed?
    a. Yes
    b. No

4. Identify the surgical procedure performed on *each* lesion present.
    a. Biopsy of specimen
    b. Bipolar cautery removal
    c. Hot-biopsy removal
    d. Snare technique removal
    e. Destruction/ablation/fulguration
    f. Submucosal injection (India ink, saline, corticosteroids, Botox)
    g. Other (specify)

5. Identify the type of instrument/approach used on *each* lesion (if applicable).
    a. Cold-biopsy forceps
    b. Hot-biopsy forceps
    c. Transendoscopic ultrasound-guided intramural fine needle aspiration/biopsy(s)
    d. Transendoscopic ultrasound-guided transmural fine needle aspiration/biopsy(s)
    e. Not documented/applicable

6. CPT surgery code(s) and modifier(s): **45384, 45385–59**

Case Study 7.2

1. Identify *each* anatomical site examined with the endoscope.
   a. Esophagus
   b. Stomach
   c. Duodenum
   d. Small intestine
   e. Anus
   f. Rectum
   g. Sigmoid colon
   h. Descending colon
   i. Transverse colon
   j. Ascending colon
   k. Cecum

2. Was an endoscopic ultrasound examination performed?
   a. Yes
   b. No

3. Was a transendoscopic device placed?
   a. Yes
   b. No

4. Identify the surgical procedure performed on *each* lesion present.
   a. Biopsy of specimen
   b. Bipolar cautery removal
   c. Hot-biopsy removal
   d. Snare technique removal
   e. Destruction/ablation/fulguration
   f. Submucosal injection (India ink, saline, corticosteroids, Botox)
   g. Other (specify)

5. Identify the type of instrument/approach used on *each* lesion (if applicable).
   a. Cold-biopsy forceps
   b. Hot-biopsy forceps
   c. Transendoscopic ultrasound-guided intramural fine needle aspiration/biopsy(s)
   d. Transendoscopic ultrasound-guided transmural fine needle aspiration/biopsy(s)
   e. Not documented/applicable

6. CPT surgery code(s) and modifier(s): **45383, 45380–59**

Case Study 7.3

1. Identify *each* anatomical site examined with the endoscope.
   a. Esophagus
   b. Stomach
   c. Duodenum
   d. Small intestine
   e. Anus
   f. Rectum
   g. Sigmoid colon
   h. Descending colon
   i. Transverse colon
   j. Ascending colon
   k. Cecum

2. Was an endoscopic ultrasound examination performed?
   a. Yes
   b. No

3. Was a transendoscopic device placed?
   a. Yes
   b. No

4. Identify the surgical procedure performed on *each* lesion present.
   a. Biopsy of specimen
   b. Bipolar cautery removal
   c. Hot-biopsy removal
   d. Snare technique removal
   e. Destruction/ablation/fulguration
   f. Submucosal injection (India ink, saline, corticosteroids, Botox)
   g. Other (specify)

5. Identify the type of instrument/approach used on *each* lesion (if applicable).
   a. Cold-biopsy forceps
   b. Hot-biopsy forceps
   c. Transendoscopic ultrasound-guided intramural fine needle aspiration/biopsy(s)
   d. Transendoscopic ultrasound-guided transmural fine needle aspiration/biopsy(s)
   e. Not documented/applicable

6. CPT surgery code(s) and modifier(s): **45380**

Case Study 7.4

1. Identify *each* anatomical site examined with the endoscope.
   a. Esophagus
   b. Stomach
   c. Duodenum
   d. Small intestine
   e. Anus
   f. Rectum
   g. Sigmoid colon
   h. Descending colon
   i. Transverse colon
   j. Ascending colon
   k. Cecum

2. Was an endoscopic ultrasound examination performed?
   a. Yes
   b. No

3. Was a transendoscopic device placed?
   a. Yes
   b. No

4. Identify the surgical procedure performed on *each* lesion present.
   a. Biopsy of specimen
   b. Bipolar cautery removal
   c. Hot-biopsy removal
   d. Snare technique removal
   e. Destruction/ablation/fulguration
   f. Submucosal injection (India ink, saline, corticosteroids, Botox)
   g. Other (specify): Dilation of colon stricture

5. Identify the type of instrument/approach used on *each* lesion (if applicable).
   a. Cold-biopsy forceps
   b. Hot-biopsy forceps
   c. Transendoscopic ultrasound-guided intramural fine needle aspiration/biopsy(s)
   d. Transendoscopic ultrasound-guided transmural fine needle aspiration/biopsy(s)
   e. Not documented/applicable

6. CPT surgery code(s) and modifier(s): **45386, 45380–59**

Case Study 7.5

1. What type of endoscopy was performed?
    a. Colonoscopy
    b. Sigmoidoscopy
    c. Esophagogastroduodenoscopy

2. Was an endoscopic ultrasound examination performed?
    a. Yes
    b. No

3. Was a transendoscopic device placed?
    a. Yes
    b. No

4. Identify the surgical procedure performed on *each* lesion present.
    a. Biopsy of specimen
    b. Bipolar cautery removal
    c. Hot-biopsy removal
    d. Snare technique removal
    e. Destruction/ablation/fulguration
    f. Submucosal injection (India ink, saline, corticosteroids, Botox)
    g. Other (specify): Dilation of colon stricture
    h. None

5. CPT surgery code(s) and modifier(s): **45341**

Case Study 7.6

1. Identify *each* anatomical site examined with the endoscope.
    a. Esophagus
    b. Stomach
    c. Duodenum
    d. Small intestine
    e. Anus
    f. Rectum
    g. Sigmoid colon
    h. Descending colon
    i. Transverse colon
    j. Ascending colon
    k. Cecum

2. Was an endoscopic ultrasound examination performed?
    a. Yes
    b. No

    If yes, list each anatomical site examined with the echoendoscope. The echoendoscope was used to examine the esophagus, the stomach, and the duodenum.

3. Was a transendoscopic device placed?
    a. Yes
    b. No

4. Identify the surgical procedure performed on *each* lesion present.
    a. Biopsy of specimen
    b. Bipolar cautery removal
    c. Hot-biopsy removal
    d. Snare technique removal
    e. Destruction/ablation/fulguration
    f. Submucosal injection (India ink, saline, corticosteroids, Botox)
    g. Other (specify): Dilation of colon stricture

5. Identify the type of instrument/approach used on *each* lesion (if applicable)
    a. Cold-biopsy forceps
    b. Hot-biopsy forceps
    c. Transendoscopic ultrasound fine needle aspiration/biopsy(s)
    d. Not documented/applicable

Case Study 7.7

1. Does the patient have a current diagnosis of achalasia?
   No

2. Was an endoscopy performed?
   Yes

3. Identify *each* anatomical site examined with the endoscope.
   a. Esophagus
   b. Stomach
   c. Duodenum
   d. All of the above

4. Identify the method of dilation utilized.
   a. Balloon (less than 30 mm in diameter)
   b. Balloon (larger than 30 mm in diameter)
   c. Insertion of guide wire followed by dilation over guide wire
   d. Unguided sound
   e. Bougie
   f. Retrograde dilators

5. CPT surgery code(s) and modifier(s): **43249, 43239**

Case Study 7.8

1. Does the patient have a current diagnosis of achalasia?
   No

2. Was an endoscopy performed?
   Yes

3. Identify *each* anatomical site examined with the endoscope.
   a. Esophagus
   b. Stomach
   c. Duodenum
   d. All of the above

4. Identify the method of dilation utilized.
   a. Balloon (less than 30 mm in diameter)
   b. Balloon (larger than 30 mm in diameter)
   c. Insertion of guide wire followed by dilation over guide wire
   d. Unguided sound
   e. Bougie
   f. Retrograde dilators

5. CPT surgery code(s) and modifier(s): **43249, 43450**

Case Study 7.9

1. Does the patient have a past history of hernia repair surgery on the left and/or right side(s)?
   a. **Yes**
   b. No

2. What is the patient's age?
   58

3. If patient is less than one year old, specify the patient's gestational age at birth.
   Not applicable

4. Identify the type of unilateral or bilateral hernia(s) currently being repaired.
   a. Inguinal
   b. Sliding inguinal
   c. Lumbar
   d. Femoral
   e. **Incisional (ventral)**
   f. Epigastric
   g. Umbilical
   h. Spigelian

5. What is the clinical presentation of *each* hernia?
   a. **Reducible**
   b. Incarcerated
   c. Strangulated

6. What surgical repair method(s) was utilized?
   a. **Open**
   b. Laparoscopic
   c. **Mesh application**

7. CPT surgery code(s) and modifier(s): **49565, 49568**

Case Study 7.10

1. Does the patient have a past history of hernia repair surgery on the left and/or right side(s)?
   a. Yes
   b. **No**

2. What is the patient's age?
   5 weeks old

3. If patient is less than one year old, specify the patient's gestational age at birth.
   38 weeks' gestation at birth

4. Identify the type of unilateral or bilateral hernia(s) currently being repaired.
   a. **Inguinal**
   b. Sliding inguinal
   c. Lumbar
   d. Femoral
   e. Incisional (ventral)
   f. Epigastric
   g. Umbilical
   h. Spigelian

5. What is the clinical presentation of *each* hernia?
   a. **Reducible**
   b. Incarcerated
   c. Strangulated

6. What surgical repair method(s) was utilized?
   a. **Open**
   b. Laparoscopic
   c. Mesh application

7. CPT surgery code(s) and modifier(s): **49495–50**

Case Study 7.11

1. Does the patient have a past history of hernia repair surgery on the left and/or right side(s)?
   a. Yes
   b. No

2. What is the patient's age?
   50

3. If patient is less than one year old, specify the patient's gestational age at birth.
   Not applicable

4. Identify the type of unilateral or bilateral hernia(s) currently being repaired.
   a. Inguinal
   b. Sliding inguinal
   c. Lumbar
   d. Femoral
   e. Incisional (ventral)
   f. Epigastric
   g. Umbilical
   h. Spigelian

5. What is the clinical presentation of *each* hernia?
   a. Reducible
   b. Incarcerated
   c. Strangulated

6. What surgical repair method(s) was utilized?
   a. Open
   b. Laparoscopic
   c. Mesh application

7. CPT surgery code(s) and modifier(s): **49587**

Case Study 7.12

1. What type if endoscopy was performed?
   a. Capsule endoscopy
   b. Flexible fiberoptic endoscopy
   c. Echoendoscopy
   d. Rigid endoscopy

2. Was the esophagus through ileum examined?
   a. Yes
   b. No

3. CPT surgery code(s) and modifier(s): **91110**

Case Study 7.13

1. What type of anal fistula procedure was performed?
   a. Fistulectomy
   b. Fistulotomy
   c. Placement of anal seton
   d. Instillation of fibrin glue
   e. Closure with rectal advancement flap
   f. Second-stage repair
   g. Removal of anal seton

2. CPT surgery code(s) and modifier(s): **46280**

Case Study 7.14

1. What type of repair was performed?
   a. Fistulectomy
   b. Fistulotomy
   c. Placement of anal seton
   d. Instillation of fibrin glue
   e. Closure with rectal advancement flap
   f. Second-stage repair
   g. Removal of anal seton

2. CPT surgery code(s) and modifier(s): **46030, 46288**

Case Study 7.15

1. What type of hemorrhoid(s) was present?
   a. Tag
   b. Internal
   c. External
   d. Internal and external
   e. Prolapsed
   f. Thrombotic

2. What surgical technique was used to repair *each* hemorrhoid?
   a. Incision
   b. Excision (hemorrhoidectomy)
   c. Enucleation
   d. Injection of sclerosing agent
   e. Destruction (for example, laser, electrocauterization)
   f. Simple ligation (for example, rubber band)
   g. Ligation (surgical)
   h. Fissurectomy
   i. Fistulectomy

3. CPT surgery code(s) and modifier(s): **46260**

Case Study 7.16

1. What type of hemorrhoid(s) was present?
   a. Tag
   b. Internal
   c. External
   d. Internal and external
   e. Prolapsed
   f. Thrombotic

2. What was the location of *each* hemorrhoid plexus?
   The hemorrhoids were located in three major quadrants: left lateral, right anterolateral, and right posterior lateral.

3. What surgical technique was used to repair *each* hemorrhoid?
   a. Incision
   b. Excision (hemorrhoidectomy)
   c. Enucleation
   d. Injection of sclerosing agent
   e. Destruction (for example, laser, electrocauterization)
   f. Simple ligation (for example, rubber band)
   g. Ligation (surgical)
   h. Fissurectomy
   i. Fistulectomy

4. CPT surgery code(s) and modifier(s): **46261, 46080**

Case Study 8.1

1. What type of endoscopy was performed?
    a. Cystoscopy
    b. Ureteroscopy
    c. Both of the above

2. What type of procedure was performed?
    Bilateral ureteral stent change

3. Was the procedure unilateral or bilateral?
    a. Unilateral
    b. Bilateral

4. CPT surgery code(s) and modifier(s): **52310, 52332–50**

Case Study 8.2

1. What type of endoscopy was performed?
    a. Cystoscopy
    b. Ureteroscopy
    c. Both of the above

2. What type of procedure was performed?
    Resection of a 6 mm x 5 mm bladder lesion

3. What was the size of the bladder lesion in centimeters?
    0.6 cm x 0.5 cm

4. CPT surgery code(s) and modifier(s): **52234**

Case Study 8.3

1. What type of endoscopy was performed?
    a. Cystoscopy
    b. Ureteroscopy
    c. Both of the above

2. What type of procedure was performed?
    Right retrograde pyelogram
    Insertion of right ureteral stent

3. Was the procedure(s) unilateral or bilateral?
    a. Unilateral
    b. Bilateral

CPT surgery code(s) and modifier(s): **52332–RT, 52005–RT**

Case Study 8.4

1. What type of endoscopy was performed?
   a. Cystoscopy
   b. Ureteroscopy
   c. Pyeloscopy
   d. All of the above

2. Which of the following procedures was performed?
   a. Removal of ureteral calculus
   b. Removal of urethral calculus
   c. Fragmentation of ureteral calculus
   d. Fragmentation of urethral calculus
   e. Treatment of ureteral stricture
   f. Treatment of ureteropelvic junction stricture
   g. Treatment of intra-renal stricture
   h. Lithotripsy
   i. Electroshock wave lithotripsy
   j. Biopsy of lesion
   k. Resection of lesion

3. Ureteral catheterization was performed.
   a. True
   b. False

4. Insertion of ureteral stent was performed.
   a. True
   b. False

5. CPT surgery code(s) and modifier(s): **52332–RT, 52005–RT, 52351, 50590–RT**

Case Study 8.5

1. What type of endoscopy was performed?
   a. Cystoscopy
   b. Ureteroscopy
   c. Pyeloscopy
   d. All of the above

2. Which of the following procedures was performed?
   a. Removal of ureteral calculus
   b. Removal of urethral calculus
   c. Fragmentation of ureteral calculus
   d. Fragmentation of urethral calculus
   e. Treatment of ureteral stricture
   f. Treatment of ureteropelvic junction stricture
   g. Treatment of intra-renal stricture
   h. Lithotripsy
   i. Electroshock wave lithotripsy
   j. Biopsy of lesion
   k. Resection of lesion

3. Ureteral catheterization was performed.
   a. True
   b. False

4. Insertion of ureteral stent was performed.
   a. True
   b. False

5. CPT surgery code(s) and modifier(s): **52345, 52005**

Case Study 8.6

1. What type of endoscopy was performed?
   a. Cystoscopy
   b. Ureteroscopy
   c. Pyeloscopy
   d. All of the above

2. Which of the following procedures was performed?
   a. Endoscopic injection of implant material into the submucosal tissues of the urethra and/or bladder neck
   b. Endoscopic subureteric injection of implant material

3. The surgical component of the intraoperative cystogram should be coded as?
   a. Code 51600, Injection procedure for cystography or voiding urethrocystography
   b. Code 51610, Injection procedure for retrograde urethrocystography

4. CPT surgery code(s) and modifier(s): **52327, 51600**

Case Study 8.7

1. What type of endoscopy was performed?
   a. Cystoscopy
   b. Ureteroscopy
   c. Pyeloscopy
   d. All of the above

2. Which of the following procedures was performed?
   a. Removal of ureteral calculus
   b. Removal of urethral calculus
   c. Fragmentation of ureteral calculus
   d. Fragmentation of urethral calculus
   e. Treatment of ureteral stricture
   f. Treatment of ureteropelvic junction stricture
   g. Treatment of intra-renal stricture
   h. Lithotripsy
   i. Electroshock wave lithotripsy
   j. Biopsy of lesion
   k. Resection of lesion

3. Ureteral catheterization was performed.
   a. True
   b. False

4. Insertion of ureteral stent was performed.
   a. True
   b. False

5. CPT surgery code(s) and modifier(s): **52344, 52332-RT**

Case Study 8.8

1. What type of orchiectomy was performed?
   a. Simple orchiectomy with testicular prosthesis
   b. Simple orchiectomy without testicular prosthesis
   c. Partial orchiectomy
   d. Radical orchiectomy, inguinal approach
   e. Radical orchiectomy, abdominal approach

2. Was the procedure unilateral or bilateral?
   a. Unilateral
   b. Bilateral

3. CPT surgery code(s) and modifier(s): **54522-RT**

Case Study 8.9

1. What type of procedure was performed on the vas deferens?
   a. Vasotomy
   b. Vasovasostomy
   c. Percutaneous suture ligation
   d. Vasectomy

2. Was the procedure unilateral or bilateral?
   a. Unilateral
   b. Bilateral

3. The correct CPT code and modifier is 55250–50. Explain your answer.
   a. True
   b. False

   Explanation: CPT code 55250 states "unilateral or bilateral," so modifier –50 is not needed.

Case Study 8.10

1. Was a cystoscopy performed?
   a. Yes
   b. No

2. Which of the following procedures was performed on the prostate?
   a. Prostatectomy
   b. Prostate biopsy
   c. Exposure of prostate for insertion of radioactive substance
   d. Transperineal placement of needles or catheters into prostate for interstitial radioelement application

3. How many needles were used in total?
   a. 18
   b. 24
   c. 6

4. How many seeds were implanted in total?
   a. 18
   b. 24
   c. 91
   d. 10

5. Which of the following codes classify this case?
   a. 55875
   b. 55875, 76965

6. Which of the following pass-through device codes are needed for the seeds and needles?
   a. C1715 (brachytherapy needle)
   b. C1728 (catheter, brachytherapy seed administration)
   c. Both of the above

Case Study 8.11

1. What type of penile prosthesis was inserted?
   a. Noninflatable (semirigid)
   b. Inflatable (self-contained)
   c. Multicomponent inflatable

2. CPT surgery code(s) and modifier(s): **54400**

Case Study 8.12

1. What type of penile prosthesis was inserted?
   a. Noninflatable (semirigid)
   b. Inflatable (self-contained)
   c. Multicomponent inflatable

2. CPT surgery code(s) and modifier(s): **54405**

Case Study 8.13

1. What type of penile prosthesis did the patient have?
   a. Noninflatable (semirigid)
   b. Inflatable (self-contained)
   c. Multicomponent inflatable

2. What type of procedure was performed?
   a. Removal of all components of a multicomponent inflatable penile prosthesis without replacement
   b. Repair of component(s) of a multicomponent inflatable penile prosthesis
   c. Removal and replacement of all components of a multicomponent inflatable penile prosthesis at the same operative session
   d. Removal and replacement of noninflatable (semirigid) penile prosthesis at the same operative session
   e. Removal and replacement of an inflatable (self-contained) penile prosthesis at the same operative session
   f. Removal and replacement of all components of a multicomponent inflatable penile prosthesis, through an infected field, at the same operative session
   g. Removal and replacement of noninflatable (semirigid) penile prosthesis, through an infected field, at the same operative session
   h. Removal and replacement of all components of an inflatable (self-contained) penile prosthesis, through an infected field, at the same operative session

3. CPT surgery code(s) and modifier(s): **54408**

Case Study 8.14

1. What type of penile prosthesis did the patient have before the surgery started?
   a. Noninflatable (semirigid)
   b. Inflatable (self-contained)
   c. Multicomponent inflatable

2. What type of procedure was performed?
   a. Removal of all components of a multicomponent inflatable penile prosthesis without replacement
   b. Repair of component(s) of a multicomponent inflatable penile prosthesis
   c. Removal and replacement of all components of a multicomponent inflatable penile prosthesis at the same operative session
   d. Removal and replacement of noninflatable (semirigid) penile prosthesis at the same operative session
   e. Removal and replacement of an inflatable (self-contained) penile prosthesis at the same operative session
   f. Removal and replacement of all components of a multicomponent inflatable penile prosthesis, through an infected field, at the same operative session
   g. Removal and replacement of noninflatable (semirigid) penile prosthesis, through an infected field, at the same operative session
   h. Removal and replacement of all components of an inflatable (self-contained) penile prosthesis, through an infected field, at the same operative session

3. CPT surgery code(s) and modifier(s): **54410**

Case Study 9.1

1. What technique was used to perform the sterilization?
   a. Fulguration
   b. Excision
   c. Occlusion

2. Was the procedure unilateral or bilateral?
   a. Unilateral
   b. Bilateral

3. What approach was used for the procedure?
   a. Open
   b. Laparoscopic

4. CPT surgery code(s) and modifier(s): **58600**

Case Study 9.2

1. What type of abortion did this patient have?
   a. Elective
   b. Missed
   c. Incomplete

2. CPT surgery code(s) and modifier(s): **59812**

Case Study 9.3

1. What type of abortion did this patient have?
   a. Elective
   b. Missed
   c. Incomplete

2. CPT surgery code(s) and modifier(s): **59820**

Case Study 9.4

1. What operative approach was used for the procedure?
   a. Open
   b. Laparoscopic

2. What was the laterality of the procedure?
   a. Unilateral
   b. Bilateral

3. What type of procedure was performed?
   a. Lysis of fallopian tube adhesions
   b. Partial salpingectomy
   c. Total salpingectomy
   d. Fulguration of fallopian tubes
   e. Occlusion of fallopian tubes
   f. Salpingostomy
   g. Salpingoneostomy

4. CPT surgery code(s) and modifier(s): **58670**

Case Study 9.5

1. What type(s) of endoscopy was/were performed?
   a. Laparoscopy
   b. Hysteroscopy

2. What surgical procedure was performed?
   a. Hysteroscopic excision of intrauterine septum
   b. Open excision of vaginal septum
   c. Open partial vaginectomy
   d. Laparoscopic excision of vaginal septum

3. CPT surgery code(s) and modifier(s): **49320, 58555, 57130**

Case Study 9.6

1. What type(s) of endoscopy was/were performed?
   a. Colposcopy
   b. Laparoscopy
   c. Hysteroscopy

2. Which of the following procedures was performed?
   a. Lysis of intrauterine adhesions
   b. Polypectomy
   c. Dilation and curettage (D&C)
   d. All of the above

3. CPT surgery code(s) and modifier(s): **58559, 58558**

Case Study 9.7

1. How many myomas/fibroid tumors were present?
   a. Two
   b. One

2. Where was the anatomical location of the myoma(s)/fibroid tumor(s)?
   a. Intramural
   b. Surface

3. What was the total weight of the myoma(s)/fibroid tumor(s)?
   a. 250 g or less
   b. Greater than 250 g

4. What surgical approach was used?
   a. Open—abdominal
   b. Open—vaginal
   c. Laparoscopic
   d. Hysteroscopic

5. Endometrial implants were also present and removed.
   a. True
   b. False

6. CPT surgery code(s) and modifier(s): **58545, 58662**

Case Study 9.8

1. What type(s) of endoscopy was/were performed?
    a. Laparoscopy
    b. Hysteroscopy

2. A dilation and curettage was performed.
    a. True
    b. False

3. Where were the adhesions located?
    a. Sigmoid colon
    b. Left fallopian tube
    c. Left ovary
    d. Round ligament
    e. Left pelvic sidewall
    f. Right ovary
    g. Right pelvic sidewall
    h. All of the above

4. How was the right ovarian cyst treated?
    a. Open drainage, vaginal approach
    b. Open drainage, abdominal approach
    c. Laparoscopic drainage

5. CPT surgery code(s) and modifier(s): **44180, 58120, 58555, 58660, 49322**

Case Study 10.1

1. What medical substance(s) were injected into the spine?
    a. Lysis solution (for example, hypertonic saline, enzyme)
    b. Anesthetic(s)
    c. Antispasmodic(s)
    d. Opioid(s)
    e. Steroid(s)
    f. Neurolytic substance(s) (for example, alcohol, phenol, iced saline solution, chemical, thermal, electrical, radiofrequency)
    g. Other solution(s)—specify (for example, narcotic)

2. Were the substances administered via an indwelling catheter?
    a. Yes
    b. No

3. What type of injection was performed?
    a. Single
    b. Multiple/regional block
    c. Differential
    d. Continuous infusion
    e. Intermittent bolus

4. Identify the anatomical site(s) of the injection(s).
    a. Lumbar subarachnoid
    b. Cervical subarachnoid
    c. Thoracic subarachnoid
    d. Sacral subarachnoid
    e. Lumbar epidural
    f. Cervical epidural
    g. Thoracic epidural
    h. Sacral epidural
    i. Lumbar paravertebral facet joint or facet joint nerve
    j. Cervical paravertebral facet joint or facet joint nerve
    k. Thoracic paravertebral facet joint or facet joint nerve
    l. Sacral paravertebral facet joint or facet joint nerve
    m. Lumbar transforaminal
    n. Cervical transforaminal
    o. Thoracic transforaminal
    p. Sacral transforaminal

q. Somatic nerve (circle one): Trigeminal facial greater occipital, vagus, phrenic, spinal accessory, cervical plexus, brachial plexus, axillary, suprascapular, intercostal, ilioinguinal, iliohypogastric, pudendal, paracervical (uterine), thoracic paravertebral, lumbar paravertebral, sacral paravertebral, coccygeal paravertebral, lumbar paravertebral facet joint, sciatic, lumbar plexus

r. Sympathetic nerve (circle one): Sphenopalatine ganglion, carotid sinus, stellate ganglion/cervical sympathetic, lumbar paravertebral sympathetic, thoracic paravertebral sympathetic, celiac plexus, superior hypogastric plexus

5. List *each* vertebral level of the spine that was injected.
    Left L3-4, Left L4-5, Left L5-S1, Right L3-4, Right L4-5, Right L5-S1

6. CPT surgery code(s) and modifier(s): **64475–50, 64476–50, 64476–50**

Case Study 10.2

1. What type of catheter was inserted?
    a. Intrathecal
    b. Epidural

2. How was the catheter inserted?
    a. Surgically implanted
    b. Percutaneous placement

3. What anatomical site was injected?
    a. Cervical
    b. Subarachnoid
    c. Thoracic
    d. Subdural
    e. Lumbar
    f. Caudal

4. What type of injection was performed?
    a. Single
    b. Differential
    c. Continuous

5. CPT surgery code(s) and modifier(s): **62310**

Case Study 10.3

1. Identify the medical substance(s) injected into the spine.
    a. Lysis solution (for example, hypertonic saline, enzyme)
    b. Anesthetic(s)
    c. Antispasmodic(s)
    d. Opioid(s)
    e. Steroid(s)
    f. Neurolytic substance(s) (for example, alcohol, phenol, iced saline solution, chemical, thermal, electrical, radiofrequency)
    g. Other solution(s)—specify (for example, narcotic)

2. Were the substances administered via an indwelling catheter?
    a. Yes
    b. No

3. What type of injection was performed?
    a. Single
    b. Multiple/regional block
    c. Differential
    d. Continuous infusion
    e. Intermittent bolus

4. Identify the anatomical site(s) of the injection (s).
    a. Lumbar subarachnoid
    b. Cervical subarachnoid
    c. Thoracic subarachnoid
    d. Sacral subarachnoid

    e.   Lumbar epidural
    f.   Cervical epidural
    g.   Thoracic epidural.
    h.   Sacral epidural
    i.   Lumbar paravertebral facet joint or facet joint nerve
    j.   Cervical paravertebral facet joint or facet joint nerve
    k.   Thoracic paravertebral facet joint or facet joint nerve
    l.   Sacral paravertebral facet joint or facet joint nerve
    m. Lumbar transforaminal
    n.   Cervical transforaminal
    o.   Thoracic transforaminal
    p.   Sacral transforaminal
    q.   Somatic nerve (circle one): Trigeminal facial greater occipital, vagus, phrenic, spinal accessory, cervical plexus, brachial plexus, axillary, suprascapular, intercostal, ilioinguinal, iliohypogastric, pudendal, paracervical (uterine), thoracic paravertebral, lumbar paravertebral, sacral paravertebral, coccygeal paravertebral, lumbar paravertebral facet joint, sciatic, lumbar plexus
    r.   Sympathetic nerve (circle one): Sphenopalatine ganglion, carotid sinus, stellate ganglion/cervical sympathetic, lumbar paravertebral sympathetic, thoracic paravertebral sympathetic, celiac plexus, superior hypogastric plexus

5.   List *each* vertebral level of the spine that was injected.
    C5-6

6.   CPT surgery code(s) and modifier(s): **64479–RT**

Case Study 10.4

1.   Identify the medical substance(s) injected into the spine.
    a.   Lysis solution (for example, hypertonic saline, enzyme)
    b.   Anesthetic(s)
    c.   Antispasmodic(s)
    d.   Opioid(s)
    e.   Steroid(s)
    f.   Neurolytic substance(s) (for example, alcohol, phenol, iced saline solution, chemical, thermal, electrical, radiofrequency)
    g.   Other solution—specify (for example, narcotic)

2.   Which of the following medial branches was/were treated?
    a.   L2
    b.   L3
    c.   L4
    d.   L5
    e.   all of the above

3.   How was the medial branch treatment performed?
    a.   unilaterally
    b.   bilaterally

4.   CPT surgery code(s) and modifier(s):
    64622-50, 64623-50, 64623-50, 64623-50

Case Study 10.5

1.   What was the surgical approach for this procedure?
    a.   Incision and subcutaneous placement
    b.   Percutaneous
    c.   Laminectomy for implantation

2.   What type of procedure was performed?
    a.   Initial placement of electrode
    b.   Initial placement of pulse generator or receiver
    c.   Replacement of electrode
    d.   Replacement of pulse generator or receiver
    e.   Removal of electrode
    f.   Removal of pulse generator or receiver
    g.   Revision of electrode
    h.   Revision of pulse generator or receiver

3. On what anatomic site was the procedure performed?
   a. Cranial nerve
   b. Epidural
   c. Peripheral nerve
   d. Autonomic nerve
   e. Sacral nerve
   f. Neuromuscular
   g. Transcutaneous
   h. Spinal cord

4. CPT surgery code(s) and modifier(s): **63650**

Case Study 10.6

1. What was the surgical approach for this procedure?
   a. Open via incision
   b. Percutaneous
   c. Laminectomy

2. What type of procedure was performed?
   a. Initial placement of electrode
   b. Initial placement of pulse generator or receiver
   c. Replacement of electrode
   d. Replacement of pulse generator or receiver
   e. Removal of electrode
   f. Removal of pulse generator or receiver
   g. Revision of electrode
   h. Revision of pulse generator or receiver

3. On what anatomic site was the procedure performed?
   a. Cranial nerve
   b. Epidural
   c. Peripheral nerve
   d. Autonomic nerve
   e. Sacral nerve
   f. Neuromuscular
   g. Transcutaneous
   h. Spinal cord

4. CPT surgery code(s) and modifier(s): **63688**

Case Study 10.7

1. What was the surgical approach for this procedure?
   a. Open via incision
   b. Percutaneous
   c. Laminectomy

2. What types of procedures were performed?
   a. Initial placement of electrode
   b. Initial placement of pulse generator or receiver
   c. Replacement of electrode
   d. Replacement of pulse generator or receiver
   e. Removal of electrode
   f. Removal of pulse generator or receiver
   g. Revision of electrode
   h. Revision of pulse generator or receiver

3. On what anatomic site was the procedure performed?
   a. Cranial nerve
   b. Epidural
   c. Peripheral nerve
   d. Autonomic nerve
   e. Sacral nerve
   f. Neuromuscular
   g. Transcutaneous
   h. Spinal cord

4. CPT surgery code(s) and modifier(s): **63660, 63688**

Case Study 10.8

1. What was the surgical approach for the electrode procedure?
   a. Incision and subcutaneous placement
   b. Percutaneous
   c. Laminectomy for implantation

2. What was the surgical approach for the generator procedure?
   a. Incision and subcutaneous placement
   b. Percutaneous
   c. Laminectomy for implantation

3. What types of procedures were performed?
   a. Initial placement of electrode
   b. Initial placement of pulse generator or receiver
   c. Replacement of electrode
   d. Replacement of pulse generator or receiver
   e. Removal of electrode
   f. Removal of pulse generator or receiver
   g. Revision of electrode
   h. Revision of pulse generator or receiver

4. On what anatomic site was the procedure performed?
   a. Cranial nerve
   b. Epidural
   c. Peripheral nerve
   d. Autonomic nerve
   e. Sacral nerve
   f. Neuromuscular
   g. Transcutaneous
   h. Spinal cord

5. CPT surgery code(s) and modifier(s): **63685, 63650**

Case Study 10.9

1. Which of the following procedures was performed?
   a. Removal of previously implanted catheter
   b. Implantation of nonprogrammable pump
   c. Implantation of programmable pump
   d. Replacement of nonprogrammable pump
   e. Replacement of programmable pump
   f. Removal of pump (nonprogrammable or programmable)
   g. Electronic analysis of programmable pump with reprogramming
   h. Electronic analysis of programmable pump without reprogramming
   i. Refilling and maintenance of implantable pump

2. CPT surgery code(s) and modifier(s): **62355, 62365**

Case Study 11.1

1. What type of procedure was performed?
   a. Insertion of the Krupin valve aqueous shunt to extraocular reservoir
   b. Revision of the Krupin valve aqueous shunt to extraocular reservoir

2. CPT surgery code(s) and modifier(s): **66185–LT, 67255–LT**

Case Study 11.2

1. What type of procedure was performed?
   a. Trabeculotomy
   b. Trabeculectomy in absence of previous surgery
   c. Trabeculectomy with scarring from previous ocular surgery or trauma
   d. Trabeculectomy with previous ocular surgery or trauma with no documentation of scarring

2. CPT surgery code(s) and modifier(s): **66170–LT**

Case Study 11.3

1. What type of vitrectomy was performed?
   a. Anterior approach
   b. Posterior/pars plana approach

2. What type of procedure was performed?
   a. Nonmechanical (that is, the use of Weck-cel sponges and scissors)
   b. Mechanical (for example, the use of vitrector, microvit, ocutome, retractor)
   c. Injection of vitreous substitute
   d. Intravitreal injection of pharmacologic agent
   e. Implantation of intravitreal drug delivery system (for example, Ganciclovir implant)
   f. Aspiration or release of vitreous
   g. Discission of vitreous strands
   h. Severing of vitreous strands
   i. Epiretinal membrane stripping
   j. Focal endolaser photocoagulation
   k. Endolaser panretinal photocoagulation
   l. Vitrectomy with pars plana lensectomy/removal of lens material
   m. Vitrectomy for retinal detachment

3. CPT surgery code(s) and modifier(s): **67040–LT**

Case Study 11.4

1. What type of vitrectomy was performed?
   a. Anterior approach
   b. Posterior/pars plana approach

2. What type of procedure was performed?
   a. Nonmechanical (that is, the use of Weck-cel sponges and scissors)
   b. Mechanical (for example, the use of vitrector, microvit, ocutome, retractor)
   c. Injection of vitreous substitute
   d. Intravitreal injection of pharmacologic agent
   e. Implantation of intravitreal drug delivery system (for example, Ganciclovir implant)
   f. Aspiration or release of vitreous
   g. Discission of vitreous strands
   h. Severing of vitreous strands
   i. Epiretinal membrane stripping (for example macular pucker)
   j. Focal endolaser photocoagulation
   k. Endolaser panretinal photocoagulation
   l. Vitrectomy with pars plana lensectomy/removal of lens material
   m. Vitrectomy for retinal detachment

3. CPT surgery code(s) and modifier(s): **67041–LT, 67039–LT**

Case Study 11.5

1. What type of vitrectomy was performed?
   a. Anterior approach
   b. Posterior/pars plana approach

2. What type of procedure was performed?
   a. Nonmechanical (that is, the use of Weck-cel sponges and scissors)
   b. Mechanical (for example, the use of vitrector, microvit, ocutome, retractor)
   c. Injection of vitreous substitute
   d. Intravitreal injection of pharmacologic
   e. Implantation of intravitreal drug delivery system (for example, Ganciclovir implant)
   f. Aspiration or release of vitreous
   g. Discission of vitreous strands
   h. Severing of vitreous strands
   i. Removal of preretinal cellular membrane
   j. Focal endolaser photocoagulation
   k. Endolaser panretinal photocoagulation
   l. Vitrectomy with pars plana lensectomy/removal of lens material
   m. Vitrectomy for retinal detachment

3. CPT surgery code(s) and modifier(s): **67041–LT**

Case Study 11.6

1. What type of cataract was removed?
   a. Nuclear cataract-Central part of the lens
   b. Cortical cataract-Peripheral part of the lens
   c. Idiopathic cataract-Posterior subcapsular part of the lens

2. What type of procedure was performed?
   a. Extracapsular cataract removal with insertion of IOL
   b. Intracapsular cataract removal with insertion of IOL
   c. Exchange of IOL only
   d. Use of ophthalmic endoscope

3. CPT surgery code(s) and modifier(s): **66984–RT**

Case Study 11.7

1. What type of vitrectomy was performed?
   a. Anterior approach
   b. Posterior/pars plana approach

2. What type of procedure was performed?
   a. Nonmechanical (that is, the use of Weck-cel sponges and scissors)
   b. Mechanical (for example, the use of vitrector, microvit, ocutome, retractor)
   c. Injection of vitreous substitute
   d. Intravitreal injection of pharmacologic agent
   e. Implantation of intravitreal drug delivery system (for example, Ganciclovir implant)
   f. Aspiration or release of vitreous
   g. Discission of vitreous strands
   h. Severing of vitreous strands
   i. Epiretinal membrane stripping
   j. Focal endolaser photocoagulation
   k. Endolaser panretinal photocoagulation
   l. Vitrectomy with pars plana lensectomy/removal of lens material
   m. Vitrectomy for retinal detachment

3. CPT surgery code(s) and modifier(s): **67027–LT**

Case Study 11.8

1. What is the diagnosis for the eyelid(s) treated?
   Dermatochalasia

2. Which eyelids were treated surgically?
   a. Left upper eyelid
   b. Right upper eyelid
   c. Left lower eyelid
   d. Right lower eyelid

3. What surgical technique was used to repair each eyelid?
   a. Implantation of upper eyelid load (for example, gold weight)
   b. Blepharoplasty
   c. Blepharoplasty with extensive lower eyelid herniated fat pad
   d. Blepharoplasty with excessive skin weighting down upper eyelid
   e. Tarsal wedge excision
   f. Extensive repair
   g. Tarsal strip operation
   h. Capsulopalpebral fascia repair
   i. Excision and repair of eyelid
   j. Transfer of tarsoconjunctival flap from opposing eyelid

4. Brow ptosis was performed.
   a. True
   b. False

5. CPT surgery code(s) and modifier(s): **15822–50, 67900–50**

Case Study 11.9

1. Which eyelid was treated surgically?
   a. Left upper eyelid
   b. Right upper eyelid
   c. Left lower eyelid
   d. Right lower eyelid

2. What percentage of the eyelid margin was resected?
   a. Up to one-fourth of lid margin
   b. Over one-fourth of lid margin

3. What surgical technique was used to repair each eyelid?
   a. Implantation of upper eyelid load (for example, gold weight)
   b. Blepharoplasty
   c. Blepharoplasty with extensive lower eyelid herniated fat pad
   d. Blepharoplasty with excessive skin weighting down upper eyelid
   e. Tarsal wedge excision
   f. Extensive repair
   g. Tarsal strip operation
   h. Capsulopalpebral fascia repair
   i. Excision and repair of eyelid
   j. Transfer of tarsoconjunctival flap from opposing eyelid

4. CPT surgery code(s) and modifier(s): **67966–E2**

Case Study 11.10

1. Which eyelids were treated surgically?
   a. Left upper eyelid
   b. Right upper eyelid
   c. Left lower eyelid
   d. Right lower eyelid

2. What percentage of the eyelid margin was resected?
   a. Up to one-fourth of lid margin
   b. Over one-fourth of lid margin

3. What surgical technique was performed on each eyelid?
   a. Implantation of upper eyelid load (for example, gold weight)
   b. Blepharoplasty
   c. Blepharoplasty with extensive lower eyelid herniated fat pad
   d. Blepharoplasty with excessive skin weighting down upper eyelid
   e. Tarsal wedge excision
   f. Extensive repair
   g. Tarsal strip operation
   h. Capsulopalpebral fascia repair
   i. Excision and repair of eyelid
   j. Transfer of tarsoconjunctival flap from opposing eyelid
   k. Shave biopsy
   l. Excision

4. CPT surgery code(s) and modifier(s): **67966–E2, 11310**

Case Study 11.11

1. What type of anesthesia was used?
   General anesthesia

2. What type of procedure was performed?
   a. Insertion of myringotomy/ventilating tube, unilateral
   b. Insertion of bilateral myringotomy/ventilating tubes
   c. Removal of unilateral myringotomy/ventilating tube
   d. Removal of bilateral myringotomy/ventilating tubes

3. CPT surgery code(s) and modifier(s): **69424–LT**

Case Study 11.12

1. What type of tympanic membrane surgery was performed?
   a. Tympanic membrane repair (with or without site preparation, perforation, or patch)
   b. Tympanoplasty without mastoidectomy
   c. Tympanoplasty with antrotomy
   d. Tympanoplasty with mastoidotomy
   e. Tympanoplasty with mastoidectomy
   f. Ossicular chain reconstruction
   g. Ossicular chain reconstruction and synthetic prosthesis (partial or total replacement).

2. Code 69424 (ventilating tube removal requiring general anesthesia) should be coded for this case.
   a. True
   b. False

   Explanation: This procedure was not performed under general anesthesia.

3. CPT surgery code(s) and modifier(s): **69610–LT**

Case Study 11.13

1. What type of mastoidectomy was performed?
   a. Simple
   b. Complete
   c. Modified radical
   d. Radical

2. What type(s) of tympanic membrane surgery was performed?
   a. Tympanic membrane repair (with or without site preparation, perforation, or patch)
   b. Tympanoplasty without mastoidectomy
   c. Tympanoplasty with antrotomy
   d. Tympanoplasty with mastoidotomy
   e. Tympanoplasty with mastoidectomy
   f. Ossicular chain reconstruction

3. What was the external auditory canal wall status?
   a. Intact
   b. Reconstructed
   c. Down

4. What was the donor site for the graft that was placed over the prosthesis?
   a. Nasal septum
   b. Areolar tissue
   c. Fascia lata

5. CPT surgery code(s) and modifier(s): **69642–LT, 15732**

Case Study 11.14

1. What type of mastoidectomy was performed?
   a. Simple
   b. Complete
   c. Modified radical
   d. Radical

2. What type(s) of tympanic membrane surgery was performed?
   a. Tympanic membrane repair (with or without site preparation, perforation, or patch)
   b. Tympanoplasty without mastoidectomy
   c. Tympanoplasty with antrotomy
   d. Tympanoplasty with mastoidotomy
   e. Tympanoplasty with mastoidectomy
   f. Ossicular chain reconstruction

3. What was the external auditory canal wall status?
   a. Intact
   b. Reconstructed
   c. Down

4. What was the donor site for the graft that was placed over the prosthesis?
   a. Nasal septum
   b. Areolar tissue
   c. Fascia lata

5. CPT surgery code(s) and modifier(s): **69644–RT, 15732**

Case Study 11.15

1. What type of anesthesia was used?
   General supplemented with local

2. What type of stapes surgery was performed?
   a. Stapedectomy
   b. Stapedotomy
   c. Stapedectomy with footplate drill-out
   d. Stapedotomy with footplate drill-out

3. What type of myringotomy procedure was performed?
   a. Myringotomy, unilateral
   b. Myringotomy, bilateral
   c. Insertion of myringotomy/ventilating tube, unilateral
   d. Insertion of bilateral myringotomy/ventilating tubes
   e. Removal of unilateral myringotomy/ventilating tube
   f. Removal of bilateral myringotomy/venitilating tubes

4. CPT surgery code(s) and modifier(s): **69661–RT, 69421–RT**

Case Study 12.1

1. Using Exhibit 1.2, assign the E/M level for this case.
   a. Low level
   b. Midlevel
   c. High level

Case Study 12.2

1. Which of the following codes correctly classify this case?
   a. 90760: Intravenous infusion, hydration; initial, 31 minutes to 1 hour
   b. 96409: Chemotherapy administration, intravenous; push technique single or initial substance/drug
   c. +96411 Chemotherapy administration, intravenous; each additional substance/drug
   d. All of the above
   e. 90760 and 96409 only

Case Study 12.3

1. Which of the following codes correctly classify this case?
   a. 90760 (Intravenous infusion, hydration; initial, 31 minutes to 1 hour)
   b. 96409 (Chemotherapy administration, intravenous; push technique single or initial substance/drug)
   c. +96411 (Chemotherapy administration, intravenous; each additional substance/drug
   d. 90772–59 (Injection, subcutaneous; Distinct procedural services)
   e. All of the above
   f. 96409 and 90772-59 only

Case Study 12.4

1. Which code correctly classifies this case?
   a. 77055
   b. 77056
   c. 77057
   d. 77057–50

Case Study 12.5

1. Which code correctly classifies this case?
    a. 70450
    b. 70460
    c. 70470

Case Study 12.6

1. Which code correctly classifies this case?
    a. 78000
    b. 78006
    c. 78007

Case Study 12.7

1. Which code pairs correctly classify both the injection and imaging components of this case?
    a. 58340 and 74742
    b. 74740 and 58340
    c. 58340 and 58340-59

Case Study 12.8

1. Which code correctly classifies this case?
    a. 76775
    b. 76770
    c. 76705
    d. 76700

Case Study 12.9

1. What type of proton beam treatment delivery was performed?
    a. 77520—Simple. Proton treatment delivery to a single treatment area utilizing a single nontangential/oblique port, custom block without compensation
    b. 77522—Simple. Proton treatment delivery to a single treatment area utilizing a single nontangential/oblique port, custom block with compensation
    c. 77523—Intermediate. Proton treatment delivery to one or more treatment areas utilizing two or more ports or one or more tangential/oblique ports, with custom blocks and compensators
    d. 77525—Complex. Proton treatment delivery to one or more treatment areas utilizing two or more ports per treatment area with matching or patching fields and/or multiple isocenters, with custom blocks and compensators

    Explanation: Code 77523 includes the two treatment areas, the use of two ports, two custom blocks, and two compensators as described in the clinical note.

Index